Biological and Pharmaceutical Applications of Nanomaterials

Edited by

Polina Prokopovich

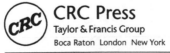

CRC Press
Taylor & Francis Group
Boca Raton London New York

CRC Press is an imprint of the
Taylor & Francis Group, an **informa** business

CRC Press
Taylor & Francis Group
6000 Broken Sound Parkway NW, Suite 300
Boca Raton, FL 33487-2742

First issued in paperback 2020

ISBN 13: 978-0-367-57564-9 (pbk)
ISBN 13: 978-1-4822-5016-9 (hbk)

Library of Congress Cataloging-in-Publication Data

Biological and pharmaceutical applications of nanomaterials / edited by Polina
    Prokopovich.
    p. ; cm.
    Includes bibliographical references and index.
    ISBN 978-1-4822-5016-9 (hardback : alk. paper)
    I. Prokopovich, Polina, editor.
    [DNLM: 1. Nanostructures--therapeutic use. 2. Anti-Infective Agents. 3. Biosensing
Techniques. 4. Drug Delivery Systems--methods. QT 36.5]

RM267
615.7'92--dc23   2015008961

Visit the Taylor & Francis Web site at
http://www.taylorandfrancis.com

and the CRC Press Web site at
http://www.crcpress.com

Contents

SECTION II   Antimicrobial Nanomaterials

SECTION III   Nanomaterials in Biosensors

SECTION IV *Safety of Nanomaterials*

Preface

This book represents recent developments and research activities in the field of nanomaterials with particular focus on biological and pharmaceutical applications.

The book is divided into four sections, each comprising chapters with a common theme. Section I contains seven chapters dealing with nanomaterials for drug delivery. Topics covered in Section I include stimuli-responsive nanostructured silica matrixes, gold nanoparticles, and liposomes for targeting drug delivery applications and dental applications. In addition, material on nanocarriers and nanoparticles as cancer therapeutics and as peptide therapeutics are covered in this section. Section II consists of two chapters dedicated to antimicrobial nanomaterials. Section II covers topics on the influence of surface characteristics on microbial adhesion and summarizes recent advances in antimicrobial nanostructured polymers for medical applications. Section III contains five chapters dealing with nanomaterials in biosensors, and Section IV consists of a single chapter on safety of nanomaterials. Section III covers recent advances in nanodiagnostic techniques for infectious agents, chromogenic biosensors for pathogen detection and electrochemical biosensors for detecting DNA damage and genotoxicity, and molecular imaging with quantum dots including surface modifications by polymers for biosensing applications.

The authors who contributed to this book are very experienced researchers with years of experience in industry and academia. All of the book contributors are experts in their field with considerable experience in researching, developing, and applying the proposed techniques. We sincerely hope that the information in this book will be a valuable resource for clinicians, microbiologists, cell biologists, pharmacists, chemists, and material scientists. This fascinating and comprehensive book will reinforce the multidisciplinary nature of the nanomaterial field.

Polina Prokopovich
Cardiff University, United Kingdom

Editor

Polina Prokopovich, BSc, MSc, PhD, CEng, CBiol, is a lecturer in the School of Pharmacy and Pharmaceutical Sciences of Cardiff University, United Kingdom.

Dr. Prokopovich holds an honorary appointment as a visiting academic in the Department of Biological Engineering of the Massachusetts Institute of Technology (USA), and she is a visiting professor at Kazakh National Technical University and a visiting lecturer at the University of Ljubljana (Slovenia).

She has published a total of 72 refereed papers, which are composed of 35 original research journal papers, 4 invited reviews, and 33 conference papers; 7 book chapters; and 1 edited book. She has given numerous invited talks at international professional meetings/conferences. Dr. Prokopovich serves on a number of editorial boards, grant panels, and scientific international committees.

Contributors

Annia Alba-Menéndez
Branch of Parasitology
Pedro Kourí Institute of Tropical
   Medicine
Havana, Cuba

Shylaja Arulkumar
Centre for Stem Cell Research
Christian Medical College Campus
Vellore, India

Yuxing Bai
Department of Orthodontics
School of Stomatology
Capital Medical University
Beijing, China

Bhubaneswari Bal
Centre of Biotechnology
Bioengineering Laboratory
Siksha O Anusandhan University
Bhubaneswar, India

Kacoli Banerjee
School of Medical Science
   and Technology
Indian Institute of Technology
Kharagpur, India

Shubhadeep Banerjee
School of Medical Science
   and Technology
Indian Institute of Technology
Kharagpur, India

Klemen Bohinc
Faculty of Health Sciences
University of Ljubljana
Ljubljana, Slovenia

Weibo Cai
Materials Science Program
Department of Radiology
Department of Medical Physics
University of Wisconsin, Madison
and
University of Wisconsin Carbone
   Cancer Center
Madison, Wisconsin

Nadia Canilho
Université de Lorraine
SRSMC
Vandoeuvre-lès-Nancy, France

Xin Cao
Chinese Academy of Sciences Key
   Laboratory for Biological Effects
   of Nanomaterials and Nanosafety
National Center for Nanoscience
   and Technology
and
School of Material Science
   and Engineering
Beihang University
Beijing, China

Lei Cheng
Biomaterials and Tissue Engineering
  Division
Department of Endodontics,
  Prosthodontics, and Operative
  Dentistry
University of Maryland Dental School
Baltimore, Maryland

and

State Key Laboratory of Oral Diseases
West China College of Stomatology
Sichuan University
Chengdu, China

Marcella Chiari
Consiglio Nazionale delle Ricerche
Istituto di Chimica del Riconoscimento
  Molecolare
Milan, Italy

Marina Cretich
Consiglio Nazionale delle Ricerche
Istituto di Chimica del Riconoscimento
  Molecolare
Milan, Italy

Alok P. Das
Centre of Biotechnology
Bioengineering Laboratory
Siksha O Anusandhan University
Bhubaneswar, India

Goran Dražić
National Institute of Chemistry
Ljubljana, Slovenia

Nelson Duran
NanoBioss
IQ-UNICAMP
and
Biological Chemistry Laboratory
Instituto de Química
Universidade Estadual de Campinas
Campinas, São Paulo, Brazil

Ali A. Ensafi
Department of Chemistry
Isfahan University of Technology
Isfahan, Iran

Chiara Finetti
Consiglio Nazionale delle Ricerche
Istituto di Chimica del Riconoscimento
  Molecolare
Milan, Italy

Rok Fink
Faculty of Health Sciences
University of Ljubljana
Ljubljana, Slovenia

Octavio Luiz Franco
Pos-Graduação em Ciências Genômicas
  e Biotecnologia
Universidade Catolica de Brasilia
Brasilia, Brazil

Paola Gagni
Consiglio Nazionale delle Ricerche
Istituto di Chimica del Riconoscimento
  Molecolare
Milan, Italy

Swapnil Gaikwad
Nanobiotechnology Laboratory
Department of Biotechnology
Sant Gadge Baba Amravati University
Amravati, Maharashtra, India

Shreya Goel
Materials Science Program
University of Wisconsin, Madison
Madison, Wisconsin

María Isabel González-Sánchez
Department of Physical Chemistry
School of Industrial Engineering
Castilla-La Mancha University
Albacete, Spain

Indarchand Gupta
Nanobiotechnology Laboratory
Department of Biotechnology
Sant Gadge Baba Amravati University
Amravati, Maharashtra, India

and

Department of Biotechnology
Institute of Science
Aurangabad, Maharashtra, India

Esmaeil Heydari-Bafrooei
Department of Chemistry
Faculty of Science
Vali-e-Asr University of Rafsanjan
Rafsanjan, Iran

Hsin-Yun Hsu
Department of Applied Chemistry
National Chiao-Tung University
and
Institute of Molecular Science
National Chiao-Tung University
Hsinchu, Taiwan

Zhongbo Hu
University of Chinese Academy
of Sciences
Beijing, China

Xin-Chun Huang
Department of Applied Chemistry
National Chiao-Tung University
Hsinchu, Taiwan

Shuaidong Huo
Chinese Academy of Sciences Key
Laboratory for Biological Effects
of Nanomaterials and Nanosafety
National Center for Nanoscience
and Technology
and
University of Chinese Academy
of Sciences
Beijing, China

Avinash Ingle
Nanobiotechnology Laboratory
Department of Biotechnology
Sant Gadge Baba Amravati University
Amravati, Maharashtra, India

Mojca Jevšnik
Faculty of Health Sciences
University of Ljubljana
Ljubljana, Slovenia

Sanghoon Kim
Université de Lorraine
SRSMC
Vandoeuvre-lès-Nancy, France

Kateryna Kon
Department of Microbiology, Virology,
and Immunology
Kharkiv National Medical University
Kharkiv, Ukraine

Xing-Jie Liang
Chinese Academy of Sciences Key
Laboratory for Biological Effects
of Nanomaterials and Nanosafety
National Center for Nanoscience
and Technology
Beijing, China

Carlos López-Abarrategui
Center for Protein Studies
Faculty of Biology
Havana University
Havana, Cuba

Yun-Ling Luo
Department of Applied Chemistry
National Chiao-Tung University
Hsinchu, Taiwan

Pragyan Smita Mahapatra
Centre of Biotechnology
Bioengineering Laboratory
Siksha O Anusandhan University
Bhubaneswar, India

Mahitosh Mandal
School of Medical Science
  and Technology
Indian Institute of Technology
Kharagpur, India

Mary Anne S. Melo
Biomaterials and Tissue Engineering
  Division
Department of Endodontics,
  Prosthodontics, and Operative
  Dentistry
University of Maryland Dental School
Baltimore, Maryland

Anselmo J. Otero-González
Center for Protein Studies
Faculty of Biology
Havana University
Havana, Cuba

Andreea Pasc
Université de Lorraine
SRSMC
Vandoeuvre-lès-Nancy, France

Stefano Perni
School of Pharmacy and
  Pharmaceutical Sciences
Cardiff University
Cardiff, Wales, United Kingdom

and

Department of Biological Engineering
Massachusetts Institute of Technology
Cambridge, Massachusetts

Polina Prokopovich
School of Pharmacy and
  Pharmaceutical Sciences
Cardiff University
Cardiff, Wales, United Kingdom

and

Department of Biological Engineering
Massachusetts Institute of Technology
Cambridge, Massachusetts

Mahendra Rai
Nanobiotechnology Laboratory
Department of Biotechnology
Sant Gadge Baba Amravati University
Amravati, Maharashtra, India

Murugan Ramalingam
Centre for Stem Cell Research
Christian Medical College Campus
Vellore, India

and

WPI-Advanced Institute for Materials
  Research
Tohoku University
Sendai, Japan

Deepti Rana
Centre for Stem Cell Research
Christian Medical College Campus
Vellore, India

Peter Raspor
Faculty of Health Sciences
University of Primorska
Izola, Slovenia

Edilso Reguera
CICATA-IPN
Unidad Legaria
México City, México

Lidiany K.A. Rodrigues
Postgraduate Program in Dentistry
Faculty of Pharmacy, Dentistry,
    and Nursing
Federal University of Ceará
Fortaleza, Brazil

Laura Sola
Consiglio Nazionale delle Ricerche
Istituto di Chimica del Riconoscimento
    Molecolare
Milan, Italy

Muhammad Ali Syed
Department of Microbiology
University of Haripur
Haripur, Khyber Pakhtunkhwa,
    Pakistan

Michael D. Weir
Biomaterials and Tissue Engineering
    Division
Department of Endodontics,
    Prosthodontics, and Operative
    Dentistry
University of Maryland Dental School
Baltimore, Maryland

Hockin H.K. Xu
Biomaterials and Tissue Engineering
    Division
Department of Endodontics,
    Prosthodontics, and Operative
    Dentistry
University of Maryland Dental School
and
Center for Stem Cell Biology
    and Regenerative Medicine
University of Maryland School
    of Medicine
and
University of Maryland Marlene and
    Stewart Greenebaum Cancer Center
University of Maryland School
    of Medicine
Baltimore, Maryland

Sarah P. Yang
Wisconsin Department of Natural
    Resources
Madison, Wisconsin

Ke Zhang
Biomaterials and Tissue Engineering
    Division
Department of Endodontics,
    Prosthodontics, and Operative
    Dentistry
University of Maryland Dental School
Baltimore, Maryland

and

Department of Orthodontics
School of Stomatology
Capital Medical University
Beijing, China

Xuedong Zhou
State Key Laboratory of Oral Diseases
West China College of Stomatology
Sichuan University
Chengdu, China

Section I

Nanomaterials for Drug Delivery

1 Stimuli-Responsive Nanostructured Silica Matrix Targeting Drug Delivery Applications

Sanghoon Kim, Nadia Canilho, and Andreea Pasc

CONTENTS

ABSTRACT

Nowadays, challenges in drug delivery include engineering intelligent vectors for simultaneous diagnosis and treatment, vectors that are safe, easily administered, and with a reduced cost. Moreover, there is an increasing need for controlling the delivery with respect to the dose and the site level, in order to decrease adverse side effects. As a matter of fact, many important site-selective drugs, such as highly toxic antitumor molecules, require "zero release" before reaching the targeted cells or tissues. This chapter underlines the latest progress made in controlled drug delivery through external stimuli such as magnetic field, irradiation, or temperature, to cite a few examples.

Keywords: Mesoporous silica, Drug delivery, Stimuli-responsive materials

1.1   SILICA RESPONDING TO CHALLENGES IN DRUG DELIVERY

The ongoing development in drug delivery technologies takes into account primary factors such as the nature of therapeutics being delivered, the mode of administration beneficial to the patient, the well-being of the employees, and cost.

1.1.1   POROUS MATERIALS

In addition, the current challenges consist of considering therapeutic and physiological criteria for the development of drug delivery devices that

- Improve drug efficiency
- Reduce drug side effects
- Control sustained drug release
- Increase drug bioavailability
- Facilitate drug administration and use compliance

Implants and cancer treatments have opened the way to new materials and biocompatible therapeutic systems.[1] Indeed, in this field, the nature of the vector is a strategic choice from a medical point of view. For a long time, biocompatible polymers, either pH or thermally sensitive, have been used as drug delivery systems (DDSs), but polymeric carriers have a limited efficacy in terms of drug loading, especially because of their low porosity, and therefore, research leaned toward porous materials with high pore volume and specific surface. One example is carbon nanotubes (i.e., single walled and multiwalled). These nanomaterials have shown interesting results as drug carriers; however, their use is rather limited owing to their lack of biodegradability and toxicity resulting from their accumulation in body tissues. Inorganic biomaterials seem to be the most advantageous type. This is attributed to their porosity (withstanding loading capacity), thermal and chemical stability, and their resistance to corrosion under physiological conditions. They are also appreciated for their good biocompatibility but present a lower degradable rate except for silica-based biomaterials. In addition, their inherent physical and chemical properties can prove beneficial to various medical applications. Hence, porous silica materials are currently the subject of great interest because of their biocompatibility and high loading drug capacity. Moreover, therapeutic drug nanoparticle carriers are mainly designed to overcome some drug constraints such as poor solubility, limited stability, rapid metabolization, drug excretion, undesired side effects, and lack of selectivity toward specific cell types.

However, in order to design a specific drug release system (DDS), the latter prerequisites must be integrated to the porous silica support through several functionalization ways that are constantly under study and that contribute to controlling the

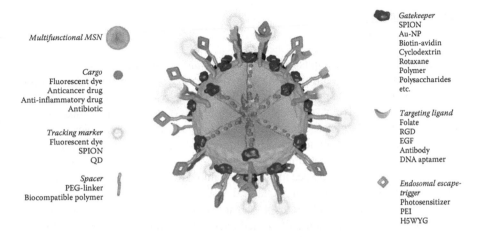

Multifunctional MSN

Cargo
Fluorescent dye
Anticancer drug
Anti-inflammatory drug
Antibiotic

Tracking marker
Fluorescent dye
SPION
QD

Spacer
PEG-linker
Biocompatible polymer

Gatekeeper
SPION
Au-NP
Biotin-avidin
Cyclodextrin
Rotaxane
Polymer
Polysaccharides
etc.

Targeting ligand
Folate
RGD
EGF
Antibody
DNA aptamer

Endosomal escape-trigger
Photosensitizer
PEI
H5WYG

FIGURE 1.1 Schematic illustration of a multifunctional MSN containing the necessary features for a stimuli-responsive controlled release of the loaded cargo into the cytosol of a targeted cell. Au-NP, gold nanoparticle; EGF, epidermal growth factor; H5WYG, endosomolytic peptide; PEG, poly(ethylene glycol); PEI, poly(ethylene imine); QD, quantum dot; RGD, Arg-Gly-Asp amino acid sequence; SPION, superparamagnetic iron oxide nanoparticle. (Reprinted with permission from C. Argyo et al., Multifunctional mesoporous silica nanoparticles as a universal platform for drug delivery, *Chem. Mater.*, 26, 435–451. Copyright 2014 American Chemical Society.)

molecular drug release at an appropriate rate.[2] Such criteria are also valid for oral drug release delivery of pharmaceutical molecules, protein, and nucleotide-based drugs.

Among silica vectors, mesoporous silica nanoparticles (MSNs) are being extensively studied to design multifunctional cargo to achieve drug release under different stimuli-responsive trigger systems (see Figure 1.1).[3] The tuning of MSNs must also improve biocompatibility and prevent endosomal escape. Thus, nanoparticles can be hybrid organic–inorganic core–shell types where targeting ligands for specific cellular recognition or markers for the particle tracking in the cells are attached on the organic shell.

Another challenge for MSN cargos is particle sizing. In fact, it is now well known that some synthesis parameters such as concentration, pH medium, chemical nature of the surfactants, temperature, and reaction time enable control of the morphology, the structure, and the pore size of the mesoporous silica material.[4–8] Nevertheless, for drug delivery into cells, particle size must be less than 120 nm to facilitate endocytic uptake.[9]

1.1.2 ADMINISTRATION ROUTE

Although the methods of treatment are relatively specific to each disease, in the case of cancer, multiple administration routes are explored:

- Intravenous injection
- Pulmonary inhalation
- Dermal application

- Oral uptake
- Local drug delivery

There are specific constraints linked to the administration route. In the case of *local DDSs*, 2D ordered nanoporous alumina with any connection between the channels and nanotubular titania are the most advanced and smart drug-releasing implants.[10] They are biocompatible materials, able to load important amounts of drug into the nanostructured matrix and release chemicals, with zero-order kinetics, under various release triggers (magnetic field, ultrasonication, and radiofrequency). Despite the continuously extending range of applications (including bone therapies, cardiovascular stents, postsurgical healing, and treatment of localized infection, inflammation, or cancer), these systems are limited to therapies in which an implantable device can be introduced.

Oral administration has been exploited for most drugs because of several great advantages such as production cost, varied packaging, and user-friendliness. Pills or capsules are general forms of drugs for the oral route. Both products in question do not need to be sterilized, hence dramatically reducing production and logistic costs for the pharmaceutical industry. Being able to use several excipients is also an advantage for drugs that are orally administered. Extended or sustained drug release can be easily achieved using specific excipients like polymeric matrix based on xanthan gum.[11] Oral drug delivery technologies have also been developed to protect the drug from the acidic environment of the digestive tract up to the gastrointestinal barrier where it should be released. However, one disadvantage, specifically in cancer therapy, is that vectors could generate side effects and have limited effectiveness mainly because of the lack of target specificity.[1] Moreover, oral administration might limit the bioavailability of the active ingredient. Some of the hydrophobic active ingredients like curcumin show extremely poor bioavailability that might be caused by its insolubility in water, poor absorption, rapid metabolism, and systemic elimination.[12] In addition, absorbed drug must pass the liver that accelerates rapid metabolism; as a result, the drug becomes less active. This phenomenon is often called *first-pass effect*.[13] Another disadvantage is that drug absorption is highly dependent on the interaction with food in the stomach. For instance, some drugs such as griseofulvin showed poor adsorption in the presence of food; however, the absorption ability of propranolol is enhanced in the presence of food. Despite this fact, the relation between drug and food has not been systematically studied; each case should be taken into consideration.[14] Additionally, the size might also cause a minor problem for patients, particularly in children, who rarely swallow sizable tablets or capsules as a whole.[15] Thus, often most ingredients for drug in tablet form are pharmaceutically inactive excipients; hence, reducing or replacing some excipients could reduce drug size and enhance user-friendliness.[16]

Actually, many studies have been conducted that tried to overcome the disadvantages concerning oral drugs. Nonetheless, no "magical" system has been proposed as a solution to the problems mentioned above, perhaps except for MSNs.

MSNs have well-ordered mesopores (2–50 nm) with high pore volume as well as large surface area. Drug molecules can be encapsulated inside mesopores without difficulty. MSN matrix can also serve as a good barrier for drug molecules; therefore, many problems concerning bioavailability or interaction with food would be resolved or have already been solved.[17]

The field of application for MSN is not limited to oral administration; it might be extended to *topical administration*. Based on the target, this administration can be divided into two general terms: (1) skin and (2) mucosal membrane system. If the target is the human skin (case 1), one of the traditional formulations of the drug is a cream or ointment for direct dermal application. Patch form formulation has also been widely used, especially for stop-smoking therapy.[18] These formulations have numerous advantages (e.g., no first-pass effect, user-friendliness). Moreover, controlled DDS could also be achieved with formulation in patch form that consists of several membrane sheets. However, the cost of production is not as low as that for the tablet or capsule formulation. In particular, for cream and ointment, highly purified water is needed because of the risk of bacterial proliferation. Furthermore, a large amount of additives (the toxicity of some of which remains controversial) should be added for the same reason.[19] In addition, for cream and ointment, drug burst release, along with the degradation of the initial formulation, is a limiting factor for certain active ingredients. Targeting the mucosal membrane system (case 2) is a more complicated challenge, compared to a direct application on skin. In general, human mucosal membranes like nasal (nose) and buccal (oral) mucosal membranes are "naked" outside and are directly affected by the external environment, owing to the lack of physical barrier (skin).[20] Thus, in terms of formulation, only few excipients are allowed and the use of irritating preservatives is strictly prohibited. Moreover, highly clean production conditions and an appropriate logistic system are required, which result in an expensive drug for the customers. Here, using MSN in formulations can also be an alternative way to overcome these issues. As explained, a drug that is encapsulated inside MSNs is not directly exposed to the external environment; thus, a well-protected drug has fewer chances of being degraded and hence additive use is considerably reduced. Additionally, the response of MSN to the pH of the skin or temperature can provide "perfect" tools for some formulations that have systematic burst release. (Note that the pH of human skin is slightly acidic [4–5],[21] and skin temperature is around 31°C.[22]) A detailed explanation on stimuli-responsive MSN strategy will be covered later in this chapter.

MSNs would also have a distinguishable position among drugs for intravascular (parenteral) administration. Taking a careful look into intravascular drug administration, multiple disadvantages have been ignored as a result of the good bioavailability of the drugs. A high concentration of the drug by injection can lead to side effects; hence, multiple injections with low concentration have been performed, causing serious discomfort for patients. For instance, during chemotherapy, antiemetic medication (ondansetron [brand name, Zofran]) should be injected several times a day to maintain therapeutic concentration in the blood. However, MSNs, the sustained release performance of which is already confirmed,[2] could be applied to intravascular administration. Only through the use of an active ingredient or with a small amount of excipients for the injection of the drug formulation have scientists confirmed that MSNs of less than 150 nm diameter have no side effects on rat cells.[9] Besides, MSN uptake rate into cells (endocytosis) and drug release rate showed that MSN might be an outstanding candidate to replace the traditional injection method.[2]

As highlighted above, MSN has revealed some advantages whatever the administration route. Yet, the first clinical tests are not planned in the near future. As of 2014, drug-MSN carriers are only at the in vivo stage in mouse or rabbit, and the first clinical tests are planned for 2017.[23] It seems that, to date, the most advanced application of MSN in vivo is in bone regeneration. Indeed, MSN embedded inside bioceramic or bioglasses could easily bypass some problems such as toxicity or bioavailability.[24]

1.2 NANOSTRUCTURED SILICA: SUITABLE MATRIX FOR LOADING AND RELEASE

In the last two decades, investigations on hollow silica structures or silica nanocapsules have been engaged in the development of chemical and physicochemical synthesis approaches via the sol-gel process,[25,26] emulsion/interfacial polymerization methods,[27-29] or colloidal templating. The most used methods are illustrated in Figure 1.2.[30]

Hard templates such as SiO_2, C spheres, polymers, or metal particle lead to good morphology and size control from microns to a few nanometers, while with soft templates such as oil and vesicles, the hollow particles usually present poor monodispersity and high deformability because of the soft core.[29,31-33]

The template-free method seems to be a new approach for the synthesis of inorganic hollow particles. This method combines the advantage of hard- and soft-template approaches, thus dodging the template-removing procedure. It is based on the Oswald ripening process where "the larger crystals grow from those of smaller size, which have higher solubility than the larger ones."[34] Then, small crystals undergoing dissolution become a nutrient supply for the growth of larger ones. Because of driving forces that tend to minimize the surface energy, particles aggregate and the larger ones continue to grow. Voids begin to appear progressively during the diffusion of solute. This solute diffusion phenomenon regulates the thickness of the shell.[35-40] As an example, Hah et al. prepared hollow silica particles in two steps: hydrolysis of phenyltrimethoxysilane under acidic conditions followed by silane condensation under basic

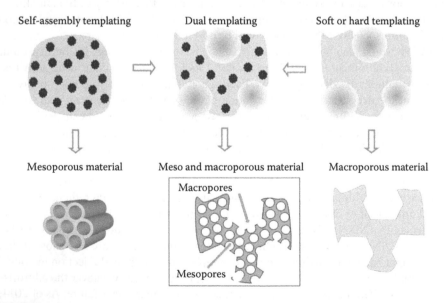

FIGURE 1.2   Schematic illustration of colloidal templating routes.

conditions resulting in monodisperse hollow silica particles. The particle sizing has been controlled through hydrolysis time and a 400-nm diameter was reached.[41]

Spherical hollow silica structures with porous shell are also extensively explored to design controlled delivery biomedical materials. They allow for larger loading capacity to encapsulate drugs, genes, or biological molecules and small molecules that are generally stimuli sensitive in the shell.[42–44] Pasc et al. prepared meso-macroporous silica hallow particles using a co-templated approach. Monodisperse-sized particles were obtained, and the porosity was controlled using solid lipid nanoparticles as soft template for macropores and a block copolymer surfactant as template for the mesoporous network.[45]

Hollow particles combining silica with inorganic composites such as TiO_2, ZnO, or polymer were also designed. In summary, silica could be used either as an adsorbent or as an anchor layer, a protective and a biocompatible shell that could be mesoporous when a controlled drug administration function is expected.

Originally, hollow particles were largely used as simple cargo for drug administration. Over time and with the development of new biomedical approaches, magnetic and fluorescent hollow spheres have been preferred for medical imaging applications as markers or trackers for tumor cells.[46–49]

Some others silica matrixes such as nanosilica fibers have been investigated to design biomaterials as well, but since there is a limitation in using simple nonporous silica fibers as drug vectors, synthesis research has been rapidly oriented to using prepared nanoporous silica. In this context, the work of Stucky et al. and Linton et al. highlighted the major synthesis parameters capable of influencing particle morphology to obtain mesoporous nanorods.

In 2000, Stucky et al. were interested in controlling the morphology of mesoporous silica materials using a combination of block copolymers, cosurfactants, cosolvents, or strong electrolytes. Under acid conditions, long mesoporous SBA-15 fibers were successfully prepared by using poly(ethylene oxide)-block–poly(propylene oxide)-block–poly(ethylene oxide) triblock copolymer ($EO_{20}PO_{70}EO_{20}$) as a structure-directing agent and tetramethyl orthosilicate as a silica source.[50] More recently, Linton et al. have investigated the mechanism for the aggregate growth of mesoporous particles in order to control particle size.[51]

Furthermore, Ding et al. succeeded in obtaining SBA-15 nanorods by adjusting the pH media in the range of 0.5 to 2.5. Through their application, they noticed that SBA-15 rod morphology improved the adsorption of enzymes when compared to conventional spheric particles.[52]

Numerous investigations through the years lead to the synthesis of porous silica nanotubes by variable templating sol-gel methods using inorganic, organic, biological templates; reverse microemulsions; or electrospinning.[53–57] The biosilicification principle inspired from various marine biological systems, such as diatoms or sponges, is also an interesting route to synthesize hollow porous silica fibers under mild conditions.[58] It was demonstrated that long-chain polyamines are intimately linked to the biosilicification process in the case of diatoms. After this finding, many efforts have been made in using organic templates such as self-assembled fibrils of polypeptides[59–61] or amine-modified polysaccharides[62] to synthesize silica nanotubes. In this way, silica with an outer diameter of 15 to 20 nm could be obtained.

As for hexagonal mesoporous silica (HMS), silica nanotubes are also designed to be stimuli responsive. The first DDS based on magnetic nanoparticles consisted of mesoporous silica nanorods where pores were end capped by magnetic Fe_3O_4 nanoparticles linked to nanorods through a chemically labile disulfide function. Human cells secrete antioxidant agents such as dihydrolipoic acid and dithiothreitol (DTT) that are capable of cleaving disulfide bonds.[63] More importantly, the silica fibers show a strong self-activated luminescence ranging from 300 to 600 nm, and centered at 405 nm, without rare earth or transition metal ions as activators. This sample could be potentially used as an environmentally friendly luminescent material.

Thereby, interesting optical properties of nanofibers have been enhanced in various researches during the last few years, including those discovered by Hou et al. with porous SiO_2 composite fibers. They are focused on developing synthetic protocols to make high-energy luminescent porous composite fibers of $NaYF_4:Yb^{3+},Er^{3+}@SiO_2$ useful for bioimaging.[64]

Concerning mesoporous silica materials (MSNs), since the discovery of the MCM-41 mesostructure (Mobil Crystalline Material), many other MSNs have been developed with different ionic or nonionic surfactants or copolymers to obtain materials combining variable pore size and morphology together with high surface area and volume.[65-68]

It is increasingly difficult to describe the entire synthetic route specific to each type of MSN, but it is well known now that mesoporous materials can be prepared from surfactant or small block copolymer templates self-assembled into liquid crystal mesophases, which tailor the arrangement of silica mesopores. Moreover, all the investigations conducted to date converge to the unanimous result that the most significant reaction parameters to tune the morphology and the size of the particles are the pH value, the temperature, the surfactant concentration, the water content, and the silica source.[69] Those latest parameters parameters have a strong impact in the silica condensation rate.[70,71]

Then, through mastering the condition of reactions, it is possible to obtain mesoporous particles at the nanoscale level. As a result, drug delivery vectors have experienced a revival with the first ibuprofen encapsulation in MCM-41 proposed by Vallet-Regí et al. in 2001.[72]

Since then, MSNs have been extensively studied to design biomaterials for controlling release delivery of pharmaceutical drugs, genes, or proteins and even biocides and nutriments to the target sites.

Compared to nonporous silica nanoparticles, mesoporous silica materials within particular hexagonally ordered pores present several advantages such as large specific area, tunable pore diameter, and surface chemistry for hosting molecules with different sizes, shapes, and functionalities.

As a drug release vector, it is much more difficult to control release in the case of hollow nanoparticles than in MSNs. In fact, HMS has many interconnected pores leading to the central reservoir. A capping of the pore openings is systematically carried out to prevent the entrapped drug leaching, whereas in the case of MSNs, end capping is much more convenient and efficient to keep the drug inside mesopores, because the pore network consists of unconnected parallel channels with only two openings.

Mesoporous silica material can be functionalized by stimulable molecules or directly by the drug molecule via two main routes. The first is by "one pot" where organic molecules are co-condensed at the same time as the silica source.[73] The second is by postsynthesis of the silica material. In the latter case, MSN is generally immersed in a solution containing the molecules to be grafted and thus attached covalently or physically (depending on the trigger release) to the silica surface and walls.[74]

As an example, Lin et al. used different chain lengths of alkyl methylimidazolium cationic surfactants as template and its antibacterial effect on *Escherichia coli* K12.[75]

Today, the challenges no longer concern the synthesis itself, but the requirements and constant adaptations imposed by the bioscience field.

1.3   STIMULI-RESPONSIVE NANOSTRUCTURED SILICA MATERIALS

Usually, the MSN functionalization process can be done following two methods: co-condensation, also called one-pot synthesis, and grafting or postsynthesis modification including the surface coating on MSN.[76-79] Co-condensation is in general interesting as it produces an inorganic–organic hybrid network, and the method allows introduction of both acidic and basic functional groups into MSN for pH stimuli.[66,80,81]

Grafting is made on free silanol groups after the synthesis of MSNs especially when external surface modification is needed[82,83] to facilitate, for example, dispersion in biological environment or to prevent particle aggregation.

Another postsynthesis functionalization is the imprint coating method where MSNs are coated with organic molecules with specific binding such as ligands for ionic complexation.[84-86]

Ideally, it is expected that DDSs are capable of sensing external environment signals and releasing the therapeutic dose through appropriate external stimuli that could induce on–off switches to the delivery mechanism.

External MSN surface functionalization with organic and inorganic moieties aims not only to exhibit, for the drug delivery, specific multifunctional interactions triggered by specific environment stimuli but also to improve specific cell targeting, prevent premature release with large molecules as pore gating, improve biocompatibility, and colloidal and chemical stability in the environment.[87-89]

Internal modification of MSN surface with organic entities is generally selected to control drug diffusion, delivery kinetics, and stability of the therapeutic molecules.[90,91]

As explained previously, stimuli-responsive MSNs are prepared via co-condensation or over a postsynthetic grafting step.[66,92] The challenge is to control the location of the functional groups in mesoporous silica particles. An example of specific functionalization is gating, an important strategy for triggered release of the drug. Entities such as large molecular groups like proteins, superparamagnetic iron oxide nanoparticles, or gold nanoparticles are used as gatekeepers to block the pore entrances for efficient sealing of the interior of the cargo.[93-96]

MSNs are sometimes directly functionalized by the molecular drug inside the pores through covalent or coordinative bonds cleavable by specific stimuli such as reducing agents, competitive binding molecules, or ultraviolet (UV) light.[97-102]

Very good pore sealing can also be achieved by a complete coating of the MSNs. For instance, polymers, oligonucleotides, or supported lipid bilayers have been shown to prevent premature cargo release.[103–112] Often, phase transitions or competitive displacement reactions lead to opening of the pores and efficient cargo delivery.[113,114]

Usually, molecules or entities used as stimuli are classified into six categories of stimuli: pH, temperature, redox, magnetic, light, and biological stimuli.[115–118] The first studies on stimuli-responsive materials focused only on pH and temperature. Now, chemical science has succeeded in combining several stimuli.

1.3.1 pH Stimuli-Responsive MSN

MSN with pH responsiveness is one of the earliest investigation of MSN in drug delivery; the first application was conducted by Vallet-Regí et al. in 2001.[72] The use of interaction between the drug and silica matrix, such as hydrogen bonding or electrostatic interaction, is a common method to load and release the "guest" drug molecule. As already known, these interactions can be more or less strong as a function of the pH. This is the basic concept of pH-responsive DDS based on MSN. However, without inner surface modification of mesoporous silica, only weak hydrogen bonding involving the silanol group could be expected. Thus, the guest drug molecule should contain a hydrogen bonding group to improve drug loading efficiency.

To overcome this disadvantage of mesoporous silica as DDS, scientists have conducted several modifications of silica nanoparticles by various functional groups such as amino[90] or carboxylate.[91] Among some outstanding results, Balas et al. showed the confinement and the controlled release of alendronate from MCM-41-type mesoporous silica.[119] Alendronate is a bisphosphonate, used as a model drug in osteoporosis treatment. It can be loaded into amino-functionalized mesoporous MCM-41 at pH 4.8 and released by increasing the pH up to 7.4 where electrostatic interaction between the guest molecule and the host mesoporous silica becomes too weak.

Metal-involved coordination bonding–based mesoporous silica is also a good approach for pH-responsive DDS. Zheng et al. reported a construction of a coordination bonding "host–metal–drug" architecture using amino-functionalized mesoporous silica (APS) and doxorubicin (DOX) as model drug.[120] As it is well known, NH_2–metal or metal–drug coordination bonding can be broken off as pH decreases such that pH can trigger drug release from mesoporous silica material in these systems. Indeed, suitable host–metal–drug matching is required for its application and the number of functionalized sites such as the amino group should be controlled to reach a maximum drug loading. For instance, the "NH_2–Cu–DOX" architecture showed a highly sensitive pH-responsive release profile compared to the "NH_2–Zn–DOX" architecture (see Figure 1.3).

Although the concept that relies on host–guest interaction showed enormous applications and its potential for pH-responsive DDS, a good matching between guest molecule and host silica matrix is always necessary; hence, wide use of this strategy is sometimes limited. The limit of host–guest interaction–based pH-responsive DDS can be overcome by the gatekeeping strategy. In fact, the gatekeeping strategy was first introduced by Lin et al. in 2003 using CdS nanoparticles that capped the

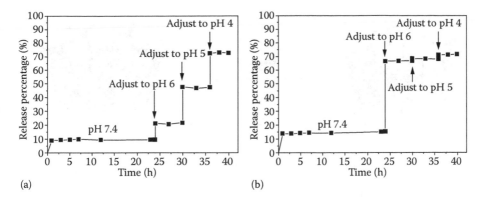

FIGURE 1.3 pH-responsive DOX release of NH_2–Cu–DOX (a) and NH_2–Zn–DOX (b) by acidification step by step. The AMS (anionic surfactant templated mesoporous silica) nanoparticle used here was synthesized with $APS/C_{18}GluA = 2.5$. $Cu(CH_3COO)_2$ and $Zn(CH_3COO)_2$ have been used as metal sources. (Reprinted with permission from H. Zheng et al., Coordination bonding-based mesoporous silica for pH-responsive anticancer drug doxorubicin delivery, *J. Phys. Chem. C*, 115, 16803–16813. Copyright 2011 American Chemical Society.)

mesopore's "gate" that contained the drug.[87] In this system, the stimulus to trigger the drug release is not pH but external magnetic field, which will be discussed later.

For pH stimuli–responsive DDS, Liu et al. developed pH-responsive gold-capped mesoporous silica through an acetal linker.[121] First, the outer surface of mesoporous silica is functionalized by a carboxylic acid group. This can react with one of the amino group of a di-amino di-acetal linker. After drug loading, the mesopore's "gates" were then capped by carboxylic acid–modified gold nanoparticles. The latest were attached to the modified silica surface via the remaining free amino side groups bared by the di-amino di-acetal linker. Thus, the acid-cleavable acetal bond linking the modified mesoporous silica to the gold nanoparticles showed an efficient gate-capping ability at neutral pH. Since the stability of acetal bonding is highly dependent on pH, drug delivery can be triggered by acidic pH and release rate can also be controlled as a function of pH (see Figure 1.4).

Another strategy for pH-responsive gatekeeping is to use a supramolecular system as capping agent.[122–124] For instance, the efficient supramolecular nanovalve based on cucurbit[6]uril (CB[6]) was developed by Zink et al.[125] The gatekeeping method aims to create a nanovalve using CB[6]-induced 1,3-cycloaddition of azidoethylamine on alkyne-functionalized MCM-41. The final material contains two amine groups and CB[6] as gatekeeper on the linker. The nanovalve can be opened by adjusting the pH at 10 where the deprotonation of amine can disrupt ion–dipole interaction between the linker and CB[6] ring, and the rhodamine B (RhB) is released as shown in Figure 1.5.

An alternative way to cap mesopore gates is to use a pH-sensitive polymer as coating agent for the outer surface of mesoporous silica. A tremendous challenge in oral drug administration is that some drugs based on proteins or peptides undergo degradation at low pH. These drugs' absorption should take place in the intestine,

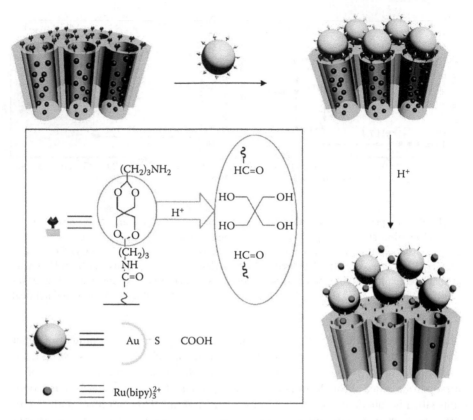

FIGURE 1.4　Schematic illustration of pH-responsive nanogated ensemble based on gold-capped mesoporous silica through acid-labile acetal linker. (Reprinted with permission from R. Liu et al., pH-responsive nanogated ensemble based on gold-capped mesoporous silica through an acid-labile acetal linker, *J. Am. Chem. Soc.*, 132, 1500–1501. Copyright 2010 American Chemical Society.)

and as such, an effective drug protection at low pH is required. Choi et al. developed polymer-coated spherical mesoporous silica for pH-controlled delivery of insulin.[126] Because of the important molecular size of insulin, the pore diameter of mesoporous silica was tuned up to 32 nm, which is 3- to 10-fold larger than classic mesoporous silica. Moreover, the inner silica surface was modified by amino groups to increase insulin loading efficiency. Eudragit L100, which has been employed in oral administration formulation, was used to coat the outer surface of mesoporous silica (see Figure 1.6). Eudragit L100 polymer coating protects mesoporous silica very efficiently under low pH, and it can be dissolved above pH 5.5–6.0 provoking drug release.

Among some biocompatible coating agents, pH-responsive nutraceuticals have attracted much attention in the scientific community. Considered as functional food in some countries such as Canada, nutraceuticals are biocompatible and biodegradable, and their production costs are much lower than classical biopolymers.[127] Guillet-Nicolas et al. prepared for oral DDS a mesoporous silica material functionalized by

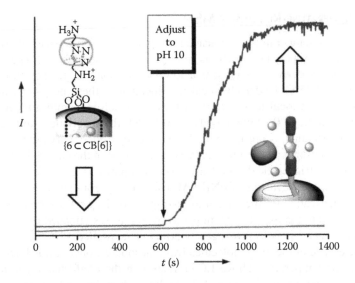

FIGURE 1.5   Release of the RhB guest molecules monitored by following the luminescence intensity of the solution of nanoparticles with shorter linkers {6 ⊂ CB[6]} (blue trace). Control experiments without changing the pH value (red trace) were also performed. There was no leakage. (S. Angelos et al.: pH-responsive supramolecular nanovalves based on cucurbit[6]uril pseudorotaxanes. *Angew. Chem. Int. Ed.* 2008. 47. 2222–2226. Copyright Wiley-VCH Verlag GmbH & Co. KGaA. Reproduced with permission.)

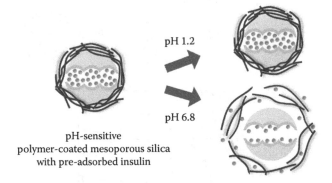

FIGURE 1.6   Schematic for the pH-controlled insulin delivery system based on pH-sensitive polymer coating of insulin-loaded spherical mesocellular foam (S-MCF) and its pH-responsive release. (S.R. Choi et al., Polymer-coated spherical mesoporous silica for pH-controlled delivery of insulin, *J. Mater. Chem. B*, 2, 616–619 (2014). Reproduced by permission of The Royal Society of Chemistry.)

succinylated β-lactoglobulin, which is a pH-responsive nutraceutical. They succeeded in preventing drug release under stomach conditions with such a biopolymer coating. In fact, below pH 5, the coated MSN keeps the drug inside of its mesopores because of gelation of the succinylated β-lactoglobulin, whose isoelectric point is at pH 5. As pH increases, the biopolymer becomes permeable, allowing the release of the drug.

1.3.2 TEMPERATURE-RESPONSIVE MSN

The synthesis of temperature-responsive mesoporous silica has been achieved using a thermosensitive polymer such as poly(N-isopropylacrylamide) (PNIPAM).[128] PNIPAM and its derivatives present a low critical solution temperature (LCST) between 30 and 35°C. Under chemical modification of these polymers, the LCST increases up to the local temperature of tumors, which is slightly higher than the normal temperature of the human body.[129] At LCST, these polymers undergo a transition of conformation, resulting in the increase of hydrophobicity owing to the loss of hydrogen bonding between the solvent (water in most of the cases). This transition could be used to trigger the drug release form mesopores.

Zhu et al. reported grafting of PNIPAM inside mesoporous silica by atom transfer radical polymerization for the temperature-responsive drug release system.[130] In this system, ibuprofen was used as the model drug, and it was attached to the PNIPAM chains inside mesopores by hydrogen bonding. The swelled PNIPAM chains prevented the escape of the drug molecules from mesopores, once it was loaded inside. Increasing the temperature above LCST results in the conformation transition of PNIPAM, causing the breaking up of the hydrogen bonding and opening the mesopores by a decrease of its own polymer chains, which can trigger the drug release.

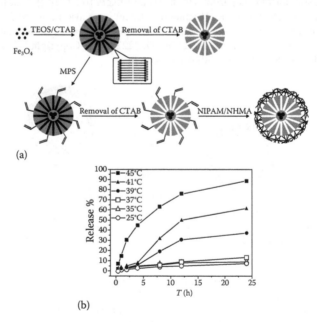

FIGURE 1.7 (a) Schematic preparation process of magnetic MSN (M-MSN) and M-MSN/P(NIPAM-co-NHMA). (b) Cumulative drug release of drug-loaded systems in PBS solution (pH 7.4): cumulative drug release from ZnPcS$_4$@M-MSN/P(NIPAM-co-NHMA)-5-10 system in PBS solution at different temperatures. CTAB, cetyltrimethylammonium bromide; MPS, 3-(trimethoxysilyl)propyl methacrylate. (C. Liu et al., Magnetic mesoporous silica microspheres with thermo-sensitive polymer shell for controlled drug release, *J. Mater. Chem.*, 19, 4764–4770 (2009). Reproduced by permission of The Royal Society of Chemistry.)

Another strategy that involves coating the outer surface of mesoporous silica by the derivatives of PNIPAM was demonstrated by Liu et al.[131] N-isopropylacrylamide (NIPA) and N-hydroxymethylacrylamide (NHMA) were copolymerized at the shell of MCM-41-type silica that already contained Fe_3O_4 as magnetic-responsive agent. The copolymer showed LCST around 38°C–42°C, a more adequate temperature for tumor-targeting drug delivery than nonmodified PNIPA. The experimental results showed a highly temperature-responsive drug release profile in which at low temperature, less than 10% of drug was "leaked" from mesopores (see Figure 1.7).

In the outer surface coating system, drug release temperature could also be easily customized using paraffins, which have various melting temperatures depending on alkyl chain length. Aznar et al. showed paraffin-capped MSNs as temperature-responsive drug cargo.[132] In this case, the outer surface of MCM-41 was functionalized with octadecyltrimethoxysilane. The alkyl chain interaction is mainly driven by London forces, which are able to form a hydrophobic layer around MCM-41. Increasing the temperature above the melting point of paraffins results in the capped mesopores opening and, thus, the release of the drug.

Schlossbauer et al. demonstrated that DNA could be used as an efficient capping agent of mesopores.[133] In their system, the main strategy relies on the DNA strand melting property at the specific temperature of the oligonucleotide, provoking the mesoporous silica cargo to open to release the drug loaded within.

1.3.3 Redox-Responsive MSN

Redox responsiveness is another powerful tool to control drug release from MSNs. Since the cleavage of disulfide bond (–S–S–) takes place in a reducing environment and most intracellular compartments can provide such a condition, the use of disulfide bond on mesoporous silica as a couple of redox stimuli is a good strategy to trigger drug release, especially inside cells. Moreover, in many tumor cells, the level of glutathione (GSH), a disulfide-reducing agent, is higher than normal cells and thus tumor-targeting drug delivery could also be achieved.[134]

Lin's group, which first introduced the gatekeeping strategy in mesoporous silica, reported CdS nanoparticle-capped mesoporous silica through linkers of disulfide and amino groups on the inner surface of mesopores.[87] Briefly, vancomycin and ATP (a neurotransmitter) were loaded into mesoporous silica, which was further capped by CdS nanoparticles. No leaking of the drugs was observed after capping mesopores. Drug release could be triggered by increasing the concentration in a disulfide-reducing agent (i.e., DTT), which cleaves disulfide bonds and unlocks the mesopores (see Figure 1.8).

Again, Lin et al. demonstrated that cysteine, which already contains a thiol group and might be toxic in an extracellular environment, could be loaded in thiol-modified MSNs without the capping method. Cysteine release can be triggered and regulated by redox stimuli, in this case, by the intracellular GSH's level.[135]

Other authors also designed redox stimuli–responsive mesoporous silica based on disulfide bond, using the gatekeeping approach with CB[6] or a-CD rings[136] or the polyethylene glycol (PEG) coating method via a cystine-based linker.[137]

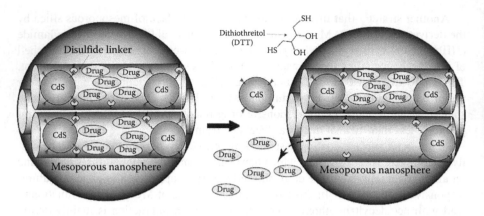

FIGURE 1.8 Schematic representation of the CdS nanoparticle-capped MSN-based drug/ neurotransmitter delivery system. The controlled-release mechanism of the system is based on chemical reduction of disulfide linkage between the CdS caps and the MSN hosts. (Reprinted with permission from C.-Y. Lai et al., A mesoporous silica nanosphere-based carrier system with chemically removable CdS nanoparticle caps for stimuli-responsive controlled release of neurotransmitters and drug molecules, *J. Am. Chem. Soc.*, 125, 4451–4459. Copyright 2003 American Chemical Society.)

1.3.4 LIGHT-RESPONSIVE MSN

Photoactive silica materials also became very useful in the control of drug delivery through organic light stimuli–sensitive molecules. Generally, they are grafted at the pore outlets and act as gatekeepers. In such systems, the drug delivery is activated by external light and usually drug molecules do not have a light absorption band overlapped with the gatekeeper molecules in order to follow the release efficiency.

In this context, Fujiwara et al. reported the first example of light stimuli–responsive MSNs, based on MCM-41, where the loading, storage, and drug release of model molecules (steroid cholestane, pyrene, phenanthrene, and progesterone) were controlled by light. To do so, they functionalized MCM-41 materials with a photosensitive coumarin derivative, the 7-[(3-triethoxysilyl)propoxy]coumarin, either by postsynthesis functionalization or by co-condensation. Then, modified MCM-41 was loaded with drug by the impregnation method. This material was irradiated under UV light (>310 nm for 30 min) in order to form the gatekeepers, namely, the cyclobutane rings, which result from the photodimerization reaction between a pair of coumarin groups. Then, the drug was easily released since cyclobutane rings are photocleavable upon UV light irradiation (around 250 nm), as shown in Figure 1.9. The release process efficiency was evaluated by UV-visible spectroscopy where the recurrence of coumarin absorption band was followed in time.[138]

MSNs modified with azobenzene moiety have also been largely investigated for their interesting photoreversibility property. As an example, Zink et al. reported light stimuli–responsive MSNs functionalized by azobenzene derivatives used as gatekeepers. They prepared two modified azobenzene molecules presenting *trans*-to-*cis*

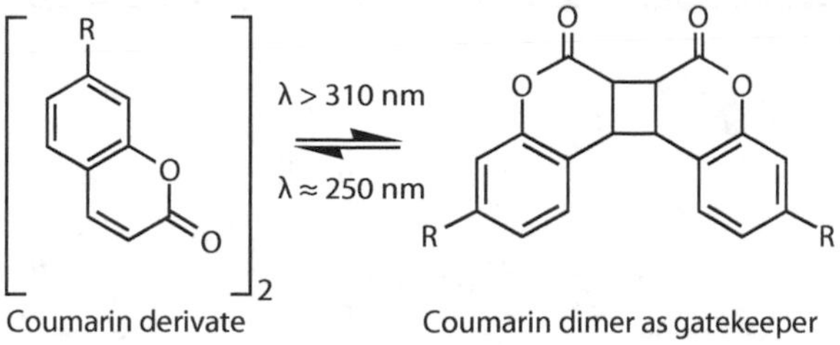

FIGURE 1.9 Coumarin photodimerization reaction to activate or deactivate gatekeeper dimer.

transition for postsynthesis functionalization of MCM-41 nanoparticles. The azobenzene derivative molecules were grafted inside the MCM-41 pores pointing straight along the channel like a thread when in the *trans* configuration. The latest conformation allowed loading RhB inside the MCM-41 porosity and either a pyrene-β-cyclodextrin or a β-cyclodextrin molecule was chosen as the sealing nanopore group. The cargo porosity was released under UV light irradiation at 351 nm where azobenzene derivative molecules adopt the *cis* configuration.[139]

In another work, Zink et al. coupled the photoisomerization property of the azobenzene derivative moiety with a pH-switchable pseudorotaxane (CB[6] rings encircling bisammonium derivative stalks) acting as nanovalves blocking the pores. Adding such pH-responsive secondary gatekeepers at the outlet of mesopores could reduce drug leaking and also design dual-controllable MSN DDS. The UV irradiation at 448 nm provokes continuous photocommutation of azobenzene moiety from *trans* to *cis* configuration inside of the pore. Moreover, under basic pH, the ion–dipole interaction between CB[6] rings and bisammonium derivative stalks is disrupted. Then, the dissociation of the rings releases guest molecules as illustrated in Figure 1.10.[140]

In some applications needing photostimulation, the encapsulated drug is sensitive to light and degrades, as is the case for DOX. Lin et al. developed MSN functionalized with aminopropyl groups protected by nitroveratryl function through a carbamate bond. When the carbamate linker is irradiated at 350 nm, DOX loaded in MSN is released. In fact, UV light triggers the deprotection of amine groups, which become positively charged when the process is done in water; thus release of DOX molecules is induced by electrostatic repulsion between the respective ammonium moieties. The mechanism was verified by zeta potential measurement that showed the increase of positive charge owing to the free amino group.[141] Lin et al. also designed lightresponsive MSNs using gold nanoparticles as gatekeepers[142] to cap outlet mesopores through a cleavable photolabile linker, named thioundecyl-tetraethyleneglycolesteronitrobenzylethyldimethyl ammonium bromide, for intracellular drug delivery. Their system was tested for photoinduced intracellular controlled release of an anticancer drug, paclitaxel, inside of human fibroblast and liver cells. According to the results, endocytosis and drug release were efficient under irradiation (λ = 365 nm), preventing zero premature release.

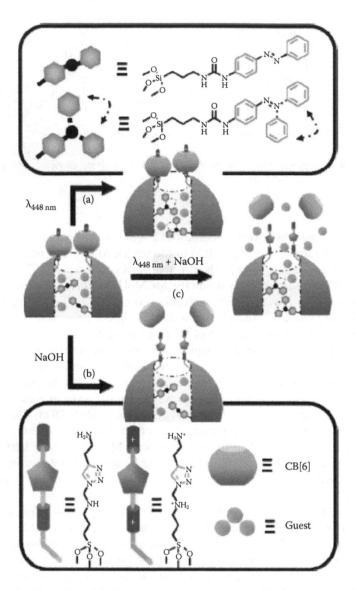

FIGURE 1.10 Operation of dual-controlled nanoparticles. (a) Excitation with 448 nm light induces the dynamic wagging motion of the nanoimpellers, but the nanovalves remain shut and the contents are contained. (b) Addition of NaOH opens the nanovalves, but the static nanoimpellers are able to keep the contents contained. (c) Simultaneous excitation with 448 nm light and addition of NaOH cause the contents to be released. (Reprinted with permission from D.P. Ferris et al., Light-operated mechanized nanoparticles, *J. Am. Chem. Soc.*, 131, 1686–1688. Copyright 2009 American Chemical Society.)

1.3.5 Magnetic-Responsive MSN

Building MSNs that respond to the magnetic field has attracted a lot of attention because of its potential applications. As DDSs, based on magnetic MSN, they could be guided to the desired site and then removed after complete release using an external magnetic field. This strategy might be of interest for cancer-targeting drugs, showing certain toxicity for organs, in order to reduce adverse side effects. Besides guiding the drug by magnetic field, magnetic MSN can be used for hyperthermia therapy.[143–145] For instance, superparamagnetic nanoparticles embedded into MSNs were already widely studied for both drug guide system and hyperthermia properties.[146] However, biocompatibility and toxicity problems are always a limiting factor; thus, only magnetite (Fe_3O_4) or maghemite (γ-Fe_2O_3) have been considered for biomedical applications. To date, more than 1700 publications (based on Web of Science) deal with magnetic MSN. We will focus on some examples that marked a turning point in the biomedical field.

For the synthesis of magnetic MSN, various designs and strategies have been proposed.[147,148] A core–shell structure with magnetic nanoparticles, proposed by Shi et al., has considered as a basic model for magnetic MSN (see Figure 1.11).[149,150] Its potential medical applications were confirmed using ibuprofen as well.

Zhao's group in Fudan University has extended the core–shell model using several iron sources and also simplified synthesis methods (see Figure 1.12).[150–152] Besides conventional drug molecules, DNA can be carried inside mesopores and delivered using magnetic field (see Figure 1.13).[153] Moreover, magnetic MSNs have been extensively tested on in vivo cells in recent years.[154] The results showed that a core–shell structure, in which nanoparticles do not have direct contact with cellular culture, is not toxic but exhibits excellent biocompatibility.

Embedding magnetic nanoparticles into MSNs has also been of interest for scientists. Magnetic nanoparticles can be easily incorporated inside mesopores or on the matrix of silica. Corriu's group reported the synthesis of magnetic silica-based nanocomposites containing magnetite (Fe_3O_4) nanoparticles using internal anchored acetylacetonate groups as a ligand.[155] Huang et al. demonstrated controlled and targeted ibuprofen release using magnetic γ-Fe_2O_3@MSN composites with different morphologies.[156]

Recently, the rattle-type hollow structure rose to the spotlight. Like in meso-macroporous materials, a hollow cavity can enhance surface area/pore volume ratio,

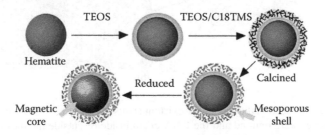

FIGURE 1.11 Illustration of synthesis of MFeCMS nanospheres. C18TMS, *n*-octadecyltrimethoxysilane. (Reprinted with permission from W. Zhao et al., Fabrication of uniform magnetic nanocomposite spheres with a magnetic core/mesoporous silica shell structure, *J. Am. Chem. Soc.*, 127, 8916–8917. Copyright 2005 American Chemical Society.)

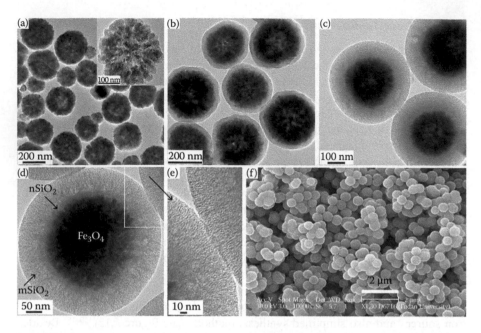

FIGURE 1.12 TEM images of (a) Fe_3O_4 particles, (b) $Fe_3O_4@SiO_2$, and (c–e) $Fe_3O_4@nSiO_2@$ $mSiO_2$ microspheres, and (f) SEM image of $Fe_3O_4@nSiO_2@mSiO_2$ microspheres. (Reprinted with permission from Y. Deng et al., Superparamagnetic high-magnetization microspheres with an $Fe_3O_4@SiO_2$ core and perpendicularly aligned mesoporous SiO_2 shell for removal of microcystins, *J. Am. Chem. Soc.*, 130, 28–29. Copyright 2008 American Chemical Society.)

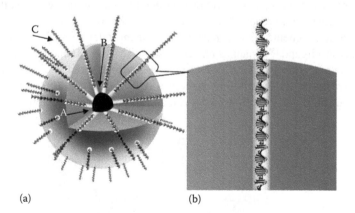

(a)   (b)

FIGURE 1.13 (a) Sectional drawing for existent status of DNA in M-MSN mesopores (the empty mesopores were omitted and the DNA chain inside or outside the mesopore was not depicted accurately). Arrow A represented the magnetic core, arrow B represented the mesopore, and arrow C represented DNA molecule. (b) An enlarged image for DNA molecule in mesopore. (Reprinted with permission from X. Li et al., Adsorption and desorption behaviors of DNA with magnetic mesoporous silica nanoparticles, *Langmuir*, 27, 6099–6106. Copyright 2011 American Chemical Society.)

which also means an increase in drug binding surface/volume. Therefore, more drug can be encapsulated than into a core–shell model. Shi's group reported rattle-type hollow-structured magnetic mesoporous silica nanocapsules as a platform for simultaneous cell imaging and anticancer drug delivery (see Figure 1.14).[48,157] As expected, these MSNs showed high DOX loading capacity and entrapment efficiency compared to the simple core–shell structure.[157]

Another type of magnetic MSNs consists of using magnetic nanoparticles as a capping agent for mesopore gates. Lin et al. reported MSN capped by Fe_3O_4 nanoparticles via disulfide linker. This double stimuli–responsive system could be used in

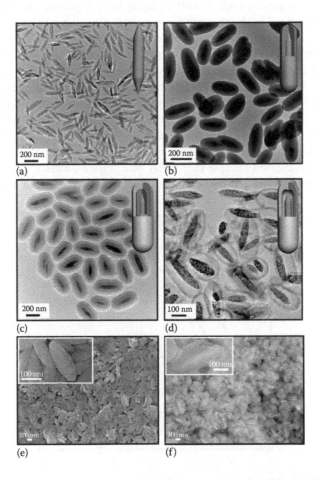

FIGURE 1.14   TEM images of ellipsoidal (a) Fe_2O_3, (b) $Fe_2O_3@SiO_2$, (c) $Fe_2O_3@SiO_2@mSiO_2$, and (d) $Fe_3O_4@mSiO_2$. Secondary electron SEM image of ellipsoidal Fe_2O_3 (e, inset: SEM image at high magnification) and backscattered electron SEM (f) image of ellipsoidal $Fe_3O_4@mSiO_2$ nanocapsules (inset: purposely selected backscattered electron image of broken nanocapsules to reveal the hollow nanostructure). (Reprinted with permission from Y. Chen et al., Core/shell structured hollow mesoporous nanocapsules: A potential platform for simultaneous cell imaging and anticancer drug delivery, *ACS Nano*, 4, 6001–6013. Copyright 2010 American Chemical Society.)

more sophisticated applications like targeting by magnetic field and drug trigger by redox condition.[63] Gate-capped MSNs with linkers, which respond to other stimuli such as light or pH, were already discussed.

1.3.6 BIOLOGICAL STIMULI-RESPONSIVE DRUG RELEASE

Recent improvements in the design of stimuli-responsive drug release systems have been employed to develop biological stimuli carriers.

For example, Yu et al. showed programmable drug release from MSNs that responded to biological stimuli.[158] Sulfasalazine (SZ), a prodrug, is encapsulated in amino-functionalized MSNs through electrostatic interactions. The material is then coated with succinylated soy protein isolate (SSPI), which is relatively affordable and considered a food additive in some countries such as Canada. This system showed no leakage of drug at low pH and in the water because hydrophobic SSPI does not undergo hydrolysis except at high pH. In the presence of pancreatin enzyme, which predominates in the intestine, SSPI is hydrolyzed and mesopore gates can be opened. Moreover, azo-reductase produced by colon microflora can cut the azo function of SZ, yielding the active metabolite 5-aminosalicylic acid (see Figure 1.15).

Qu et al. reported DNA-capped MSN for which pores can be opened upon treatment with deoxyribonuclease I (DNase I).[159] DNA was grafted on the surface of MSN via the click conjugating method between azide-functionalized MSN and aryl-modified

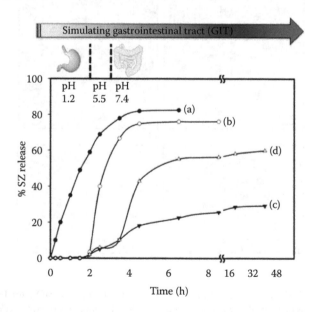

FIGURE 1.15 Release of profiles of SZ from (a) MCM-48-SZ, (b) MSN-NH2-SZ, (c) MSN-NH2-SZ@SSPI without enzyme, and (d) MSN-NH2-SZ@SSPI in the presence of enzymes (pepsin at pH 1.2 and pancreatin at pH 7.4) present in simulated GIT fluids. (Reprinted with permission from A. Popat et al., Programmable drug release using bioresponsive mesoporous silica nanoparticles for site-specific oral drug delivery, *Chem. Commun.*, 50, 5547–5550. Copyright 2014 Royal Chemical Society.)

DNA sequence. The duplex DNA is a highly effective capping method; less than 10% of the drug is leaked without external stimuli. When this system is exposed to DNase I, the duplex DNA could be hydrolyzed, opening the mesopores and releasing the drug.

Adenosine triphosphate (ATP) can also be used as biological stimuli for controlled drug release. Gooding et al. designed an MSN-based drug release system containing ATP-responsive gold nanoparticles as capping agent. Indeed, mesopore capping is achieved by the complexation of Cu^{2+} between amino-functionalized MSN and L-cysteine-modified gold nanoparticles (AuNP) under acid pH.[160] ATP, which contains a more effective complexation site than a single amino group, was shown to be a biological stimulus to detach gold nanoparticles from mesopore gates through Cu^{2+} complexation. In this investigation, low pH and ATP have been used as biological stimuli for drug release within either the lysosome in the case of low pH or the cytosol, which contains a high concentration of ATP.

Using the US Food and Drug Administration (FDA)–approved peptide drug protamine as coating agent of MSN is an effective way of making a biological stimuli–responsive DDS, as demonstrated by Raichur et al.[161] Indeed, like other coating agents, protamine can effectively protect the encapsulated drug from burst or undesired release. Coating is conducted on amino-functionalized MSNs using glutaraldehyde as coupling agent. In the presence of enzyme (such as trypsin) that recognizes and cuts arginine or lysine sites, the protamine coating can dissolve, opening the mesopores and releasing the drug.

1.4 SILICA: SUITABLE MATRIX FOR BIOMEDICAL APPLICATIONS (TOXICITY, BIOCOMPATIBILITY)

For a long time, the definition of *biocompatibility* was reduced to a basic criterion stating exhaustively that medical devices would be nontoxic, nonimmunogenic, nonthrombogenic, noncarcinogenic, and nonirritant and should not harm the patient.[162] However, medical devices should meet increasingly specific therapeutic demands that they are now becoming less and less inert but designed to interact with particular human tissues and body environment. Thus, today, the new definition of *biocompatibility* suggested in 2008 by William involves the fact that "biomaterials with all their specific functions must perform their desired function with respect to a medical therapy, without eliciting any undesirable local or systemic effects in the recipient or beneficiary of that therapy, but generating the most appropriate beneficial cellular or tissue response in that specific situation, and optimising the clinically relevant performance of that therapy."[162]

Today, many biomaterials are based on silicon, one of the most abundant elements in nature that also contributes to human needs. Moreover, the FDA decreed amorphous silicon dioxide as "Generally Recognized As Safe (GRAS)."[16] For all these reasons, numerous investigations have been done for the development of silicon-based biomaterials for DDSs, probes for diagnosis, and materials for tissue engineering. The weak bonds between silicon atoms themselves or with oxygen make Si-based materials biodegradable and biocompatible, but even if a large number of in vitro assays showed encouraging results, the probable in vivo behavior remains difficult to deduce from these evaluations, mainly because of the physiological and environmental complexities not reproducible in vitro.[163]

Many therapeutic treatments or medical devices under in vitro assessment take the long road to a potential medical application. Interactions between nanoparticles and cells are the topic of many investigations. In general, local drug delivery needs to have an efferent cellular uptake, which depends strongly on the targeting strategy. The latter is classified into two categories called *passive targeting* and *active targeting* according to the literature. Passive targeting relies on the accumulation of nanoparticles in tumor tissues through an enhanced permeability and retention (EPR) effect. In fact, tumor vasculature is highly permeable to modified nanoparticles with, for example, positively charged groups.[164] Unfortunately, an EPR effect is not generalized to all tumor cells. Active targeting uses, for example, folic acid, peptides, or macromolecules (PEG, DNA) as ligands that are able to bind to certain overexpressed receptors on tumor cell surfaces and to promote the cellular uptake of the nanocargo. Thus, it is possible to improve targeting specificity and then improve drug delivery while evading nonspecific binding and activation of immunogenic effects.[103]

An efficient delivery process is often confronted by entrapment of endosomes, which favor nanocarriers, and by drug molecule degradation by specific digestive enzymes present in lysosomes. Natural systems such as bacteria and viruses have developed ingenious strategies to penetrate membranes and reach the target sites while escaping endosomal entrapment.

The mechanisms that have been developed so far are intended to penetrate the endosomal barrier. Different mechanisms such as pore formation in the endosomal membrane, pH-buffering effects of protonatable groups ("proton sponge"), or fusion into the lipid bilayer of endosomes have been proposed to facilitate endosomal escape.[165] In addition, photochemical methods to rupture the endosomal membrane have been introduced to MSNs.[104,166]

Nevertheless, by combining several recent in vitro and in vivo evaluations, it seems that nanoparticle silica toxicity is strongly related to their physicochemical parameters such as particle size, shape, surface chemistry, and charges.[23] It was found that the shape of particles could modify the cell behavior. In fact, Huang et al. demonstrate in vitro that MSNs with variable aspect ratio (1, 2, and 4) and length (100, 240, and 450 nm) could influence the cellular uptake.[167] They compared the transport of the different MSNs to an A375 model of malignant melanoma cells and they investigated the shape effect on cell proliferation, apoptosis, adhesion, migration, and cytoskeleton formation. They demonstrated that the MSNs' shape modifies cellular responses and regulation cell functions. However, the results showed that MSNs with a smaller aspect ratio had a minor effect on cell operation.

Biocompatibility and stability are usually improved through the chemical modification of the nanoparticle shell. Since the efficiency of the cellular uptake is enhanced for nanocargos smaller than 120 nm, to avoid thrombogenic effects, it is essential to prevent nanoparticle aggregation with polymer coatings, charged groups, or supported lipid bilayers.[168–170] Thus, better stability has been observed for silica nanoparticles, while preventing premature dissolution of silica in the biological media.[171–177]

In general, MSNs coated with a protective organic shell improved biocompatibility and hemocompatibility and can be potentially used for intravenous drug delivery.[178]

For example, He et al. proceed to in vivo assays on ICR mice to compare the biodistribution and excretion of MSNs and PEG-coated MSN nanoparticles, all sized from 80 to 360 nm.[179] Nanoparticles have been injected through the tail vein of the mice. They analyzed liver, spleen, and lung tissues and noticed that smaller particles escaped easily from those organs, in particular those coated with PEG. However, it was noticed that PEGylated MSNs were slowly biodegraded and correspondingly had a lower excreted amount of degradation products in the urine because of a longer blood circulation lifetime. However, neither MSNs nor PEGylated MSNs caused tissue toxicity after 1 month in vivo.

1.5 CONCLUSION AND PERSPECTIVES

This chapter demonstrates that MSNs have been intensively employed to design efficient DDSs especially because of their high loading capacity, high stability, and the ability to protect the guest molecules from various biochemical attacks. Indeed, what encourages many research groups to design MSN drug carriers are the biocompatibility and biodegradability of these materials. In addition, MSNs offer a multitude of functionalization routes that allow decorating either the inner or the outer surface, with pH, thermal, light, and magnetic stimuli–responsive molecules, polymers, metallic nanoparticles, and targeting ligands. The latest functionalization strategies have been tailored to control the drug delivery kinetics at the appropriate place with zero premature release together with preventing undesired side effects. That leaves the door open for researchers to build fascinating and efficient multifunctional nanocarriers for targeted disease treatment and bioimaging devices. For the moment, most in vitro studies helped in the evaluation of the cytotoxicity, biocompatibility, biodegradability, and retention of MSN nanocarriers and in the understanding of some cellular uptake mechanisms. However, toxicity and intracellular uptake results reported in the literature are specific to each DDS developed up to now. Moreover, in vitro diagnostics could not be systematically representative of the in vivo assays because of the complexity of the body environment. Thereby, in vivo studies that demonstrate the potential of MSNs as DDSs or biosensors in therapeutic applications remain one of the biggest challenges today.[180,181]

ACKNOWLEDGMENT

The authors would like to acknowledge the French Ministry for Research and Education for the PhD grant attributed to Sanghoon Kim.

REFERENCES

1. C.S. Brunner, Challenges and Opportunities in Emerging Drug Delivery Technologies, *Product Genesis* (2004).
2. I. Slowing, J. Vivero-Escoto, C. Wu, and V. Lin, Mesoporous Silica Nanoparticles as Controlled Release Drug Delivery and Gene Transfection Carriers, *Adv. Drug Deliv. Rev.*, 60, 1278–1288 (2008).
3. C. Argyo, V. Weiss, V.C. Bräuchle, and T. Bein, Multifunctional Mesoporous Silica Nanoparticles as a Universal Platform for Drug Delivery, *Chem. Mater.*, 26, 435–451 (2014).

4. A. Popat, J. Liu, G.Q.M. Lu, and S.Z. Qiao, A pH-Responsive Drug Delivery System Based on Chitosan Coated Mesoporous Silica Nanoparticles, *J. Mater. Chem.*, 22, 11173–11178 (2012).
5. Y.S. Lin, N. Abadeer, K.R. Hurley, and C.L. Haynes, Ultrastable, Redispersible, Small, and Highly Organomodified Mesoporous Silica Nanotherapeutics, *J. Am. Chem. Soc.*, 133, 20444–20457 (2011).
6. K. Ma, U. Werner-Zwanziger, J. Zwanziger, and U. Wiesner, Controlling Growth of Ultrasmall Sub-10 nm Fluorescent Mesoporous Silica Nanoparticles, *Chem. Mater.*, 25, 677–691 (2013).
7. J. Kobler, K. Möller, and T. Bein, Colloidal Suspensions of Functionalized Mesoporous Silica Nanoparticles, *ACS Nano*, 2, 791–799 (2008).
8. M.-H. Kim, H.-K. Na, Y.-K. Kim, S.-R. Ryoo, H.S. Cho, K.E. Lee, H. Jeon, R. Ryoo, and D.-H. Min, Facile Synthesis of Monodispersed Mesoporous Silica Nanoparticles with Ultralarge Pores and Their Application in Gene Delivery, *ACS Nano*, 5, 3568–3576 (2011).
9. S.P. Hudson, R.F. Padera, R. Langer, and D.S. Kohane, The Biocompatibility of Mesoporous Silicates, *Biomaterials*, 29, 4045–4055 (2008).
10. M. Sinn Aw, M. Kurian, and D. Losic, Non-Eroding Drug-Releasing Implants with Ordered Nanoporous and Nanotubular Structures: Concepts for Controlling Drug Release, *Biomater. Sci.*, 9, 9243–9257 (2014).
11. M.G. Pankhania, C.D. Melia, and J.F. Lampard, Sustained-Release Pharmaceutical Formulation Containing Xanthan Gum, EP 0234670 B1.
12. B.B. Aggarwal, A. Kumar, and A.C. Bharti, Anticancer Potential of Curcumin: Preclinical and Clinical Studies, *Anticancer Res.*, 23, 363–398 (2003).
13. K.C. Kwan, Oral Bioavailability and First-Pass Effects, *Drug Metab. Dispos.*, 25, 1329–1336 (1997).
14. U.S. Food and Drug Administration, Avoid Food-Drug Interactions (2010).
15. E.O. Meltzer, M.J. Welch, and N.K. Ostrom, Pill Swallowing Ability and Training in Children 6 to 11 Years of Age, *Clin. Pediatr.*, 45, 725–733 (2006).
16. U.S. Food and Drug Administration, Inactive Ingredient Database. Available at http://www.accessdata.fda.gov/scripts/cder/iig/index.Cfm.
17. S. Jambhrunkar, S. Karmakar, A. Popat, M. Yu, and C. Yu, Mesoporous Silica Nanoparticles Enhance the Cytotoxicity of Curcumin, *RSC Adv.*, 4, 709–712 (2013).
18. Schering Corporation A Corp. of NJ, Transdermal Delivery of Nicotine, US 4908213A.
19. S.K. Niazi, *Handbook of Pharmaceutical Manufacturing Formulations*, Informa Healthcare, Switzerland (2009).
20. D. Harris, and J.R. Robinson, Drug Delivery via the Mucous Membranes of the Oral Cavity, *J. Pharm. Sci.*, 81, 1–10 (1992).
21. H. Lambers, S. Piessens, A. Bloem, H. Pronk, and P. Finkel, Natural Skin Surface pH is on Average below 5, which is Beneficial for Its Resident Flora, *Int. J. Cosmet. Sci.*, 28, 359–370 (2006).
22. D.I. Sessler, and A. Moayeri, Skin-Surface Warming: Heat Flux and Central Temperature, *Anesthesiology*, 73, 218–224 (1990).
23. Y. Chen, H. Chen, and J. Shi, In Vivo Bio-Safety Evaluations and Diagnostic/Therapeutic Applications of Chemically Designed Mesoporous Silica Nanoparticles, *Adv. Mater.*, 25, 3144–3176 (2013).
24. D. Arcos, and M. Vallet-Regí, Bioceramics for Drug Delivery, *Acta Mater.*, 61, 890–911 (2013).
25. W. Stober, A. Fink, and E. Bohn, Controlled Growth of Monodisperse Silica Spheres in the Micron Size Range, *J. Colloid Interface Sci.*, 26, 62–69 (1968).
26. I. Tissot, J.P. Reymond, F. Lefebvre, and E. Bourgeat-Lami, SiOH-Functionalized Polystyrene Latexes. A Step toward the Synthesis of Hollow Silica Nanoparticles, *Chem. Mater.*, 14, 1325–1331 (2002).

27. C.E. Fowler, D. Khushalani, and S. Mann, Interfacial Synthesis of Hollow Microspheres of Mesostructured Silica, *Chem. Commun.*, 2028–2029 (2001).
28. G. Aharon, M. Yizhak, and R. Rohit Kumar, Acoustic Cavitation Leading to the Morphosynthesis of Mesoporous Silica Vesicles, *Adv. Mater.*, 14, 1414–1418 (2002).
29. A. Stein, S.G. Rudisill, and N.D. Petkovich, Perspective on the Influence of Interactions Between Hard and Soft Templates and Precursors on Morphology of Hierarchically Structured Porous Materials, *Chem. Mater.*, 26, 259–276 (2014).
30. Y.D. Liu, J. Goebl, and Y.D. Yin, Templated Synthesis of Nanostructured Materials, *Chem. Soc. Rev.*, 42, 2610–2653 (2013).
31. B. Tan, and S.E. Rankin, Dual Latex/Surfactant Templating of Hollow Spherical Silica Particles with Ordered Mesoporous Shells, *Langmuir*, 21, 8180–8187 (2005).
32. J. Čejková, and F. Štěpánek, Compartmentalized and Internally Structured Particles for Drug Delivery—A Review, *Curr. Pharm. Des.*, 19, 6298–6314 (2013).
33. A. Pasc, J.-L. Blin, M.J. Stébé, and J. Ghanbajab, Solid Lipid Nanoparticles (SLN) Templating of Macroporous Silica Beads, *RCS Adv.*, 1, 1204–1206 (2012).
34. P.W. Voorhees, The Theory of Ostwald Ripening, *J. Stat. Phys.*, 38, 231–235 (1985).
35. J. Liu, F. Liu, K. Gao, J. Wu, and D. Xue, Recent Developments in the Chemical Synthesis of Inorganic Porous Capsules, *J. Mater. Chem.*, 19, 6073–6084 (2009).
36. G. Réthoré, and A. Pandit, Use of Templates to Fabricate Nanoscale Spherical Structures for Defined Architectural Control, *Small*, 6, 488–498 (2010).
37. X.W.D. Lou, L.A. Archer, and Z. Yang, Hollow Micro-/Nanostructures: Synthesis and Applications, *Adv. Mater.*, 20, 3987–4019 (2008).
38. Y. Zhao, and L. Jiang, Hollow Micro/Nanomaterials with Multilevel Interior Structures, *Adv. Mater.*, 21, 3621–3638 (2009).
39. H.C. Zeng, Synthesis and Self-Assembly of Complex Hollow Materials, *J. Mater. Chem.*, 21, 7511–7526 (2011).
40. Y. Ma, and L. Qi, Solution-Phase Synthesis of Inorganic Hollow Structures by Templating Strategies, *J. Colloid Interface Sci.*, 335, 1–10 (2009).
41. H.J. Hah, J.S. Kim, B.J. Jeon, S.M. Koo, and Y.E. Lee, Simple Preparation of Monodisperse Hollow Silica Particles without Using Templates, *Chem. Commun.*, 1712–1713 (2003).
42. Y. Zhu, J. Shi, W. Shen, X. Dong, J. Feng, M. Ruan, and Y. Li, Stimuli-Responsive Controlled Drug Release from a Hollow Mesoporous Silica Sphere/Poly-Electrolyte Multilayer Core–Shell Structure. *Angew. Chem. Int. Ed.*, 44, 5083–5087 (2005).
43. J. Hu, M. Chen, X. Fang, and L. Wu, Fabrication and Application of Inorganic Hollow Spheres, *Chem. Soc. Rev.*, 40, 5472–5491 (2011).
44. D.A. Wheeler, R.J. Newhouse, H. Wang, S. Zou, and J.Z. Zhang, Optical Properties and Persistent Spectral Hole Burning of Near Infrared-Absorbing Hollow Gold Nanospheres, *J. Phys. Chem. C*, 114, 18126–18133 (2010).
45. R. Ravetti-Duran, J.-L. Blin, M.J. Stébé, C. Castel, and A. Pasc, Tuning the Morphology and the Structure of Hierarchical Meso–Macroporous Silica by Dual Templating with Micelles and Solid Lipid Nanoparticles (SLN), *J. Mater. Chem.*, 22, 21540–21548 (2012).
46. J.Z. Zhang, Biomedical Applications of Shape-Controlled Plasmonic Nanostructures: A Case Study of Hollow Gold Nanospheres for Photothermal Ablation Therapy of Cancer, *J. Phys. Chem. Lett.*, 1, 686–695 (2010).
47. X. Jiang, T.L. Ward, Y.-S. Cheng, J. Liu, and C.J. Brinker, Aerosol Fabrication of Hollow Mesoporous Silica Nanoparticles and Encapsulation of L-Methionine as a Candidate Drug Cargo, *Chem. Commun.*, 46, 3019–3021 (2010).
48. Y. Zhu, Y. Fang, and S. Kaskel, Folate-Conjugated $Fe_3O_4@SiO_2$ Hollow Mesoporous Spheres for Targeted Anticancer Drug Delivery, *J. Phys. Chem. C*, 114, 16382–16388 (2010).

49. F. Lu, A. Popa, S. Zhou, J.-J. Zhu, and A.C.S. Samia, Iron Oxide-Loaded Hollow Mesoporous Silica Nanocapsules for Controlled Drug Release and Hyperthermia, *Chem. Commun.*, 49, 11436–11438 (2013).

50. D. Zhao, J. Sun, Q. Li, and G.D. Stucky, Morphological Control of Highly Ordered Mesoporous Silica SBA-15, *Chem. Mater.*, 12, 275–279 (2000).

51. P. Linton, and V. Alfredsson, Growth and Morphology of Mesoporous SBA-15 Particles, *Chem. Mater.*, 20, 2878–2880 (2008).

52. Y. Ding, G. Yin, X. Liao, Z. Huang, X. Chen, Y. Yao, and J. Li, A Convenient Route to Synthesize SBA-15 Rods with Tunable Pore Length for Lysozyme Adsorption, *Micropor. Mesopor. Mater.*, 170, 45–51 (2013).

53. W. Shenton, T. Douglas, M. Young, G. Stubbs, and S. Mann, Inorganic Organic Nanotube Composites from Template Mineralization of Tobacco Mosaic Virus, *Adv. Mater.*, 11, 253–256 (1999).

54. S.B. Lee, Antibody-Based Bio-Nanotube Membranes for Enantiomeric Drug Separations, *Science*, 296, 2198–2000 (2002).

55. K.J.C. van Bommel, A. Friggeri, and S. Shinkai, Organic Templates for the Generation of Inorganic Materials, *Angew. Chem. Int. Ed.*, 42, 980–999 (2003).

56. J. Jang, and H. Yoon, Novel Fabrication of Size-Tunable Silica Nanotubes Using a Reverse- Microemulsion-Mediated Sol-Gel Method, *Adv. Mater.*, 16, 799–802 (2004).

57. W. Wang, J. Zhou, S. Zhang, J. Song, H. Duan, M. Zhou, C. Gong, Z. Bao, B. Lu, X. Li, W. Lan, and E. Xie, A Novel Method to Fabricate Silica Nanotubes Based on Phase Separation Effect, *J. Mater. Chem.*, 20, 9068–9072 (2010).

58. M. Sumper, and E. Brunner, Learning from Diatoms: Nature's Tools for the Production of Nanostructured Silica, *Adv. Funct. Mater.*, 16, 17–26 (2006).

59. S.C. Holmström, P.J.S. King, M.G. Ryadnov, M.F. Butler, S. Mann, and D.N. Woolfson, Templating Silica Nanostructures on Rationally Designed Self-Assembled Peptide Fibers, *Langmuir*, 24, 11778–11783 (2008).

60. A. Altunbas, N. Sharma, M.S. Lamm, C. Yan, R.P. Nagarkar, J.P. Schneider, and D.J. Pochan, Peptide–Silica Hybrid Networks: Biomimetic Control of Network Mechanical Behavior, *ACS Nano*, 4, 181–188 (2010).

61. S. Wang, X. Ge, J. Xue, H. Fan, L. Mu, Y. Li, H. Xu, and J.R. Lu, Mechanistic Processes Underlying Biomimetic Synthesis of Silica Nanotubes from Self-Assembled Ultrashort Peptide Templates, *Chem. Mater.*, 23, 2466–2472 (2011).

62. C. Zollfrank, H. Scheel, and P. Greil, Regioselectively Ordered Silica Nanotubes by Molecular Templating, *Adv. Mater.*, 19, 984–987 (2007).

63. S. Giri, B.G. Trewyn, M.P. Stellmaker, and V. Lin, Stimuli-Responsive Controlled-Release Delivery System Based on Mesoporous Silica Nanorods Capped with Magnetic Nanoparticles, *Angew. Chem. Int. Ed.*, 44, 5039–5044 (2005).

64. Z. Hou, C. Li, P. Ma, Z. Cheng, X. Li, Y. Zhang, Y. Dai, D. Yang, H. Lian, and J. Lin, Up-Conversion Luminescent and Porous NaYF4:Yb3+, Er3+@SiO2 Nanocomposite Fibers for Anti-Cancer Drug Delivery and Cell Imaging, *Adv. Funct. Mater.*, 22, 2713–2722 (2012).

65. C.T. Kersge, M.E. Leonowicz, W.J. Roth, J.C. Vartuli, and J.S. Beck, Ordered Mesoporous Molecular Sieves Synthesized by a Liquid-Crystal Template Mechanism, *Nature*, 359, 710–712 (1992).

66. F. Hoffmann, M. Cornelius, J. Morell, and M. Fröba, Silica-Based Mesoporous Organic–Inorganic Hybrid Materials, *Angew. Chem. Int. Ed.*, 45, 3217–3251 (2006).

67. Y. Wan, and D. Zhao, On the Controllable Soft-Templating Approach to Mesoporous Silicates, *Chem. Rev.*, 107, 2821–2860 (2007).

68. I. Slowing, J. Vivero-Escoto, B.G. Trewyn, and V. Lin, Mesoporous Silica Nanoparticles: Structural Design and Applications, *J. Mater. Chem.*, 20, 7924–7937 (2010).

69. S.-H. Wu, C.-Y. Mou, and H.-P. Lin, Synthesis of Mesoporous Silica Nanoparticles, *Chem. Soc. Rev.*, 42, 3862–3875 (2013).
70. C.J. Brinker, *Advances in Chemistry*, vol. 234, American Chemical Society: Washington DC, 361–401 (1994).
71. J. Sefcik, and A.V. McCormick, Kinetic and Thermodynamic Issues in the Early Stages of Sol-Gel Processes Using Silicon Alkoxides, *Catal. Today*, 35, 205–223 (1997).
72. M. Vallet-Regi, A. Rámila, R.P. del Real, and J. Pérez-Pariente, A New Property of MCM-41: Drug Delivery System, *Chem. Mater.*, 13, 308–311 (2001).
73. C.H. Tsai, J.L. Vivero-Escoto, I.I. Slowing, I.J. Fang, B.G. Trewyn, and V.S.Y. Lin, Surfactant-Assisted Controlled Release of Hydrophobic Drugs Using Anionic Surfactant Templated Mesoporous Silica Nanoparticles, *Biomaterials*, 32, 6234–6244 (2011).
74. G. Wang, A. N. Otuonye, E. A. Blair, K. Denton, Z. Tao, and T. Asefa, Functionalized Mesoporous Materials for Adsorption and Release of Different Drug Molecules: A Comparative Study, *J. Solid State Chem.*, 182, 1649–1660 (2009).
75. B.G. Trewyn, C.M. Whitman, and V. Lin, Morphological Control of Room-Temperature Ionic Liquid Templated Mesoporous Silica Nanoparticles for Controlled Release of Antibacterial Agents, *Nano Lett.*, 4, 2139–2143 (2004).
76. M.M. Wan, W.J. Qian, W.G. Lin, Y. Zhou, and J.H. Zhu, Multiple Functionalization of SBA-15 Mesoporous Silica in One-Pot: Fabricating an Aluminum-Containing Plugged Composite for Sustained Heparin Release, *J. Mater. Chem. B*, 1, 3897–3905 (2013).
77. D. Brühwiler, Postsynthetic Functionalization of Mesoporous Silica, *Nanoscale*, 2, 887–892 (2010).
78. P. Yang, S. Gai, and J. Lin, Functionalized Mesoporous Silica Materials for Controlled Drug Delivery, *Chem. Soc. Rev.*, 41, 3679–3698 (2012).
79. A. Vinu, K.Z. Hossain, and K. Ariga, Recent Advances in Functionalization of Mesoporous Silica, *J. Nanosci. Nanotechnol.*, 5, 347–371 (2005).
80. S.L. Burkett, S.D. Sims, and S. Mann, Synthesis of Hybrid Inorganic-Organic Mesoporous Silica by Co-Condensation of Siloxane and Organosiloxane Precursors, *Chem. Commun.*, 1367–1368 (1996).
81. A.P. Wight, and M.E. Davis, Design and Preparation of Organic–Inorganic Hybrid Catalysts, *Chem. Rev.*, 102, 3589–3614 (2012).
82. M.H. Lim, and A. Stein, Comparative Studies of Grafting and Direct Syntheses of Inorganic-Organic Hybrid Mesoporous Materials, *Chem. Mater.*, 11, 3285–3295 (1999).
83. A. Walcarius, M. Etienne, and B. Lebeau, Rate of Access to the Binding Sites in Organically Modified Silicates. 2. Ordered Mesoporous Silicas Grafted with Amine or Thiol Groups, *Chem. Mater.*, 15, 2161–2173 (2003).
84. P. Banet, N. Marcotte, D.A. Lerner, and D. Brunel, Single-Step Dispersion of Functionalities on a Silica Surface, *Langmuir*, 24, 9030–9037 (2008).
85. E.A. Kadib, N. Katir, M. Bousmina, and J.P. Majoral, Dendrimer–Silica Hybrid Mesoporous Materials, *New J. Chem.*, 36, 241–255 (2012).
86. M. Hebrant, M. Rose-Helene, J.-P. Joly, and A. Walcarius, Kinetics of the Complexation of Ni^{2+} ions by 5-phenyl-azo-8-hydroxyquinoline Grafted on Colloidal Silica Particles, *Colloids Surf. A*, 380, 261–269 (2011).
87. C.-Y. Lai, B.G. Trewyn, D.M. Jeftinija, K. Jeftinija, S. Xu, S. Jeftinija, and V. Lin, A Mesoporous Silica Nanosphere-Based Carrier System with Chemically Removable CdS Nanoparticle Caps for Stimuli-Responsive Controlled Release of Neurotransmitters and Drug Molecules, *J. Am. Chem. Soc.*, 125, 4451–4459 (2003).
88. C. Park, K. Oh, S.C. Lee, and C. Kim, Controlled Release of Guest Molecules from Mesoporous Silica Particles Based on a pH-Responsive Polypseudorotaxane Motif, *Angew. Chem. Int. Ed.*, 46, 1455–1457 (2007).

89. X. Huang, L. Li, T. Liu, N. Hao, H. Liu, D. Chen, and F. Tang, The Shape Effect of Mesoporous Silica Nanoparticles on Biodistribution, Clearance, and Biocompatibility in Vivo, *ACS Nano*, 5, 5390–5399 (2011).
90. J.M. Rosenholm, and M. Lindén, Towards Establishing Structure–Activity Relationships for Mesoporous Silica in Drug Delivery Applications, *J. Control. Release*, 128, 157–164 (2008).
91. Q. Yang, S. Wang, P. Fan, L. Wang, Y. Di, K. Lin, and F.-S. Xiao, pH-Responsive Carrier System Based on Carboxylic Acid Modified Mesoporous Silica and Polyelectrolyte for Drug Delivery, *Chem. Mater.*, 17, 5999–6003 (2005).
92. J. Kecht, and T. Bein, Functionalization of Colloidal Mesoporous Silica by Metalorganic Reagents, *Langmuir*, 24, 14209–14214 (2009).
93. A. Schlossbauer, J. Kecht, and T. Bein, Biotin–Avidin as a Protease-Responsive Cap System for Controlled Guest Release from Colloidal Mesoporous Silica, *Angew. Chem. Int. Ed.*, 48, 3092–3095 (2009).
94. L. Chen, Y. Wen, B. Su, J. Di, Y. Song, and L. Jiang, Programmable DNA Switch for Bioresponsive Controlled Release, *J. Mater. Chem.*, 21, 13811–13816 (2011).
95. Y. Cui, H. Dong, X. Cai, D. Wang, and Y. Li, Mesoporous Silica Nanoparticles Capped with Disulfide-Linked PEG Gatekeepers for Glutathione-Mediated Controlled Release, *ACS Appl. Mater. Interfaces*, 4, 3177–3183 (2012).
96. P. Nadrah, U. Maver, A. Jemec, T. Tišler, M. Bele, G. Dražić, M. Benčina, A. Pintar, O. Planinšek, and M. Gaberšček, Hindered Disulfide Bonds to Regulate Release Rate of Model Drug from Mesoporous Silica, *ACS Appl. Mater. Interfaces*, 5, 3908–3915 (2013).
97. J. Lu, E. Choi, F. Tamanoi, and J.I. Zink, Light-Activated Nanoimpeller-Controlled Drug Release in Cancer Cells, *Small*, 4, 421–426 (2008).
98. J. Méndez, A. Monteagudo, and K. Griebenow, Stimulus-Responsive Controlled Release System by Covalent Immobilization of an Enzyme into Mesoporous Silica Nanoparticles, *Bioconjug. Chem.*, 23, 698–704 (2012).
99. W. Fang, J. Yang, J. Gong, and N. Zheng, Photo- and pH-Triggered Release of Anticancer Drugs from Mesoporous Silica-Coated Pd@Ag Nanoparticles, *Adv. Funct. Mater.*, 22, 842–848 (2012).
100. N.Ž. Knežević, B.G. Trewyn, and V. Lin, Functionalized Mesoporous Silica Nanoparticle-Based Visible Light Responsive Controlled Release Delivery System, *Chem. Commun.*, 47, 2817–2819 (2011).
101. Z. Zhang, L. Wang, J. Wang, X. Jiang, X. Li, Z. Hu, Y. Ji, X. Wu, and C. Chen, Mesoporous Silica-Coated Gold Nanorods as a Light-Mediated Multifunctional Theranostic Platform for Cancer Treatment, *Adv. Mater.*, 24, 1418–1423 (2012).
102. Z. Xiao, C. Ji, J. Shi, E.M. Pridgen, J. Frieder, J. Wu, and O.C. Farokhzad, DNA Self-Assembly of Targeted Near-Infrared-Responsive Gold Nanoparticles for Cancer Thermo-Chemotherapy, *Angew. Chem. Int. Ed.*, 51, 11853–11857 (2012).
103. C.E. Ashley, E.C. Carnes, G.K. Phillips, D. Padilla, P.N. Durfee, P.A. Brown, T.N. Hanna, J. Liu, B. Phillips, M.B. Carter, N.J. Carroll, X. Jiang, D.R. Dunphy, C.L. Willman, D.N. Petsev, D.G. Evans, A.N. Parikh, B. Chackerian, W. Wharton, D.S. Peabody, and C.J. Brinker, The Targeted Delivery of Multicomponent Cargos to Cancer Cells by Nanoporous Particle-Supported Lipid Bilayers, *Nat. Mater.*, 10, 389–397 (2011).
104. V. Cauda, H. Engelke, A. Sauer, D. Arcizet, J. Rädler, and T. Bein, Colchicine-Loaded Lipid Bilayer-Coated 50 nm Mesoporous Nanoparticles Efficiently Induce Microtubule Depolymerization upon Cell Uptake, *Nano Lett.*, 10, 2484–2492 (2010).
105. S.A. Mackowiak, A. Schmidt, V. Weiss, C. Argyo, C. von Schirnding, T. Bein, and C. Bräuchle, Targeted Drug Delivery in Cancer Cells with Red-Light Photoactivated Mesoporous Silica Nanoparticles, *Nano Lett.*, 13, 2576–2583 (2013).
106. R. Liu, P. Liao, J. Liu, and P. Feng, Responsive Polymer-Coated Mesoporous Silica as a pH-Sensitive Nanocarrier for Controlled Release, *Langmuir*, 27, 3095–3099 (2011).

107. X. Yang, X. Liu, Z. Liu, F. Pu, J. Ren, and X. Qu, Near-Infrared Light-Triggered, Targeted Drug Delivery to Cancer Cells by Aptamer Gated Nanovehicles, *Adv. Mater.*, 24, 2890–2895 (2012).

108. L.-S. Wang, L.-C. Wu, S.-Y. Lu, L.-L. Chang, I.-T. Teng, C.-M. Yang, and J.-A. Ho, Biofunctionalized Phospholipid-Capped Mesoporous Silica Nanoshuttles for Targeted Drug Delivery: Improved Water Suspensibility and Decreased Nonspecific Protein Binding, *ACS Nano*, 4, 4371–4379 (2010).

109. G. Nordlund, J.B. Sing Ng, L. Bergström, and P. Brzezinski, A Membrane-Reconstituted Multisubunit Functional Proton Pump on Mesoporous Silica Particles, *ACS Nano*, 3, 2639–2646 (2009).

110. J. Liu, X. Jiang, C. Ashley, and C.J. Brinker, Electrostatically Mediated Liposome Fusion and Lipid Exchange with a Nanoparticle-Supported Bilayer for Control of Surface Charge, Drug Containment, and Delivery, *J. Am. Chem. Soc.*, 131, 7567–7569 (2009).

111. J. Liu, A. Stace-Naughton, X. Jiang, and C.J. Brinker, Porous Nanoparticle Supported Lipid Bilayers (Protocells) as Delivery Vehicles, *J. Am. Chem. Soc.*, 131, 1354–1355 (2009).

112. C.E. Ashley, E.C. Carnes, K.E. Epler, D.P. Padilla, G.K. Phillips, R.E. Castillo, D.C. Wilkinson, B.S. Wilkinson, C.A. Burgard, R.M. Kalinich, J.L. Townson, B. Chackerian, C.L. Willman, D.S. Peabody, W. Wharton, and C.J. Brinker, Delivery of Small Interfering RNA by Peptide-Targeted Mesoporous Silica Nanoparticle-Supported Lipid Bilayers, *ACS Nano*, 6, 2174–2188 (2012).

113. X. Hu, X. Hao, Y. Wu, J. Zhang, X. Zhang, P.C. Wang, G. Zou, and X.-J. Liang, Multifunctional hybrid silica nanoparticles for controlled doxorubicin loading and release with thermal and pH dual response, *J. Mater. Chem. B*, 1, 1109–1118 (2013).

114. E. Climent, A. Bernardos, R. Martínez-Máñez, A. Maqueira, M.D. Marcos, N. Pastor-Navarro, R. Puchades, F. Sancenón, J. Soto, and P. Amorós, Controlled Delivery Systems Using Antibody-Capped Mesoporous Nanocontainers, *J. Am. Chem. Soc.*, 131, 14075–14080 (2009).

115. X. Wu, Z. Wang, D. Zhu, S. Zong, L. Yang, Y. Zhong, and Y. Cui, pH and Thermo Dual-Stimuli-Responsive Drug Carrier Based on Mesoporous Silica Nanoparticles Encapsulated in a Copolymer–Lipid Bilayer, *ACS Appl. Mater. Interfaces*, 5, 10895–10903 (2013).

116. C. Chen, J. Geng, F. Pu, X. Yang, J. Ren, and X. Qu, Polyvalent Nucleic Acid/ Mesoporous Silica Nanoparticle Conjugates: Dual Stimuli-Responsive Vehicles for Intracellular Drug Delivery, *Angew. Chem. Int. Ed.*, 50, 882–886 (2010).

117. P. Zhang, F. Cheng, R. Zhou, J. Cao, J. Li, C. Burda, Q. Min, and J.-J. Zhu, DNA-Hybrid-Gated Multifunctional Mesoporous Silica Nanocarriers for Dual-Targeted and MicroRNA-Responsive Controlled Drug Delivery, *Angew. Chem. Int. Ed.*, 53, 2371–2375 (2014).

118. S. Zhou, X. Du, F. Cui, and X. Zhang, Multi-Responsive and Logic Controlled Release of DNA- Gated Mesoporous Silica Vehicles Functionalized with Intercalators for Multiple Delivery, *Small*, 10, 980–988 (2014).

119. F. Balas, M. Manzano, P. Horcajada, and M. Vallet-Regí, Confinement and Controlled Release of Bisphosphonates on Ordered Mesoporous Silica-Based Materials, *J. Am. Chem. Soc.*, 128, 8116–8117 (2006).

120. H. Zheng, Y. Wang, and S. Che, Coordination Bonding-Based Mesoporous Silica for pH-Responsive Anticancer Drug Doxorubicin Delivery, *J. Phys. Chem. C*, 115, 16803–16813 (2011).

121. R. Liu, Y. Zhang, X. Zhao, A. Agarwal, L.J. Mueller, and P. Feng, pH-Responsive Nanogated Ensemble Based on Gold-Capped Mesoporous Silica through an Acid-Labile Acetal Linker, *J. Am. Chem. Soc.*, 132, 1500–1501 (2010).

122. C. Yu, M. Luo, F. Zeng, F. Zheng, and S. Wu, Mesoporous Silica Particles for Selective Detection of Dopamine with β-cyclodextrin as the Selective Barricade, *Chem. Commun.*, 47, 9086–9088 (2010).

123. H. Kim, S. Kim, C. Park, H. Lee, H.J. Park, and C. Kim, Glutathione-Induced Intracellular Release of Guests from Mesoporous Silica Nanocontainers with Cyclodextrin Gatekeepers, *Adv. Mater.*, 22, 4280–4283 (2010).

124. J. Croissant, and J.I. Zink, Nanovalve-Controlled Cargo Release Activated by Plasmonic Heating, *J. Am. Chem. Soc.*, 134, 7628–7631 (2012).

125. S. Angelos, Y.-W. Yang, K. Patel, J.F. Stoddart, and J.I. Zink, pH-Responsive Supramolecular Nanovalves Based on Cucurbit[6]uril Pseudorotaxanes, *Angew. Chem. Int. Ed.*, 47, 2222–2226 (2008).

126. S.R. Choi, D.-J. Jang, S. Kim, S. An, J. Lee, E. Oh, and J. Kim, Polymer-Coated Spherical Mesoporous Silica for pH-Controlled Delivery of Insulin, *J. Mater. Chem. B*, 2, 616–619 (2014).

127. R. Guillet-Nicolas, A. Popat, J.-L. Bridot, G. Monteith, S.Z. Qiao, and F. Kleitz, pH-Responsive Nutraceutical-Mesoporous Silica Nanoconjugates with Enhanced Colloidal Stability, *Angew. Chem. Int. Ed.*, 52, 2318–2322 (2013).

128. K. Murakami, X. Yu, S. Watanabe, T. Kato, Y. Inoue, and K. Sugawara, Synthesis of Thermosensitive Polymer/Mesoporous Silica Composite and its Temperature Dependence of Anion Exchange Property, *J. Colloid Interface Sci.*, 354, 771–776 (2011).

129. D.E. Thrall, R.L. Page, M.W. Dewhirst, R.E. Meyer, P.J. Hoopes, and J.N. Kornegay, Temperature Measurements in Normal and Tumor Tissue of Dogs Undergoing whole Body Hyperthermia, *Cancer Res.*, 46, 6229–6235 (1986).

130. Z. Zhou, S. Zhu, and D. Zhang, Grafting of Thermo-Responsive Polymer inside Mesoporous Silica with Large Pore Size using ATRP and Investigation of its use in Drug Release, *J. Mater. Chem.*, 17, 2428–2433 (2007).

131. C. Liu, J. Guo, W. Yang, J. Hu, C. Wang, and S. Fu, Magnetic Mesoporous Silica Microspheres with Thermo-Sensitive Polymer Shell for Controlled Drug Release, *J. Mater. Chem.*, 19, 4764–4770 (2009).

132. E. Aznar, L. Mondragón, J.V. Ros-Lis, F. Sancenón, M.D. Marcos, R. Martínez-Máñez, J. Soto, E. Pérez-Payá, and P. Amorós, Finely Tuned Temperature-Controlled Cargo Release Using Paraffin-Capped Mesoporous Silica Nanoparticles, *Angew. Chem. Int. Ed.*, 50, 11172–11175 (2011).

133. A. Schlossbauer, S. Warncke, P.M.E. Gramlich, J. Kecht, A. Manetto, T. Carell, and T. Bein, A Programmable DNA-Based Molecular Valve for Colloidal Mesoporous Silica, *Angew. Chem. Int. Ed.*, 49, 4734–4737 (2010).

134. G. K. Balendiran, R. Dabur, and D. Fraser, The Role of Glutathione in Cancer, *Cell Biochem. Funct.*, 22, 343–352 (2004).

135. R. Mortera, J. Vivero-Escoto, I. Slowing, E. Garrone, B. Onida, and V. Lin, Cell-Induced Intracellular Controlled Release of Membrane Impermeable Cysteine from a Mesoporous Silica Nanoparticle-Based Drug Delivery System, *Chem. Commun.*, 3219–3221 (2009).

136. T.D. Nguyen, Y. Liu, S. Saha, K.C.F. Leung, J.F. Stoddart, and J.I. Zink, Design and Optimization of Molecular Nanovalves Based on Redox-Switchable Bistable Rotaxanes, *J. Am. Chem. Soc.*, 129, 626–634 (2007).

137. L. Chen, Z. Zheng, J. Wang, and X. Wang, Mesoporous SBA-15 End-Capped by PEG via L-cystine Based Linker for Redox Responsive Controlled Release, *Micropor. Mesopor. Mater.*, 185, 7–15 (2014).

138. N.K. Mal, M. Fujiwara, and Y. Tanaka, Photocontrolled Reversible Release of Guest Molecules from Coumarin-Modified Mesoporous Silica, *Nature*, 421, 350–353 (2003).

139. S. Angelos, Y.-W. Yang, N.M. Khashab, J.F. Stoddart, and J.I. Zink, Dual-Controlled Nanoparticles Exhibiting AND Logic, *J. Am. Chem. Soc.*, 131, 11344–11346 (2009).

140. D.P. Ferris, Y.-L. Zhao, N.M. Khashab, H.A. Khatib, J.F. Stoddart, and J.I. Zink, Light-Operated Mechanized Nanoparticles, *J. Am. Chem. Soc.*, 131, 1686–1688 (2009).
141. N.Ž. Knežević, B.G. Trewyn, and V. Lin, Light- and pH-Responsive Release of Doxorubicin from a Mesoporous Silica-Based Nanocarrier, *Chem. Eur. J.*, 17, 3338–3342 (2011).
142. J.L. Vivero-Escoto, I. Slowing, C.-W. Wu, and V. Lin, Photoinduced Intracellular Controlled Release Drug Delivery in Human Cells by Gold-Capped Mesoporous Silica Nanosphere, *J. Am. Chem. Soc.*, 131, 3462–3463 (2009).
143. S.P. Mornet, S.B. Vasseur, F. Grasset, and E. Duguet, Magnetic Nanoparticle Design for Medical Diagnosis and Therapy, *J. Mater. Chem.*, 14, 2161–2175 (2004).
144. M. Mahmoudi, S. Sant, B. Wang, S. Laurent, and T. Sen, Superparamagnetic Iron Oxide Nanoparticles (SPIONs): Development, Surface Modification and Applications in Chemotherapy, *Adv. Drug Deliv. Rev.*, 63, 24–46 (2011).
145. S. Kim, C. Bellouard, A. Pasc, E. Lamouroux, J.-L. Blin, C. Carteret, Y. Fort, M. Emo, P. Durand, and M.J. Stébé, Nanoparticle-Free Magnetic Mesoporous Silica with Magneto-Responsive Surfactants, *J. Mater. Chem. C*, 1, 6930–6934 (2013).
146. D. Arcos, V. Fal-Miyar, E. Ruiz-Hernández, M. Garcia-Hernández, M.L. Ruiz-González, J. González-Calbet, and M. Vallet-Regí, Supramolecular Mechanisms in the Synthesis of Mesoporous Magnetic Nanospheres for Hyperthermia, *J. Mater. Chem.*, 22, 64–72 (2011).
147. N.Ž. Knežević, E. Ruiz-Hernández, W.E. Hennink, and M. Vallet-Regí, Magnetic Mesoporous Silica-based Core/Shell Nanoparticles for Biomedical Applications, *RSC Adv.*, 3, 9584–9593 (2013).
148. T. Sen, A. Sebastianelli, and I.J. Bruce, Mesoporous Silica–Magnetite Nanocomposite: Fabrication and Applications in Magnetic Bioseparations, *J. Am. Chem. Soc.*, 128, 7130–7131 (2006).
149. W. Zhao, J. Gu, L. Zhang, H. Chen, and J. Shi, Fabrication of Uniform Magnetic Nanocomposite Spheres with a Magnetic Core/Mesoporous Silica Shell Structure, *J. Am. Chem. Soc.*, 127, 8916–8917 (2005).
150. W. Zhao, J. Shi, H. Chen, and L. Zhang, Particle size, Uniformity, and Mesostructure Control of Magnetic Core/Mesoporous Silica Shell Nanocomposite Spheres, *J. Mater. Res.*, 21, 3080–3089 (2011).
151. Y. Deng, D. Qi, C. Deng, X. Zhang, and D. Zhao, Superparamagnetic High-Magnetization Microspheres with an $Fe_3O_4@SiO_2$ Core and Perpendicularly Aligned Mesoporous SiO_2 Shell for Removal of Microcystins, *J. Am. Chem. Soc.*, 130, 28–29 (2008).
152. L. Zhang, S.Z. Qiao, Y.G. Jin, Z.G. Chen, H.C. Gu, and G.Q. Lu, Magnetic Hollow Spheres of Periodic Mesoporous Organosilica and Fe_3O_4 Nanocrystals: Fabrication and Structure Control, *Adv. Mater.*, 20, 805–809 (2008).
153. X. Li, J. Zhang, and H. Gu, Adsorption and Desorption Behaviors of DNA with Magnetic Mesoporous Silica Nanoparticles, *Langmuir*, 27, 6099–6106 (2011).
154. C.-C. Huang, C.-Y. Tsai, H.-S. Sheu, K.-Y. Chuang, C.-H. Su, U.-S. Jeng, F.-Y. Cheng, C.-H. Su, H.-Y. Lei, and C.-S. Yeh, Enhancing Transversal Relaxation for Magnetite Nanoparticles in MR Imaging Using Gd 3^+-Chelated Mesoporous Silica Shells, *ACS Nano*, 5, 3905–3916 (2011).
155. V. Matsura, Y. Guari, J. Larionova, C. Guérin, A. Caneschi, C. Sangregorio, E. Lancelle-Beltran, A. Mehdi, and R.J.P. Corriu, Synthesis of Magnetic Silica-Based Nanocomposites Containing Fe_3O_4 Nanoparticles, *J. Mater. Chem.*, 14, 3026–3033 (2004).
156. S. Huang, P. Yang, Z. Cheng, C. Li, Y. Fan, D. Kong, and J. Lin, Synthesis and Characterization of Magnetic $Fe_xO_y@SBA$-15 Composites with Different Morphologies for Controlled Drug Release and Targeting, *J. Phys. Chem. C*, 112, 7130–7137 (2008).
157. Y. Chen, H. Chen, D. Zeng, Y. Tian, F. Chen, J. Feng, and J. Shi, Core/Shell Structured Hollow Mesoporous Nanocapsules: A Potential Platform for Simultaneous Cell Imaging and Anticancer Drug Delivery, *ACS Nano*, 4, 6001–6013 (2010).

158. A. Popat, S. Jambhrunkar, J. Zhang, J. Yang, H. Zhang, A. Meka, and C. Yu, Programmable Drug Release Using Bioresponsive Mesoporous Silica Nanoparticles for Site-Specific Oral Drug Delivery, *Chem. Commun.*, 50, 5547–5550 (2014).
159. C. Chen, F. Pu, Z. Huang, Z. Liu, J. Ren, and X. Qu, Stimuli-Responsive Controlled-Release System Using Quadruplex DNA-Capped Silica Nanocontainers, *Nucleic Acids Res.*, 39, 1638–1644 (2011).
160. X. Chen, X. Cheng, A.H. Soeriyadi, S.M. Sagnella, X. Lu, J.A. Scott, S.B. Lowe, M. Kavallaris, and J.J. Gooding, Stimuli-Responsive Functionalized Mesoporous Silica Nanoparticles for Drug Release in Response to Various Biological Stimuli, *Biomater. Sci.*, 2, 121–130 (2013).
161. K. Radhakrishnan, S. Gupta, D.P. Gnanadhas, P.C. Ramamurthy, D. Chakravortty, and A.M. Raichur, Protamine-Capped Mesoporous Silica Nanoparticles for Biologically Triggered Drug Release, *Part. Part. Syst. Charact.*, 31, 449–458 (2013).
162. D.F. Williams, On the Mechanisms of Biocompatibility, *Biomaterials*, 29, 2941–2953 (2008).
163. B.J. Marquis, S.A. Love, K.L. Braun, and C.L. Haynes, Analytical Methods to Assess Nanoparticle Toxicity, *Analyst*, 134, 425–439 (2009).
164. D. Tarn, C.E. Ashley, M. Xue, E.C. Carnes, J.I. Zink, and C.J. Brinker, Mesoporous Silica Nanoparticle Nanocarriers: Biofunctionality and Biocompatibility, *Acc. Chem. Res.*, 46, 792–801 (2013).
165. A.K. Varkouhi, M. Scholte, G. Storm, and H.J. Haisma, Endosomal Escape Pathways for Delivery of Biologicals, *J. Control. Release*, 151, 220–228 (2011).
166. A. Schlossbauer, A.M. Sauer, V. Cauda, A. Schmidt, H. Engelke, U. Rothbauer, K. Zolghadr, H. Leonhardt, C. Bräuchle, and T. Bein, Cascaded Photoinduced Drug Delivery to Cells from Multifunctional Core-Shell Mesoporous Silica, *Adv Healthcare Mater.*, 1, 316–320 (2012).
167. X. Huang, X. Teng, D. Chen, F. Tang, and J. He, The Effect of the Shape of Mesoporous Silica Nanoparticles on Cellular Uptake and Cell Function, *Biomaterials*, 31, 438–448 (2010).
168. A. Yildirim, E. Ozgur, and M. Bayindir, Impact of Mesoporous Silica Nanoparticle Surface Functionality on Hemolytic Activity, Thrombogenicity and Non-Specific Protein Adsorption, *J. Mater. Chem. B*, 1, 1909–1920 (2013).
169. C. Argyo, V. Cauda, H. Engelke, J. Rädler, G. Bein, and T. Bein, Heparin-Coated Colloidal Mesoporous Silica Nanoparticles Efficiently Bind to Antithrombin as an Anticoagulant Drug-Delivery System, *Chem. Eur. J.*, 18, 428–432 (2011).
170. M. Liong, J. Lu, M. Kovochich, T. Xia, S.G. Ruehm, A.E. Nel, F. Tamanoi, and J.I. Zink, Multifunctional Inorganic Nanoparticles for Imaging, Targeting, and Drug Delivery, *ACS Nano*, 2, 889–896 (2008).
171. S.-H. Wu, Y. Hung, and C.-Y. Mou, Mesoporous Silica Nanoparticles as Nanocarriers, *Chem. Commun.*, 47, 9972–9985 (2011).
172. H. Meng, M. Liong, T. Xia, Z. Li, Z. Ji, J.I. Zink, and A.E. Nel, Engineered Design of Mesoporous Silica Nanoparticles to Deliver Doxorubicin and P-Glycoprotein siRNA to Overcome Drug Resistance in a Cancer Cell Line, *ACS Nano*, 4, 4539–4550 (2010).
173. Q. He, J. Shi, M. Zhu, Y. Chen, and F. Chen, The Three-Stage in Vitro Degradation Behavior of Mesoporous Silica in Simulated Body Fluid, *Micropor. Mesopor. Mater.*, 131, 314–320 (2010).
174. T. Maldiney, B. Ballet, M. Bessodes, D. Scherman, and C. Richard, Mesoporous Persistent Nanophosphorus for In Vivo Optical Bioimaging and Drug-Delivery, *Nanoscale*, 6, 13970–13976 (2014).
175. M. A. Wuillemin, W. T. Stuber, T. Fox, M. J. Reber, D. Brühwiler, R. Alberto, and H. Braband, A Novel99mTc Labelling Strategy for the Development of Silica Based Particles for Medical Applications, *Dalton Trans.*, 43, 4260–4263 (2014).

176. M. Colilla, B. González, and M. Vallet-Regí, Mesoporous Silica Nanoparticles for the Design of Smart Delivery Nanodevices, *Biomater. Sci.*, 1, 114–134 (2013).
177. V. Cauda, A. Schlossbauer, and T. Bein, Bio-Degradation Study of Colloidal Mesoporous Silica Nanoparticles: Effect of Surface Functionalization with Organo-Silanes and Poly(ethylene glycol), *Micropor. Mesopor. Mater.*, 132, 60–71 (2010).
178. V. Cauda, C. Argyo and T. Bein, Impact of Different PEGylation Patterns on the Long-Term Bio-Stability of Colloidal Mesoporous Silica Nanoparticles, *J. Mater. Chem.*, 20, 8693–8699 (2010).
179. Q. He, Z. Zhang, F. Gao, Y. Li, and J. Shi, In Vivo Biodistribution and Urinary Excretion of Mesoporous Silica Nanoparticles: Effects of Particle Size and PEGylation, *Small*, 7, 271–280 (2010).
180. Y.-S. Lin, K.R. Hurley, and C.L. Haynes, Critical Considerations in the Biomedical Use of Mesoporous Silica Nanoparticles, *J. Phys. Chem. Lett.*, 3, 364–374 (2012).
181. V. Mamaeva, C. Sahlgren, and M. Lindén, Mesoporous Silica Nanoparticles in Medicine-Recent Advances, *Adv. Drug Deliv. Rev.*, 65, 689–702 (2013).

2 Gold Nanoparticles
A Novel and Promising Avenue for Drug Delivery

Shuaidong Huo, Xin Cao,
Zhongbo Hu, and Xing-Jie Liang

CONTENTS

ABSTRACT

As one of the most attractive candidates for drug delivery, gold nanoparticles (Au NPs) exhibit many unique physical and chemical properties for their potential use in the biomedical field. From different sizes to a variety of surface modifications, Au NPs can be selected to carry drugs with different properties and those with a specific purpose. Drug loading mechanisms, as well as the toxicity of Au NPs, will be mainly introduced in this chapter.

Keywords: Gold nanopartciles, Synthesis, Modifications, Toxicity, Drug delivery

2.1 INTRODUCTION

With the booming development of nanoscience and nanotechnology, more and more nanoscale materials, such as nanoparticles (NPs), nanorods (NRs), liposomes, micelles, and dendrimers, have been used for different biomedical purposes [1–5]. In order to improve the efficiency and effectiveness of payloads to the targets, several nanomaterials have been designed as delivery vehicles. NPs have been applied to drug delivery because of the following features: first, the high surface area of NPs provides enough sites and space for drug loading and enhances the stability and solubility of loaded drugs. Second, the NPs that can be modified by various targeting ligands or surface receptors enhance the specific efficiency of the expected drugs. Third, compared with free drugs in molecule, these drug-loaded NPs accumulate preferentially at sites of tumor growth or inflammation so that they can enter cells much more rapidly through different mechanisms [6].

As one of the most attractive candidates for drug delivery and other applications in the biomedical field, gold nanoparticles (Au NPs) exhibit many unique physical and chemical properties. Because of their intense optical and photo-physical properties, Au NPs are used for biodiagnostic assays of cancer, HIV-AIDS, and other diseases [7]; they have also been used in pregnancy tests for several decades [8]. Because of their facile surface chemical property, Au NPs can be used as artificial antibodies. Usually, gold nanorods (Au NRs) are applied in highly specific thermal ablation of infected or diseased tissues, owing to their efficient conversion of light into heat [9]. Moreover, Au NPs can be used to enhance cancer radiation therapy or increase imaging contrast in diagnostic computed tomography scans by exploiting their ability to absorb abundant amounts of x-ray radiation [10]. Importantly, the functionalized Au NPs can be employed to facilitate the efficient delivery of poorly soluble drugs, fluorescence imaging probes, and contrast agents by the use of their multivalency [6,11–13].

Because of their easy fabrication, controllable size and shape, tunable surface functionalization, and good biocompatibility, many efforts have been made to develop Au NP–based therapeutic approaches over the last decades, including drug and gene delivery vehicles, diagnostic tools, imaging agent in therapy, and biomarkers in the pharmaceutical field [14–16].

2.2   SYNTHESIS OF Au NPs

Au NPs are the first nanomaterial that people used, which can be traced back to the 5th or 4th century BC in ancient Egypt and China [17], while the actual scientific research on Au NPs was conducted approximately 150 years ago by Michael Faraday who first came up with the idea that there might be gold particles in the colloidal gold solution [18]. Afterward, with the development of scientific research and technology, especially the invention of electronic microscope, researchers have understand properties and other aspects of Au NPs more clearly and thoroughly. In addition, various fabrication methods have been developed, many of which are still used nowadays. Generally speaking, common methods of fabrication of Au NPs include the reverse micelle method, the aqueous-phase reduction method, and the hydrothermal method. Further classification includes reduction by sodium citrate, reduction of white phosphorus, reduction of ascorbic acid, and so on. Since there are so many preparation methods [19], in order to elaborate systematically, we will illustrate different methods of Au NPs with different sizes as well as different surface modifications in Table 2.1.

TABLE 2.1

Synthetic Method of Au NPs with Different Sizes or Surface Modifications

Core Size (d), nm	Synthetic Method	Reducing Agent	Capping Agent	Year	References
1.4 ± 0.4	Reduction of PPh_3AuCl	Diborane and sodium borohydride	Phosphine	1981	[20]
1.5 ± 0.4	Reduction of PPh_3AuCl and ligand exchange	Sodium borohydride	Phosphine	2000	[21]
1–3	Reduction of $HAuCl_4$ in a two-phase system	Sodium borohydride	Dodecanethiol	1994	[22]
3–10	Heat-induced size ripening method	Sodium borohydride	Alkanethiol	2001	[23]
16–150	Reduction of $HAuCl_4$	Sodium citrate	Citrate	1972	[24]
5–250	Slow coagulation of colloidal gold	Citrate	Citrate	1963	[25]
13	Ligand displace	Citrate	DNA	1996	[27]
34	Oligonucleotide-directed immobilization	Citrate	Antibody	2001	[28]
20	Nuclear translocation	Citrate	Peptide and bovine serum albumin	2002	[29]
5 ± 0.75	Au NP core serves as a size- and shape-controllable scaffold	Citrate	Phospholipids and apolipoprotein A-I	2009	[30]

2.2.1 SYNTHESIS OF AU NPS WITH DIFFERENT SIZES

In 1981, Schmid et al. fabricated 1.4 ± 0.4 nm Au NPs ($Au_{55}(PPh_3)_{12}Cl_6$) by means of reduction of $AuCl(PPh_3)$ with diborane of sodium borohydride [20]. It was the first time that researchers synthesized such small size and narrow disparity. However, since this reaction required strictly anaerobic conditions and diborane gas should be used as reducing agent, it was quite difficult to synthesize such Au NPs. Then, Weare et al. improved this method. They eliminated the use of diborane, and through ligand exchange, they fabricated $Au_{101}(PPh_3)_{21}Cl_5$, which was more convenient and safer [21]. Characterized by transmission electron microscope, the Au NPs that they synthesized were 1.5 ± 0.4 nm in diameter. In 1994, Brust et al. prepared thiol-derivatized Au NPs in a two-phase liquid–liquid system [22]. In that system, the gold chloride was transferred to toluene by way of a phase-transfer reagent, tetraoctylammonium bromide, and reduced in the presence of tert-dodecyl mercaptan ($C_{12}H_{25}SH$), which was used as a stabilizer. When the reaction condition changed, the ratio of thiol to gold in the product changed as well. In addition, the Au NPs' diameter ranged from 1 to 3 nm. In 2001, Teranishi et al. used heat treatment in the solid-state method to formulate the size of Au NPs of 3–10 nm at the temperature between 150°C and 250°C [23]. In their experiment, dodecanethiol-protected Au NPs that were prepared by using Brust's method (two-phase reaction procedure) were used as a source for the heat treatment while octadecanethiol was used as a protective ligand as well as a protective agent taking the place of dodecanethiol. In 1972, Frens synthesized Au NPs with 16–150 nm in diameter through reduction of $HAuCl_4$, with sodium citrate as reducing agent [24]. All other factors being equal, the diameter of the Au NPs could be changed by altering the concentration of sodium citrate. The higher the concentration of sodium citrate, the smaller the diameter and vice versa.

2.2.2 SYNTHESIS OF AU NPS WITH DIFFERENT SURFACE MODIFICATIONS

In addition to the methods of fabrication of Au NPs with different sizes, many other alternative ways of synthesis of Au NPs with different surface functionalizations have been used by researchers. In 1963, Enustun and Turkevich synthesized citrated-capped Au NPs in the way that colloidal gold was stabilized by citrate ions and $NaClO_4$ was used as coagulating agent [25]. In another study, transferrin-coated citrate-functionalized Au NPs were fabricated by Yang et al. [26]. They reported that those Au NPs could be absorbed by cells very well. However, they were susceptible to the environment and prone to aggregate. Many researchers tried to improve the above method or tried alternative surface functionalizations. Mirkin et al. found a way to synthesize Au NPs that could be controlled and reversibly assembled through an oligonucleotide-based method [27]. Since DNA oligonucleotides had the property of molecular recognition, they could be used as the trigger of NPs' self-assembly progress. By changing the sequence and length of the oligonucleotides, various stable structures could be attained. In 2001, Niemever and Ceyhan fabricated antibody-gold nanoconjugates through the method of oligonucleotide-directed immobilization [28]. At first, they combined the covalent DNA-streptavidin with mouse IgG or rabbit IgG, and then these conjugates were bonded with Au NPs. The fabrication method was simple and efficient. The following year, Tkachenko et al. found a good approach to nuclear translocation, in which several different peptides were combined on a 20-nm-diameter Au NP [29]. Although there would be obstacles of different cell membranes in the process of nuclear translocation, each of the peptides had a very good ability to cross different cellular membrane barriers so that they could translocate nuclei well. In recent years, lipids have also been used to modify Au NPs. Through adsorbing lipids and proteins to the surface of Au NPs, Thaxton et al. synthesized biomimetic high-density lipoprotein (HDL) nanostructures [30]. Au NPs adsorbed apolipoprotein and A-I phospholipids (APOA1) to their surface and then phospholipids were combined on those conjugates. Since such nanostructure could mimic other biological HDL counterparts, they could be used to bind cholesterol as biomimetic materials.

2.3 TOXICITY OF Au NPs

As a drug delivery system, one of the most concerning aspects of Au NPs is their possible toxicity. Until now, comprehensive *in vitro* and *in vivo* toxicological evaluations were performed on various types of Au NPs, and cell/animal models were used to evaluate these effects [17,31]. The general conclusion from these studies is that the Au NPs are biologically inert and almost had no toxicity. However, this is not absolutely true when the size of gold core decreases below 2 nm, where the surface of the Au NPs shows unusual and high chemical reactivity [31]. The high surface reactivity of this size can also be the source of unwanted reactions/side effects in biological systems [31,32].

Most studies were conducted using *in vitro* models (cultured cells) to evaluate the safety of Au NP solutions. Toxicological effects of Au NPs on culture cells, such as viability assays, reactive oxygen species analysis, gene expression analysis, cell substrate impedance and micro-motility analysis (electric cell-substrate impedance sensing), and cellular morphology assays, have been assessed by researchers [33–36]. At the cellular level, there is no standard dose that is known to be safe or toxic. However, one thing that has been generally agreed upon is that cellular uptake of Au NPs occurs as a function of size, shape, surface charge, functionalization, aggregation state of NPs, concentration of NPs, the type of cell, incubation conditions, and type of culture media [13,37]. Despite the fact that the Au NP core is considered inert and nontoxic, the stabilizer or its degradation products, leftover chemicals from the synthesis, as well as remnants from inadequate purification can induce toxicity [38]. One of the common examples is Au NRs. Because of the presence of free cetyltrimethyl ammonium bromide (CTAB) (capping agent) in the solution, apparent toxicity is shown at nanomolar concentrations [38–40]. In this case, the toxicity is not attributed to the Au NR core itself. One way to reduce the acute toxicity of Au NRs in cell culture is by replacing CTAB with another nontoxic capping agent or by preventing CTAB desorption from the surface of Au NRs [31,38].

Compared to *in vitro* toxicological studies, few studies focus on evaluating the toxicity of NPs *in vivo* until now. In order to apply Au NPs as drug carriers, their side effects should be evaluated, as well as the pharmacokinetic parameters of Au NPs *in vivo*, such as absorption, distribution, metabolism, and elimination [17]. Among these, the clearance of NPs from tissues after injection is of paramount importance to the evaluation of local inflammation and toxicity. There are various routes of clearance of small-molecule organic drugs from the body such as the kidneys (renal/urinary excretion), the hepatobiliary system, the skin, and the lungs. However, the case for NPs is not the same since they are larger in size and in many cases cannot cross filtration barriers such as the glomeruli in kidneys (6–8 nm) [41,42]. Most studies have suggested that safety in the intravenous administration of Au NPs can be based on general assessments such as animal average weight, loss of appetite, mortality rates, or other gross visual observations [17].

In summary, although most studies suggest that the gold core itself is biologically inert and safe, a great deal of work is also needed to evaluate and reduce the toxicity of the Au NPs.

2.4 Au NPs FOR DRUG DELIVERY

2.4.1 Loading as Capping Agents

As shown in Figure 2.1a, it has been reported that the thiols or amines can be anchored to the surface of Au NPs through Au–S or Au–N bonds [43,44]. By this way, drugs [45,46], DNA [47–49], and siRNA can be loaded on the surface of Au

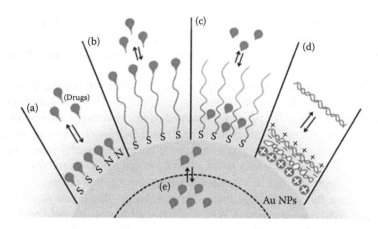

FIGURE 2.1 Illustration of various methods of loading/unloading therapeutics into/from Au NPs. (a) Anchoring drugs directly to the surfaces of Au NPs through Au–S or Au–N bonds. (b) Drugs are coupled or attached to the terminal functional groups of the capping agent via a cleavable linker. (c) Partitioning and diffusion-driven release of hydrophobic drug molecules in an amphiphilic corona layer. (d) Loading charged biomolecules (e.g., DNA or siRNA) onto the surfaces of Au NPs by electrostatic layer-by-layer assembly. (e) Loading into the hollow Au NPs and released out by external stimuli.

NPs. Because the Au–S bond is stronger than the Au–N bond, the release of drugs with the Au–S bond needs more energy than those with the Au–N bond. The common methods of drug release include diffusion to cellular membrane, thiol exchange, and external light stimulus, to name a few. Because the Au–N bond is relatively weaker, in the cases of amines, they can release simply by diffusion [50], while for thiolated drugs, they release through thiol exchange or external light stimulus [51]. When Au NPs absorb light and then convert light into heat, the Au–S bond can be broken or NP itself may be melted to release drugs.

2.4.2 LOADING BY ATTACHMENT TO CAPPING AGENTS

As capping agents, organic compounds can be attached to the surface of Au NPs via covalent bonding, Au–S or Au–N bond, which prevents NPs aggregating. To take advantage of this, therapeutic drugs are coupled to the terminal of the capping agents through cleavable linkers as shown in Figure 2.1b. For instance, Brown et al. capped Au NPs with thiolated poly(ethylene glycol) (PEG) and they added the anticancer drug oxaliplatin to the surface of PEG through covalent bonding [52]. Dhar et al. coupled cisplatin Pt(IV) to the terminal of amine functionalized DNA-Au NPs via the formation of amide bonds [53]. Pt(IV) can be reduced to Pt(II) in the intercellular milieu. Because Pt(IV) is very inert and has low side effects, it has become a valuable alternative to Pt(II) complexes. Schoenfisch et al. functionalized Au NPs with bromo-terminated alkanethiols and then attached amine compounds via ligand exchange so that –CH$_2$Br was eliminated [54,55]. The amine compounds they synthesized could release nitric oxide, which could be potentially used in vasodilation.

Agasti et al. used a monolayer of photocleavable and zwitterionic thiol ligands as capping agents, and 5-fluorouracil, an anticancer drug, was attached to the mono-layer with terminal carboxylic acids through a photosensitive *o*-nitrobenzyl linkage [56]. With irradiation of UV light, the photosensitive linkage could be broken and could be observed through UV-vis spectral.

However, the capping drugs on the surface of Au NPs, especially hydrophobic ones, often aggregate after coupling reactions. For instance, Gibson et al. found that a chemotherapeutic drug, paclitaxel, capped on NP via esterification with hexaethyl-ene glycol linker, which was used as capping agent, aggregated to the extent of ~70 paclitaxel molecules per NP [57]. Because of this aggregation, the solubility of these nanoclusters decreased in aqueous media whereas it increased in organic matters.

2.4.3 LOADING BY PARTITIONING

When preparing Au NPs, capping agents are used to stabilize Au NPs against aggregation or sometimes used as shape-directing agents during the growth of NPs; thus, as-prepared Au NPs have a mono- or bilayer of capping agents on the surface [6]. In some cases, the existence of such mono- or bilayer is very useful to load drugs and release them in the diseased site. This mono- or bilayer, consisting of organic compounds, can be considered as a thin layer of organic solution, as shown in Figure 2.1c, in which hydrophobic drugs can be partitioned from the surround-ing medium [58]. For instance, Kim et al. synthesized Au NPs with a monolayer of polymer as capping agents, which had both a hydrophobic alkanethiol interior and a hydrophilic organic compound exterior [59]. The hydrophobic nature of interior ligands can load hydrophobic drugs and the exterior region can stabilize the Au NPs in the aqueous media. With this structure, the Au NPs are more likely to bind specific biomacromolecules. The hydrophobic drugs are partitioned in the organic solution and released when the NPs interact with specific cell membrane while the NPs do not enter the cell. Hydrophobic drugs are released into the cell via membrane-mediated diffusion.

2.4.4 LOADING BY LAYER-BY-LAYER ASSEMBLY

Au NPs are usually synthesized in a water medium, which is a strong polar solvent. In water media, many charged capping agents are coupled on the surface of Au NPs so that these NPs are high charged as well. Based on this, as shown in Figure 2.1d, Murphy et al. fabricated gold cores with charged drugs via electrostatic conjugation or the related layer-by-layer coating [60,61]. In addition, because nucleic acids— DNA or siRNA—are highly negative charged, DNA or siRNA molecules can be coupled on the surface of cationic Au NPs. Huang et al. and Bonoiu et al. applied this method for gene delivery and gene silencing [62,63]. However, in some cases, the electrostatic interaction between Au NPs and nucleic acids was so strong that it could retard the release of DNA or siRNA. In order to solve this problem, Guo et al. found that charge-reversal functional Au NPs could improve the nucleic acids' delivery efficiency [64]. In their research, they used a charge-reversal copolymer that could change charge nature according to pH. When the polymers were in acidic pH, such as endosome or lysosome, they became positive charged so that DNA or siRNA would dissociate from Au NPs. When in neutral pH, the polymers remained negative charged. Lee et al. found another method to release complexed DNA or siRNA [65]. They synthesized Au NPs using four layers of poly-L-lysine (PLL), which were protease-degradable, and three layers of siRNA as capping agents. With the degradation of PLL, siRNA could be released and extended gene-silencing effect could be observed.

2.4.5   LOADING INSIDE THE NPs

Not only can drugs be coupled to the exterior surface of Au NPs, they can also be loaded into the hollow gold nanospheres as shown in Figure 2.1e, such as nanocages and nanoshells. Xia et al. developed gold nanocages that were porous in structure [14]. The interior surfaces of the gold nanocages had unique optical/photothermal properties so that they could absorb and scatter near-infrared (NIR) light. Drugs were loaded into the gold nanocages through two steps [66]. First, drugs attached gold nanocages through thiol–gold bonds. After that, they entered the cages via simple inward diffusion from aqueous media. The release of these drugs was quite easy. By absorbing NIR light, the interior thermosensitive polymers could convert light into heat so that the gold nanocages would melt and then drugs were released out. Based on this, drug release could be controlled through changing the NIR light intensity or irradiation time. Similar to gold nanocages, gold nanoshells can also load drugs in the nanostructure. But one important difference between the two is that gold nanoshells are not porous so that drugs should be capped before the formation of nanoshells. Troutman et al. prepared a degradable sphere template, which was formed by liposomes and then gold nanodots capped on the template [67]. By absorbing visible or NIR light, gold nanostructure would degrade and drugs would be released. The release could also be controlled by changing the irradiation time or light intensity as stated above. Such gold nanostructure has a great potential use.

2.5   OUTLOOK AND CONCLUSIONS

Gold-based therapeutics have a long history in medicine [43]. For a long time, gold compounds (such as Auranofin, with brand name Ridura) had been used in anti-arthritic medications [68]. Recently, gold-based molecular compounds have been found to significantly restrict the viral reservoir in primate AIDS models [69]. Huge number of studies and clinical research demonstrated that Au NPs had great potential in biomedicine, especially used as drug carriers. Because of their easy fabrication with controllable size and shape, very low toxicity, functional flexibility, and ability to control the release of drugs, Au NPs offer many possibilities for further development of drug delivery systems. Comprehensive and exhaustive research into these nanoscale delivery vehicles should be continued to fully understand their pharmacokinetics and interaction in living biological systems. Furthermore, more effort should be required to engineer new surface-functionalized and bioavailable Au NPs for drug delivery.

ACKNOWLEDGMENTS

This work was supported by the Chinese Natural Science Foundation project (No. 30970784 and No. 81171455), a National Distinguished Young Scholars grant (31225009) from the National Natural Science Foundation of China, the National Key Basic Research Program of China (2009CB930200), the Chinese Academy of Sciences (CAS) "Hundred Talents Program" (07165111ZX), the CAS Knowledge Innovation Program, and the State High-Tech Development Plan (2012AA020804). This work was also supported in part by NIH/NIMHD 8 G12 MD007597 and USAMRMC W81XWH-10-1-0767 grants. The authors also appreciate the support given by the "Strategic Priority Research Program" of the Chinese Academy of Sciences (XDA09030301).

REFERENCES

1. E.T. Kisak, B. Coldren, C.A. Evans, C. Boyer and J.A. Zasadzinski, The Vesosome—A Multicompartment Drug Delivery Vehicle, *Current Medicinal Chemistry*, 11(2), 199–219 (2004).
2. C.M. Paleos, D. Tsiourvas, Z. Sideratou and L. Tziveleka, Acid- and Salt-Triggered Multifunctional Poly(propylene imine) Dendrimer as A Prospective Drug Delivery System, *Biomacromolecules*, 5(2), 524–529 (2004).
3. A.K. Salem, P.C. Searson and K.W. Leong, Multifunctional Nanorods for Gene Delivery, *Nature Materials*, 2(10), 668–671 (2003).
4. W. Wu, S. Wieckowski, G. Pastorin, M. Benincasa, C. Klumpp, J.P. Briand, R. Gennaro, M. Prato and A. Bianco, Targeted Delivery of Amphotericin B to Cells by Using Functionalized Carbon Nanotubes, *Angewandte Chemie-International Edition*, 44(39), 6358–6362 (2005).
5. P.S. Xu, E.A.V. Kirk, Y.H. Zhan, W.J. Murdoch, M. Radosz and Y.Q. Shen, Targeted Charge-Reversal Nanoparticles for Nuclear Drug Delivery, *Angewandte Chemie-International Edition*, 46(26), 4999–5002 (2007).
6. E.C. Dreaden, A.M. Alkilany, X.H. Huang, C.J. Murphy and M.A. El-Sayed, The Golden Age: Gold Nanoparticles for Biomedicine, *Chemical Society Reviews*, 41(7), 2740–2779 (2012).
7. A. Kumar, B.M. Boruah and X.J. Liang, Gold Nanoparticles: Promising Nanomaterials for the Diagnosis of Cancer and HIV/AIDS, *Journal of Nanomaterials*, 2011, 202187. doi:10.1155/2011/202187 (2011).
8. R. Rojanathanes, A. Sereemaspun, N. Pimpha, V. Buasorn, P. Ekawong and V. Wiwanitkit, Gold Nanoparticle as an Alternative Tool for a Urine Pregnancy Test, *Taiwan J Obstet Gynecol*, 47(3), 296–299 (2008).
9. H.H. Richardson, M.T. Carlson, P.J. Tandler, P. Hernandez and A.O. Govorov, Experimental and Theoretical Studies of Light-to-Heat Conversion and Collective Heating Effects in Metal Nanoparticle Solutions, *Nano Letters*, 9(3), 1139–1146 (2009).
10. R. Kunzel, E. Okuno, R.S. Levenhagen and N.K. Umisedo, Evaluation of the X-Ray Absorption by Gold Nanoparticles Solutions, *ISRN Nanotechnology*, 2013, 865283. doi:10.1155/2013/865283 (2013).
11. V.P. Chauhan, Z. Popovic, O. Chen, J. Cui, D. Fukumura, M.G. Bawendi and R.K. Jain, Fluorescent Nanorods and Nanospheres for Real-Time In Vivo Probing of Nanoparticle Shape-Dependent Tumor Penetration, *Angewandte Chemie-International Edition*, 50(48), 11417–11420 (2011).

12. B. Kim, G. Han, B.J. Toley, C.K. Kim, V.M. Rotello and N.S. Fprbes, Tuning Payload Delivery in Tumour Cylindroids Using Gold Nanoparticles, *Nature Nanotechnology*, 5(6), 465–472 (2010).

13. B.D. Chithrani, A.A. Ghazani and W.C.W. Chan, Determining the Size and Shape Dependence of Gold Nanoparticle Uptake Into Mammalian Cells, *Nano Letters*, 6(4), 662–668 (2006).

14. J.Y. Chen, F. Saeki, B.J. Wiley, H. Cang, M.J. Cobb, Z.Y. Li, L. Au, H. Zhang, M.B. Kimmey, X.D. Li and Y.N. Xia, Gold Nanocages: Bioconjugation and Their Potential Use as Optical Imaging Contrast Agents, *Nano Letters*, 5(3), 473–477 (2005).

15. L.R. Hirsch, R.J. Stafford, J.A. Bankson, S.R. Sershen, B. Rivera, R.E. Price, J.D. Hazie, N.J. Halas and J.L. West, Nanoshell-Mediated Near-Infrared Thermal Therapy of Tumors Under Magnetic Resonance Guidance, *Proceedings of the National Academy of Sciences of the United States of America*, 100(23), 13549–13554 (2003).

16. L. Dykman and N. Khlebtsov, Gold Nanoparticles in Biomedical Applications: Recent Advances and Perspectives, *Chemical Society Reviews*, 41(6), 2256–2282 (2012).

17. N. Khlebtsov and L. Dykman, Biodistribution and Toxicity of Engineered Gold Nanoparticles: A Review of In Vitro and In Vivo Studies, *Chemical Society Reviews*, 40(3), 1647–1671 (2011).

18. M. Faraday, The Bakerian Lecture: Experimental Relations of Gold (and Other Metals) to Light, *Philosophical Transactions of the Royal Society of London*, 147, 145–181 (1857).

19. B. Ducan, C. Kim and V.M. Rotello, Gold Nanoparticle Platforms as Drug and Biomacromolecule Delivery Systems, *Journal of Controlled Release*, 148(1), 122–127 (2010).

20. G. Schmid, R. Pfell, R. Boese, F. Bandermann, S. Meyer, G.H.M. Calis and J.W.V.D. Velden, Au55[P(C6H5)3]12Cl6—Ein Goldcluster ungewöhnlicher Größe, *Chemische Berichte*, 114(11), 3634–3642 (1981).

21. W.W. Weare, S.M. Reed, M.G. Warner and J.E. Hutchison, Improved Synthesis of Small (d(CORE) approximate to 1.5 nm) Phosphine-Stabilized Gold Nanoparticles, *Journal of the American Chemical Society*, 122(51), 12890–12891 (2000).

22. M. Brust, M. Walker, D. Bethell, D.J. Schiffrin and R. Whyman, Synthesis of Thiol-Derivatised Gold Nanoparticles in a Two-Phase Liquid-Liquid system, *Journal of the Chemical Society, Chemical Communications*, 801–802 (1994).

23. T. Teranishi, S. Hasegawa, T. Shimizu and M. Miyake, Heat-Induced Size Evolution of Gold Nanoparticles in the Solid State, *Advanced Materials*, 13(22), 1699–1701 (2001).

24. G. Frens, Controlled Nucleation for the Regulation of the Particle Size in Monodisperse Gold Suspensions, *Nature*, 241(105), 20–22 (1973).

25. B.V. Enustun and J. Turkevich, Coagulation of Colloidal Gold, *Journal of the American Chemical Society*, 85(21), 3317 (1963).

26. P.H. Yang, X. Sun, J.F. Chiu, H. Sun and Q.Y. He, Transferrin-Mediated Gold Nanoparticle Cellular Uptake, *Bioconjugate Chemistry*, 16(3), 494–496 (2005).

27. C.A. Mirkin, R.L. Letsinger, R.C. Mucic and J.J. Storhoff, A DNA-Based Method for Rationally Assembling Nanoparticles into Macroscopic Materials, *Nature*, 382(6592), 607–609 (1996).

28. C.M. Niemever and B. Ceyhan, DNA-Directed Functionalization of Colloidal Gold with Proteins, *Angewandte Chemie-International Edition*, 40(19), 3685–3688 (2001).

29. A.G. Tkachenko, H. Xie, D. Coleman, W. Glomm, J. Ryan, M.F. Anderson, S. Franzen and D.L. Feldheim, Multifunctional Gold Nanoparticle-Peptide Complexes for Nuclear Targeting, *Journal of the American Chemical Society*, 125(16), 4700–4701 (2003).

30. C.S. Thaxton, W.L. Daniel, D.A. Giljohann, A.D. Thomas and C.A. Mirkin, Templated Spherical High Density Lipoprotein Nanoparticles, *Journal of the American Chemical Society*, 131(4), 1384–1385 (2009).

31. A.M. Alkilany and C.J. Murphy, Toxicity and Cellular Uptake of Gold Nanoparticles: What We Have Learned So Far? *Journal of Nanoparticle Research*, 12(7), 2313–2333 (2010).
32. M. Turner, V.B. Golovko, O.P.H. Vaughan, P. Abdulkin, A.B. Murcia, M.S. Tikhov, B.F.G. Johnson and R.M. Lambert, Selective Oxidation with Dioxygen by Gold Nanoparticle Catalysts Derived from 55-Atom Clusters, *Nature*, 454(7207), 981–983 (2008).
33. A.E. Nel, L. Madler, D. Velegol, T. Xia, E.M.V. Hoek, P. Somasundaran, F. Klaessig, V. Castranova and M. Thompson, Understanding Biophysicochemical Interactions at the Nano-Bio Interface, *Nature Materials*, 8(7), 543–557 (2009).
34. B.J. Marquis, S.A. Love, K.L. Braun and C.L. Haynes, Analytical Methods to Assess Nanoparticle Toxicity, *Analyst*, 134(3), 425–439 (2009).
35. K. Kandasamy, C.S. Choi and S. Kim, An Efficient Analysis of Nanomaterial Cytotoxicity Based on Bioimpedance, *Nanotechnology*, 21(37), 375501 (2010).
36. K.B. Male, B. Lachance, S. Hrapovic, G. Sunahara and J.H. Luong, Assessment of Cytotoxicity of Quantum Dots and Gold Nanoparticles Using Cell-Based Impedance Spectroscopy, *Analytical Chemistry*, 80(14), 5487–5493 (2008).
37. W. Jiang, B.Y.S. Kim, J.T. Rutka and W.C.W. Chan, Nanoparticle-Mediated Cellular Response is Size-Dependent, *Nature Nanotechnology*, 3(3), 145–150 (2008).
38. A.M. Alkilany, P.K. Nagaria, C.R. Hexel, T.J. Shaw, C.J. Murphy and M.D. Wyatt, Cellular Uptake and Cytotoxicity of Gold Nanorods: Molecular Origin of Cytotoxicity and Surface Effects, *Small*, 5(6), 701–708 (2009).
39. T. Niidome, M. Yamagata, Y. Okamoto, Y. Akiyama, H. Takahashi, T. Kawano, Y. Katayama and Y. Niidome, PEG-Modified Gold Nanorods with a Stealth Character for In Vivo Applications, *Journal of Controlled Release*, 114(3), 343–347 (2006).
40. T.S. Hauck, A.A. Ghazani and W.C.W. Chan, Assessing the Effect of Surface Chemistry on Gold Nanorod Uptake, Toxicity, and Gene Expression in Mammalian Cells, *Small*, 4(1), 153–159 (2008).
41. H.S. Choi, W.H. Liu, P. Misra, E. Tanaka, J.P. Zimmer, B.I. Ipe, M.G. Bawendi and J.V. Frangioni, Renal Clearance of Quantum Dots, *Nature Biotechnology*, 25(10), 1165–1170 (2007).
42. J.P. Caulfield and M.G. Farquhar, The Permeability of Glomerular Capillaries to Graded Dextrans Identification of the Basement Membrane as the Primary Filtration Barrier, *The Journal of Cell Biology*, 63(3), 883–903 (1974).
43. E.C. Dreaden, M.A. Mackey, X. Huang, B. Kang and M.A. El-Sayed, Beating Cancer in Multiple Ways Using Nanogold, *Chemical Society Reviews*, 40(7), 3391–3404 (2011).
44. E.C. Dreaden, S.C. Mwakwari, Q.H. Oyelere and M.A. El-Sayed, Tamoxifen-Poly(ethylene glycol)-Thiol Gold Nanoparticle Conjugates: Enhanced Potency and Selective Delivery for Breast Cancer Treatment, *Bioconjugate Chemistry*, 20(12), 2247–2253 (2009).
45. Y. Cheng, J.D. Meyers, A.M. Broome, M.E. Kenney, J.P. Basilion and C. Burda, Deep Penetration of a PDT Drug into Tumors by Noncovalent Drug-Gold Nanoparticle Conjugates, *Journal of the American Chemical Society*, 133(8), 2583–2591 (2011).
46. Y. Cheng, A.C. Samia, J.D. Meyers, I. Panagopoulos, B. Fei and C. Burda, Highly Efficient Drug Delivery with Gold Nanoparticle Vectors for In Vivo Photodynamic Therapy of Cancer, *Journal of the American Chemical Society*, 130(32), 10643–10647 (2008).
47. N.L. Rosi, D.A. Giljohann, C.S. Thaxton, A.K.R. Lytton-Jean, M.S. Han and C.A. Mirkin, Oligonucleotide-Modified Gold Nanoparticles for Intracellular Gene Regulation, *Science*, 312(5776), 1027–1030 (2006).
48. D.A. Giljohann, D.S. Seferos, A.E. Prigodich, P.C. Patel and C.A. Mirkin, Gene Regulation with Polyvalent siRNA-Nanoparticle Conjugates, *Journal of the American Chemical Society*, 131(6), 2072–2073 (2009).

49. L. Poon, W. Zandberg, Z. Erno, D. Sen, B.D. Gates and N.R. Branda, Photothermal Release of Single-Stranded DNA from the Surface of Gold Nanoparticles Through Controlled Denaturing and Au-S Bond Breaking, *ACS Nano*, 4(11), 6395–6403 (2010).

50. Y. Cheng, A.C. Samia, J. Li, M.E. Kenney, A. Resnick and C. Burda, Delivery and Efficacy of a Cancer Drug as a Function of the Bond to the Gold Nanoparticle Surface, *Langmuir*, 26(4), 2248–2255 (2010).

51. P.K. Jain, W. Qian and M.A. El-Sayed, Ultrafast Cooling of Photoexcited Electrons in Gold Nanoparticle-Thiolated DNA Conjugates Involves the Dissociation of the Gold-Thiol Bond, *Journal of the American Chemical Society*, 128(7), 2426–2433 (2006).

52. S.D. Brown, P. Nativo, J. Smith, D. Stirling, P.R. Edwards, B. Venugopal, D.J. Flint, J.A. Plumb, D. Graham and N.J. Wheate, Gold Nanoparticles for the Improved Anticancer Drug Delivery of the Active Component of Oxaliplatin, *Journal of the American Chemical Society*, 132(13), 4678–4684 (2010).

53. S. Dhar, W.L. Daniel, D.A. Giljohann, C. Mirkin and S.J. Lippard, Polyvalent Oligonucleotide Gold Nanoparticle Conjugates as Delivery Vehicles for Platinum(IV) Warheads, *Journal of the American Chemical Society*, 132(48), 17335 (2010).

54. A.R. Rothrock, R.L. Donkers and M.H. Schoenfisch, Synthesis of Nitric Oxide-Releasing Gold Nanoparticles, *Journal of the American Chemical Society*, 127(26), 9362–9363 (2005).

55. M.A. Polizzi, N.A. Stasko and M.H. Schoenfisch, Water-Soluble Nitric Oxide-Releasing Gold Nanoparticles, *Langmuir*, 23(9), 4938–4943 (2007).

56. S.S. Agasti, A. Chompoosor, C.C. You, P. Ghosh, C.K. Kim and V.M. Rotello, Photoregulated Release of Caged Anticancer Drugs from Gold Nanoparticles, *Journal of the American Chemical Society*, 131(16), 5728–5729 (2009).

57. J.D. Gibson, B.P. Khanal and E.R. Zubarev, Paclitaxel-Functionalized Gold Nanoparticles, *Journal of the American Chemical Society*, 129(37), 11653–11661 (2007).

58. A.M. Alkilany, R.L. Frey, J.L. Ferry and C.J. Murphy, Gold Nanorods as Nanoadmicelles: 1-Naphthol Partitioning into a Nanorod-Bound Surfactant Bilayer, *Langmuir*, 24(18), 10235–10239 (2008).

59. C.K. Kim, P. Ghosh, C. Pagliuca, Z.J. Zhu, S. Menichetti and V.M. Rotello, Entrapment of Hydrophobic Drugs in Nanoparticle Monolayers with Efficient Release into Cancer Cells, *Journal of the American Chemical Society*, 131(4), 1360–1361 (2009).

60. C.J. Murphy, L.B. Thompson, A.M. Alklany, P.N. Sisco, S.P. Boulos, S.T. Sivapalan, J.A. Yang, D.J. Chernak and J.Y. Huang, The Many Faces of Gold Nanorods, *Journal of Physical Chemistry Letters*, 1(19), 2867–2875 (2010).

61. A. Gole and C.J. Murphy, Seed-Mediated Synthesis of Gold Nanorods: Role of the Size and Nature of the Seed, *Chemistry of Materials*, 16(19), 3633–3640 (2004).

62. H.C. Huang, S. Barua, D.B. Kay and K. Rege, Simultaneous Enhancement of Photothermal Stability and Gene Delivery Efficacy of Gold Nanorods Using Polyelectrolytes, *ACS Nano*, 3(10), 2941–2952 (2009).

63. A.C. Bonoiu, S.D. Mahajan, H. Ding, I. Roy, K.T. Yong, R. Kumar, R. Hu, E.J. Bergey, S.A. Schwartz and P.N. Prasad, Nanotechnology Approach for Drug Addiction Therapy: Gene Silencing Using Delivery of Gold Nanorod-siRNA Nanoplex in Dopaminergic Neurons, *Proceedings of the National Academy of Sciences of the United States of America*, 106(14), 5546–5550 (2009).

64. S.T. Guo, Y.Y. Huang, Q. Jiang, Y. Sun, L.D. Deng, Z.C. Liang, Q. Du, J.F. Xing, Y.L. Zhao, P.C. Wang, A.J. Dong and X.J. Liang, Enhanced Gene Delivery and siRNA Silencing by Gold Nanoparticles Coated with Charge-Reversal Polyelectrolyte, *ACS Nano*, 4(9), 5505–5511 (2010).

65. S.K. Lee, M.S. Han, S. Asokan and C.H. Tung, Effective Gene Silencing by Multilayered siRNA-Coated Gold Nanoparticles, *Small*, 7(3), 364–370 (2011).

66. X.C. Yang, B. Samanta, S.S. Agasti, Y. Jeong, Z.J. Zhu, S. Rana, O.R. Miranda and V.M. Rotello, Drug Delivery Using Nanoparticle-Stabilized Nanocapsules, *Angewandte Chemie-International Edition*, 50(2), 477–481 (2011).
67. T.S. Troutman, J.K. Barton and M. Romanowski, Biodegradable Plasmon Resonant Nanoshells, *Advanced Materials*, 20(13), 2604–2605 (2008).
68. G. Borg, E. Allander, B. Lund, U. Brodin, H. Pettersson and L. Trang, Auranofin Improves Outcome in Early Rheumatoid-Arthritis—Results from a 2-Year, Double-Blind, Placebo Controlled-Study, *Journal of Rheumatology*, 15(12), 1747–1754 (1988).
69. M.G. Lewis, S. DaFonseca, N. Chomont, A.T. Palamara, M. Tarduqno, A. Mai, M. Collins, W.L. Wagner, I. Yalley-Oqunro, B. Chirullo, S. Norelli, E. Garaci and A. Savarino, Gold Drug Auranofin Restricts the Viral Reservoir in the Monkey AIDS Model and Induces Containment of Viral Load Following ART Suspension, *AIDS*, 25(11), 1347–1356 (2011).

3 Liposomes as a Drug Delivery System

Kacoli Banerjee,* Shubhadeep Banerjee,*
and Mahitosh Mandal

CONTENTS

ABSTRACT

The discovery of phospholipids spontaneously forming spherical, self-closed bubbles known as liposomes, upon dispersion in water, ushered a new era in drug delivery technology. Continuous and systematic research over the last few decades has resulted in the development of tailor-made liposomal formulations

---

* Authors contributed equally.

53

primarily for the treatment of cancer and gene therapy. The availability of a large array of vesicular systems differing in composition and applications has led to the effective delivery of bioactive molecules either by passive targeting through enhanced permeation and retention phenomena or by active binding to specific target cells and subsequent delivery of cargo. Coupled with the increased blood circulation time through the development of stealth technology, various liposomal formulations have already been approved for clinical use while others are in various stages of clinical trials across the globe. Recent advances in nanotherapeutics have resulted in engineered liposomes emerging as workhorses in nanomedicine, providing better therapeutic control of pathological states through enhanced enrichment of therapeutic or diagnostic agents in diseased tissues. This has paved the way for the development of second-generation liposomes with theranostic utilities for enhanced benefit and could ultimately lead to a paradigm shift from the conventional drug delivery technologies.

Keywords: Liposomes, Drug delivery, Therapeutics, Targeting

3.1 INTRODUCTION

3.1.1 History of Liposomes

The discovery of phospholipids spontaneously forming spherical, self-closed bubbles consisting of one or several concentric lipid bilayers with an aqueous phase inside and between lipid bilayers upon dispersion in water was made by A.D. Bangham in 1961 (Bangham et al. 1965a). He and his colleagues observed that smears of egg lecithin reacted with water to form quite intricate structures, and the strong positive birefringence of lecithin dispersions in water was lost, or even reversed in sign, upon incorporation into the lipid lamellae of increasing amounts of long-chain anions or cations (Duzgunes and Gregoriadis 2005). Electron microscopy demonstrated the formation of a multitude of lipid spherules, which entrapped ionic species dissolved in the aqueous phase at the time of their formation. These lipid vesicles initially called "smectic mesophases" were later renamed as "liposomes" (Figure 3.1) (Sessa and Weissman 1968).

The recognition of the biological cells exploiting surface-active properties of lipids to define anatomical membranes led to the development of model systems based on the orientation of lipids at the interfaces for the investigation of transport functions and mechanisms, permeation properties, as well as adhesion and fusion kinetics. Model lipid membranes that mimic many aspects of cell membranes have been very useful in helping investigations to discern the mechanism of interaction between bioactive molecules and lipids (Banerjee et al. 2012a). The lipid organization in these model systems bears a close resemblance to the arrangement of lipids in natural cell membranes (Seddon et al. 2009). Simplified artificial membrane systems provide a suitable platform for investigation of biophysical interactions of drugs and drug delivery systems bypassing the intricacies

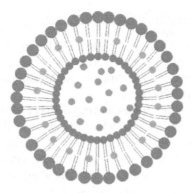

Liposome bearing hydrophilic and hydrophobic drug

Phospholipid molecule

Hydrophilic drug

Hydrophobic drug

FIGURE 3.1 Schematic representation of a liposome. Liposomes are able to entrap both hydrophilic and hydrophobic drugs, thus making them attractive drug delivery vehicles.

of cell membrane structures and associated dynamic nature of lipid–lipid and lipid–protein interactions in cell membranes and also allow experimentation to be performed under conditions that living cells may not be able to withstand and remain viable (Peetla et al. 2009).

The diffusion of univalent cations and anions out of the liposomes was observed to be remarkably similar to the diffusion of such ions across biological membranes (Sessa and Weissman 1968). In fact, the rate of leakage of sequestered ions formed a good measure of the overall permeability of the structures, each containing several lamellae (Bangham et al. 1965a,b). Since these measurements were analogous to the determination of ion efflux from cells or organelles, liposomes started to attract attention as an artificial model membrane (Huang 1969) to determine the modes of action of toxins, drugs, hormones, and anesthetics, as well for studies of the permeability of lipid membranes.

The resemblance of their lamellar structure with natural membranes, the capability to discriminate ions (cations diffuse poorly from membranes that are permeable to univalent anions and water), and susceptibility to stabilization or labilization by bioactive molecules similar to biological membranes have rendered liposomes a versatile tool in the field of biology, biochemistry, and medicine (Bangham et al. 1965a). The ability of the vesicles to swell osmotically, the possibility to vary membrane composition and surface potential, and availability of several analytical techniques to study these systems have made liposomes a preferred lipid matrix model of living cells (Bangham et al. 1965b).

With the recognition of the biocompatibility, biodegradability, low toxicity and immunogenicity, and the capability to entrap molecules, liposomes have moved a long way from being just another exotic object of biophysical research to becoming a pharmaceutical carrier of choice for numerous practical applications (Black and Gregoriadis 1976; Gregoriadis 1976; Juliano and McCullough 1980; Neerunjun and Gregoriadis 1976; Torchilin 2005).

The initial excitement of liposomes as drug delivery vehicles was, however, short lived because of insufficient understanding of liposome disposition and clearance *in vivo*, inaccurate extrapolation of *in vitro* liposome–cell interactions or liposome targeting data, and pronounced instability and reduced circulation time of liposome-based drugs *in vivo* (Lian and Ho 2001). Substantial advances in the late 1980s and early 1990s, including detailed understanding of lipid polymorphisms, physiological mechanisms of *in vivo* liposome disposition, and lipid–drug and lipid–protein interactions, overcame many of the early disappointments (Torchilin 2005). However, the major breakthrough came with the realization that steric stabilization can significantly increase liposome stability and prolong, by several orders of magnitude, their persistence in the blood circulation system after administration (Immordino et al. 2006). These resulted in the development of tailor-made liposomal formulations with increased stability both *in vitro* and *in vivo*, improved biodistribution, and optimized resident time in systemic (or blood) circulation (Allen et al. 1991; Klibanov et al. 1990). The goal of liposomes as drug carriers in pharmaceutical applications was realized in the mid-1990s with the approval of liposomal formulations of anticancer drugs Doxil (Sequus Pharmaceuticals, Inc.) and DaunoXome (Gilead, Nexstar) by the US Food and Drug Administration for clinical use (Lian and Ho 2001).

3.1.2 COMPONENTS OF LIPOSOMES

3.1.2.1 Phospholipids

The general chemical structure of phospholipids has two acyl chains linked to a headgroup by means of a glycerol backbone. Figure 3.2 shows the structural formula of a phospholipid, where R_1 and R_2 are saturated or unsaturated acyl chains and R_3 is the polar headgroup, while Figure 3.3 represents the chemical structures of lipids in liposome formulations. The lipid nature of the phospholipid is attributed to the long-chain fatty acids that are esterified with the hydroxyl groups of the glycerol (Lian and Ho 2001). The polar headgroups such as glycerol, choline, ethanolamine,

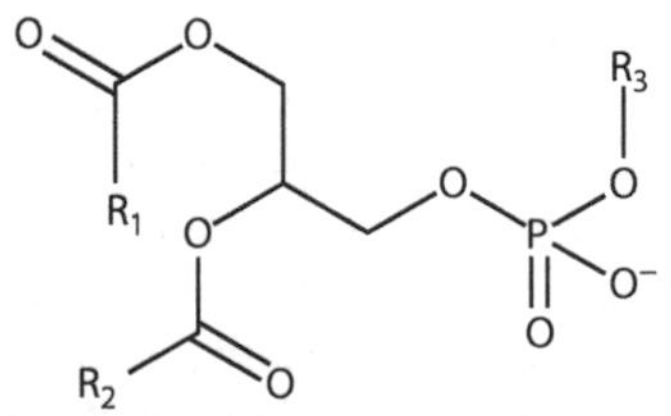

FIGURE 3.2 Structural formula of phospholipids. R_1, R_2 are the tail group–fatty acyl chains and R_3 represent the various headgroups.

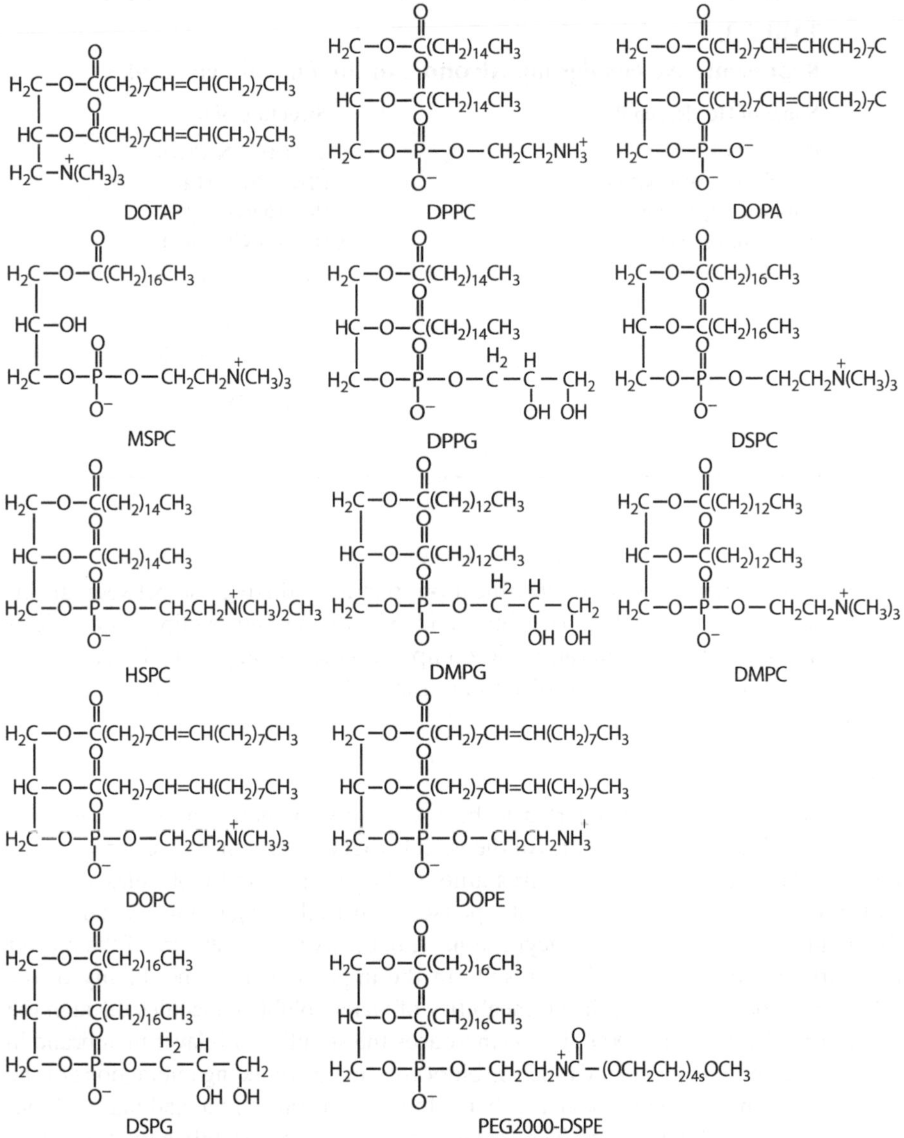

$$H_2C-O-\overset{\overset{\displaystyle O}{\|}}{C}(CH_2)_7CH=CH(CH_2)_7CH_3$$
$$HC-O-\overset{\overset{\displaystyle O}{\|}}{C}(CH_2)_7CH=CH(CH_2)_7CH_3$$
$$H_2C-\overset{+}{N}(CH_3)_3$$

DOTAP

$$H_2C-O-\overset{\overset{\displaystyle O}{\|}}{C}(CH_2)_{14}CH_3$$
$$HC-O-\overset{\overset{\displaystyle O}{\|}}{C}(CH_2)_{14}CH_3$$
$$H_2C-O-\overset{\overset{\displaystyle O}{\|}}{P}-O-CH_2CH_2NH_3^+$$
$$O^-$$

DPPC

$$H_2C-O-\overset{\overset{\displaystyle O}{\|}}{C}(CH_2)_7CH=CH(CH_2)_7C$$
$$HC-O-\overset{\overset{\displaystyle O}{\|}}{C}(CH_2)_7CH=CH(CH_2)_7C$$
$$H_2C-O-\overset{\overset{\displaystyle O}{\|}}{P}-O^-$$
$$O^-$$

DOPA

$$H_2C-O-\overset{\overset{\displaystyle O}{\|}}{C}(CH_2)_{16}CH_3$$
$$HC-OH$$
$$H_2C-O-\overset{\overset{\displaystyle O}{\|}}{P}-O-CH_2CH_2\overset{+}{N}(CH_3)_3$$
$$O^-$$

MSPC

$$H_2C-O-\overset{\overset{\displaystyle O}{\|}}{C}(CH_2)_{14}CH_3$$
$$HC-O-\overset{\overset{\displaystyle O}{\|}}{C}(CH_2)_{14}CH_3$$
$$H_2C-O-\overset{\overset{\displaystyle O}{\|}}{P}-O-\overset{H_2}{C}-\overset{H}{\underset{OH}{C}}-\underset{OH}{CH_2}$$
$$O^-$$

DPPG

$$H_2C-O-\overset{\overset{\displaystyle O}{\|}}{C}(CH_2)_{16}CH_3$$
$$HC-O-\overset{\overset{\displaystyle O}{\|}}{C}(CH_2)_{16}CH_3$$
$$H_2C-O-\overset{\overset{\displaystyle O}{\|}}{P}-O-CH_2CH_2\overset{+}{N}(CH_3)_3$$
$$O^-$$

DSPC

$$H_2C-O-\overset{\overset{\displaystyle O}{\|}}{C}(CH_2)_{14}CH_3$$
$$HC-O-\overset{\overset{\displaystyle O}{\|}}{C}(CH_2)_{14}CH_3$$
$$H_2C-O-\overset{\overset{\displaystyle O}{\|}}{P}-O-CH_2CH_2\overset{+}{N}(CH_3)_2CH_3$$
$$O^-$$

HSPC

$$H_2C-O-\overset{\overset{\displaystyle O}{\|}}{C}(CH_2)_{12}CH_3$$
$$HC-O-\overset{\overset{\displaystyle O}{\|}}{C}(CH_2)_{12}CH_3$$
$$H_2C-O-\overset{\overset{\displaystyle O}{\|}}{P}-O-\overset{H_2}{C}-\overset{H}{\underset{OH}{C}}-\underset{OH}{CH_2}$$
$$O^-$$

DMPG

$$H_2C-O-\overset{\overset{\displaystyle O}{\|}}{C}(CH_2)_{12}CH_3$$
$$HC-O-\overset{\overset{\displaystyle O}{\|}}{C}(CH_2)_{12}CH_3$$
$$H_2C-O-\overset{\overset{\displaystyle O}{\|}}{P}-O-CH_2CH_2\overset{+}{N}(CH_3)_3$$
$$O^-$$

DMPC

$$H_2C-O-\overset{\overset{\displaystyle O}{\|}}{C}(CH_2)_7CH=CH(CH_2)_7CH_3$$
$$HC-O-\overset{\overset{\displaystyle O}{\|}}{C}(CH_2)_7CH=CH(CH_2)_7CH_3$$
$$H_2C-O-\overset{\overset{\displaystyle O}{\|}}{P}-O-CH_2CH_2\overset{+}{N}(CH_3)_3$$
$$O^-$$

DOPC

$$H_2C-O-\overset{\overset{\displaystyle O}{\|}}{C}(CH_2)_7CH=CH(CH_2)_7CH_3$$
$$HC-O-\overset{\overset{\displaystyle O}{\|}}{C}(CH_2)_7CH=CH(CH_2)_7CH_3$$
$$H_2C-O-\overset{\overset{\displaystyle O}{\|}}{P}-O-CH_2CH_2NH_3^+$$
$$O^-$$

DOPE

$$H_2C-O-\overset{\overset{\displaystyle O}{\|}}{C}(CH_2)_{16}CH_3$$
$$HC-O-\overset{\overset{\displaystyle O}{\|}}{C}(CH_2)_{16}CH_3$$
$$H_2C-O-\overset{\overset{\displaystyle O}{\|}}{P}-O-\overset{H_2}{C}-\overset{H}{\underset{OH}{C}}-\underset{OH}{CH_2}$$
$$O^-$$

DSPG

$$H_2C-O-\overset{\overset{\displaystyle O}{\|}}{C}(CH_2)_{16}CH_3$$
$$HC-O-\overset{\overset{\displaystyle O}{\|}}{C}(CH_2)_{16}CH_3$$
$$H_2C-O-\overset{\overset{\displaystyle O}{\|}}{P}-O-CH_2CH_2\overset{+}{N}\overset{\overset{\displaystyle O}{\|}}{C}-(OCH_2CH_2)_{45}OCH_3$$
$$O^-$$

PEG2000-DSPE

FIGURE 3.3 Chemical structures of lipids in liposome formulations. Abbreviations: DOTAP, 1,2-dioleoyl-3-trimethylammonium propane; DPPC, dipalmitoylphosphatidylcholine; DOPA, 1,2-dioleoyl-sn-glycero-3-phosphate; MSPC, monostearoylphosphatidylcholine; DPPG, dipalmitoylphosphatidylglycerol; DSPC, distearoylphosphatidylcholine; HSPC, hydrogenated soy PC; DMPG, l-α-dimyristoylphosphatidylglycerol; DMPC, l-α-dimyristo ylphosphatidylcholine; DOPC, 1,2-dioleoyl-sn-glycero-3-phosphocholine; DOPE, dioleoyl phosphatidylethanolamine; DSPG, distearoylphosphatidylglycerol; PEG2000-DSPE, polyethylene glycol 2000-distearoylphosphatidylethanolamine. (Reproduced from H. I. Chang and M. K. Yeh, *Int J Nanomed*, 7, 49–60, 2012.)

TABLE 3.1

Representative Headgroup Alcohols of the Phosphoglycerides

Name of Headgroup R_3	Structure of R_3
Phosphatidylcholine	$-CH_2-CH_2-N(CH_3)_3^+$
Phosphatidylethanolamine	$-CH_2-CH_2-NH_3^+$
Phosphatidylglycerol	$-CH_2-CHOH-CH_2OH$
Phosphatidylserine	$-CH_2-CH-NH_2COOH$
Phosphatidylinositol	

serine, and inositol are used for classification, that is, to distinguish between different phospholipids (Table 3.1). The fatty acid part of the phospholipid molecule is important and differences in fatty acid composition can change the characteristics of the phospholipids. Fatty acids differ in number of carbon atom chains and degree of unsaturation.

3.1.2.2 Sterols

Cholesterol has also been reported to be used in the preparation of liposomes to improve the bilayer characteristics of the vesicles. Cholesterol molecules (possessing a steroid backbone) orient themselves among the phospholipid molecules with the hydroxyl group facing toward the water phase, the tricyclic ring sandwiched between the first few carbons of the fatty acyl chains, into the hydrocarbon core of the bilayer (Vemuri and Rhodes 1995). This results in the improvement of the fluidity of the bilayer and the reduction of the permeability of water-soluble molecules through the membrane (Peetla et al. 2009). It also increases the stability of bilayer membrane in the presence of biological fluids such as blood/plasma by reducing interactions of the liposomes with the blood proteins such as albumin, m-transferrin, and macroglobulin (Vemuri and Rhodes 1995). These components tend to destabilize the liposomes and reduce the utility of liposomes as drug delivery systems. However, the presence of a large quantity of cholesterol in a vesicle results in the loss of liposomal phospholipid (Damen et al. 1981).

3.1.3 SELF-ASSEMBLY OF PHOSPHOLIPIDS

The ability of the phospholipids to spontaneously aggregate into liposomes is attributed to the dual preference of the amphiphiles for solvent. Since the hydrophobic and hydrophilic components of amphiphiles are soluble in nonpolar and polar solvents, respectively, the presence of water causes self-assembly of the phospholipids above a certain concentration, to minimize unfavorable hydrophobic interactions. This self-organization is usually accompanied by increased entropy of the system (Finney and Soper 1994), which originates from the water–hydrocarbon interactions that force the water molecules into an ordered structure around the hydrophobic part when the amphiphiles are freely suspended as monomers. Release of the ordered water is achieved by driving the hydrophobic parts out of the aqueous solution and sequestering them within the interior of the aggregate. The increase in entropy gained by the water molecules will lead to an overall gain in free energy and result in spontaneous aggregation (Blokzijl and Engberts 1993).

The spontaneous aggregation of the phospholipids into bilayer structures is not only determined by the hydrophobic contribution mentioned earlier but also related to the molecular parameters of the amphiphile. The aggregate structure for amphiphiles is predicted by the "surfactant parameter" (S), which in turn takes into account parameters such as the hydrophobic volume, chain length, and headgroup area that contain information about the geometrical shape of the molecule (Israelachvili et al. 1976). The surfactant parameter is defined as follows:

$$S = v/(l \times a_0), \tag{3.1}$$

where v, l, and a_0 are the volume of the hydrophobic portion of the amphiphile, the length of the hydrocarbon chains, and the effective area per headgroup, respectively. The value of the surfactant parameter relates the properties of the molecule to the mean curvature of the formed aggregates. By convention, the curvature of an aggregate is positive if the aggregate is curved around the hydrophobic part and negative if it is curved toward the polar part (Seddon et al. 2009). The former is also said to form normal aggregates and phases, while the latter forms reversed ones. It has already been reported that while small values of S imply highly curved aggregates such as micelles, $S \sim 1$ represent planar bilayers (Israelachvili et al. 1976).

The geometry of the phospholipid molecules composed of two hydrocarbon chains attached to a polar headgroup has been approximated as cylinders. According to the geometrical packing concept described above, phospholipids prefer to self-assemble into bilayers. At higher lipid concentrations, these molecules usually form lamellar phases where two-dimensional planar lipid bilayers alternate with water layers (Israelachvili et al. 1976).

3.1.4 Classification of Liposomes

The liposome family comprises different types of vesicles that vary in size, structure, composition, method of preparation, application, and novelty. Although systematic classification of this wide range of varying colloidal particles is quite cumbersome, a simplified classification on the basis of structure (Table 3.2), method of preparation (Table 3.3) (Samad et al. 2007), and composition and application (Table 3.4) (Wagner and Vorauer-Uhl 2011) is attempted in this chapter.

TABLE 3.2

Classification of Liposomes Based on Structure

Vesicle Type	Abbreviation	Hydrodynamic Diameter	No. of Lipid Bilayers	Reference
Small unilamellar vesicles	SUV	20–50 nm	1	Iqbal et al. 2011
Large unilamellar vesicles	LUV	100–1000 nm	1	Sharma and Sharma 1997
Giant unilamellar vesicles	GUV	>1000 nm	1	Tomsie et al. 2005
Multilamellar vesicles	MLV	>500 nm	5–25	Banerjee et al. 2012a,b
Oligolamellar vesicles	OLV	100–1000 nm	~5	Goren et al. 1990
Multivesicular vesicles	MVL	>1000 nm	Multicompartmental structure	Grant et al. 2004

TABLE 3.3

Classification of Liposomes Based on the Method of Preparation

Preparation Method	Abbreviation	Reference
Thin film hydration	MLV	Roux et al. 2003
Frozen and thawed multilamellar vesicles	FAT-MLV	Maestrelli et al. 2009
Extrusion technique	VET (LUVET/SUVET)	Mayer et al. 1986
Multilamellar vesicles by reverse-phase evaporation	MLV-REV	Taylor et al. 1990
Single- or oligolamellar vesicles by reverse-phase evaporation	REV	Szoka and Papahadjopoulos 1978
Dehydration–rehydration	DRV	Kirby and Gregoriadis 1984
Stable plurilamellar vesicles	SPLV	Gruner et al. 1985

3.2 LIPOSOMES AS DRUG DELIVERY VEHICLES

3.2.1 LIPOSOMAL DRUG DELIVERY: PASSIVE AND ACTIVE TARGETING

In order to circumvent the problems associated with conventional drug delivery, which includes inefficient biodistribution throughout the body and lack of specific delivery and passively targeting tissues and organs that have discontinuous endothelium (e.g., liver, spleen, and bone marrow), liposomal formulations of several key active molecules were developed (Immordino et al. 2006). The chaotic tumor-vessel architecture characterizing any solid tumor facilitates passive targeting. Leaky vasculature and dysfunctional lymphatic drainage characterize any solid tumor

TABLE 3.4
Classification of Commonly Known Lipid Vesicles according to Their Composition and Application

Identification	Definition	Reference
Stealth liposomes	Liposomes coated with polyethylene glycol (PEG), a synthetic hydrophilic polymer, have improved stability and enhanced half-life in circulation by avoiding or retarding liposome recognition by the reticuloendothelial system (RES). The PEG-stabilizing effect results from local surface concentration of highly hydrated groups that sterically inhibit both hydrophobic and electrostatic interactions of a variety of blood components (e.g., albumin) at the liposome surface.	Allen et al. 1991; Klibanov et al. 1990
Niosomes	Small unilamellar vesicles made from nonionic surfactants. These vesicles are also known as novasomes.	Brewer and Alexander 1994
Archeosomes	Vesicles consisting of archaebacteria lipids, which are chemically distinct from eukaryotes and prokaryotes. These vesicles are less sensitive to oxidative stress, high temperature, and alkaline pH. Their chemical stability is comparable to niosomes.	Conlan et al. 2001; Krishnan et al. 2000
Ethosomes	Multilamellar vesicles composed of phosphatidylcholine and approximately 30% of ethanol. They are used mainly for efficient delivery of drugs to the skin in terms of both quantity and depth compared to conventional liposomes.	Touitou et al. 2000
Transfersomes	Ultradeformable vesicles composed of phosphatidylcholine and cholate with enhanced skin-penetrating properties.	Jain et al. 2003
Proliposomes	Dry, free-flowing particles that immediately form a liposomal dispersion on contact with water.	Jung et al. 2002; Payne et al. 1986
Proteosomes	Immunogenic vesicles of bacterial origin, prepared by solubilizing, ammonium sulfate precipitation, and dialysis against detergent buffer, have proteins and peptides noncovalently complexed to the membranes.	Lowell et al. 1988
Immunoliposomes	Liposomes modified with antibodies, Fab's, or peptide structures on the bilayer surface for recognizing and binding to cells of interest and thereby increasing liposomal drug accumulation in the desired tissues and organs.	Huang et al. 1983; Sullivan et al. 1986
Immunosomes	Glycoprotein molecules anchored to preformed liposomes with structural and immunogen characteristics closer to purified and inactivated viruses unlike other forms of glycoprotein–lipid association.	Perrin et al. 1985

(Continued)

TABLE 3.4 (CONTINUED)
Classification of Commonly Known Lipid Vesicles according to Their Composition and Application

Identification	Definition	Reference
Immune stimulating complex	Spherical, lipid assemblies made of the saponin mixture Quil A, cholesterol, and phospholipids containing amphiphilic antigens like membrane proteins and have a built-in adjuvant, *Quillaja* saponin, which is a structural part of the vehicle.	Kersten and Crommelin 2003
Lipoplexes	Cationic lipid–DNA complexes that are efficient carriers for cell transfection. However, associated toxicity is a major drawback.	Audouy and Hoekstra 2001; Khalil et al. 2006
Virosomes	Small unilamellar vesicles containing influenza hemagglutinin, by which they become fusogenic with endocytic membranes. Co-incorporation of other membrane antigens induces enhanced immune responses.	Gluck 1999
Dendrosomes	A family of novel, nontoxic, neutral, biodegradable, covalent, or self-assembled, hyperbranched, dendritic, spheroidal nanoparticles that are easy to prepare, inexpensive, and highly stable. Predominantly used for gene delivery.	Sarbolouki et al. 2000
Polymerized liposomes	Polymerized phosphatidylcholine vesicles composed of lipids bearing one or two methacrylate groups per monomer. Compared to nonpolymeric analogs, these vesicles exhibit improved stability and controllable time-release properties.	Regen et al. 1981
Temperature-sensitive liposomes	Liposomes composed of lipids that undergo a gel-to-liquid crystalline phase transition a few degrees above physiological temperature have thermosensitive polymers anchored to the bilayers that render vesicle temperature sensitive. These vesicles are typically used to achieve site-specific delivery of drugs and can be modified in a temperature-dependent manner to control content release behavior, surface properties, and affinity to cell surface.	Kono 2001; Needham and Dewhirst 2001
pH-sensitive liposomes	Liposomes that respond to local pH changes and undergo conformational transition to release the encapsulated cargo. These types of liposomes are further subdivided into four subclasses: (a) vesicles composed of polymorphic lipids and mild acidic amphiphiles that act as stabilizers at neutral pH (extensively investigated); (b) vesicles composed of caged lipid derivatives that results in increased permeability to encapsulated solutes; (c) vesicles utilizing pH-sensitive peptides or reconstituted fusion proteins to destabilize membranes at low pH; and (d) pH-sensitive polymers to destabilize membranes after change of the polymer conformation at low pH (most recent). Mainly used for enhanced delivery of drugs within cells by fusing with endovascular membranes under low pH condition.	Drummond et al. 2000

(Underwood and Carr 1972). The fenestrations of the leaky vasculature allow the liposomes to escape into the tumor tissue. Extravasation is successively followed by increased retention of the drug-loaded nanocarrier in the tumor tissue (Peer et al. 2007; Phillips et al. 2010) leading to enhanced drug delivery at the diseased region. Maeda and Matsumura (1989) first termed this phenomenon as *enhanced permeation and retention* (EPR) effect (Figure 3.4).

High interstitial fluid pressure (IFP) in most solid tumors (Jain 1987) reduces significantly the anticancer drug delivery (Jain 1987, 1994). Unlike low-molecular-weight drugs, the movement of high-molecular-weight anticancer drugs/nanoparticles takes place by convection rather than by diffusion from the circulatory system through the interstitial space. Convection is inhibited by increased IFP, which in turn results in decreased uptake of drugs into tumor. Moreover, in comparison to its periphery, IFP at the center of the solid tumor is higher (Danhier et al. 2010). High IFP barrier within tumors may be overcome by adopting active targeting strategies (Chang et al. 2009). An important active targeting strategy involves the use of ligands with affinity for the receptors expressed on the plasma membrane of cancer cells or tumor neovasculature, to increase the accumulation of anticancer drugs even with high IFP environment of the tumor tissues and improve the therapeutic efficacy (Lee et al. 2007). In conjugation with nanotherapeutics, therapeutic interventions designed to reduce IFP could be applied to augment the treatment of cancer (Cairns et al. 2006).

The problems associated with passive targeting include increased toxicity in normal cells, decreased retention of drug-loaded nanocarriers owing to higher IFP, and development of drug resistance can be overcome by explicitly directing liposomes

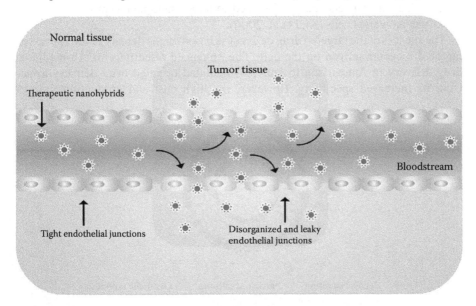

FIGURE 3.4 Schematic representation of tumor targeting by nanohybrids via the EPR effect. (Reproduced with permission from S. Prakash et al., *Advanced Drug Delivery Reviews*, 63, 1340–1351, 2011.)

to bind to specific target cells (Medina et al. 2004; Sapra and Allen 2003). Major active drug delivery strategies involve ligand-mediated or antibody (Ab)-mediated targeting of the therapeutics to the cancer cell. Ligand-targeting therapeutics leads to increased drug efficacy (therapeutic effect) and reduced drug toxicity (side effects) (Juliano and Daoud 1990; Lian and Ho 2001; Malam et al. 2009; Perumal et al. 2011), resulting in improved therapeutic index of the drug. Recent reports describe the use of ligand-targeting agents such as protein (Ab or Ab fragments) (Heath et al. 1983), peptides (arginine–glycine–aspartic acid or RGD) (Schiffelers et al. 2003), vitamin (folic acid) (Rui et al. 1998), nucleic acid (aptamer) (Brody and Gold 2000; Floege et al. 1999; White et al. 2000), and glycoprotein (transferrin) (Juliano and Stamp 1976). While RGD targets cellular adhesion molecules important in cancer progression (Cooper et al. 2002) like integrin $\alpha_v\beta_3$ (Suri et al. 2007), growth factor receptors are specifically targeted by transferrin (Weinzimer et al. 2001) and folate ligands (Herbert et al. 1962).

Non-Ab ligand-targeted delivery like folate and transferrin-mediated drug delivery systems are being reported lately (Figure 3.5). Folate-mediated liposome targeting is increasingly gaining importance because of the frequent overexpression of folate receptors in a wide variety of tumor cells (Lu and Low 2002). Similarly, targeting tumors with transferrin-modified liposomes also provides a suitable approach owing to the increased frequency of transferrin receptors in cancer cells (Gowda 2013; Hatakeyama et al. 2004). Peptides (RGD) (Schiffelers et al. 2003), glycan (Xie et al. 2012), and nucleic acid (aptamer) (Leamon et al. 2003) have also been reported as other forms of non-Ab ligand liposome-based targeted drug delivery systems. Second-generation liposomes bearing dual ligands enhance targeting selectivity of drug-loaded nanocarriers and are designed to target multiple receptors for reduced toxicity on nontarget cells (Saul et al. 2006).

The success of the targeted drug delivery is based on the density of the expressed targeted receptor/antigen on the cell. The enhanced effectivity of Ab-mediated drug delivery in comparison to non–Ab-mediated targeted drug delivery arises from its increased specificity. However, the high cost and production time of

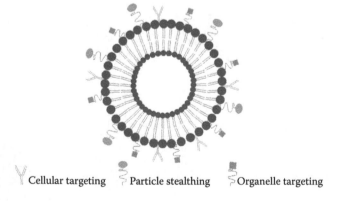

Cellular targeting   Particle stealthing   Organelle targeting

FIGURE 3.5 Schematic representation of an engineered liposome for long circulation and ligand/Ab-mediated targeted delivery. (Reproduced with permission from K. Sen and M. Mandal, *Int J Pharmaceut*, 448, 28–43, 2013.)

Ab-anchored liposomes significantly limit its application in targeted delivery (Allen 2002).

3.2.2 LIPOSOME-BASED THERAPEUTICS

Gregoriadis et al. (1974) first proposed liposomes for delivery of cancer therapeutics. Liposomes have been widely reported to be a therapeutic tool of choice since they have numerous advantages as pharmaceutical carriers (Table 3.5). However, the major associated limitation of conventional liposomes (Table 3.6) for therapeutic use lies in its fast elimination from the blood and recognition by the reticuloendothelial system (RES) (Torchilin 2005).

The efficient uptake of liposomes by macrophages and subsequent removal from systemic circulation upon intravenous administration are, however, severely affected when the target site is beyond the mononuclear phagocyte system (MPS). The binding of opsonins (such as immunoglobulins, fibronectin, and C-reactive protein) (Falcone 1986; Patel 1992; Volanakis and Narkates 1981) on the surface of liposomes results in MPS recognizing these serum proteins rather than the vesicles and translates into removal of the liposomes from the circulation. Complement components such as C5b-9 complexes (membrane attack complex [MAC]), which

---

TABLE 3.5
Advantages of Liposomes as Pharmaceutical Carriers

Biocompatibility (Mufamadi et al. 2011)

Prevents premature degradation of encapsulated cargo (Goyal et al. 2005; Petros and DeSimone 2010)

Entrapment of both hydrophilic and hydrophobic drugs (Medina et al. 2004; Zhang et al. 2008)

Targeted delivery—Can be functionalized with ligands to deliver therapeutic agents into cells or cellular components (Torchilin 2005)

Site avoidance—The entrapped drug is prevented from reaching the healthy tissue (Hofheinz et al. 2005)

Size or lipid component variation helps in regulating biodistribution of liposomes (Iinuma et al. 2002)

Source: K. Sen and M. Mandal, *Int J Pharmaceut,* 448, 28–43, 2013.

TABLE 3.6
Limitations of Liposomes in Drug/Gene Delivery

High production cost—raw material (lipids) cost is high (Barenholz 2001; Peer et al. 2007)

Oxidation of some phospholipids (Peer et al. 2007)

Rapid clearance by the reticuloendothelial system (Mufamadi et al. 2011)

Removal from the circulatory system (Peer et al. 2007)

Nonspecific uptake (Peer et al. 2007)

Physiochemical instability (aggregation, sedimentation, hydrolysis) (Gurley 2011)

Source: K. Sen and M. Mandal, *Int J Pharmaceut,* 448, 28–43, 2013.

act as an immediate host defense against invading foreign particles, also recognize liposomes (Hamaguchi et al. 2007; Wilson et al. 2008) and initiate membrane lysis through pore formation and enhance uptake by neutrophils, monocytes, and macrophages (MPS cells) (Immordino et al. 2006). However, the presence of dysopsonins such as human serum albumin and IgA on the vesicle surface reduces recognition and inhibits phagocytosis of liposomes (Petros et al. 2010). In fact, a fine balance between the blood opsonic and suppressive proteins regulates the rate of liposome clearance (Wilson et al. 2008). The conventional liposomes were also observed to demonstrate profound instability in plasma, which resulted in the rapid release of the encapsulated cargo owing to their interactions with both high- and low-density lipoproteins (HDL and LDL, respectively) (Immordino et al. 2006).

In order to bypass the low-systemic circulation time of conventional liposomes, synthesis of long circulating liposomes (Stealth liposomes) has been attempted by coating the liposome surface with polymers, such as polyethylene glycol (PEG) (Klibanov et al. 1990), poly(vinyl pyrrolidone) (PVP), poly(acryl amide) (PAA) (Torchilin et al. 1994), poly[N-(2-hydroxypropyl)methacrylamide], and amphiphilic poly-N-vinylpyrrolidones (Torchilin et al. 2001) (Figure 3.5). This resulted in significantly increased liposome stability, which prolonged, by several orders of magnitude, their blood circulation times after systemic administration (Immordino et al. 2006) and ultimately led to the development of tailor-made liposomal formulations with increased stability both *in vitro* and *in vivo*, improved biodistribution, and optimized residence time in systemic circulation (Allen et al. 1991; Klibanov et al. 1990).

Repeated injections of sterically stabilized liposomes over a short duration leads to their rapid elimination from the system. This reduction in half-life of PEG liposomes has been termed *accelerated blood clearance* (ABC) (Ishida et al. 2003b, 2004). The ABC effect has been observed in animal models (rat, rabbit, mouse, Rhesus monkey, and Beagle dog) and reflects a major change in pharmacokinetics of consecutive injections of PEG liposomes (Dams et al. 2000; Ishida et al. 2003a; Zhao et al. 2012). Repeated injections of PEGylated liposomes elicit immune response and lead to production of anti-PEG IgM, which enhances blood clearance of subsequently injected PEGylated liposomes via anti-PEG IgM-mediated complement activation under certain conditions (Ishida et al. 2005, 2006b). However, it has been recently reported that encapsulated Doxorubicin in drug-loaded PEGylated liposomes causes selective damage of T cell–independent B cell–mediated ABC phenomenon (Koide et al. 2010).

However, these pharmacokinetic changes were most distinct at dosing frequencies (1–3 weeks) that are higher than those used in current clinical practice of approved formulation (e.g., Doxil 180, 3–6 weeks). PEG liposomal doxorubicin formulation has a recommended low injection frequency of 3–6 weeks in order to prevent the occurrence of cutaneous toxicity (Muggia et al. 1997); thus, the occurrence of ABC effect has not yet been reported in humans (Dams et al. 2000).

The magnitude of the induction of the ABC phenomenon is directly dependent on the interval between injections (Dams et al. 2000) and inversely related to the dose (Ishida et al. 2005). Thus, it is very important to design optimal dosing schedules in order to enhance the therapeutic efficacy and reduce the induced toxicity or immunological responses (Ishida et al. 2006a).

Recent combinatorial approaches aim to achieve greater circulation time of the vesicles (via PEGylation), specific delivery of encapsulated payload, and synergistic uptake via dual-ligand targeting (Takara et al. 2010). *In vitro* and *in vivo* intracellular delivery of doxorubicin with RGD-modified PEGylated liposomes exhibited increased cytotoxicity against melanoma (Xiong et al. 2005). Cationic liposomes have been effectively utilized in the treatment of resistant forms of cancer, which have been unresponsive to conventional chemotherapy and other forms of treatment (Campbell et al. 2009). Combinatorial treatment regimens involving cationic nanosystems and other cancer therapeutic approaches such as hyperthermia or application of magnetic fields are currently assessed (Campbell et al. 2009) for enhanced cancer chemotherapy. Cationic liposomes are effective, but they strongly interact with the blood components before they can reach the therapeutic target (Nicolazzi et al. 2003). Latest second-generation liposomal strategy aiming at conjugating lipoplex technology that involves catonic lipid-based vesicles bearing oligonucleotide with PEGylation has been reported to have substantial increase in circulation time. While this succeeds in enhancing the effectivity of these formulations (Nicolazzi et al. 2003), its limitation lies in reduced transfection rates (Xu et al. 2011).

Recent advances report the emergence of a new class of liposomes for cancer-specific therapy, which successfully overcomes the limitations of conventional liposomes. In contrast to conventional liposomes, stimuli-responsive vesicles undergo relatively large and abrupt physical and chemical changes in sharp response to applied stimuli. This becomes of particular interest when the stimuli to which these vesicles react are disease or systemic-biochemistry specific (such as pH). Solid tumors are characterized by poor vasculature, which causes prevalence of anaerobic conditions, and the extracellular pH is also significantly acidic (~6–7) than systemic pH (7.4). The pH shift of the specific tissues can act as internal stimuli of chemical and biochemical origin that trigger drug release from the stimuli-responsive nanocarriers. External physical stimuli triggering release of encapsulated cargo include heat, light, and magnetic field (Fleige et al. 2012; Kato 2012; Scheel and Weinberg 2011). With primary cancer prevention being the goal of the present-day cancer chemotherapy, cancer vaccines have been developed to significantly reduce the incidence of cancer caused by microorganisms such as hepatocellular carcinoma (hepatitis B virus) and cervical carcinoma (human papilloma viruses) (Goymer 2005; Villa et al. 2005). However, the antitumor vaccine studies have been limited to *in vivo* models, and transition to the clinical trials have not been very fulfilling (Lollini et al. 2006). Liposomal vaccine formulation bearing antigenic peptide derived from choriomeningitis virus and immune-stimulatory oligonucleotides has been reported to elicit antiviral and antitumor immunity (Ludewig et al. 2000). One of the most recent additions to the repertoire of liposomes is the multifunctional theranostic liposomes, which can be considered as a key advancement in nanomedicine and has opened up a plethora of possibilities for simultaneous cancer therapy and diagnosis.

Approved liposomal drug formulations in cancer therapeutics have gone a long way and evolved from classical conventional liposomes (Myocet/DaunoXome) (Batist et al. 2001; Petre and Dittmer 2007) to PEGylated forms (Doxil and

Lipo-Dox) (Barenholz 2012). Second-generation liposomal drug delivery system endeavors for clinic use range from dual drug–loaded liposomes (CPX-1/CPX-351) (Dicko et al. 2010; Riviere et al. 2011) to stimuli-sensitive liposomes (ThermoDox) (Poon and Borys 2011). The current focus of drug delivery research in clinical trials has been on active targeted drug delivery (MM-302/MBP-436) (Drummond et al. 2006; McDonagh et al. 2012) or utilization of cationic liposomes for drug delivery (EndoTAG-1) (Fasol et al. 2012). Liposomal cancer vaccines being tested clinically include the Anti-MUC1 cancer vaccine (Bradbury and Shepherd 2008) and L-BLP25 (Butts et al. 2005). Other approaches include RNA interference (RNAi)–based therapies that involve the delivery of siRNA (ALN-VSP/TKM-PLK1/TKM-ApoB) (Semple et al. 2010). By tracking the evolution of liposomes as potent pharmaceutical carriers for anticancer drugs, one can assimilate that liposomes have gone a long way and currently numerous attractive and diversified strategies are being successfully applied preclinically or clinically for enhanced and effective delivery of drugs.

3.2.3 ROUTE OF ADMINISTRATION OF LIPOSOMES

The parenteral route, in particular intravenous administration, is the preferred route of administration for most clinically approved liposomal and lipid-based products (Allen and Cullis 2013). The other routes that are being successfully clinically applied include the ocular route (for the product Visudyne) (Bochot and Fattal 2012) and the transdermal route (Schroeter et al. 2010). The advantages of the intravitreal liposomal drug delivery include limited obstruction of vision owing to the small size of liposomes, controlled drug release, and improved vitreous half-life (Table 3.7). Moreover, it eliminates the problem of increased intraocular pressure since the volume to be administered is reduced. Poor bioavailability of associated drugs owing to gastrointestinal degradation of the carrier poses a major impediment in oral delivery of liposomal products (Allen and Cullis 2013). Drug delivery to the brain after parenteral administration is low, which has been reportedly enhanced by the use of convection and retro-convection (Krauze et al. 2007; Motion et al. 2011).

TABLE 3.7
Advantages and Drawbacks of Liposomes for Intravitreal Administration

Advantages	Drawbacks
Increase the stability of entrapped drugs	Blurring the vision
Increase the drug half-life in the vitreous	Cationic surface charge might induce inflammation
Reduce the drug toxicity	Possibility of aggregation during storage or *in vivo* when colloidal stability is poor
Possibility of ligands attachment	
Reduce the number of administrations	

Source: A. Bochot and E. Fattal, *J Control Release*, 161, 628–634, 2013.

3.2.4 Liposomes in Clinical Use

Liposomes act as reservoirs encapsulating the drug, protecting it from degradation (Goyal et al. 2005) and reducing the unintended side effects such as cardiotoxicity (Forssen and Tokes 1981), nephrotoxicity (Smeesters et al. 1988), neurotoxicity (Park et al. 2008; Rosentha and Kaufman 1974), or dermal toxicity (Boman et al. 1996). Numerous liposomal formulations bearing cancer therapeutics have been approved or are currently undergoing clinical trials (Tables 3.8 and 3.9).

Liposomal formulation of doxorubicin, an anthracycline-class drug and topo-isomerase inhibitor with reported irreversible cardiotoxicity (Lipshultz et al. 1995; Vonhoff et al. 1979), has been successfully developed to effectively treat cancers with much lesser-associated side effects. Other noted examples of conventional liposomes in clinical use include Myocet (Sopherion Therapeutics or Cephalon in the United States and Europe, respectively) loaded with doxorubicin (Alberts et al. 2004), DaunoXome (Galen) encapsulating daunorubicin (Allen et al. 1991), and Marqibo (Talon Therapeutics) carrying vincristine sulfate (Boehlke and Winter 2006; Rodriguez et al. 2009). Liposomal daunorubicin formulation DaunoXome is a pure lipid formulation that efficiently bypasses the RES and has reduced cardiotoxicity (Batist et al. 2001).

TABLE 3.8
Approved Liposomal Formulations in the Market

Product	Company	Drug	Disease
AmBisome	Gilead Sciences Ltd.	Amphotericin B	Severe fungal infections
DaunoXome	Galen	Daunorubicin	Advanced Kaposi's sarcoma
DepoCyt	DepoTech Corporation	Cytarabine	Lymphomatous meningitis
DepoDur	Pacira Pharmaceuticals	Epidural morphine sulfate	Pain management
Doxil/Caelyx	Johnson&Johnson	Doxorubicin	Metastatic ovarian cancer and advanced Kaposi's sarcoma
Epaxal	Crucell Company, Berna Biotech	Inactivated hepatitis A virus (strain RG-SB)	Hepatitis A
Inflexal V	Crucell Company, Berna Biotech	Inactivated hemagglutinin of influenza virus strains A and B	Influenza
Lipo-Dox	Taiwan Liposome Company	Doxorubicin	Kaposi's sarcoma, breast and ovarian cancer
Marqibo	Talon Therapeutics	Vincristine sulfate	Philadelphia chromosome negative (Ph−) acute lymphoblastic leukemia
Myocet	Cephalon/Sopherion Therapeutics	Doxorubicin	Metastatic breast cancer
Visudyne	Valeant Pharmaceuticals International, Inc.	Verteporfin	Age-related macular degeneration, pathologic myopia, ocular histoplasmosis

TABLE 3.9

Liposome-Based Therapeutics Undergoing Clinical Trials

Product	Company/ Organization	Drug	Disease
Annamycin	Aronex Pharmaceuticals	Annamycin	Breast cancer
Aroplatin	Antigenics Inc.	*cis*-bis-neodeca-noato-*trans-R,R*-1,2-diaminocyclohexane platinum(II) [analog of oxaliplatin]	Advanced solid malignancies, B-cell lymphoma
Atragen	Aronex Pharmaceuticals	All-*trans*-retinoic acid (tretinoin)	Leukemia
CPX-1	Celator Pharmaceuticals	Fixed combination of irinotecan and floxuridine	Advanced colorectal cancer
CPX-351	Celator Pharmaceuticals	Fixed combination of cytarabine and daunorubicin	Advanced hematologic cancer
IHL-305	Yakult Honsha Co., Ltd.	Irinotecan	Treat advanced solid tumors
INX-0125	Inex Pharm	Vinorelbine	Advanced breast cancer
JNS002	Janssen Pharmaceutical K.K.	Doxorubicin	Epithelial ovarian carcinoma, primary carcinoma of fallopian tube, peritoneal carcinoma
L9NC	University of New Mexico	9-nitro-20(*S*)-camptothecin	Metastatic or recurrent cancer of the endometrium or the lung
LEM	Insys Therapeutics Inc.	Mitoxantrone	Advanced cancer
LEP-ETU	NeoPharm	Paclitaxel	Ovarian, breast, and lung cancer
LE-SN38	NeoPharm	SN-38 active metabolite of irinotecan	Advanced colorectal cancer
Lipoplatin	Regulon	Cisplatin	Colon cancer, gastric tumor
Lipoxal	Regulon	Oxaliplatin	Colorectal cancer
Liprostin	Endovasc Inc.	Prostaglandin E1	Peripheral vascular disease
L-NDDP	New York University School of Medicine and National Cancer Institute	Cisplatin analog—aroplatin	Malignant mesothelioma
MBP-426	Mebiopharm Co., Ltd.	Oxaliplatin	Treat advanced or metastatic solid tumors
NL CPT-11	University of California, San Francisco	CPT-11	Recurrent high-grade gliomas
Nyotran	Aronex Pharmaceuticals	Nystatin	Systemic fungal infections

(Continued)

TABLE 3.9 (CONTINUED)
Liposome-Based Therapeutics Undergoing Clinical Trials

Product	Company/ Organization	Drug	Disease
OSI-211	OSI Pharmaceuticals	Lurtotecan	Ovarian cancer
OSI-7904L	OSI Pharmaceuticals	(S-2-[-5-[[[1,2-dihydro-3-methyl-1-oxobenzo[f]-quinazolin-9-yl]methyl] amino]-1-oxo-2-isoinso-linyl] glutaric acid) [thymidylate synthase inhibitor]	Gastric or gastroesophageal cancer
PEP02	PharmaEngine	Irinotecan	Metastatic pancreatic cancer
PNU-93914	Memorial Sloan-Kettering Cancer Center and National Cancer Institute	Paclitaxel	Locally advanced or metastatic cancer of the esophagus
S-CKD602	Johnson&Johnson	CKD-602 [semisynthetic analog of camptothecin]	Advanced malignancies
SPI-77	New York University School of Medicine and National Cancer Institute	Cisplatin	Recurrent ovarian cancer
Stimuvax	Oncothyreon	BLP25 lipopeptide (MUC1-targeted peptide)	Cancer vaccine for multiple myeloma developed encephalitis
Telcyta	Telik, Inc.	Canfosfamide HCl	Advanced ovarian, non–small cell lung, colon and breast cancers
ThermoDox	Celsion	Doxorubicin	Hepatocellular carcinoma
TLC ELL-12	The Liposome Company	L-O-octadecyl-2-O-methyl-sn-glycero-3-phosphocholine [L-ET-18-OCH3 (EL)]	Advanced solid tumors, including non–small cell lung, prostate cancer, and melanoma
TLI	Talon Therapeutics, Inc.	Topotecan	Small cell lung cancer, ovarian cancer, and other advanced solid tumors
T4N5 liposome lotion	AGI Dermatics	Bacteriophage T4 endonuclease 5	Xeroderma pigmentosum
VLI	Talon Therapeutics, Inc.	Vinorelbine	Advanced solid tumors, non-Hodgkin's lymphoma or Hodgkin's disease

Vincristine sulfate has been successfully used in the treatment of childhood and adolescent leukemia (Crom et al. 1994) and lymphoma (Jackson et al. 1984). However, the associated toxicity of vincristine sulfate is clinically manifested by mixed senso-rimotor neuropathy. Other side effects include seizures, mental changes, orthostatic hypotension, and inappropriate secretion of antidiuretic hormone (Rosentha and Kaufman 1974). Vincristine-induced dermal toxicity is significantly reduced when the drug is delivered via liposomes (Boman et al. 1996).

Aroplatin (Antigenics Inc., Lexington, MA, USA), a multilamellar liposomal formulation of saturated phospholipids dimyristoyl phosphatidylcholine (DMPC) and dimyristoyl phosphatidylglycerol (DMPG) bearing the oxaliplatin analog, is undergoing clinical trials (Immordino et al. 2006) and has been reported to have reduced nephrotoxicity (Farrell 2011), a side effect attributed to the drug, without compromising its tumoricidal activity.

Liposomal annamycin (3'-deamino-4'-epi-3'-hydroxy-2'-iodo-4-demethoxy doxorubicin), composed of DMPC and DMPG (Wasan and Kwong 1997), exhibited increased encapsulation of the drug within the vesicles and increased its therapeutic potential (Priebe and Perez-Soler 1993).

AmBisome, the liposomal formulation of amphotericin B used for treatment of invasive fungal infections, has reduced acute and chronic side effects like fever, chills, and renal toxicity with respect to the parent drug (Heinemann et al. 1997).

Extended-release epidural morphine (DepoDur) is an effective postoperative analgesia that is administered into the lumbar epidural space for lower abdominal and lower extremity surgery–associated moderate-to-severe pain (Hartrick and Hartrick 2008).

Virosome-based antigen delivery systems Epaxal and Inflexal V are two vaccines currently being utilized to potentiate cell-mediated and humoral immune response and generate immunity against hepatitis A and influenza, respectively (Chang and Yeh 2012).

One of the sole liposomal formulations with ophthalmic applications includes Visudyne, which is utilized for photodynamic treatment of age-related macular degeneration. Visudyne is used for intravenous drug delivery of the monomeric form Verteporfin, a hydrophobic chlorin-like photosensitizer, which tends to undergo self-aggregation in aqueous media (Bochot and Fattal 2012; Bressler and Bressler 2000).

3.2.5 CONVENTIONAL LIPOSOMES

Conventional drug-bearing liposomes have only been described to be loaded with single drugs previously; however, second-generation liposomes have been reported to be loaded with two or more different drugs simultaneously for enhanced therapeutic effects or cytotoxicity in cancer cells (Agrawal et al. 2005; Cosco et al. 2012). This strategy aims at association of two or more compounds for reduced effective dosages and associated side effects (Figure 3.6) (Colomer 2005; Theodossiou et al. 1998). The liposomal multidrug carrier (MDC) can either be loaded with both water-soluble (in the aqueous core) and lipophilic (entrapped in the bilayers) (Cosco et al. 2012) drugs or multiple drugs with the same affinity (hydrophilic/hydrophobic) without any interactions between the two compounds (Tardi et al. 2007).

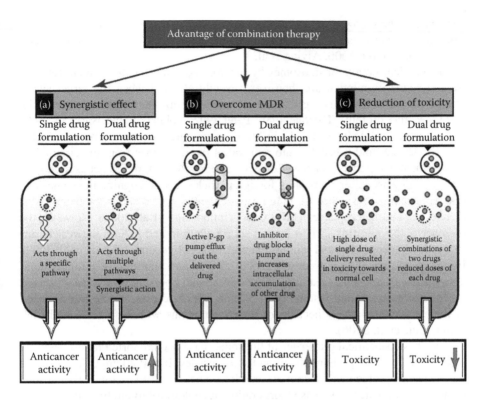

FIGURE 3.6 Schematic representation depicting numerous advantages of combination drug delivery for cancer therapy. (a) Single drug acts through a particular pathway, whereas multiple drugs can show enhanced anticancer activity by acting through several pathways. (b) In the case of single drug treatment, MDR proteins such as P-gp efflux drug out of the cell, whereas for dual formulations, the P-gp inhibitor blocks the role of MDR proteins and increases the intracellular concentration of other coadministered drugs resulting in higher efficacy by overcoming the MDR phenotype. (c) High dose is required for single drug treatment and consequently results in toxicity to normal cells, whereas treatment with different drug combinations leads to synergistic action, which can reduce the dose of each single drug and thereby decrease the toxicity. (Reproduced with permission from P. Parhi et al., *Drug Discovery Today*, 17, 1044–1052, 2012.)

3.2.6 STEALTH LIPOSOMES: PEG-COATED LIPOSOMES

Liposomal formulations of several key active molecules were developed in order to overcome the problems associated with conventional drug therapy such as inefficient biodistribution throughout the body and target-specific delivery by encapsulating the molecules within the vesicles to prevent degradation and passively targeting tissues and organs that have discontinuous endothelium (e.g., liver, spleen, and bone marrow) (Immordino et al. 2006). The capability of the liposomal formulations to efficiently deliver antiparasitic and antimicrobial drugs to treat infections localized in the mononuclear phagocytic system and the ability to encapsulate immune modulators in activated macrophages in cancer models to produce tumoricidal agents were attributed to the recognition and subsequent capture and removal of the liposomes from the blood circulation by MPS upon intravenous administration of the vesicles (Agrawal and Gupta 2000; Alving et al. 1978).

The efficient uptake of liposomes by macrophages and the consequent removal from systemic circulation are, however, severely affected when the target site is beyond the MPS. The binding of opsonins (such as immunoglobulins, fibronectin, and C-reactive protein) (Falcone 1986; Patel 1992; Volanakis and Narkates 1981) on the surface of liposomes results in MPS recognizing these serum proteins rather than the vesicles and translates into removal of the liposomes from the circulation. Complement components such as C5b-9 complexes (MAC), which act as an immediate host defense against invading foreign particles, also recognize liposomes and initiate membrane lysis through pore formation and enhance uptake by neutrophils, monocytes, and macrophages (MPS cells) (Immordino et al. 2006). However, the presence of dysopsonins such as human serum albumin and IgA on the vesicle surface reduces recognition and inhibits phagocytosis of liposomes (Ishida et al. 2002). In fact, a fine balance between the blood opsonic and suppressive proteins regulates the rate of liposome clearance. The conventional liposomes were also observed to demonstrate profound instability in plasma, which resulted in the rapid release of the encapsulated cargo because of their interactions with both HDL and LDL (Immordino et al. 2006).

The physicochemical properties of liposomes have been reported to influence the stability and type of proteins that bind to the vesicles. Initial attempts to overcome the associated problems with conventional liposomes involved manipulation of lipid membrane components such as incorporation of cholesterol to modify bilayer fluidity through increased packing of the phospholipid molecules in the lipid bilayers to reduce transfer of phospholipids to HDL (Damen et al. 1981). Further attempts to bypass these problems included utilization of phosphatidylcholine with saturated fatty acyl chains (with a high liquid crystalline transition temperature) rather than phosphatidylcholine with unsaturated fatty acyl chains to increase the stability and modulate the size and charge of the vesicles to reduce systemic clearance (Senior and Gregoriadis 1982). However, the serious associated limitations such as low entrapment volume, toxicity, and incomplete inhibition of binding with serum components resulted in the development of novel strategies involving the use of inert molecules to coat the surface of the vesicles to form a spatial barrier (Allen et al. 1989; Gabizon and Papahadjopoulos 1988).

Liposomes mimicking erythrocyte membranes with the bilayer surface modified with gangliosides and sialic acid derivatives such as monosialoganglioside (GM1) were developed, which significantly decreased MPS uptake and remained in blood circulation for several hours (Liu et al. 1992). This was possibly attributed to the ability of these moieties to reduce opsonization and the potential to bind with dysopsonins, which reduced recognition by MPS. However, the ganglioside- and sialic acid–modified liposomes have only been observed to have prolonged half-life in a few animal models (rats and mice) (Immordino et al. 2006). Furthermore, the high cost of sialic acid has also prevented its extensive use (Park et al. 1992).

The strategy of using hydrophilic polymers to increase the hydrophilicity of liposomal surface was exploited to increase the longevity of the vesicles in circulation. Although various polymers were investigated, PEG has been widely used as the polymeric steric stabilizer (Allen et al. 1991, 2002). PEG, a linear polyether diol possessing excellent biocompatibility, solubility in both aqueous and organic solvents, lack of toxicity, very low immunogenicity and antigenicity, and good excretion kinetics, can be easily modulated for specific purposes such as molecular weight and chemical structure manipulation and is much easier and cheaper to conjugate with lipids (Dreborg and Akerblom 1990; Monfardini and Veronese 1998). PEGylated vesicles are characterized by strongly reduced MPS uptake, prolonged blood circulation, and improved distribution in perfused tissues (Caliceti and Veronese 2003). The presence of PEG chains on the liposome surface prevents vesicle aggregation and enhances the stability of the vesicles by providing strong interbilayer repulsion that overcomes attractive Van der Waals forces (Needham et al. 1992).

The presence of PEG molecules on the liposome surface results in the exclusion of other macromolecules from the "periliposomal layer" by occupying the space immediately adjacent to the vesicles through its flexible chains. The access and binding of the opsonins to the liposome surface become considerably reduced and ultimately result in inhibiting interactions with the macrophages (Drummond et al. 1999). The reduced MPS uptake causes the long circulating vesicles to passively accumulate within tissues and organs, specifically within solid tumors undergoing angiogenesis through a process known as the EPR effect, and function as a sustained drug release system (Maeda 2001). However, the presence of tight junctions between capillary endothelial cells in the normal tissues prevents extravasation of the liposomes from the bloodstream. This results in the enhancement of the therapeutic activity of liposomal cancer chemotherapeutic agents with respect to free drugs.

The success of PEGylated vesicles in cancer treatment was achieved with the approval of the stealth liposomal formulation of doxorubicin for the treatment of Kaposi's sarcoma (Krown et al. 2004) and recurrent ovarian cancer (Rose 2005) in the United States and Europe. Currently, many other formulations are undergoing clinical trials and a few more formulations are expected to be available in the market very soon (Hau et al. 2004; Katsaros et al. 2005). Recent research initiatives have yielded newer polymers like PVP, PAA (Torchilin et al. 1994), poly[N-(2-hydroxypropyl) methacrylamide], amphiphilic poly-N-vinylpyrrolidones (Torchilin et al. 2001), L-amino acid–based biodegradable polymer–lipid conjugate (Metselaar et al. 2003), and polyvinyl alcohol, which achieved even better control over the properties of liposomes leading to extended blood circulation time, better passive targeting of the encapsulated cargo to the site of action, and reduction in general drug toxicity (Immordino et al. 2006).

3.2.7 STIMULI-RESPONSIVE LIPOSOMES: THE ROLE OF "SMART" POLYMERS

Liposome-mediated delivery of therapeutic agents has made rapid progress in the transition from the laboratory to the clinic. The significant advances in liposome technology have resulted in increased circulation lifetimes, enhanced drug loading efficiency, more stable drug formulations, and greater efficacy of liposomal drugs. This has brightened the prospects for future liposome-based therapies (Torchilin 2005).

However, the ability to selectively increase the bioavailability of the drugs at the target tissue while maintaining stability in the circulation remained an elusive problem. Specific delivery of bioactive molecules to a target site is essential to increase their efficacy and decrease the associated side effects. Extensive studies have been performed to develop liposomes that release their contents at specific sites in response to external physical or chemical stimuli (Drummond et al. 2000; Kono 2001).

Engineered liposomes that provide therapeutic control of pathological states by an enhanced enrichment of therapeutic or diagnostic agents in diseased tissues have currently emerged as workhorses in nanomedicine (Fleige et al. 2012). Stimuli-responsive liposomes are active delivery vehicles that evolve with an external signal and are equipped with "load-and-release" modalities within their constituting units. The central operating principle lies in the fact that a specific cellular/extracellular stimulus of chemical, biochemical, or physical origin can modify the structural composition or conformation of the liposomes, thereby promoting release of the active species to a specific biological environment (Calderon et al. 2010; Kost and Langer 2001). In contrast to conventional liposomes, stimuli-responsive vesicles undergo relatively large and abrupt physical and chemical changes in sharp response to applied stimuli. This becomes of particular interest when the stimuli to which these vesicles act are disease or systemic-biochemistry specific (as pH). The specificity allows liposomes to release the encapsulated cargo in a temporal or spatial pattern in response to particular pathological triggers present in the diseased tissues (Ganta et al. 2008) with substantially reduced side effects (Drummond et al. 2000). These liposomes mimic numerous feedback controlled biological events prevailing in nature where the enrichment or absence of any physical, chemical, or physicochemical factors regulates a series of biochemical processes (Fleige et al. 2012).

Stimuli-sensitive liposomes, especially temperature-sensitive (Kono 2001) and pH-sensitive vesicles (Drummond et al. 2000), have started to attract attention since the former is useful for tumor targeting in conjunction with hyperthermia and the latter is useful for cytoplasmic delivery of membrane-impermeable molecules. Temperature-sensitive liposomes relying on a relatively sharp phase transition in the lipid phase at temperatures only a few degrees above body temperature display lipid-packing defects at the gel-to-liquid crystalline phase transition and result in increased permeability to entrapped cargo (Fleige et al. 2012; Henry et al. 2006; Magin et al. 1979; Weinstein et al. 1979; Yatvin et al. 1978). However, these liposomes require the addition of an external heat stimulus in a spatially well-defined region, surrounding and including the tumor (Drummond et al. 2000). pH-sensitive liposomes that release their contents into the cytoplasm after endocytosis rely on selective destabilization of liposomes after acidification of the surrounding medium (Yatvin et al. 1980). Although the initial rationale for the design of pH-sensitive liposomes was to exploit the acidic environment of tumors to trigger destabilization of liposomal membranes, cytoplasmic release provided a more suitable target to achieve (Dellian et al. 1996; Huang et al. 1992). Since the sites of greatest acidity in tumors are distant from the tumor microvasculature (Drummond et al. 2000) and the pH of the tumor interstitium rarely declines below pH 6.5 unlike endosomes and lysosomes where pH reaches values below 5.0 (Ohkuma and Poole 1978), development of pH-sensitive vesicles for tumor targeting was technically difficult because of the narrow pH window available to engineer liposomes (Roux et al. 2003).

While various phospholipids, such as dipalmitoylphosphatidylcholine (Papahadjopoulos et al. 1973) and unsaturated dioleoylphosphatidylethanolamine (Drummond and Daleke 1997; Gerasimov et al. 1997; Litzinger and Huang 1992), have been studied to prepare temperature-sensitive and pH-sensitive vesicles, respectively, the recent initiative of incorporation of stimuli-sensitive molecules to liposomal membranes has started to generate interest (Chen et al. 1999; Meyer et al. 1998). Modification of vesicles with stimuli-responsive polymers offers an effective method to prepare functional liposomes. These polymers change their conformation and physicochemical properties in response to various stimuli and environmental conditions (Tonge and Tighe 2001) and interact with lipid membranes differently in response to these stimuli and changes in the environment conditions when conjugated with liposomes.

3.2.7.1 Thermosensitive Polymer-Based Temperature-Sensitive Liposomes

Temperature sensitization of liposomes has been attempted with many thermosensitive synthetic and natural polymers that exhibit a lower critical solution temperature (LCST) in aqueous solutions (Schild and Tirrell 1990; Winnik 1987). The chains of these polymers undergo a coil-to-globule transition as the temperature increases through the LCST. The polymers that are soluble in water below LCST become insoluble in water above LCST since they change their nature from hydrophilic to hydrophobic around LCST (Urry 1993). The change in nature affects the stabilization/destabilization of vesicles that have thermoresponsive polymers anchored on the membrane and results in the regulation of content release and fusion in a temperature-dependent manner. These polymers that are highly hydrated below their LCST cover the entire liposome surface and suppress their interactions with proteins and cells. However, they are fully dehydrated and contracted above LCST, which leads to an increase in the hydrophobicity of the liposome surface and exposure of the bare lipid membrane surface and allows liposome–cell interactions in a temperature-dependent manner (Kono 2001).

Poly(N-isopropylacrylamide) (p-NIPAM), a thermosensitive polymer, has been extensively exploited to render vesicles temperature sensitive (Ringsdorf et al. 1991; Schild 1992). p-NIPAM exhibits a drastic thermoreversible change in water solubility in a very narrow temperature window (Schild and Tirrell 1990), which can be further modulated by co-polymerization with co-monomers with varying hydrophilicity or hydrophobicity (Feil et al. 1993; Shibayama et al. 1996). Recent initiatives have shown the importance of hydrophobic groups that strongly anchor the hydrated polymer chain on to the liposome surface (Ringsdorf et al. 1991). For effective fixation of the thermosensitive polymers, two types of anchor-bearing polymers have been developed: (i) polymers with anchors at random positions in the polymer backbone (Kim et al. 1997) and (ii) polymers having an anchor at the chain end (Kono et al. 1999d). While the former class of polymers has been synthesized by free radical co-polymerization using monomers having hydrophobic side groups such as octadecylacrylate (ODA) (Meyer et al. 1998) and N,N-didodecylacrylamide (Kono et al. 1999b), the latter class comprises polymers obtained by combining an anchor to the polymers that have an amino group at the chain end (Kono et al. 1999a).

Previous studies on the effect of the position of anchors in the polymer chain on the binding to liposomal membranes have reported that polymers with anchors at the chain end have a greater binding constant to the liposomes (Polozova et al. 1999). However, the prediction of the best type of anchors for fixation is a difficult proposition since the binding ability of the anchor-bearing polymers would be affected by a number of factors ranging from molecular weight, monomer unit/anchor ratio, and the number of anchors per chain (Kono et al. 1999d). These differences have been found to affect the temperature-induced transition of the thermosensitive polymers. Furthermore, the fluidity of the liposomal membranes also plays an important role in the determination of the degree of fixation of these polymers (Polozova and Winnik 1997; Polozova et al. 1999).

Anchorage of thermoresponsive polymers onto liposomal surfaces offers the possibility of temperature-controlled destabilization of the vesicles and release of encapsulated cargo through induction of structural defects (Kitano et al. 1994). In relation to drug delivery applications, liposomes are required to exhibit thermoresponsiveness at temperatures slightly higher than physiological temperature (Hayashi et al. 1998). Precise control of LCST has allowed polymer modification of liposomal surfaces especially in the case of cationic liposomes, which resulted in the regulation of the nature of interactions around LCST (Kono et al. 1999a). The thermosensitive polymer-modified liposomes offer an attractive strategy for accurate drug delivery within the target site by temperature-induced control of affinity of liposomes to the cell surface (Kono et al. 1999c).

3.2.7.2 pH-Responsive Polymer-Based pH-Sensitive Liposomes

pH-responsive polymers offer a promising alternative to both phosphatidylethanolamine (PE)-based formulations and pH-sensitive fusogenic peptides for rendering liposomes pH sensitive (Akinc et al. 2005; El-Sayed et al. 2005a,b; Pack et al. 2000). Synthetic polymers, which can be conveniently synthesized in large scales at low cost, have low immunogenic potential and can easily be used to prepare pH-sensitive liposomes of almost any composition because of their structure versatility and easy association to the vesicular surface (Drummond et al. 2000).

The ability of certain polymers to hypercoil or associate hydrophobically to form extensive compact molecules can be exploited to change the conformation and subsequent function of these polymers in response to local stimuli. Polymers with weakly charged (positive/negative) groups form extended structures owing to mutual repulsion between the charged groups (Tonge and Tighe 2001). The additional presence of alkyl pendant groups in the polymer would subject the pendant groups to hydrophobic interactions, which would tend to restrict the alkyl side chains to minimal volume within an aqueous environment. This would allow maximum hydrogen bonding between water molecules. The hydrophobic effect observed in the case of hypercoiling polymers is also evident as the driving force in the formation of lipid assemblies in biological membranes and in defining the conformation of native proteins (Bienvenue et al. 1977).

Acid-triggered polymer-based liposome destabilization/fusion is usually accompanied by a modification of the polymer conformation or association with the liposome bilayer, which results in its destabilization (Oku et al. 1987; Richardson et al.

1999). The mechanism of membrane destabilization varies depending on whether the polyelectrolyte is a weak base (polycation) or a weak acid (polyanion). Polymers with weakly ionizable cationic pendant groups such as pyridine or imidazole are substantially charged below their pK_b value. The resulting ionic repulsion overcomes hydrophobic interactions between alkyl side chains within such polymers and leads to uncoiling of the polymer chain. However, as the pH is raised, the proportion of charged pendant group decreases and the hydrophobic interactions between the alkyl side chains become predominant. This results in the progressive collapse of the polymer chain into distinct hydrophobic microdomains, which ultimately results in the formation of compact, insoluble globular molecules that subsequently precipitate from the aqueous solution. In the case of polymers bearing weakly acidic pendant groups such as carboxylic acids, although the macromer exhibits an extended chain form above the pK_a value, it progressively collapses as the pH is lowered and finally precipitates below its pK_a (Tonge and Tighe 2001).

The progressive and nonuniform loss of charge during the hypercoiling process transforms the polymer into an amphipathic molecule that possesses surface-active properties. This results in switching on or off of the surface activity and related functional properties in response to subtle variations in the external pH. The mechanism of response to surrounding pH observed in the case of hypercoiling polymers is similar to the behavior of responsive macromolecules found in nature (Fichtner and Schonert 1977).

The conformation of hypercoiling polymers that undergo drastic changes in solution is governed by solvent–polymer interaction. The conformation of solvated molecules depends on the balance between electrostatic repulsion between charged subgroups, Van der Waals cohesion of uncharged side groups, hydrogen bonds, and interactions with solvent and acts both within the molecule and between the molecule and surrounding solution. However, charge and hydrophobic effect are the principal driving forces behind hydrophobic association of these polymers (Tonge and Tighe 2001).

Both polycationic and anionic hypercoiling polymers have been synthesized and examined for their pH-responsive properties. Synthetic cationic polypeptides such as poly(L-lysine) (Gad et al. 1982; Hong et al. 1983) or poly(L-histidine) (Uster and Deamer 1985; Wang and Huang 1984) were examined for their pH-dependent fusogenic properties. Poly(4-vinylpyridine) (Tonge and Tighe 2001), poly(tertiary amines) such as poly[thio-1-(N,N-diethyl)aminoethylethylene], and poly(vinylimidazole) such as poly(styrene-imidazole) (Handel et al. 1987; Sutton et al. 1988) have also been reported as cationic hypercoilers that exhibit profound conformational changes in response to surrounding pH variations. Recent reports indicated the pH-dependent membrane destabilization behavior of poly(amidoamines) (Richardson et al. 1999). Furthermore, the utility of these polymers is also restricted because of adverse cytotoxicity (Drummond et al. 2000).

Acidic hypercoilers are able to trigger content leakage from both neutral and charged vesicles unlike their cationic counterparts. The mechanism of leakage is governed by the structure of the polymer and does not always involve fusion in the destabilization process. Anionic polymers exhibiting hypercoiling behavior are invariably composed of carboxylic acid pendant groups commonly in the form of acrylic acid or maleic acid in both homo-polymers and alternating co-polymers (Drummond et al. 2000; Tonge and Tighe 2001). In the case of alternating co-polymers, the hydrophobic moieties are generally methyl or ethyl acrylates, alkyl vinyl ethers, styrene co-monomers, and alkyl acrylamides. While the hydrophobicity of these polymers is regulated by the alkyl chain length (Needham et al. 1998; Schroeder and Tirrell 1989; Thomas et al. 1995), the charge density variation is controlled by pH. The ability of these polymers to interact and destabilize lipid bilayers depends on the ionization state of the carboxylic acid groups. While homo-polymers of methacrylic and ethacrylic acids (Joyce and Kurucsev 1981; Kay et al. 1976), co-polymers of acrylic acid and ethyl acrylate (Tan and Gasper 1974), maleic anhydride and alkyl vinyl ethers (Dubin and Strauss 1967), and maleic anhydride/acid and styrene (Banerjee et al. 2012b; Okuda et al. 1977) have been reported to display hypercoiling behavior, the major systems that have been extensively studied to destabilize membranes are poly(acrylic acid) derivatives (Seki and Tirrell 1984; Thomas et al. 1996), succinylated poly(glycidols) (Kono et al. 1994), and copolymers of N-isopropylacrylamide (NIPAM) (Chen and Hoffman 1995; Hirotsu et al. 1987).

Poly(2-ethylacrylic acid) (PEAA) was demonstrated to bind to a variety of multilamellar vesicles including anionic vesicles (Seki and Tirrell 1984) and induce destabilization under acidic conditions either through micellization at higher concentrations (Tirrell et al. 1985) or through pore formation in the bilayer at lower concentrations (Kitano et al. 1994). The pH at which permeabilization occurred was found to be modulated by adjusting the molecular weight (Schroeder and Tirrell 1989) or by substituting PEAA with a more hydrophilic/hydrophobic acrylic acid derivative (Needham et al. 1998; Thomas et al. 1995). Poly(acrylic acid) derivatives have recently been investigated to trigger endosomal release of drugs and eventual transfer to the cytoplasm (Lackey et al. 1999). However, the strong negative zeta potential values of PEAA-anchored liposomes attributed to significant ionization of the carboxylic groups of the polymer at physiological pH would seriously compromise their blood circulation time (Drummond et al. 2000). Succinylated poly(glycidols) with hydroxyl and carboxylic acid groups (succinic acid) on the side chain are structurally related to PEG. Previous studies have reported that the presence of succinylated poly(glycidols), with long alkyl chains in egg phosphatidylcholine small unilamellar vesicles, induced content leakage and intermembrane mixing at pH <5.5 (Kono et al. 1994, 1997).

The LCST of poly(NIPAM) co-polymers, which have earlier been reported for their thermosensitivity, can be modified as a function of pH by introducing a small proportion of charged groups (Chen and Hoffman 1995). The incorporation of carboxylic acid group such as methylacrylic acid and hydrophobic anchor ODA into NIPAM could trigger, under physiological acidic conditions (pH 4.9–5.5), the release of entrapped cargo from large unilamellar vesicles (Drummond et al. 2000). NIPAM copolymers are able to destabilize high-temperature phase transition phospholipid vesicles at physiological temperature and trigger the release of drugs unlike poly(acrylic acid) derivatives (Zignani et al. 2000). Although the development of pH-sensitive liposomes based on NIPAM co-polymers is being actively pursued, the instability of these vesicles in systemic circulation remains a concern, along with a partial loss of pH sensitivity after incubation with serum (Roux et al. 2004).

Development and evaluation of new pH-responsive polymers are thus required to develop clinically viable pH-responsive liposomes.

3.2.8 Cationic Liposomes

One of the most effective nonviral systems for oligonucleotide or gene delivery is the cationic lipid–based liposomes. The resulting complex of cationic lipid–based vesicles with oligonucleotides is termed *lipoplex*. Lipoplexes have been described to treat cancer efficiently (Table 3.10) and are reported to encapsulate large amounts of nucleotides (Felgner and Ringold 1989). Cationic liposome bearing paclitaxel (MBT-0206) showed selective uptake by angiogenic tumoral endothelial cells abundant in solid tumor and metastases (Immordino et al. 2006). EndoTAG-1 initially developed by MediGene (MediGene A.G., Martinsried, Germany) is currently undergoing Phase III clinical trial designed and financed by SynCore Biotechnology Co. Ltd. (Taipei, Taiwan) (Field et al. 2014). Recent research initiatives have reported lipoplexes to effectively transfect cells with DNA (Neves et al. 2009) or microRNAs (Malone et al. 1989; Wu et al. 2011). Moreover, the transfection efficiency of cationic liposomes has been known to increase when their surface is tagged with a ligand that is recognized by a cell surface receptor through the initial binding of the ligand to the cell (Pirollo et al. 2000). Cationic liposomes target the anionic functional groups that line the tumor vasculature and ultimately help in arresting tumor angiogenesis (Figures 3.7 and 3.8). Although RNAi therapeutics is an emerging novel approach against cancer, the key challenge lies in effective delivery to target tissues. The preclinical development and toxicological profiling of lipid nanoparticle–formulated siRNA chemotherapeutic has thus been a major thrust area of investigation recently (Barros and Gollob 2012; Ozpolat et al. 2010).

The combination of stealth and ligand-targeted therapeutics with antisense delivery has proved to be a promising strategy. Conjugating stealth liposomal technology with Tf-mediated delivery of drug has been described for the delivery of a

TABLE 3.10
Lipoplexes Undergoing Clinical Trials

Product	Company	Description
SGT-53	SynerGene Therapeutics, Inc.	Liposome encapsulates plasmid DNA coding for p53 wild-type gene
FANG vaccine	Gradalis, Inc.	Expresses rhGMCSF, bifunctional RNAi effector, and bi-shRNAfurin
Pbi-shRNA STMN1 LP	Gradalis, Inc.	Encapsulates bifunctional short hairpin RNAs (shRNA) against human stathmin 1 (STMN1)
BP-100-1.01	Bio-Path Holdings, Inc.	Delivers antisense oligodeoxynucleotide (ODN) growth factor receptor-bound protein 2 (Grb2), with potential antineoplastic activity

Source: K. Sen and M. Mandal, *Int J Pharmaceut*, 448, 28–43, 2013.

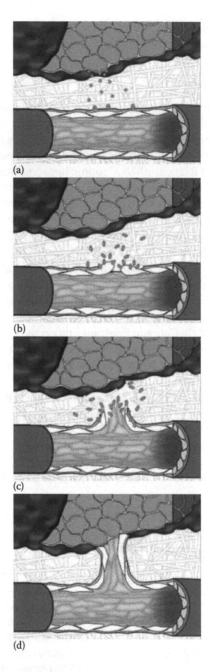

(a)

(b)

(c)

(d)

FIGURE 3.7 Tumor angiogenesis: a step-by-step approach: An angiogenic stimulus is secreted by a developing tumor and a vessel sprouts in the direction of the stimulus (a), proteases begin to degrade the basement membrane (b), while endothelial cells migrate in the direction of the stimulus formed through the newly formed openings in the basement membrane (c), and a new vessel sprout forms (d). (Reproduced with permission from R. B. Campbell et al., *Journal of Pharmaceutical Sciences*, 98, 411–429, 2009.)

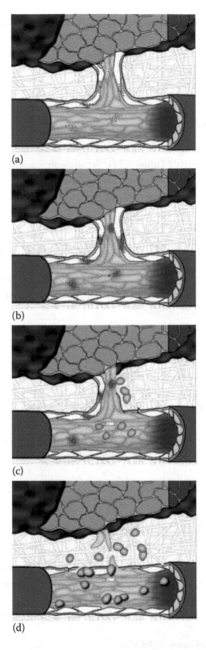

(a)

(b)

(c)

(d)

FIGURE 3.8 Vascular targeting with cationic liposomal therapeutics: The tumor vasculature is lined with an overexpression of anionic functional groups (a), cationic liposomal therapeutics interact with tumor vessels (b), injury to the tumor microvasculature results in damage to the endothelial cells (c), and eventual loss of tumor vessel function results in the death of thousands of cancer cells owing to severe oxygen and nutrient deprivation (d). (Reproduced with permission from R. B. Campbell et al., *Journal of Pharmaceutical Sciences*, 98, 411–429, 2009.)

phosphorothioate antisense oligodeoxyribonucleotide (G3139, oblimersen sodium, or Genasense) in leukemia cells *in vitro* for effective treatment via Bcl-2 regulation (Chiu et al. 2006). *In vivo* combination treatment of PEGylated siBcl-2-lipoplex and S-1(5-FU) prodrug has been reported to exhibit enhanced antineoplastic activity in a DLD-1 xenograft model (Nakamura et al. 2011).

3.2.9 Immunoliposomes

Immunoliposomes are considered to be a promising new candidate for targeted delivery of anticancer drugs (Table 3.11). Immunoliposomes have monoclonal Abs (mAbs) or Ab fragments conjugated to their surface. Conjugation with whole mAb leads to greater binding avidity and higher stability. However, the increased immunogenicity of whole mAb owing to the presence of the fragment crystallizable (F_c) domain (Allen 2002) severely limits its application.

Targeted drug delivery utilizing immunoliposomes involves two phases: the transport phase, where the immunoliposomes traverse from the site of administration to the target cells, and the effector phase, which includes specific binding of immunoliposomes to the target cells and the subsequent delivery of encapsulated cargo (Mastrobattista et al. 1999).

The immunoliposome preparation is based on the following chemical strategies: (i) use of free functional groups like amino groups, carboxyl groups, and carbohydrate chains present in the Ab molecule; (ii) modification of existing functional groups (disulfide, amine, carboxyl, and carbohydrate groups) in the Abs with appropriate cross-linking reagents bearing reactive functional groups; (iii) utilization of free functional groups present in phospholipids (like hydroxyl and amine groups); (iv) modification of the existing functional groups of the phospholipids using suitable cross-linking reagents containing reactive functionalities; and (v) utilization of various functionalized PEG derivatives, which act as a linker between Abs and

TABLE 3.11
Antibody-Mediated Drug Delivery Using Liposomes

Ligand	Cancer	Reference
Anti-CD74 antibody	Malignant B lymphoma	Lundberg et al. 2004
Monoclonal nucleosome–specific 2C5 antibody (mAb 2C5)	Mammary adenocarcinoma	Lukyanov et al. 2004
F(ab')2 fragment of human monoclonal antibody GAH	Metastatic stomach cancer	Matsumura 2004
Fab' fragments of a humanized anti-p185HER2 monoclonal antibody (rhuMAbHER2)	Breast cancer	Park et al. 1995
Anti-transferrin receptor single-chain antibody fragment (TfRscFv)	Advanced solid tumors	Xu et al. 2002

Source: K. Sen and M. Mandal, *Int J Pharmaceut*, 448, 28–43, 2013.

liposomes (Manjappa et al. 2011). An interesting example relates to monoclonal nucleosome–specific Ab 2C5, which has been modified with poly(ethylene glycol)-phosphatidylethanolamine conjugate (PEG-PE) with the free PEG terminus activated by *p*-nitrophenylcarbonyl group (pNP-PEG-PE) for incorporation onto the liposomal surface (Lukyanov et al. 2004).

Long-circulating liposomes coated with hydrophilic polymer PEG conjugated with mAbs (mAb N-12A5) directed against erbB-2 oncoprotein, a functional surface antigen in breast cancer, have been reported (Goren et al. 1996). Another study reports the production of sterically stabilized immunoliposomal drugs useful in "mix and match" combinatorial applications of a variety of anticancer drugs (Ishida et al. 1999). Sterically stabilized liposomes containing doxorubicin (Doxil, Johnson&Johnson) modified with monoclonal nucleosome–specific 2C5 Ab (mAb 2C5) showed improved antitumor efficacy *in vitro* in comparison to nontargeted conventional doxorubicin-loaded liposomes (Lukyanov et al. 2004).

3.2.10 VIROSOMES

Virosomes are reconstituted virus liposomes that contain viral membrane proteins or peptide antigens incorporated into the liposomes. Epaxal is a virosomal vaccine that prevents hepatitis A infection, utilizing virosomes as adjuvants in place of aluminum salts, to elicit cell-mediated and humoral immune responses (Bovier 2008). Inflexal V is a novel virosome-based trivalent influenza vaccine that delivers influenza antigens to the endosome and stimulates a strong immune response by immunocompetent cells. The major highlight of Inflexal V is its high immunogenicity and tolerance in a wide age group including children, young adults, and the elderly (Mischler and Metcalfe 2002).

3.3 CONCLUSIONS

The evolution of new-generation pharmaceutical liposomes has marked a new era in drug delivery systems in cancer therapeutics. Liposomes are versatile drug delivery systems that can be designed and modified in order to enhance the effectivity of the therapeutic drug. The wide array of liposomal drug formulations approved and undergoing clinical trials (Tables 3.6 and 3.7) points to the translation of liposomes from an object of research to preferred pharmaceutical carriers for clinical applications. Other important liposomal formulations approved for use in applications other than tumorigenic therapy include AmBisome (fungal infections and leishmaniasis), Amphotec (invasive aspergillosis), Abelcet (aspergillosis), DepoDur (pain after surgery), Diprivan (anesthesia), Estrasorb (menopausal therapy), and Visudyne (wet macular degeneration). A better understanding of liposomal drug interaction with the biological system will facilitate the emergence of a novel class of anticancer therapeutics with improved efficacy and safety. The vast array of liposome-based therapeutics in preclinical/clinical trials and marketed formulations provide a new paradigm in nanotherapeutics with focus toward diagnosis, treatment, and prevention.

REFERENCES

Agrawal A. K. and C. M. Gupta, Tuftsin-bearing liposomes in treatment of macrophage-based infections, *Adv Drug Deliv Rev*, 41, 135–146 (2000).

Agrawal V., M. K. Paul and A. K. Mukhopadhyay, 6-mercaptopurine and daunorubicin double drug liposomes—Preparation, drug-drug interaction and characterization, *J Liposome Res*, 15, 141–155 (2005).

Akinc A., M. Thomas, A. M. Klibanov and R. Langer, Exploring polyethylenimine-mediated DNA transfection and the proton sponge hypothesis, *J Gene Med*, 7, 657–663 (2005).

Alberts D. S., F. M. Muggia, J. Carmichael, E. P. Winer, M. Jahanzeb, A. P. Venook, K. M. Skubitz, E. Rivera, J. A. Sparano, N. J. Dibella, S. J. Stewart, J. J. Kavanagh and A. A. Gabizon, Efficacy and safety of liposomal anthracyclines in phase I/II clinical trials, *Semin Oncol*, 31, 53–90 (2004).

Allen C., N. Dos Santos, R. Gallagher, G. N. C. Chiu, Y. Shu, W. M. Li, S. A. Johnstone, A. S. Janoff, L. D. Mayer, M. S. Webb and M. B. Bally, Controlling the physical behavior and biological performance of liposome formulations through use of surface grafted poly(ethylene glycol), *Biosci Rep*, 22, 225–250 (2002).

Allen T. M., Ligand-targeted therapeutics in anticancer therapy, *Nat Rev Cancer*, 2, 750–763 (2002).

Allen T. M. and P. R. Cullis, Liposomal drug delivery systems: From concept to clinical applications, *Adv Drug Deliv Rev*, 65, 36–48 (2013).

Allen T. M., C. Hansen and J. Rutledge, Liposomes with prolonged circulation times—Factors affecting uptake by reticuloendothelial and other tissues, *Biochim Biophys Acta*, 981, 27–35 (1989).

Allen T. M., C. Hansen, F. Martin, C. Redemann and A. Yauyoung, Liposomes containing synthetic lipid derivatives of poly(ethylene glycol) show prolonged circulation half-lives in vivo, *Biochim Biophys Acta*, 1066, 29–36 (1991).

Alving C. R., E. A. Steck, W. L. Chapman, V. B. Waits, L. D. Hendricks, G. M. Swartz and W. L. Hanson, Therapy of leishmaniasis—Superior efficacies of liposome-encapsulated drugs, *Proc Natl Acad Sci U S A*, 75, 2959–2963 (1978).

Audouy S. and D. Hoekstra, Cationic lipid-mediated transfection in vitro and in vivo, *Mol Membr Biol*, 18, 129–143 (2001).

Banerjee S., T. K. Pal and S. K. Guha, Probing molecular interactions of poly(styrene-co-maleic acid) with lipid matrix models to interpret the therapeutic potential of the co-polymer, *Biochim Biophys Acta-Biomembranes*, 1818, 537–550 (2012a).

Banerjee S., K. Sen, T. K. Pal and S. K. Guha, Poly(styrene-co-maleic acid)-based pH-sensitive liposomes mediate cytosolic delivery of drugs for enhanced cancer chemotherapy, *Int J Pharm*, 436, 786–797 (2012b).

Bangham A. D., M. M. Standish and J. C. Watkins, Diffusion of univalent ions across the lamellae of swollen phospholipids, *J Mol Biol*, 13, 238–252 (1965a).

Bangham A. D., M. M. Standish and G. Weissman, Action of steroids and streptolysin s on permeability of phospholipid structures to cations, *J Mol Biol*, 13, 253–259 (1965b).

Barenholz Y., Liposome application: Problems and prospects, *Curr Opin Colloid In*, 6, 66–77 (2001).

Barenholz Y., Doxil (R)—The first FDA-approved nano-drug: Lessons learned, *J Control Rel*, 160, 117–134 (2012).

Barros S. A. and J. A. Gollob, Safety profile of RNAi nanomedicines, *Adv Drug Deliv Rev*, 64, 1730–1737 (2012).

Batist G., G. Ramakrishnan, C. S. Rao, A. Chandrasekharan, J. Gutheil, T. Guthrie, P. Shah, A. Khojasteh, M. K. Nair, K. Hoelzer, K. Tkaczuk, Y. C. Park and L. W. Lee, Reduced cardiotoxicity and preserved antitumor efficacy of liposome-encapsulated doxorubicin and cyclophosphamide compared with conventional doxorubicin and cyclophosphamide in a randomized, multicenter trial of metastatic breast cancer, *J Clin Oncol*, 19, 1444–1454 (2001).

Bienvenue A., A. Rousselet, G. Kato and P. F. Devaux, Fluidity of lipids next to acetylcholine-receptor protein of torpedo membrane fragments—Use of amphiphilic reversible spin-labels, *Biochemistry*, 16, 841–848 (1977).

Black C. D. V. and G. Gregoriadis, Interaction of liposomes with blood-plasma proteins, *Biochem Soc Trans*, 4, 253–256 (1976).

Blokzijl W. and J. B. F. N. Engberts, Hydrophobic effects—Opinions and facts, *Angew Chem Int Edit*, 32, 1545–1579 (1993).

Bochot A. and E. Fattal, Liposomes for intravitreal drug delivery: A state of the art, *J Control Rel*, 161, 628–634 (2012).

Boehlke L. and J. N. Winter, Sphingomyelin/cholesterol liposomal vincristine: A new formulation for an old drug, *Expert Opin Biol Ther*, 6, 409–415 (2006).

Boman N. L., V. A. Tron, M. B. Bally and P. R. Cullis, Vincristine-induced dermal toxicity is significantly reduced when the drug is given in liposomes, *Cancer Chemother Pharmacol*, 37, 351–355 (1996).

Bovier P. A., Epaxal®: A virosomal vaccine to prevent hepatitis A infection, *Expert Review of Vaccines*, 7, 1141–1150 (2008).

Bradbury P. A. and F. A. Shepherd, Immunotherapy for lung cancer, *J Thorac Oncol*, 3, S164–S170 (2008).

Bressler N. M. and S. B. Bressler, Photodynamic therapy with verteporfin (visudyne): Impact on ophthalmology and visual sciences, *Invest Ophthalmol Vis Sci*, 41, 624–628 (2000).

Brewer J. M. and J. Alexander, Studies on the adjuvant activity of nonionic surfactant vesicles—Adjuvant-driven Igg2a production independent of Mhc control, *Vaccine*, 12, 613–619 (1994).

Brody E. N. and L. Gold, Aptamers as therapeutic and diagnostic agents, *J Biotechnol*, 74, 5–13 (2000).

Butts C., N. Murray, A. Maksymiuk, G. Goss, E. Marshall, D. Soulieres, Y. Cormier, P. Ellis, A. Price, R. Sawhney, M. Davis, J. Mansi, C. Smith, D. Vergidis, M. MacNeil and M. Palmer, Randomized phase IIB trial of BLP25 liposome vaccine in stage IIIB and IV non-small-cell lung cancer, *J Clin Oncol*, 23, 6674–6681 (2005).

Cairns R., I. Papandreou and N. Denko, Overcoming physiologic barriers to cancer treatment by molecularly targeting the tumor microenvironment, *Mol Cancer Res*, 4, 61–70 (2006).

Calderon M., M. A. Quadir, M. Strumia and R. Haag, Functional dendritic polymer architectures as stimuli-responsive nanocarriers, *Biochimie*, 92, 1242–1251 (2010).

Caliceti P. and F. M. Veronese, Pharmacokinetic and biodistribution properties of poly(ethylene glycol)-protein conjugates, *Adv Drug Deliv Rev*, 55, 1261–1277 (2003).

Campbell R. B., B. Ying, G. M. Kuesters and R. Hemphill, Fighting cancer: From the bench to bedside using second generation cationic liposomal therapeutics, *J Pharm Sci*, 98, 411–429 (2009).

Chang D. K., C. Y. Chiu, S. Y. Kuo, W. C. Lin, A. Lo, Y. P. Wang, P. C. Li and H. C. Wu, Antiangiogenic targeting liposomes increase therapeutic efficacy for solid tumors, *J Biol Chem*, 284, 12905–12916 (2009).

Chang H. I. and M. K. Yeh, Clinical development of liposome-based drugs: Formulation, characterization, and therapeutic efficacy, *Int J Nanomed*, 7, 49–60 (2012).

Chen G. and A. S. Hoffman, Graft copolymers that exhibit temperature-induced phase transitions over a wide range of pH, *Nature*, 373, 49–52 (1995).

Chen T., L. S. Choi, S. Einstein, M. A. Klippenstein, P. Scherrer and P. R. Cullis, Proton-induced permeability and fusion of large unilamellar vesicles by covalently conjugated poly(2-ethylacrylic acid), *J Liposome Res*, 9, 387–405 (1999).

Chiu S. J., S. Liu, D. Perrotti, G. Marcucci and R. J. Lee, Efficient delivery of a Bcl-2-specific antisense oligodeoxyribonucleotide (G3139) via transferrin receptor-targeted liposomes, *J Control Release*, 112, 199–207 (2006).

Colomer R., What is the best schedule for administration of gemcitabine-taxane? *Cancer Treat Rev*, 31, S23–S28 (2005).

Conlan J. W., L. Krishnan, G. E. Willick, G. B. Patel and G. D. Sprott, Immunization of mice with lipopeptide antigens encapsulated in novel liposomes prepared from the polar lipids of various Archaeobacteria elicits rapid and prolonged specific protective immunity against infection with the facultative intracellular pathogen, Listeria monocytogenes, *Vaccine*, 19, 3509–3517 (2001).

Cooper C. R., C. H. Chay and K. J. Pienta, The role of alpha(v)beta(3) in prostate cancer progression, *Neoplasia*, 4, 191–194 (2002).

Cosco D., D. Paolino, F. Cilurzo, F. Casale and M. Fresta, Gemcitabine and tamoxifen-loaded liposomes as multidrug carriers for the treatment of breast cancer diseases, *Int J Pharm*, 422, 229–237 (2012).

Crom W. R., S. S. N. Degraaf, T. Synold, D. R. A. Uges, H. Bloemhof, G. Rivera, M. L. Christensen, H. Mahmoud and W. E. Evans, Pharmacokinetics of vincristine in children and adolescents with acute lymphocytic-leukemia, *J Pediatr*, 125, 642–649 (1994).

Damen J., J. Regts and G. Scherphof, Transfer and exchange of phospholipid between small unilamellar liposomes and rat plasma high-density lipoproteins—Dependence on cholesterol content and phospholipid-composition, *Biochim Biophys Acta*, 665, 538–545 (1981).

Dams E. T. M., P. Laverman, W. J. G. Oyen, G. Storm, G. L. Scherphof, J. W. M. Van der Meer, F. H. M. Corstens and O. C. Boerman, Accelerated blood clearance and altered biodistribution of repeated injections of sterically stabilized liposomes, *J Pharmacol Exp Ther*, 292, 1071–1079 (2000).

Danhier F., O. Feron and V. Preat, To exploit the tumor microenvironment: Passive and active tumor targeting of nanocarriers for anti-cancer drug delivery, *J Control Release*, 148, 135–146 (2010).

Dellian M., G. Helmlinger, F. Yuan and R. K. Jain, Fluorescence ratio imaging of interstitial pH in solid tumours: Effect of glucose on spatial and temporal gradients, *Brit J Cancer*, 74, 1206–1215 (1996).

Dicko A., L. D. Mayer and P. G. Tardi, Use of nanoscale delivery systems to maintain synergistic drug ratios in vivo, *Expert Opin Drug Deliv*, 7, 1329–1341 (2010).

Dreborg S. and E. B. Akerblom, Immunotherapy with monomethoxypolyethylene glycol modified allergens, *Crit Rev Ther Drug*, 6, 315–365 (1990).

Drummond D. C. and D. L. Daleke, Development of pH-sensitive liposomes composed of a novel "caged" dioleoylphosphatidylethanolamine, *Biophys J*, 72, Mami1–Mami1 (1997).

Drummond D. C., O. Meyer, K. L. Hong, D. B. Kirpotin and D. Papahadjopoulos, Optimizing liposomes for delivery of chemotherapeutic agents to solid tumors, *Pharmacol Rev*, 51, 691–743 (1999).

Drummond D. C., C. O. Noble, Z. X. Guo, K. Hong, J. W. Park and D. B. Kirpotin, Development of a highly active nanoliposomal irinotecan using a novel intraliposomal stabilization strategy, *Cancer Res*, 66, 3271–3277 (2006).

Drummond D. C., M. Zignani and J. C. Leroux, Current status of pH-sensitive liposomes in drug delivery, *Prog Lipid Res*, 39, 409–460 (2000).

Dubin P. and U. P. Strauss, Hydrophobic hypercoiling in copolymers of maleic acid and alkyl vinyl ethers, *J Phys Chem*, 71, 2757–2759 (1967).

Duzgunes N. and G. Gregoriadis, Introduction: The origins of liposomes: Alec Bangham at Babraham, *Liposomes, Pt E*, 391, 1–3 (2005).

El-Sayed M. E., A. S. Hoffman and P. S. Stayton, Rational design of composition and activity correlations for pH-sensitive and glutathione-reactive polymer therapeutics, *J Control Release*, 101, 47–58 (2005a).

El-Sayed M. E., A. S. Hoffman and P. S. Stayton, Smart polymeric carriers for enhanced intracellular delivery of therapeutic macromolecules, *Expert Opin Biol Ther*, 5, 23–32 (2005b).

Falcone D. J., Fluorescent opsonization assay—Binding of plasma fibronectin to fibrin-derivatized fluorescent particles does not enhance their uptake by macrophages, *J Leukocyte Biol*, 39, 1–12 (1986).

Farrell N. P., Platinum formulations as anticancer drugs clinical and pre-clinical studies, *Curr Top Med Chem*, 11, 2623–2631 (2011).

Fasol U., A. Frost, M. Buchert, J. Arends, U. Fiedler, D. Schan, J. Scheuenpflug and K. Mross, Vascular and pharmacokinetic effects of EndoTAG-1 in patients with advanced cancer and liver metastasis, *Ann Oncol*, 23, 1030–1036 (2012).

Feil H., Y. H. Bae, J. Feijen and S. W. Kim, Effect of comonomer hydrophilicity and ionization on the lower critical solution temperature of N-Isopropylacrylamide copolymers, *Macromolecules*, 26, 2496–2500 (1993).

Felgner P. L. and G. M. Ringold, Cationic liposome-mediated transfection, *Nature*, 337, 387–388 (1989).

Fichtner F. and H. Schonert, Cooperative Change in status of polyethylacrylic acid in aqueous-solution, *Colloid Polym Sci*, 255, 230–232 (1977).

Field J. J., A. Kanakkanthara and J. H. Miller, Microtubule-targeting agents are clinically successful due to both mitotic and interphase impairment of microtubule function, *Bioorg Med Chem*, 22, 5050–5059 (2014).

Finney J. L. and A. K. Soper, Solvent structure and perturbations in solutions of chemical and biological importance, *Chem Soc Rev*, 23, 1–10 (1994).

Fleige E., M. A. Quadir and R. Haag, Stimuli-responsive polymeric nanocarriers for the controlled transport of active compounds: Concepts and applications, *Adv Drug Deliv Rev*, 64, 866–884 (2012).

Floege J., T. Ostendorf, U. Janssen, M. Burg, H. H. Radeke, C. Vargeese, S. C. Gill, L. S. Green and N. Janjic, Novel approach to specific growth factor inhibition in vivo—Antagonism of platelet-derived growth factor in glomerulonephritis by aptamers, *Am J Pathol*, 154, 169–179 (1999).

Forssen E. A. and Z. A. Tokes, Use of anionic liposomes for the reduction of chronic doxorubicin-induced cardiotoxicity, *Proc Natl Acad Sci-Biol*, 78, 1873–1877 (1981).

Gabizon A. and D. Papahadjopoulos, Liposome formulations with prolonged circulation time in blood and enhanced uptake by tumors, *Proc Natl Acad Sci U S A*, 85, 6949–6953 (1988).

Gad A. E., B. L. Silver and G. D. Eytan, Polycation-induced fusion of negatively-charged vesicles, *Biochim Biophys Acta*, 690, 124–132 (1982).

Ganta S., H. Devalapally, A. Shahiwala and M. Amiji, A review of stimuli-responsive nanocarriers for drug and gene delivery, *J Control Release*, 126, 187–204 (2008).

Gerasimov O. V., A. Schwan and D. H. Thompson, Acid-catalyzed plasmenylcholine hydrolysis and its effect on bilayer permeability: A quantitative study, *Biochim Biophys Acta*, 1324, 200–214 (1997).

Gluck R., Adjuvant activity of immunopotentiating reconstituted influenza virosomes (IRIVs), *Vaccine*, 17, 1782–1787 (1999).

Goren D., A. Gabizon and Y. Barenholz, The influence of physical characteristics of liposomes containing doxorubicin on their pharmacological behavior, *Biochim Biophys Acta*, 1029, 285–294 (1990).

Goren D., A. T. Horowitz, S. Zalipsky, M. C. Woodle, Y. Yarden and A. Gabizon, Targeting of stealth liposomes to erbB-2 (Her/2) receptor: In vitro and in vivo studies, *Br J Cancer*, 74, 1749–1756 (1996).

Gowda R., Use of nanotechnology to develop multi-drug inhibitors for cancer therapy, *J Nanomed Nanotechnol*, 4, 1–16 (2013).

Goyal P., K. Goyal, S. G. Vijaya Kumar, A. Singh, O. P. Katare and D. N. Mishra, Liposomal drug delivery systems—Clinical applications, *Acta Pharm*, 55, 1–25 (2005).

Goymer P., In the news—Gardasil—The perfect guard? *Nat Rev Cancer*, 5, 840 (2005).

Grant G. J., Y. Barenholz, E. M. Bolotin, M. Bansinath, H. Turndoft, B. Piskoun and E. M. Davidson, A novel liposomal bupivacaine formulation to produce ultralong-acting analgesia, *Anesthesiology*, 101, 133–137 (2004).

Gregoriadis G., Carrier potential of liposomes in biology and medicine (first of two parts), *N Engl J Med*, 295, 704–710 (1976).

Gregoriadis G., E. J. Wills, C. P. Swain and A. S. Tavill, Drug-carrier potential of liposomes in cancer chemotherapy, *Lancet*, 1, 1313–1316 (1974).

Gruner S. M., R. P. Lenk, A. S. Janoff and M. J. Ostro, Novel multilayered lipid vesicles—Comparison of physical characteristics of multilamellar liposomes and stable plurilamellar vesicles, *Biochemistry-Us*, 24, 2833–2842 (1985).

Gurley B. J., Emerging technologies for improving phytochemical bioavailability: Benefits and risks, *Clin Pharmacol Ther*, 89, 915–919 (2011).

Hamaguchi T., K. Kato, H. Yasui, C. Morizane, M. Ikeda, H. Ueno, K. Muro, Y. Yamada, T. Okusaka, K. Shirao, Y. Shimada, H. Nakahama and Y. Matsumura, A phase I and pharmacokinetic study of NK105, a paclitaxel-incorporating micellar nanoparticle formulation, *Brit J Cancer*, 97, 170–176 (2007).

Handel T. M., I. S. Ponticello and J. S. Tan, Effects of side-chain structure on polymer conformation—Synthesis and dilute-solution properties, *Macromolecules*, 20, 264–267 (1987).

Hartrick C. T. and K. A. Hartrick, Extended-release epidural morphine (DepoDur): Review and safety analysis, *Expert Rev Neurother*, 8, 1641–1648 (2008).

Hatakeyama H., H. Akita, K. Maruyama, T. Suhara and H. Harashima, Factors governing the in vivo tissue uptake of transferrin-coupled polyethylene glycol liposomes in vivo, *Int J Pharm*, 281, 25–33 (2004).

Hau P., K. Fabel, U. Baumgart, P. Rummele, O. Grauer, A. Bock, C. Dietmaier, W. Dietmaier, J. Dietrich, C. Dudel, F. Hubner, T. Jauch, E. Drechsel, I. Kleiter, G. Wismeth, A. Zellner, A. Brawanski, A. Steinbrecher, J. Marienhagen and U. Bogdahn, Pegylated liposomal doxorubicin-efficacy in patients with recurrent high-grade glioma, *Cancer*, 100, 1199–1207 (2004).

Hayashi H., K. Kono and T. Takagishi, Temperature-dependent associating property of liposomes modified with a thermosensitive polymer, *Bioconjug Chem*, 9, 382–389 (1998).

Heath T. D., J. A. Montgomery, J. R. Piper and D. Papahadjopoulos, Antibody-targeted liposomes: Increase in specific toxicity of methotrexate-gamma-aspartate, *Proc Natl Acad Sci U S A*, 80, 1377–1381 (1983).

Heinemann V., D. Bosse, U. Jehn, B. Kahny, K. Wachholz, A. Debus, P. Scholz, H. J. Kolb and W. Wilmanns, Pharmacokinetics of liposomal amphotericin B (AmBisome) in critically ill patients, *Antimicrob Agents Chemother*, 41, 1275–1280 (1997).

Henry S. M., M. E. El-Sayed, C. M. Pirie, A. S. Hoffman and P. S. Stayton, pH-responsive poly(styrene-alt-maleic anhydride) alkylamide copolymers for intracellular drug delivery, *Biomacromolecules*, 7, 2407–2414 (2006).

Herbert V., A. R. Larrabee and J. M. Buchanan, Studies on the identification of a folate compound of human serum, *J Clin Invest*, 41, 1134–1138 (1962).

Hirotsu S., Y. Hirokawa and T. Tanaka, Volume-phase transitions of ionized N-Isopropylacrylamide gels, *J Chem Phys*, 87, 1392–1395 (1987).

Hofheinz R. D., S. U. Gnad-Vogt, U. Beyer and A. Hochhaus, Liposomal encapsulated anticancer drugs, *Anti-Cancer Drug*, 16, 691–707 (2005).

Hong K., F. Schuber and D. Papahadjopoulos, Polyamines—Biological modulators of membrane-fusion, *Biochim Biophys Acta*, 732, 469–472 (1983).

Huang A., S. J. Kennel and L. Huang, Interactions of immunoliposomes with target-cells, *J Biol Chem*, 258, 4034–4040 (1983).

Huang C., Studies on phosphatidylcholine vesicles. Formation and physical characteristics, *Biochemistry*, 8, 344–352 (1969).

Huang S. K., E. Mayhew, S. Gilani, D. D. Lasic, F. J. Martin and D. Papahadjopoulos, Pharmacokinetics and therapeutics of sterically stabilized liposomes in mice bearing C-26 colon-carcinoma, *Cancer Res*, 52, 6774–6781 (1992).

Iinuma H., K. Maruyama, K. Okinaga, K. Sasaki, T. Sekine, O. Ishida, N. Ogiwara, K. Johkura and Y. Yonemura, Intracellular targeting therapy of cisplatin-encapsulated transferrin-polyethylene glycol liposome on peritoneal dissemination of gastric cancer, *Int J Cancer*, 99, 130–137 (2002).

Immordino M. L., F. Dosio and L. Cattel, Stealth liposomes: Review of the basic science, rationale, and clinical applications, existing and potential, *Int J Nanomed*, 1, 297–315 (2006).

Iqbal U., H. Albaghdadi, M. P. Nieh, U. I. Tuor, Z. Mester, D. Stanimirovic, J. Katsaras and A. Abulrob, Small unilamellar vesicles: A platform technology for molecular imaging of brain tumors, *Nanotechnology*, 22, (2011).

Ishida T., H. Harashima and H. Kiwada, Liposome clearance, *Bioscience Rep*, 22, 197–224 (2002).

Ishida T., D. L. Iden and T. M. Allen, A combinatorial approach to producing sterically stabilized (Stealth) immunoliposomal drugs, *FEBS Lett*, 460, 129–133 (1999).

Ishida T., R. Maeda, M. Ichihara, K. Irimura and H. Kiwada, Accelerated clearance of PEGylated liposomes in rats after repeated injections, *J Controlled Release*, 88, 35–42 (2003a).

Ishida T., K. Masuda, T. Ichikawa, M. Ichihara, K. Irimura and H. Kiwada, Accelerated clearance of a second injection of PEGylated liposomes in mice, *Int J Pharm*, 255, 167–174 (2003b).

Ishida T., T. Ichikawa, M. Ichihara, Y. Sadzuka and H. Kiwada, Effect of the physicochemical properties of initially injected liposomes on the clearance of subsequently injected PEGylated liposomes in mice, *J Controlled Release*, 95, 403–412 (2004).

Ishida T., M. Harada, X. Y. Wang, M. Ichihara, K. Irimura and H. Kiwada, Accelerated blood clearance of PEGylated liposomes following preceding liposome injection: Effects of lipid dose and PEG surface-density and chain length of the first-dose liposomes, *J Controlled Release*, 105, 305–317 (2005).

Ishida T., K. Atobe, X. Wang and H. Kiwada, Accelerated blood clearance of PEGylated liposomes upon repeated injections: Effect of doxorubicin-encapsulation and high-dose first injection, *J Controlled Release*, 115, 251–258 (2006a).

Ishida T., M. Ichihara, X. Wang, K. Yamamoto, J. Kimura, E. Majima and H. Kiwada, Injection of PEGylated liposomes in rats elicits PEG-specific IgM, which is responsible for rapid elimination of a second dose of PEGylated liposomes, *J Controlled Release*, 112, 15–25 (2006b).

Israelachvili J. N., D. J. Mitchell and B. W. Ninham, Theory of self-assembly of hydrocarbon amphiphiles into micelles and bilayers, *J Chem Soc, Faraday Trans 2*, 72, 1525–1568 (1976).

Jackson D. V., E. H. Paschold, C. L. Spurr, H. B. Muss, F. Richards, M. R. Cooper, D. R. White, J. J. Stuart, J. O. Hopkins, R. Rich and H. B. Wells, Treatment of advanced non-hodgkins lymphoma with vincristine infusion, *Cancer*, 53, 2601–2606 (1984).

Jain R. K., Barriers to drug-delivery in solid tumors, *Sci Am*, 271, 58–65 (1994).

Jain R. K., Transport of molecules in the tumor interstitium—A review, *Cancer Res*, 47, 3039–3051 (1987).

Jain S., P. Jain, R. B. Umamaheshwari and N. K. Jain, Transfersomes—A novel vesicular carrier for enhanced transdermal delivery: Development, characterization, and performance evaluation, *Drug Dev Ind Pharm*, 29, 1013–1026 (2003).

Joyce D. E. and T. Kurucsev, Hydrogen-ion equilibria in poly(methacrylic acid) and poly(ethacrylic acid) solutions, *Polymer*, 22, 415–417 (1981).

Juliano R. L. and S. S. Daoud, Liposomes as a delivery system for membrane-active antitumor drugs, *J Control Release*, 11, 225–232 (1990).

Juliano R. L. and H. N. McCullough, Controlled delivery of an anti-tumor drug—Localized action of liposome encapsulated cytosine-arabinoside administered via the respiratory system, *J Pharmacol Exp Ther*, 214, 381–387 (1980).

Juliano R. L. and D. Stamp, Lectin-mediated attachment of glycoprotein-bearing liposomes to cells, *Nature*, 261, 235–238 (1976).

Jung B. H., S. J. Chung and C. K. Shim, Proliposomes as prolonged intranasal drug delivery systems, *Stp Pharma Sci*, 12, 33–38 (2002).

Kato K., Stem cells in human normal endometrium and endometrial cancer cells: Characterization of side population cells, *Kaohsiung J Med Sci*, 28, 63–71 (2012).

Katsaros D., M. V. Oletti, I. A. R. de la Longrais, A. Ferrero, A. Celano, S. Fracchioli, M. Donadio, R. Passera, L. Cattel and C. Bumma, Clinical and pharmacokinetic phase II study of pegylated liposomal doxorubicin and vinorelbine in heavily pretreated recurrent ovarian carcinoma, *Ann Oncol*, 16, 300–306 (2005).

Kay P. J., D. P. Kelly, G. I. Milgate and F. E. Treloar, Conformational transition in poly(methacrylic acid) and butyl vinyl ether-maleic anhydride copolymers studied by H-1 Nmr linewidth measurements, *Macromol Chem*, 177, 885–893 (1976).

Kersten G. F. A. and D. J. A. Crommelin, Liposomes and ISCOMs, *Vaccine*, 21, 915–920 (2003).

Khalil I. A., K. Kogure, H. Akita and H. Harashima, Uptake pathways and subsequent intracellular trafficking in nonviral gene delivery, *Pharmacol Rev*, 58, 32–45 (2006).

Kim J. C., S. K. Bae and J. D. Kim, Temperature-sensitivity of liposomal lipid bilayers mixed with poly(N-isopropylacrylamide-co-acrylic acid), *J Biochem-Tokyo*, 121, 15–19 (1997).

Kirby C. and G. Gregoriadis, Dehydration-rehydration vesicles—A simple method for high-yield drug entrapment in liposomes, *Bio-Technol*, 2, 979–984 (1984).

Kitano H., Y. Maeda, S. Takeuchi, K. Ieda and Y. Aizu, Liposomes containing amphiphiles prepared by using a lipophilic chain transfer reagent—Responsiveness to external stimuli, *Langmuir*, 10, 403–406 (1994).

Klibanov A. L., K. Maruyama, V. P. Torchilin and L. Huang, Amphipathic polyethyleneglycols effectively prolong the circulation time of liposomes, *FEBS Lett*, 268, 235–237 (1990).

Koide H., T. Asai, K. Hatanaka, S. Akai, T. Ishii, E. Kenjo, T. Ishida, H. Kiwada, H. Tsukada and N. Oku, T cell-independent B cell response is responsible for ABC phenomenon induced by repeated injection of PEGylated liposomes, *Int J Pharm*, 392, 218–223 (2010).

Kono K., Thermosensitive polymer-modified liposomes, *Adv Drug Deliv Rev*, 53, 307–319 (2001).

Kono K., A. Henmi and T. Takagishi, Temperature-controlled interaction of thermosensitive polymer-modified cationic liposomes with negatively charged phospholipid membranes, *Biochim Biophys Acta-Biomembranes*, 1421, 183–197 (1999a).

Kono K., A. Henmi, H. Yamashita, H. Hayashi and T. Takagishi, Improvement of temperature-sensitivity of poly(N-isopropylacrylamide)-modified liposomes, *J Control Release*, 59, 63–75 (1999b).

Kono K., T. Igawa and T. Takagishi, Cytoplasmic delivery of calcein mediated by liposomes modified with a pH-sensitive poly(ethylene glycol) derivative, *Biochim Biophys Acta*, 1325, 143–154 (1997).

Kono K., R. Nakai, K. Morimoto and T. Takagishi, Temperature-dependent interaction of thermosensitive polymer-modified liposomes with CV1 cells, *FEBS Lett*, 456, 306–310 (1999c).

Kono K., R. Nakai, K. Morimoto and T. Takagishi, Thermosensitive polymer-modified liposomes that release contents around physiological temperature, *Biochim Biophys Acta-Biomembranes*, 1416, 239–250 (1999d).

Kono K., K. Zenitani and T. Takagishi, Novel pH-sensitive liposomes: Liposomes bearing a poly(ethylene glycol) derivative with carboxyl groups, *Biochim Biophys Acta*, 1193, 1–9 (1994).

Kost J. and R. Langer, Responsive polymeric delivery systems, *Adv Drug Deliv Rev*, 46, 125–148 (2001).

Krauze M. T., C. O. Noble, T. Kawaguchi, D. Drummond, D. B. Kirpotin, Y. Yamashita, E. Kullberg, J. Forsayeth, J. W. Park and K. S. Bankiewicz, Convection-enhanced delivery of nanoliposomal CPT-11 (irinotecan) and PEGylated liposomal doxorubicin (Doxil) in rodent intracranial brain tumor xenografts, *Neuro Oncol*, 9, 393–403 (2007).

Krishnan L., C. J. Dicaire, G. B. Patel and G. D. Sprott, Archaeosome vaccine adjuvants induce strong humoral, cell-mediated, and memory responses: Comparison to conventional liposomes and alum, *Infect Immun*, 68, 54–63 (2000).

Krown S. E., D. W. Northfelt, D. Osoba and J. S. Stewart, Use of liposomal anthracyclines in Kaposi's sarcoma, *Semin Oncol*, 31, 36–52 (2004).

Lackey C. A., N. Murthy, O. W. Press, D. A. Tirrell, A. S. Hoffman and P. S. Stayton, Hemolytic activity of pH-responsive polymer-streptavidin bioconjugates, *Bioconjug Chem*, 10, 401–405 (1999).

Leamon C. P., S. R. Cooper and G. E. Hardee, Folate-liposome-mediated antisense oligodeoxynucleotide targeting to cancer cells: Evaluation in vitro and in vivo, *Bioconjug Chem*, 14, 738–747 (2003).

Lee T. Y., C. T. Lin, S. Y. Kuo, D. K. Chang and H. C. Wu, Peptide-mediated targeting to tumor blood vessels of lung cancer for drug delivery, *Cancer Res*, 67, 10958–10965 (2007).

Lian T. and R. J. Ho, Trends and developments in liposome drug delivery systems, *J Pharm Sci*, 90, 667–680 (2001).

Lipshultz S. E., S. R. Lipsitz, S. M. Mone, A. M. Goorin, S. E. Sallan, S. P. Sanders, E. J. Orav, R. D. Gelber and S. D. Colan, Female sex and higher drug dose as risk-factors for late cardiotoxic effects of doxorubicin therapy for childhood-cancer, *New Engl J Med*, 332, 1738–1743 (1995).

Litzinger D. C. and L. Huang, Phosphatodylethanolamine liposomes: Drug delivery, gene transfer and immunodiagnostic applications, *Biochim Biophys Acta—Rev Biomembranes*, 1113, 201–227 (1992).

Liu D., A. Mori and L. Huang, Role of liposome size and RES blockade in controlling biodistribution and tumor uptake of GM1-containing liposomes, *Biochim Biophys Acta*, 1104, 95–101 (1992).

Lollini P. L., F. Cavallo, P. Nanni and G. Forni, Vaccines for tumour prevention, *Nat Rev Cancer*, 6, 204–216 (2006).

Lowell G. H., L. F. Smith, R. C. Seid and W. D. Zollinger, Peptides bound to proteosomes via hydrophobic feet become highly immunogenic without adjuvants, *J Exp Med*, 167, 658–663 (1988).

Lu Y. J. and P. S. Low, Folate-mediated delivery of macromolecular anticancer therapeutic agents, *Adv Drug Deliv Rev*, 54, 675–693 (2002).

Ludewig B., F. Barchiesi, M. Pericin, R. M. Zinkernagel, H. Hengartner and R. A. Schwendener, In vivo antigen loading and activation of dendritic cells via a liposomal peptide vaccine mediates protective antiviral and anti-tumour immunity, *Vaccine*, 19, 23–32 (2000).

Lukyanov A. N., T. A. Elbayoumi, A. R. Chakilam and V. P. Torchilin, Tumor-targeted liposomes: Doxorubicin-loaded long-circulating liposomes modified with anti-cancer antibody, *J Control Release*, 100, 135–144 (2004).

Lundberg B. B., G. Griffiths and H. J. Hansen, Cellular association and cytotoxicity of anti-CD74-targeted lipid drug-carriers in B lymphoma cells, *J Controlled Release*, 94, 155–161 (2004).

Maeda H., The enhanced permeability and retention (EPR) effect in tumor vasculature: The key role of tumor-selective macromolecular drug targeting, *Adv Enzyme Regul*, 41, 189–207 (2001).

Maeda H. and Y. Matsumura, Tumoritropic and lymphotropic principles of macromolecular drugs, *Crit Rev Ther Drug*, 6, 193–210 (1989).

Maestrelli F., G. Capasso, M. L. Gonzalez-Rodriguez, A. M. Rabasco, C. Ghelardini and P. Mura, Effect of preparation technique on the properties and in vivo efficacy of benzocaine-loaded ethosomes, *J Liposome Res*, 19, 253–260 (2009).

Magin R. L., J. N. Weinstein, M. B. Yatvin and R. Blumenthal, Selective localization of liposomal encapsulated methotrexate in locally heated murine tumors, *Proc Am Assoc Cancer Res*, 20, 280 (1979).

Malam Y., M. Loizidou and A. M. Seifalian, Liposomes and nanoparticles: Nanosized vehicles for drug delivery in cancer, *Trends Pharmacol Sci*, 30, 592–599 (2009).

Malone R. W., P. L. Felgner and I. M. Verma, Cationic liposome-mediated RNA transfection, *Proc Natl Acad Sci U S A*, 86, 6077–6081 (1989).

Manjappa A. S., K. R. Chaudhari, M. P. Venkataraju, P. Dantuluri, B. Nanda, C. Sidda, K. K. Sawant and R. S. Murthy, Antibody derivatization and conjugation strategies: Application in preparation of stealth immunoliposome to target chemotherapeutics to tumor, *J Control Release*, 150, 2–22 (2011).

Mastrobattista E., G. A. Koning and G. Storm, Immunoliposomes for the targeted delivery of antitumor drugs, *Adv Drug Deliv Rev*, 40, 103–127 (1999).

Matsumura Y., Phase I and pharmacokinetic study of MCC-465, a doxorubicin (DXR) encapsulated in PEG immunoliposome, in patients with metastatic stomach cancer, *Ann Oncol*, 15, 517–525 (2004).

Mayer L. D., M. J. Hope and P. R. Cullis, Vesicles of variable sizes produced by a rapid extrusion procedure, *Biochim Biophys Acta*, 858, 161–168 (1986).

McDonagh C. F., A. Huhalov, B. D. Harms, S. Adams, V. Paragas, S. Oyama, B. Zhang, L. Luus, R. Overland, S. Nguyen, J. M. Gu, N. Kohli, M. Wallace, M. J. Feldhaus, A. J. Kudla, B. Schoeberl and U. B. Nielsen, Antitumor activity of a novel bispecific antibody that targets the ErbB2/ErbB3 oncogenic unit and inhibits heregulin-induced activation of ErbB3, *Mol Cancer Ther*, 11, 582–593 (2012).

Medina O. P., Y. Zhu and K. Kairemo, Targeted liposomal drug delivery in cancer, *Curr Pharm Design*, 10, 2981–2989 (2004).

Metselaar J. M., P. Bruin, L. W. T. de Boer, T. de Vringer, C. Snel, C. Oussoren, M. H. M. Wauben, D. J. A. Crommelin, G. Storm and W. E. Hennink, A novel family of L-amino acid-based biodegradable polymer-lipid conjugates for the development of long-circulating liposomes with effective drug-targeting capacity, *Bioconjug Chem*, 14, 1156–1164 (2003).

Meyer O., D. Papahadjopoulos and J. C. Leroux, Copolymers of N-isopropylacrylamide can trigger pH sensitivity to stable liposomes, *FEBS Lett*, 421, 61–64 (1998).

Mischler R. and I. C. Metcalfe, Inflexal (R) V a trivalent virosome subunit influenza vaccine: Production, *Vaccine*, 20, B17–B23 (2002).

Monfardini C. and F. M. Veronese, Stabilization of substances in circulation, *Bioconjug Chem*, 9, 418–450 (1998).

Motion J. P., G. H. Huynh, F. C. Szoka and R. A. Siegel, Convection and retro-convection enhanced delivery: Some theoretical considerations related to drug targeting, *Pharm Res*, 28, 472–479 (2011).

Mufamadi M. S., V. Pillay, Y. E. Choonara, L. C. Du Toit, G. Modi, D. Naidoo and V. M. Ndesendo, A review on composite liposomal technologies for specialized drug delivery, *J Drug Deliv*, 2011, 939851 (2011).

Muggia F. M., J. D. Hainsworth, S. Jeffers, P. Miller, S. Groshen, M. Tan, L. Roman, B. Uziely, L. Muderspach, A. Garcia, A. Burnett, F. A. Greco, C. P. Morrow, L. J. Paradiso and L. J. Liang, Phase II study of liposomal doxorubicin in refractory ovarian cancer: Antitumor activity and toxicity modification by liposomal encapsulation, *J Clin Oncol*, 15, 987–993 (1997).

Nakamura K., A. S. Abu Lila, M. Matsunaga, Y. Doi, T. Ishida and H. Kiwada, A double-modulation strategy in cancer treatment with a chemotherapeutic agent and siRNA, *Mol Ther*, 19, 2040–2047 (2011).

Needham D. and M. W. Dewhirst, The development and testing of a new temperature-sensitive drug delivery system for the treatment of solid tumors, *Adv Drug Deliver Rev*, 53, 285–305 (2001).

Needham D., T. J. McIntosh and D. D. Lasic, Repulsive interactions and mechanical stability of polymer-grafted lipid-membranes, *Biochim Biophys Acta*, 1108, 40–48 (1992).

Needham D., J. Mills and G. Eichenbaum, Interactions between poly(2-ethylacrylic acid) and lipid bilayer membranes: Effects of cholesterol and grafted poly(ethylene glycol), *Faraday Discuss*, 103–110, discussion 137–157 (1998).

Neerunjun E. D. and G. Gregoriadis, Tumor regression with liposome-entrapped asparaginase—Some immunological advantages, *Biochem Soc Trans*, 4, 133–134 (1976).

Neves S., H. Faneca, S. Bertin, K. Konopka, N. Duzgunes, V. Pierrefite-Carle, S. Simoes and M. C. Pedroso de Lima, Transferrin lipoplex-mediated suicide gene therapy of oral squamous cell carcinoma in an immunocompetent murine model and mechanisms involved in the antitumoral response, *Cancer Gene Ther*, 16, 91–101 (2009).

Nicolazzi C., N. Mignet, N. de la Figuera, M. Cadet, R. T. Ibad, J. Seguin, D. Scherman and M. Bessodes, Anionic polyethyleneglycol lipids added to cationic lipoplexes increase their plasmatic circulation time, *J Control Release*, 88, 429–443 (2003).

Ohkuma S. and B. Poole, Fluorescence probe measurement of intralysosomal pH in living cells and perturbation of pH by various agents, *Proc Natl Acad Sci U S A*, 75, 3327–3331 (1978).

Oku N., S. Shibamoto, F. Ito, H. Gondo and M. Nango, Low pH induced membrane-fusion of lipid vesicles containing proton-sensitive polymer, *Biochemistry*, 26, 8145–8150 (1987).

Okuda T., N. Ohno, K. Nitta and S. Sugai, Conformational transition of copolymer of maleic-acid and styrene in aqueous-solution II., *J Polym Sci: Polym Phys*, 15, 749–755 (1977).

Ozpolat B., A. K. Sood and G. Lopez-Berestein, Nanomedicine based approaches for the delivery of siRNA in cancer, *J Int Med*, 267, 44–53 (2010).

Pack D. W., D. Putnam and R. Langer, Design of imidazole-containing endosomolytic bio-polymers for gene delivery, *Biotechnol Bio Eng*, 67, 217–223 (2000).

Papahadjopoulos D., K. Jacobson, S. Nir and T. Isac, Phase-transitions in phospholipid vesicles—Fluorescence polarization and permeability measurements concerning effect of temperature and cholesterol, *Biochim Biophys Acta*, 311, 330–348 (1973).

Parhi P., C. Mohanty and S. K. Sahoo, Nanotechnology-based combinational drug delivery: An emerging approach for cancer therapy, *Drug Discov Today*, 17, 1044–1052 (2012).

Park J. W., K. Hong, P. Carter, H. Asgari, L. Y. Guo, G. A. Keller, C. Wirth, R. Shalaby, C. Kotts and W. I. Wood, Development of anti-p185HER2 immunoliposomes for cancer therapy, *Proc Natl Acad Sci*, 92, 1327–1331 (1995).

Park S. B., A. V. Krishnan, C. S. Y. Lin, D. Goldstein, M. Friedlander and M. C. Kiernan, Mechanisms underlying chemotherapy-induced neurotoxicity and the potential for neuroprotective strategies, *Curr Med Chem*, 15, 3081–3094 (2008).

Park Y. S., K. Maruyama and L. Huang, Some negatively charged phospholipid derivatives prolong the liposome circulation in vivo, *Biochim Biophys Acta*, 1108, 257–260 (1992).

Patel H. M., Serum opsonins and liposomes—Their interaction and opsonophagocytosis, *Crit Rev Ther Drug*, 9, 39–90 (1992).

Payne N. I., P. Timmins, C. V. Ambrose, M. D. Ward and F. Ridgway, Proliposomes—A novel solution to an old problem, *J Pharm Sci*, 75, 325–329 (1986).

Peer D., J. M. Karp, S. Hong, O. C. Farokhzad, R. Margalit and R. Langer, Nanocarriers as an emerging platform for cancer therapy, *Nat Nanotechnol*, 2, 751–760 (2007).

Peetla C., A. Stine and V. Labhasetwar, Biophysical interactions with model lipid membranes: Applications in drug discovery and drug delivery, *Mol Pharm*, 6, 1264–1276 (2009).

Perrin P., P. Sureau and L. Thibodeau, Structural and immunogenic characteristics of rabies immunosomes, *Dev Biol Stand*, 60, 483–491 (1985).

Perumal V., S. Banerjee, S. Das, R. Sen and M. Mandal, Effect of liposomal celecoxib on proliferation of colon cancer cell and inhibition of DMBA-induced tumor in rat model, *Cancer Nano*, 2, 67–79 (2011).

Petre C. E. and D. P. Dittmer, Liposomal daunorubicin as treatment for Kaposi's sarcoma, *Int J Nanomed*, 2, 277–288 (2007).

Petros R. A. and J. M. DeSimone, Strategies in the design of nanoparticles for therapeutic applications, *Nat Rev Drug Discov*, 9, 615–627 (2010).

Petros A. M., J. R. Huth, T. Oost, C. M. Park, H. Ding, X. L. Wang, H. C. Zhang, P. Nimmer, R. Mendoza, C. H. Sun, J. Mack, K. Walter, S. Dorwin, E. Gramling, U. Ladror, S. H. Rosenberg, S. W. Elmore, S. W. Fesik and P. J. Hajduk, Discovery of a potent and selective Bcl-2 inhibitor using SAR by NMR, *Bioorg Med Chem Lett*, 20, 6587–6591 (2010).

Phillips M. A., M. L. Gran and N. A. Peppas, Targeted nanodelivery of drugs and diagnostics, *Nano Today*, 5, 143–159 (2010).

Pirollo K. F., L. Xu and E. H. Chang, Non-viral gene delivery for p53, *Curr Opin Mol Ther*, 2, 168–175 (2000).

Polozova A. and F. M. Winnik, Mechanism of the interaction of hydrophobically-modified poly-(N-isopropylacrylamides) with liposomes, *Biochim Biophys Acta-Biomembranes*, 1326, 213–224 (1997).

Polozova A., A. Yamazaki, J. L. Brash and F. M. Winnik, Effect of polymer architecture on the interactions of hydrophobically-modified poly-(N-isopropylamides) and liposomes, *Colloid Surf, A*, 147, 17–25 (1999).

Poon R. T. P. and N. Borys, Lyso-thermosensitive liposomal doxorubicin: An adjuvant to increase the cure rate of radiofrequency ablation in liver cancer, *Future Oncol*, 7, 937–945 (2011).

Prakash S., M. Malhotra, W. Shao, C. Tomaro-Duchesneau and S. Abbasi, Polymeric nanohybrids and functionalized carbon nanotubes as drug delivery carriers for cancer therapy, *Adv Drug Deliv Rev*, 63, 1340–1351 (2011).

Priebe W. and R. Perez-Soler, Design and tumor targeting of anthracyclines able to overcome multidrug resistance: A double-advantage approach, *Pharmacol Ther*, 60, 215–234 (1993).

Regen S. L., A. Singh, G. Oehme and M. Singh, Polymerized phosphatidyl choline vesicles— Stabilized and controllable time-release carriers, *Biochem Biophys Res Com*, 101, 131–136 (1981).

Richardson S., P. Ferruti and R. Duncan, Poly(amidoamine)s as potential endosomolytic polymers: Evaluation in vitro and body distribution in normal and tumour-bearing animals, *J Drug Target*, 6, 391–404 (1999).

Ringsdorf H., J. Venzmer and F. M. Winnik, Interaction of hydrophobically-modified poly-N-isopropylacrylamides with model membranes—Or playing a molecular accordion, *Angew Chem Int Ed*, 30, 315–318 (1991).

Riviere K., H. M. Kieler-Ferguson, K. Jerger and F. C. Szoka, Anti-tumor activity of liposome encapsulated fluoroorotic acid as a single agent and in combination with liposome irinotecan, *J Control Release*, 153, 288–296 (2011).

Rodriguez M. A., R. Pytlik, T. Kozak, M. Chhanabhai, R. Gascoyne, B. Lu, S. R. Deitcher, J. N. Winter and M. Investigators, Vincristine sulfate liposomes injection (Marqibo) in heavily pretreated patients with refractory aggressive non-hodgkin lymphoma report of the pivotal phase 2 study, *Cancer*, 115, 3475–3482 (2009).

Rose P. G., Pegylated liposomal doxorubicin: Optimizing the dosing schedule in ovarian cancer, *Oncologist*, 10, 205–214 (2005).

Rosentha S. and S. Kaufman, Vincristine neurotoxicity, *Ann Intern Med*, 80, 733–737 (1974).

Roux E., M. Lafleur, E. Lataste, P. Moreau and J. C. Leroux, On the characterization of pH-sensitive liposome/polymer complexes, *Biomacromolecules*, 4, 240–248 (2003).

Roux E., C. Passirani, S. Scheffold, J. P. Benoit and J. C. Leroux, Serum-stable and long-circulating, PEGylated, pH-sensitive liposomes, *J Control Release*, 94, 447–451 (2004).

Rui Y. J., S. Wang, P. S. Low and D. H. Thompson, Diplasmenylcholine-folate liposomes: An efficient vehicle for intracellular drug delivery, *J Am Chem Soc*, 120, 11213–11218 (1998).

Samad A., Y. Sultana and M. Aqil, Liposomal drug delivery systems: An update review, *Curr Drug Deliv*, 4, 297–305 (2007).

Sapra P. and T. M. Allen, Ligand-targeted liposomal anticancer drugs, *Prog Lipid Res*, 42, 439–462 (2003).

Sarbolouki M. N., M. Sadeghizadeh, M. M. Yaghoobi, A. Karami and T. Lohrasbi, Dendrosomes: A novel family of vehicles for transfection and therapy, *J Chem Technol Biotechnol*, 75, 919–922 (2000).

Saul J. M., A. V. Annapragada and R. V. Bellamkonda, A dual-ligand approach for enhancing targeting selectivity of therapeutic nanocarriers, *J Control Release*, 114, 277–287 (2006).

Scheel C. and R. A. Weinberg, Phenotypic plasticity and epithelial-mesenchymal transitions in cancer and normal stem cells? *Int J Cancer*, 129, 2310–2314 (2011).

Schiffelers R. M., G. A. Koning, T. L. ten Hagen, M. H. Fens, A. J. Schraa, A. P. Janssen, R. J. Kok, G. Molema and G. Storm, Anti-tumor efficacy of tumor vasculature-targeted liposomal doxorubicin, *J Control Release*, 91, 115–122 (2003).

Schild H. G., Poly (N-isopropylacrylamide)—Experiment, theory and application, *Prog Polym Sci*, 17, 163–249 (1992).

Schild H. G. and D. A. Tirrell, Microcalorimetric detection of lower critical solution temperatures in aqueous polymer-solutions, *J Phys Chem*, 94, 4352–4356 (1990).

Schroeder U. K. O. and D. A. Tirrell, Structural reorganization of phosphatidylcholine vesicle membranes by poly(2-ethylacrylic acid)—Influence of the molecular-weight of the polymer, *Macromolecules*, 22, 765–769 (1989).

Schroeter A., T. Engelbrecht, R. H. Neubert and A. S. Goebel, New nanosized technologies for dermal and transdermal drug delivery. A review, *J Biomed Nanotechnol*, 6, 511–528 (2010).

Seddon A. M., D. Casey, R. V. Law, A. Gee, R. H. Templer and O. Ces, Drug interactions with lipid membranes, *Chem Soc Rev*, 38, 2509–2519 (2009).

Seki K. and D. A. Tirrell, Interactions of synthetic-polymers with cell-membranes and model membrane systems V. pH-dependent complexation of poly(acrylic acid) derivatives with phospholipid vesicle membranes, *Macromolecules*, 17, 1692–1698 (1984).

Semple S. C., A. Akinc, J. X. Chen, A. P. Sandhu, B. L. Mui, C. K. Cho, D. W. Y. Sah, D. Stebbing, E. J. Crosley, E. Yaworski, I. M. Hafez, J. R. Dorkin, J. Qin, K. Lam, K. G. Rajeev, K. F. Wong, L. B. Jeffs, L. Nechev, M. L. Eisenhardt, M. Jayaraman, M. Kazem, M. A. Maier, M. Srinivasulu, M. J. Weinstein, Q. M. Chen, R. Alvarez, S. A. Barros, S. De, S. K. Klimuk, T. Borland, V. Kosovrasti, W. L. Cantley, Y. K. Tam, M. Manoharan, M. A. Ciufolini, M. A. Tracy, A. de Fougerolles, I. MacLachlan, P. R. Cullis, T. D. Madden and M. J. Hope, Rational design of cationic lipids for siRNA delivery, *Nat Biotechnol*, 28, 172–176 (2010).

Sen K. and M. Mandal, Second generation liposomal cancer therapeutics: Transition from laboratory to clinic, *Int J Pharm*, 448, 28–43 (2013).

Senior J. and G. Gregoriadis, Is half-life of circulating liposomes determined by changes in their permeability, *FEBS Lett*, 145, 109–114 (1982).

Sessa G. and G. Weissman, Phospholipid spherules (liposomes) as a model for biological membranes, *J Lipid Res*, 9, 310–318 (1968).

Sharma A. and U. S. Sharma, Liposomes in drug delivery: Progress and limitations, *Int J Pharm*, 154, 123–140 (1997).

Shibayama M., S. Mizutani and S. Nomura, Thermal properties of copolymer gels containing N-isopropylacrylamide, *Macromolecules*, 29, 2019–2024 (1996).

Smeesters C., L. Giroux, B. Vinet, R. Arnoux, P. Chaland, J. Corman, G. Stlouis and P. Daloze, Efficacy of incorporating cyclosporine into liposomes to reduce its nephrotoxicity, *Can J Surg*, 31, 34–36 (1988).

Suri S. S., H. Fenniri and B. Singh, Nanotechnology-based drug delivery systems, *J Occup Med Toxicol*, 2, 16 (2007).

Sutton R. C., L. Thai, J. M. Hewitt, C. L. Voycheck and J. S. Tan, Microdomain characterization of styrene imidazole copolymers, *Macromolecules*, 21, 2432–2439 (1988).

Sullivan S. M., J. Connor and L. Huang, Immunoliposomes—Preparation, properties, and applications, *Med Res Rev*, 6, 171–195 (1986).

Szoka F. and D. Papahadjopoulos, Procedure for preparation of liposomes with large internal aqueous space and high capture by reverse-phase evaporation, *Proc Natl Acad Sci USA*, 75, 4194–4198 (1978).

Takara K., H. Hatakeyama, N. Ohga, K. Hida and H. Harashima, Design of a dual-ligand system using a specific ligand and cell penetrating peptide, resulting in a synergistic effect on selectivity and cellular uptake, *Int J Pharm*, 396, 143–148 (2010).

Tan J. S. and S. P. Gasper, Dilute-solution behavior of polyelectrolytes. Intrinsic-viscosity and light-scattering studies, *J Polym Sci: Polym Phys*, 12, 1785–1804 (1974).

Tardi P. G., R. C. Gallagher, S. Johnstone, N. Harasym, M. Webb, M. B. Bally and L. D. Mayer, Coencapsulation of irinotecan and floxuridine into low cholesterol-containing liposomes that coordinate drug release in vivo, *Biochim Biophys Acta*, 1768, 678–687 (2007).

Taylor K. M. G., G. Taylor, I. W. Kellaway and J. Stevens, Drug entrapment and release from multilamellar and reverse-phase evaporation liposomes, *Int J Pharm*, 58, 49–55 (1990).

Theodossiou C., J. A. Cook, J. Fisher, D. Teague, J. E. Liebmann, A. Russo and J. B. Mitchell, Interaction of gemcitabine with paclitaxel and cisplatin in human tumor cell lines, *Int J Oncol*, 12, 825–832 (1998).

Thomas J. L., B. P. Devlin and D. A. Tirrell, Kinetics of membrane micellization by the hydrophobic polyelectrolyte poly(2-ethylacrylic acid), *Biochim Biophys Acta*, 1278, 73–78 (1996).

Thomas J. L., H. You and D. A. Tirrell, Tuning the response of a pH-sensitive membrane switch, *J Am Chem Soc*, 117, 2949–2950 (1995).

Tirrell D. A., D. Y. Takigawa and K. Seki, Interactions of synthetic-polymers with cell-membranes and model membrane systems VII. pH sensitization of phospholipid-vesicles via complexation with synthetic poly(carboxylic acid)s, *Ann N Y Acad Sci*, 446, 237–248 (1985).

Tomsie N., B. Babnik, D. Lombardo, B. Mavcic, M. Kanduser, A. Iglic and V. Kralj-Iglic, Shape and size of giant unilamellar phospholipid vesicles containing cardiolipin, *J Chem Inf Model*, 45, 1676–1679 (2005).

Tonge S. R. and B. J. Tighe, Responsive hydrophobically associating polymers: A review of structure and properties, *Adv Drug Deliv Rev*, 53, 109–122 (2001).

Torchilin V. P., Recent advances with liposomes as pharmaceutical carriers, *Nat Rev Drug Discov*, 4, 145–160 (2005).

Torchilin V. P., T. S. Levchenko, K. R. Whiteman, A. A. Yaroslavov, A. M. Tsatsakis, A. K. Rizos, E. V. Michailova and M. I. Shtilman, Amphiphilic poly-N-vinylpyrrolidones: Synthesis, properties and liposome surface modification, *Biomaterials*, 22, 3035–3044 (2001).

Torchilin V. P., M. I. Shtilman, V. S. Trubetskoy, K. Whiteman and A. M. Milstein, Amphiphilic vinyl-polymers effectively prolong liposome circulation time in-vivo, *Biochim Biophys Acta-Biomembranes*, 1195, 181–184 (1994).

Touitou E., N. Dayan, L. Bergelson, B. Godin and M. Eliaz, Ethosomes—Novel vesicular carriers for enhanced delivery: Characterization and skin penetration properties, *J Controlled Release*, 65, 403–418 (2000).

Underwood J. C. and I. Carr, The ultrastructure and permeability characteristics of the blood vessels of a transplantable rat sarcoma, *J Pathol*, 107, 157–166 (1972).

Urry D. W., Molecular machines—How motion and other functions of living organisms can result from reversible chemical-changes, *Angew Chem Int Ed*, 32, 819–841 (1993).

Uster P. S. and D. W. Deamer, pH-dependent fusion of liposomes using titratable polycations, *Biochemistry*, 24, 1–8 (1985).

Vemuri S. and C. T. Rhodes, Preparation and characterization of liposomes as therapeutic delivery systems: A review, *Pharm Acta Helv*, 70, 95–111 (1995).

Villa L. L., R. L. Costa, C. A. Petta, R. P. Andrade, K. A. Ault, A. R. Giuliano, C. M. Wheeler, L. A. Koutsky, C. Malm, M. Lehtinen, F. E. Skjeldestad, S. E. Olsson, M. Steinwall, D. R. Brown, R. J. Kurman, B. M. Ronnett, M. H. Stoler, A. Ferenczy, D. M. Harper, G. M. Tamms, J. Yu, L. Lupinacci, R. Railkar, F. J. Taddeo, K. U. Jansen, M. T. Esser, H. L. Sings, A. J. Saah and E. Barr, Prophylactic quadrivalent human papillomavirus (types 6, 11, 16, and 18) L1 virus-like particle vaccine in young women: A randomised double-blind placebo-controlled multicentre phase II efficacy trial, *Lancet Oncol*, 6, 271–278 (2005).

Volanakis J. E. and A. J. Narkates, Interaction of C-reactive protein with artificial phosphatidylcholine bilayers and complement, *J Immunol*, 126, 1820–1825 (1981).

Vonhoff D. D., M. W. Layard, P. Basa, H. L. Davis, A. L. Vonhoff, M. Rozencweig and F. M. Muggia, Risk-Factors for doxorubicin-induced congestive heart-failure, *Ann Intern Med*, 91, 710–717 (1979).

Wagner A. and K. Vorauer-Uhl, Liposome technology for industrial purposes, *J Drug Deliv*, 2011, 591325 (2011).

Wang C. Y. and L. Huang, Polyhistidine mediates an acid-dependent fusion of negatively charged liposomes, *Biochemistry*, 23, 4409–4416 (1984).

Wasan K. M. and M. Kwong, Blood and plasma lipoprotein distribution and gender differences in the plasma pharmacokinetics of lipid-associated annamycin, *Pharmacol Toxicol*, 80, 301–307 (1997).

Weinstein J. N., R. L. Magin, M. B. Yatvin and D. S. Zaharko, Liposomes and local hyperthermia—Selective delivery of methotrexate to heated tumors, *Science*, 204, 188–191 (1979).

Weinzimer S. A., T. B. Gibson, P. F. Collett-Solberg, A. Khare, B. R. Liu and P. Cohen, Transferrin is an insulin-like growth factor-binding protein-3 binding protein, *J Clin Endocrinol Metab*, 86, 1806–1813 (2001).

White R. R., B. A. Sullenger and C. P. Rusconi, Developing aptamers into therapeutics, *J Clin Invest*, 106, 929–934 (2000).

Wilson R., R. Plummer, J. Adam, M. Eatock, A. Boddy, M. Griffin, R. Miller, Y. Matsumura, T. Shimizu and H. Calvert, Phase I and pharmacokinetic study of NC-6004, a new platinum entity of cisplatin-conjugated polymer forming micelles, *ASCO annual meeting proceedings*, 26, 2573 (2008).

Winnik F. M., Effect of temperature on aqueous-solutions of pyrene-labeled (hydroxypropyl) cellulose, *Macromolecules*, 20, 2745–2750 (1987).

Wu Y., M. Crawford, B. Yu, Y. Mao, S. P. Nana-Sinkam and L. J. Lee, MicroRNA delivery by cationic lipoplexes for lung cancer therapy, *Mol Pharm*, 8, 1381–1389 (2011).

Xie R., S. Hong, L. Feng, J. Rong and X. Chen, Cell-selective metabolic glycan labeling based on ligand-targeted liposomes, *J Am Chem Soc*, 134, 9914–9917 (2012).

Xiong X. B., Y. Huang, W. L. Lu, X. Zhang, H. Zhang, T. Nagai and Q. Zhang, Intracellular delivery of doxorubicin with RGD-modified sterically stabilized liposomes for an improved antitumor efficacy: In vitro and in vivo, *J Pharm Sci*, 94, 1782–1793 (2005).

Xu L., C. C. Huang, W. Q. Huang, W. H. Tang, A. Rait, Y. Z. Yin, I. Cruz, L. M. Xiang, K. F. Pirollo and E. H. Chang, Systemic tumor-targeted gene delivery by anti-transferrin receptor scFv-immunoliposomes, *Mol Cancer Ther*, 1, 337–346 (2002).

Xu L., M. F. Wempe and T. J. Anchordoquy, The effect of cholesterol domains on PEGylated liposomal gene delivery in vitro, *Ther Deliv*, 2, 451–460 (2011).

Yatvin M. B., W. Kreutz, B. A. Horwitz and M. Shinitzky, pH-sensitive liposomes—Possible clinical implications, *Science*, 210, 1253–1254 (1980).

Yatvin M. B., J. N. Weinstein, W. H. Dennis and R. Blumenthal, Design of liposomes for enhanced local release of drugs by hyperthermia, *Science*, 202, 1290–1293 (1978).

Zhang L., F. X. Gu, J. M. Chan, A. Z. Wang, R. S. Langer and O. C. Farokhzad, Nanoparticles in Medicine: Therapeutic applications and developments, *Clinical Pharmacology & Therapeutics*, 83, 761–769 (2008).

Zhao Y. X., L. Wang, M. N. Yan, Y. L. Ma, G. X. Zang, Z. N. She and Y. H. Deng, Repeated injection of PEGylated solid lipid nanoparticles induces accelerated blood clearance in mice and beagles, *Int J Nanomed*, 7, 2891–2900 (2012).

Zignani M., D. C. Drummond, O. Meyer, K. Hong and J. C. Leroux, In vitro characterization of a novel polymeric-based pH-sensitive liposome system, *Biochim Biophys Acta-Biomembranes*, 1463, 383–394 (2000).

4 Nanocarriers for Breast Cancer Therapeutics

*Deepti Rana, Shylaja Arulkumar,
and Murugan Ramalingam*

CONTENTS

ABSTRACT

Cancer is one of the most lethal diseases, and breast cancer ranks as the second leading cause of cancer-related death among women. Every year, more than 1 million women are diagnosed as having breast cancer worldwide. The mortality rate of cancer has been increasing significantly, with a projection of approximately 12 million deaths in 2030. Although cancer therapy using conventional methods such as surgery, radiotherapy, and chemotherapy has saved millions of lives around the world, the rate of mortality still drastically increases because of the nonspecific actions and side effects attributed to such methods. This can be overcome by the recent advancements in nanotechnology, which help transform cancer therapeutics to a new dimension. Nanomedicine is one of the most rapidly growing biomedical research fields in the 21st century, which gives rise to new possibilities in the detection, diagnosis, and treatment of breast cancer. Nanomaterials with increased surface properties and tunable size and shape possess high selectivity to tumor cells, and their microenvironment and their greater diffusivity into tumor cells with reduced toxicity help overcome the existing limitations in conventional therapy. Keeping these points in view, this chapter reviews the state of the art of nanocarriers for use in breast cancer therapeutics.

Keywords: Nanocarriers, Microenvironment, Drugs, Tumor Cells, Breast Carcer

4.1 INTRODUCTION

Breast cancer is one of the most common invasive cancers among women around the world, and it is the second leading cause of death after lung cancer (DeSantis et al. 2011). According to the American Cancer Society, it is estimated that 465,000 women die from this disease annually and approximately 1.3 million women are being diagnosed with breast cancer (Jemal et al. 2007). Particularly in the United States, 178,480 new cases are estimated to be diagnosed and 40,460 women are expected to die from breast cancer (Canadian Cancer Statistics 2013). It was also observed that the 20-year relative survival is only around 70% after successful treatment (Canadian Cancer Statistics 2013). The breast cancer rate around the world is shown in Figure 4.1. It is expected that the breast cancer rate will increase drastically in the next few decades because of the increase in the life span of women. Therefore, it is necessary to pay much attention to breast cancer research and therapy. The exact cause of breast cancer is still largely unknown (Bassiouni and Faddah 2012). The different lifestyles and food habits of women along with environmental and genetic factors are the predicted causes of breast cancer (Bassiouni and Faddah 2012). Gene mutations (Nelson et al. 2005; Wooster and Weber 2003), prolonged exposure to estrogen (García-Closas et al. 2006), alcohol consumption, use of oral contraceptives, and chest irradiation are other factors that influence breast cancer (John et al. 2003).

Breast cancer is a type of cancer in which certain cells in the breast become abnormal and proliferate without control to form a tumor. In breast cancer, 90% of deaths

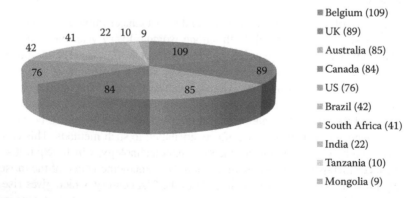

FIGURE 4.1 Chart showing statistical data (in percentage) of global breast cancer scenario. (From World Health Organization Globocan 2008, http://globocan.iarc.fr/factsheets/cancers /breast.asp.)

are attributed to malignant tumors that show metastasis (Boyle and Levin 2008; Mehlen and Puisieux 2006). Cancer cells have the potential to move from their initial site of origin to other tissues in the body, which is termed *metastasis*. Benign tumors are mild and lack malignancy, which affects only the surrounding tissues without causing severe damage to them. Women who have certain kinds of benign tumors are prone to develop malignant breast cancer (Bleyer et al. 2006). Malignant cancer is difficult to treat even if it is diagnosed early (Dhaheri et al. 2013). The metastasis of breast cancer may start at any time followed by the detection of primary breast cancer. The most common sites of breast cancer metastasis are the lungs, liver, bone, and lymph nodes (Johnston et al. 2013). The median time to metastatic recurrence in patients varies from 21 to 38 months, depending on the subtype of breast cancer (Noh et al. 2011).

The conventional methods used in breast cancer therapy include surgery, radiotherapy, and chemotherapy. Chemotherapeutic agents used in breast cancer therapy have certain characteristics such as nonspecific targeting and biodistribution, water insolubility, and systemic toxicity, which limit chemotherapy from totally curing cancer. After the initial treatment, drug resistance may develop, limiting the efficiency of therapy (Chen 2010). To overcome the lack of specificity associated with conventional therapies, several ligand-targeted therapeutic strategies such as radioimmunotherapeutics, immunotoxins, and drug immunoconjugates have been developed, but limitations still exist in their efficiency in delivering drugs (Tanaka et al. 2009). The clinical management of breast cancer has made considerable progress over the past few decades, resulting in an increase in the life expectancy of patients owing to better methods of early detection, screening, and novel therapeutic approaches.

The application of nanotechnology in medicine, also referred to as nanomedicine, creates an interdisciplinary field that has the potential to improve the treatment of many diseases including cancer (Ferrari 2005). Nanotechnology offers novel materials with unique properties, which can be utilized as a carrier system to deliver anticancer drugs. In addition, it offers new techniques to improve the detection and diagnosis of breast cancer at the molecular level (Yezhelyev et al. 2009). It involves the use of nanosized materials that will be used to carry the anticancer drugs and deliver them specifically at the tumor site, resulting in killing cancerous cells without affecting the normal cells (Chen et al. 2009). Being a nanoengineered material, the characteristics of nanocarriers can be tailored. Some of the common characteristics of nanocarriers include ease for control over system size, surface functionalization, high stability, feasibility of incorporating both hydrophobic and hydrophilic substances, and site specific delivery of drugs (Wang et al. 2009). The development of nanocarriers in different forms has resulted in unique magnetic, optic, structural, and other properties, which makes them the suitable carrier for delivery of drugs in a targeted manner (Nie et al. 2007). For example, the albumin nanocarrier bound to paclitaxel was used for the treatment of metastatic breast cancer (Miele et al. 2009). The advantages observed using this system are site-specific drug delivery and the capability of the nanocarrier to actively bind to cancer cells (Miele et al. 2009). To increase the efficiency of the drug and to decrease the requirement of the dosage, the site-specific delivery of the drugs is preferred and has always been a field of active research in nanomedicine. Keeping the above points in view, this chapter reviews the state of the art of the different types of nanocarriers, namely, metallic carrier, polymeric carrier, ceramic carrier, carbon nanotube (CNT)–based carriers, nanofiber-based carriers, nanogel-based carriers, quantum dots, and protein carriers for the application in breast cancer therapeutics and their impact on cancer cells.

4.2   BASICS OF BREAST CANCER BIOLOGY

Breast cancer is the most frequent diagnostic disease among women. Approximately up to 7% of breast cancers are being diagnosed in women below 40 years and less than 4% in women below 35 years (Brinton et al. 2008); young women have a lower risk of being diagnosed with the disease (Bleyer et al. 2006). Since breast tissues are more prone to divide throughout life, they have a higher risk of mutation than any other type of tissue. Breast tissues divide frequently from puberty till first pregnancy with an inefficient mutation repairing system, especially during the developing stages of immature breasts. It is evident that, at puberty, hormones like estrogen stimulate breast cell division, which increases the risk of permanent DNA damage in breast tissues. Because of these frequently occurring division cycles, cells override the normal cell growth control mechanisms and gain oncogenic features whenever they are exposed to carcinogens. Characteristics commonly attributed to cancer cells include the following: extensive vascularization properties (Carmeliet and Jain 2000), resistance to apoptosis and body immune system (Elnemr et al. 2001; Hannun 1997; Zhou 2000), increased expression of proteins, neighboring normal cells being induced for growth factor synthesis, and sustained renewal, which ultimately causes genetic instability and mutations in tumor suppressor genes and proto-oncogenes (Cho and Kwon 2012). Carcinogens have more affinity toward immature breast cells with an inefficient mutation repair system to cause DNA damage during the rapid breast development phase. Breast cancer stem cells possess self-renewal and regeneration properties but are not tightly controlled by the factors that control the proliferation of a stem cell and can give rise to heterogeneous cancer cell lineages that can assist in the formation of bulk tumor cells. Breast cancer stem cells make up a small part of most tumors, whereas in melanoma, they comprise 25% of the total mass (Shackleton et al. 2009).

There are four stages in the development of breast cancer tumor as shown in Figure 4.2. Stage 0 is classified into three major types of breast carcinoma: (1) ductal carcinoma in situ, which is noninvasive, wherein the abnormal cells appear in the breast duct lining; (2) lobular carcinoma in situ, which is rarely invasive, wherein the abnormal cells appear in the lobules of the breast; and (3) Paget disease of the nipple, where the abnormal cells are found in the nipple only. Stage 1 is the initial stage where the tumor starts to grow to 2 cm, which may or may not be present in the breast (Stage 1a), and the formation of small clusters can be seen in the lymph nodes (Stage 1b). In Stage 2, the breast cancer tumor starts to enlarge (larger than 2 cm but not more than 5 cm), and cancer may not spread to the lymph nodes (Stage 2a) or it may spread to the axillary lymph nodes or to the breast bone lymph nodes (Stage 2b). This is followed by further growth of the tumor (larger than 5 cm), which occurs in Stage 3, and it starts to spread to one to three axillary lymph nodes (Stage 3a) or nine axillary lymph nodes (Stage 3b). In certain cases, the tumor may be operable or inoperable where the tumor size is larger than 5 cm, which could cause swelling

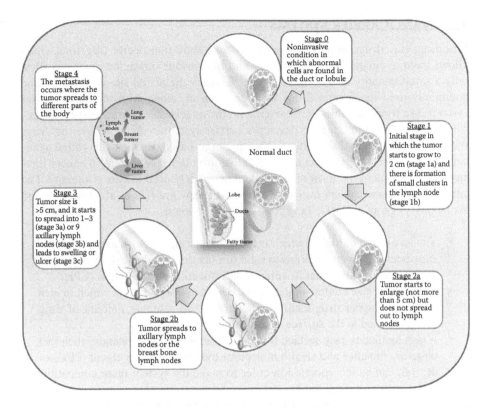

FIGURE 4.2 Pictorial representation of different stages involved in the development of breast cancer.

or ulcer, and it starts to spread to the breast skin, chest wall, or internal mammary lymph nodes (Stage 3c). The final stage of breast cancer is Stage 4 where metastasis occurs and the tumor spreads to different parts of the body such as the lungs, liver, and bone (Sharma et al. 2013).

Conventionally, anticancer drugs have been used to induce apoptosis in damaged cells to control tumor progression. These anticancer drugs act by targeting the active proliferation of cancer cells, but it is evident that they are also targeting other normal cells such as blood cells, wherein such drugs exploit and limit normal cells' functions such as folic acid synthesis or growth factor uptake. Chemotherapeutic anticancer drugs act systemically and have numerous side effects, thus creating an urgent need for improved cancer treatment.

A new approach involves site-specific and controlled delivery of drug on the site of action. Nanotechnology has provided the means to achieve high precision and efficiency to destroy cancer cells without affecting the neighboring healthy cells. With the use of multiple drug delivery carrier systems, it is now possible to specifically target cancer cells in vivo and treat them at a minimal drug dosage, thus avoiding systemic drug exposure for the whole body and preventing additional side effects from occurring. In this chapter, we have discussed different nanocarrier systems that can be used for cancer cell therapy, with special concern for breast cancer.

4.3   NANOCARRIER SYSTEMS

Free drugs (i.e., drugs without any carrier system) show nonspecific targeting, which allows them to circulate the whole body and thus invade unwanted organs or sites; only a small quantity of the drug manages to reach the actual site of action. Some commonly used therapeutic drugs for breast cancer, along with their nanocarrier systems, are listed in Table 4.1. To overcome the undesirable characteristics of anticancer drugs, it is important to develop a carrier system that can deliver the drugs with no or with minimal side effects. Nanomaterial-based carriers, also called nanocarriers, have the ability to act as an effective drug delivery system in cancer therapy. Nanocarriers in the form of particulate are widely used in cancer therapy. The advantages of nanocarriers over conventional therapy are (Hu et al. 2010; Lee and Wong 2011; Peer et al. 2007; Tang et al. 2010) as follows:

*   The size of the particles (which is in the nanoscale range) is appropriate for site-specific delivery of drugs to solid tumors through the leaky vasculature by passive targeting, that is, enhanced permeation and retention (EPR).
*   The smaller size confers higher surface area-to-volume ratio, which in turn allows for higher drug-loading efficiencies and a higher amount of drug being attached to the surface of the carrier.
*   It also facilitates easy surface functionalization and modification, such that targeting moieties and stealth molecules like polyethylene glycol (PEG) or dextran can be incorporated in order to make the system more compatible with the in vivo conditions.
*   Nanocarriers with smaller size and functional groups attached can alter the drug pharmacokinetics such as increasing the half-life of a drug and making it resistant to the reticuloendothelial system (RES).

In this chapter, nanocarriers are broadly classified into metallic carriers, polymeric carriers, ceramic carriers, CNT-based carriers, nanofiber-based carriers, nanogel-based carriers, quantum dots, and protein carriers as shown in Figure 4.3. Some of these carriers, which are being studied extensively to achieve the above-mentioned goals, are discussed in the following sections with emphasis on breast cancer.

4.3.1   METALLIC NANOCARRIERS

Metal nanoparticles as nanocarriers are increasingly being used in cancer therapy. When the metal particles are in the nanosize range, the surface properties become more pronounced and thus they can be utilized for surface functionalization of therapeutic biomolecules (Lim et al. 2011). Metallic nanoparticles are inorganic in nature and can have a high monodispersity index (Morawski et al. 2005). Among the metallic nanocarriers, gold nanoparticles and iron-oxide nanoparticles are widely used in breast cancer treatment. It has been observed that gold nanoparticles have unique physicochemical properties such as surface plasmon resonance and canal low surface modification through amine-thiol group linkage (Morawski et al. 2005).

TABLE 4.1
List of Anticancer Drugs with Their Nanocarrier Systems for Cancer Therapeutics

Nanocarrier Systems	Drug	Chemical Structure/Formula	Brand Name	Clinical Use[a]	Year of Clinical Use
PEG-targeted PLGA immunocarriers	Docetaxel	1,7β,10β-Trihydroxy-9-oxo-5β,20-epoxytax-11-ene-2α,4,13α-triyl 4-acetate 2-benzoate 13-[(2R,3S)-3-[(tert-butoxycarbonyl) amino]-2-hydroxy-3-phenylpropanoate)	Taxotere	Non–small cell lung cancer Gastric cancer Prostate cancer Squamous cell carcinoma of the head and neck that is locally being advanced	2004
Magnetic stealth nanoliposomes, PLGA: PCL nanoparticles	Gemcitabine hydrochloride	4-Amino-1-(2-deoxy-2,2-difluoro-β-D-erythro-pentofuranosyl) pyrimidin-2(1H)-on	Gemzar	Ovarian cancer Pancreatic cancer Non–small cell lung cancer	2004
PLGA nanoparticles and PLGA/MMT (montmorillonite) nanoparticles	Exemestane	6-Methylideneandrosta-1,4-diene-3,17-dione	Aromasin	Breast cancer that is advanced and also early-stage estrogen receptor positive	2005
PLGA nanoparticle, nanoliposomes	Paclitaxel	(2α,4α,5β,10β,13α)-4,10-bis(acetyloxy)-13-[[(2R,3S)-3-(benzoylamino)-2-hydroxy-3-phenylpropanoyl]oxy]-1,7-dihydroxy-9-oxo-5,20-epoxytax-11-en-2-yl benzoate	Taxol	Non–small cell lung cancer AIDS-related Kaposi's sarcoma Ovarian cancer	2006
Citrate-coated gold nanoparticles	Trastuzumab	—	Herceptin	Adenocarcinoma of the stomach or gastroesophageal junction Breast cancer that is HER2+	2006
Water-soluble polymers, dendrimers	Ixabepilone	(1R,5S,6S,7R,10S,14S,16S)-6,10-dihydroxy-1,5,7,9,9-pentamethyl-14-[(E)-1-(2-methyl-1,3-thiazol-4-yl)prop-1-en-2-yl]-17-oxa-13-azabicyclo[14.1.0]heptadecane-8,12-dione	Ixempra	Only breast cancer	2007

(Continued)

TABLE 4.1 (CONTINUED)
List of Anticancer Drugs with Their Nanocarrier Systems for Cancer Therapeutics

Nanocarrier Systems	Drug	Chemical Structure/Formula	Brand Name	Clinical Use[a]	Year of Clinical Use
Albumin–stabilized nanoparticle	Lapatinib ditosylate	N-[3-chloro-4-[(3-fluorophenyl)methoxy]phenyl]-6-[5-[(2-methylsulfonylethylamino)methyl]-2-furyl]quinazolin-4-amine	Tykerb	Breast cancer that is advanced or metastasized. It is used with: Capecitabine in women with HER2+ breast cancer Letrozole in postmenopausal women with HER2+ and hormone receptor positive breast cancer who need hormone therapy	2010
Polyethylene glycol–attached poly(β-L-malic acid)	Doxorubicin hydrochloride	(7S,9S)-7-[(2R,4S,5S,6S)-4-amino-5-hydroxy-6-methyloxan-2-yl]oxy-6,9,11-trihydroxy-9-(2-hydroxyacetyl)-4-methoxy-8,10-dihydro-7H-tetracene-5,12-dione	Adriamycin RDF Adriamycin PFS	Ovarian cancer, non-Hodgkin's lymphoma, ovarian cancer, small cell lung cancer, soft tissue and bone sarcomas, thyroid cancer, transitional cell bladder cancer, Wilms tumor, acute lymphoblastic leukemia, acute myelogenous leukemia, gastric (stomach) cancer, neuroblastoma, Hodgkin's lymphoma	–
PLGA nanoparticle, curcumin nanoparticles	Anastrozole	2,2′-[5-(1H-1,2,4-triazol-1-ylmethyl)-1,3-phenylene]bis(2-methylpropanenitrile)	Arimidex	Only breast cancer in postmenopausal women	–
Layered double hydroxides	Pamidronate disodium	(3-Amino-1-hydroxypropane-1,1-diyl)bis(phosphonic acid)	Aredia	Multiple myeloma Hypercalcemia (high blood levels of calcium) caused by malignant tumors	–
Quantum dots, solid lipid nanoparticles	Capecitabine	Pentyl [1-(3,4-dihydroxy-5-methyltetrahydrofuran-2-yl)-5-fluoro-2-oxo-1H-pyrimidin-4-yl]carbamate	Xeloda	Stage III colon cancer	–

(Continued)

TABLE 4.1 (CONTINUED)
List of Anticancer Drugs with Their Nanocarrier Systems for Cancer Therapeutics

Nanocarrier Systems	Drug	Chemical Structure/Formula	Brand Name	Clinical Use[a]	Year of Clinical Use
Liposome	Cyclophosphamide	(RS)-N,N-bis(2-chloroethyl)-1,3,2-oxazaphosphinan-2-amine 2-oxide	Clafen, Neosar, Cytoxan	Acute myeloid leukemia, acute lymphoblastic leukemia in children, chronic lymphoblastic leukemia, chronic myelogenous leukemia, Hodgkin's lymphoma, multiple myeloma, mycosis fungoides, neuroblastoma, non-Hodgkin's lymphoma, ovarian cancer, retinoblastoma	–
Poly(butyl cyanoacrylate) nanoparticles, polyvinyl pyrrolidone–loaded magnetic nanoparticles	Epirubicin hydrochloride	(8R,10S)-10-((2S,4S,5R,6S)-4-amino-5-hydroxy-6-methyltetrahydro-2H-pyran-2-yl)-6,8,11-trihydroxy-8-(2-hydroxyacetyl)-1-methoxy-7,8,9,10-tetrahydrotetracene-5,12-dione	Ellence	Only breast cancer	–
Silica xerogel	Toremifene	2-{4-[(1Z)-4-chloro-1,2-diphenyl-but-1-en-1-yl]phenoxy}-N,N-dimethylethanamine	Fareston	Breast cancer in postmenopausal women whose cancer is estrogen receptor positive or when it is not known if the cancer is ER+ or ER–	–

(Continued)

TABLE 4.1 (CONTINUED)
List of Anticancer Drugs with Their Nanocarrier Systems for Cancer Therapeutics

Nanocarrier Systems	Drug	Chemical Structure/Formula	Brand Name	Clinical Use[a]	Year of Clinical Use
Stealth liposomes, (G5) polyamidoamine dendrimer	Methotrexate	(2S)-2-[(4-[[(2,4-diaminopteridin-6-yl)methyl](methyl)amino] benzoyl)amino]pentanedioic acid	Abitrexate, Folex PFS, Methotrexate, Mexate-AQ, Mexate	Acute lymphoblastic leukemia; Gestational trophoblastic disease; Head and neck cancer; Lung cancer; Mycosis fungoides; Non-Hodgkin's lymphoma; Osteosarcoma that has not spread to other parts of the body. It is used after surgery to remove the primary tumor	—
Oil-in-water nanoemulsions	Tamoxifen citrate	(Z)-2-[4-(1,2-diphenylbut-1-enyl)phenoxy]-N,N-dimethylethanamine	Nolvadex	Breast cancer in women and men; Breast cancer in women who are at high risk for the disease	—

Source: http://www.cancer.gov/cancertopics/druginfo/breastcancer.

[a] All the drugs listed here are commonly used in breast cancer therapy and the same has also been used in other cancers, which are highlighted in the table.

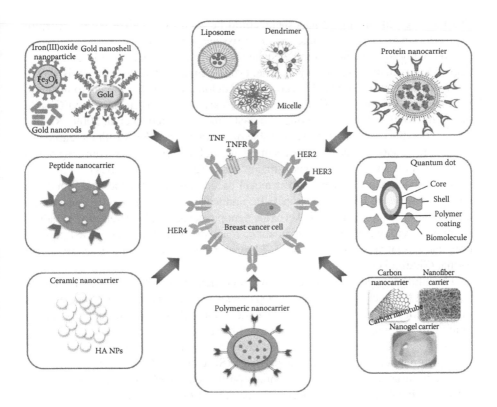

FIGURE 4.3 Classification of nanocarriers used in breast cancer therapy.

In breast cancer, approximately 15%–20% of tumors strongly overexpress HER-2, and this is known as HER-2-positive breast cancer. Citrate-coated gold nanoparticles ranging from 2 to 100 nm bounded with multiple trastuzumab antibodies were formulated in such a way that it is suitable for the efficient targeting and cross-linking of human epidermal growth factor receptor (EGFR) (HER)-2 in human SK-BR-3 breast cancer cells (Jiang et al. 2008). In this study, it was found that optimally sized nanoparticles (40–50 nm) were able to enter the cells, whereas the smaller particles tend to be dissociated from the membrane and the larger particles appeared to be taken up by the cells through receptor-mediated endocytosis. It has been specifically observed that 40-nm gold nanoparticles attached to HER were internalized, leading to a twofold increase in cytotoxicity owing to trastuzumab and the reduced expression of downstream kinases such as protein kinase B (Akt) and mitogen-activated protein kinase. It can be concluded that gold nanoparticles not only act as a passive drug carrier but also help enhance drug–cell interactions and therapeutic effects (Jiang et al. 2008).

The different forms of metallic nanocarriers have different impact over the treatment of breast cancer. *Nanorods* and *nanoshells* are the notable examples of different forms of metallic nanocarriers. HER-2-targeted silica-gold nanoshells have been formulated to discern HER-2-overexpressing breast tissue from normal tissue using two-photon microscopy and stereomicroscopy (Bickford et al. 2012). It is reported that the targeted silica-gold nanoshells could be used to visualize HER-2 receptor expression in an effective manner in breast tissue specimens.

The nanorods attached to targeted ligands help in the site-specific delivery of drugs. A schematic representation of nanorods conjugated with antibody is shown in Figure 4.4. In one study, Herceptin, a monoclonal antibody, is made to attach to gold nanorods through PEG, thus creating a carrier system, Herceptin–PEG–gold nanorods, for the efficient targeting of breast cancer (Eghtedari et al. 2009). Results showed that the carrier system was capable of escaping from RES with increased circulation time and had successfully accumulated in HER-2/neu-overexpressing breast tumor cells for application in cancer diagnostics (Eghtedari et al. 2009).

Metal oxide nanoparticles such as nickel oxide, titanium dioxide, and iron oxide nanoparticles have been used as metallic nanocarriers for therapeutic intervention and biomedical applications. Nickel oxide nanoparticles have been reported to induce apoptosis, cytotoxicity, lipid peroxidation, reactive oxygen species (ROS) production, and oxidative stress in the MCF-7 breast cancer cell line in a dose-dependent format (Siddiqui et al. 2012).

Titanium dioxide nanoparticles have considerable cytotoxic effect in human breast cells (Yoo et al. 2012). The nanoparticles of titanium dioxide, which are less than 100 nm in size, triggered ROS-dependent upregulation of FAS and Bax activation; thereby, it induces apoptosis in normal breast epithelial cells (Yoo et al. 2012). In a study, a breast tumor–targeted nanodrug has been designed, which consists of superparamagnetic iron oxide nanoparticles (SPIONs), Cy5.5 fluorescent dye, and siRNA, to target the tumor-specific antiapoptotic gene BIRC5 to shuttle specifically between siRNA and breast cancer cells as well as to monitor the siRNA delivery process noninvasively (Kumar et al. 2010). Magnetic iron oxide nanoparticles associated with optical fluorescence dyes were used as multimodal imaging probes to

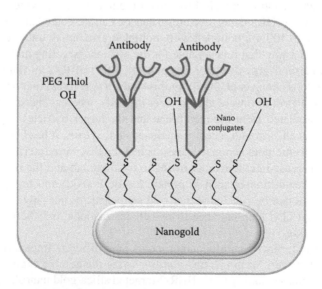

FIGURE 4.4 Schematic representation of nanorod-based carrier systems conjugated with antibody for drug delivery applications.

take advantage of the merits of optical imaging such as rapid screening and high sensitivity.

Another interesting approach is the use of water-soluble iron oxide (WSIO) nanocrystals in breast cancer treatment as a targeted magnetic resonance imaging (MRI) contrast agent for diagnostic application. WSIO nanocrystals with dimercaptosuccinic acid (DMSA) as coating material have been synthesized by cross-linking carboxylic chelating bonds and intermolecular disulfide, which is then linked to Herceptin through free DMSA thiol groups (Jun et al. 2005).

Commercially available streptavidin-conjugated SPIONs have been used as a targeted MRI contrast agent to determine the expression levels of HER-2/neu, which is overexpressed in breast cancer cells (Artemov et al. 2003). Breast cancer cells expressing various levels of receptors of HER-2/neu were pretreated with biotinylated Herceptin, which is followed by nanoparticles targeted to receptors. The contrast observed in magnetic resonance images was found to be proportional to the expression level of HER-2/neu receptors, which was 5×10^4 receptors per cell (Artemov et al. 2003). These experimental examples, in addition to others, prove the efficacy of metallic nanoparticles for use in breast cancer therapeutics.

4.3.2 POLYMERIC NANOCARRIERS

Polymers are one of the widely used carrier systems for the delivery of cancer drugs because of their functional properties that are favorable for loading and release of therapeutic molecules. Polymers that are used in drug delivery can be broadly classified into two groups: natural and synthetic polymers. The choice of polymer for use in cancer therapeutics highly depends on the mode of drug loading/delivery and site of application. Generally, the drug molecules are either physically entrapped or covalently bonded to the polymer backbone (Rawat et al. 2006). The widely used natural polymers for the design of cancer drug delivery system are albumin, chitosan, and heparin. For example, paclitaxel with serum albumin has been conjugated to form a drug polymer conjugate as formulation for the eradication of breast cancer cells (Gradishar et al. 2005). The widely used synthetic polymers for the design of cancer drug delivery system are PEG and poly(lactic-co-glycolic acid) (PLGA). The other form of delivery system for cancer treatment includes liposomes, micelles, and dendrimers. Figure 4.5 shows a schematic representation of nanocarriers being used in cancer therapeutics. Some of the common drug carriers approved by the US Food and Drug Administration (FDA) for treatment of metastatic breast cancer are Doxil (PEGylated liposomal system for doxorubicin [DOX] delivery) and Abraxane (albumin-bound paclitaxel nanoparticles). These drug conjugates have a half-life period 100 times greater than that of their free drug counterparts (Allen and Martin 2004; Desai et al. 2006; Gabizon and Martin 1997; Gabizon et al. 2003).

Polymeric nanoparticles play an important role in reducing the systemic toxicity of an anticancer drug, which is delivered to the targeted site for breast cancer treatment (Ashley et al. 2011; Min et al. 2010; Sethuraman et al. 2006). Rapamycin-loaded PLGA nanoparticles conjugated with antibodies have been used for targeting EGFR in breast cancer cells in order to observe the efficient delivery of anticancer drugs (Ashley et al. 2011). The long circulation and the ability of nanoparticles to

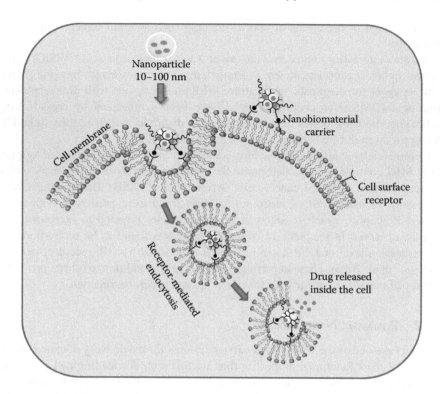

FIGURE 4.5 Schematic illustration of the nanocarrier uptake mechanism by cells.

extravasate through "leaky" tumor vasculature result in the localization of rapamy-cin in tumor tissue, thus promoting its efficiency in eradicating cancer cells (Ashley et al. 2011). It has been observed that polymeric nanocarriers associated with the drug tamoxifen have greater tissue penetration in breast cancer treatment of mice when compared to the liposomal delivery of DOX, which causes cardiological and neurological side effects (Yezhelyev et al. 2006). Albumin-bound (nab)-paclitaxel (Abraxane) (particle size, 130 nm) exhibited higher efficacy when compared with solvent-based paclitaxel (Taxol) and docetaxel (Taxotere) in metastatic breast cancer (Desai et al. 2008). It was found that the nab-paclitaxel enhanced tumor targeting through gp60 and caveolae-mediated endothelial transcytosis, and it was also associ-ated with the albumin-binding protein SPARC (secreted protein acidic and rich in cysteine) in the tumor microenvironment. The overexpression of HER-2 in breast cancer has been shown to correlate with the resistance to paclitaxel. The solvent-free formulation of nab-paclitaxel is also approved by the FDA for use in the treatment of metastatic breast cancer (Gradishar 2006). Karmali et al. (2009) demonstrated that the peptide Lyp-1 that recognizes tumor lymphatics was conjugated to nab-paclitaxel (Karmali et al. 2009). When compared to untargeted nab-paclitaxel, the Lyp-1–nab-paclitaxel conjugate produced a significantly higher inhibition of tumor growth. It has also been increasingly understood that the versatility of nab-paclitaxel is limited on the basis of drug release kinetics, drug chemotypes that can be loaded, and the ability of incorporating surface modifications (Karmali et al. 2009).

The liposome used for the targeted delivery of drug attains the efficient localization of drug inside the infected cells when compared to nontargeted drug delivery as shown in Figure 4.6. The combinatorial delivery of drugs and genes for breast cancer treatment has been attractive in recent years, and it was shown that in vivo studies for breast cancer treatment have been carried out by multitherapy carriers using combinatorial delivery of daunorubicin and tamoxifen of stealth liposomes (Mastrotto et al. 2013) and RGD-based co-delivery of siRNA and DOX (Jiang et al. 2010). Wang et al. reported that the combinatorial delivery of drugs and genes to MDA-MB-231 breast cancer cells is possible with high efficiency of drug delivery and high gene transfection (Wang et al. 2010a). The authors formulated PLGA/folate-coated PEGylated

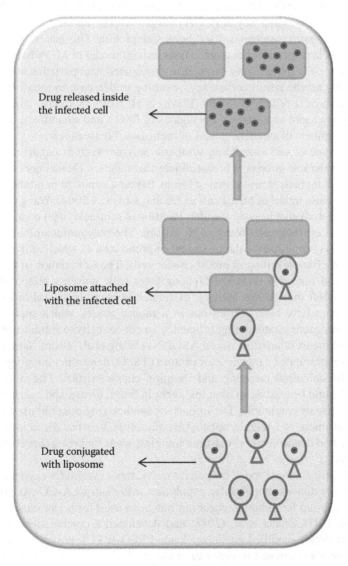

Drug released inside the infected cell

Liposome attached with the infected cell

Drug conjugated with liposome

FIGURE 4.6 Schematic of liposome-based targeted and nontargeted drug delivery systems.

polymeric liposome core–shell nanoparticles for the delivery of drug and genes. In this system, PLGA is the core, which helps entrap hydrophobic drugs such as DOX, and DNA binding on the hydrophilic cationic lipid shell has been carried out.

The recent advancement of a lipid-coated targeted nanogel drug delivery platform over polymeric nanocarriers helps encapsulate a wide range of drug chemotherapeutics, to display targeting ligands, to enhance drug retention within the nanogel core after photo-cross-linking, and to retain therapeutic activity after lyophilization for long-term storage (Murphy et al. 2011). This study has been carried out in taxane-loaded nanogels with human serum albumin (HSA) as the core where 15-fold increment in antitumor activity was observed by blocking primary tumor growth and spontaneous metastasis when compared to nab-paclitaxel (Murphy et al. 2011).

Sustained release efficiency of PLGA nanoparticles containing antisense has been demonstrated against osteopontin and bone sialoprotein. This has been evaluated in vitro and in a breast cancer bone metastasis animal model of MDA-MB-231 human breast cancer cells in nude rats. Antisense-conjugated nanoparticles were observed to exhibit higher therapeutic efficiency, resulting in decrease in tumor bone metastasis and in the size of lesions in rats (Elazar et al. 2010). In another study, the same group has developed nanoparticle conjugates of PLGA and alendronate for reducing osteoclast numbers in a murine model of metastatic breast cancer.

Another type of self-assembling synthetic polymer such as dendrimers has also been of considerable interest in breast cancer therapeutics. Dendrimers were used in the MRI of lymphatic drainage using G6 as the new nanosize paramagnetic molecule in the mouse model of breast cancer (Kobayashi et al. 2004). Wang et al. (2010b) formulated a study that helps in the identification of sentinel lymph node localization in breast cancer treatment (Wang et al. 2010b). The poly(amidoamine) (PAMAM) dendrimer has been used for the treatment of breast cancer, specifically for targeted delivery and efficient killing of breast cancer cells. The formulation of G4 polyamidoamine dendrimer (G4 PAMAM-D) conjugates with antisense oligodeoxynucleotides (ASODNs) showed less toxicity, more stability, and increased bioavailability. In vivo studies have been carried out in a mouse model, which showed that the conjugate has more accumulating efficiency in cancer cells to inhibit tumor vascularization of breast tumor than naked ASODNs (Wang et al. 2010b). Samuelson et al. (2009) have formulated a translocator protein (TSPO) dendrimer imaging agent with significantly enhanced targeting and imaging characteristics. The study revealed that TSPO could be used as an imaging agent in brain, breast, and ovarian cancer as well as in prostate carcinoma. The important synthesizing material used to produce TSPO dendrimers is 1-(2-chlorophenyl)isoquinoline-3-carboxylic acid. Hence, the TSPO-targeted dendrimer is a real-time imaging agent for breast cancer (Samuelson et al. 2009).

Micelles are another type of polymeric nanocarrier system for cancer drugs. The biodegradable diblock amphiphilic copolymer mPEG-b-p(LA-CO-MCG) having a carboxylate group for platinum chelation has been used for breast cancer treatment (Xue et al. 2011). Zhang et al. (2012) had developed a combination of salinomycin and octreotide-modified paclitaxel-loaded PEG-B-PCL polymer micelles. This combination was designed in order to eradicate both breast cancer stem cells and breast cancer cells that cannot be eradicated by conventional chemotherapy (Zhang et al. 2012). Curcumin polymeric micelles have good water solubility and potential to meet intravenous administration requirements.

4.3.3 CERAMIC NANOCARRIERS

Ceramics are polycrystalline inorganic nonmetallic compounds including silicates, carbides, sulfides, and various refractory hydrides. The ceramics that are used for biomedical applications are commonly called bioceramics. Bioceramics are subcategorized into three types: (i) nearly bioinert (e.g., alumina and zirconia), (ii) bioactive (e.g., hydroxyapatite [HA] and bioglass), and (iii) bioresorbable (e.g., tricalcium phosphate). Among them, calcium phosphate ceramics such as HA are often used in breast cancer therapy. Vechasilp et al. investigated the efficacy of HA with a binder of either alginate or chitosan impregnated with methotrexate on human mammary carcinoma cells (Vechasilp et al. 2007). The experimental results showed that both composites (HA–methotrexate–alginate and HA–methotrexate–chitosan) could release methotrexate for over a month. The striking finding of the work was that the composite using alginate as a binder released a significantly greater amount of methotrexate than that using chitosan as a binder ($p < 0.05$). The elution of both composites showed favorable cytotoxicity (to have a cytotoxic effect of >80%) when the concentration was greater than 5 µg/ml.

Ciocca et al. (2007) optimized an approach to produce an autologous therapeutic antitumor vaccine using HA for vaccinating cancer patients (Ciocca et al. 2007). The novel approach involved (i) the purification of part of the self-tumor antigens/adjuvants using column chromatography with HA, (ii) the use of HA as a medium to attract antigen-presenting cells (APCs) to the vaccination site, and (iii) the use of HA as a vector to present in vivo the tumor antigens and adjuvants to the patient's APCs. The vaccine was prepared by combining HA particles with at least three heat shock proteins and with proteins from the cell membrane system (including Hsp70, Hsp27, and membrane proteins). The work concluded that therapeutic vaccines based on HA ceramic particles and self-antigens can be safely administered and have shown encouraging clinical results in cancer patients.

4.3.4 CNT-BASED NANOCARRIERS

CNTs have generated great interest in biology, where suitably modified CNTs can serve as vaccine delivery systems or protein transporters because CNTs are noted ideal materials for several applications, ranging from ultrastrong fibers to field emission displays (Bianco et al. 2005). A notable characteristic of fluorescent-labeled CNTs (f-CNTs) is their high propensity to cross cell membrane. f-CNT was easily internalized and could be tracked into the cytoplasm or the nucleus of fibroblasts using epifluorescence and confocal microscopy through the mechanism of passive and endocytosis-independent uptake. Organic functionalization has led to the advancement in the study of the biological properties of CNTs. In an interesting study, Shao et al. (2007) hypothesized that monoclonal antibodies that are specific to the IGF1 receptor and HER-2 cell surface antigens could be bound to single-walled CNTs (SWCNTs) in order to concentrate SWCNTs on breast cancer cells for specific near-infrared phototherapy (Shao et al. 2007). Human MCF7 ER+ breast cancer cells exhibit high expression of IGF1R and thus were concluded to be a relevant surface marker for molecular targeting. SWCNTs functionalized with HER-2- and IGF1R-specific antibodies showed selective attachment to breast cancer cells compared to SWCNTs functionalized with nonspecific antibodies.

In vivo SWNT drug delivery has been demonstrated for tumor suppression in mice by conjugating paclitaxel (PTX) to branched PEG chains on SWNTs via a cleavable ester bond to obtain a water-soluble SWNT–PTX conjugate (Liu et al. 2008). In cell toxicity assay, the 4T1 murine breast cancer cell line was cultured in standard medium and treated with different concentrations of SWNT–PTX, PEG–PTX, or Taxol for 3 days. It was found that SWNT–PTX exhibited similar toxicity to Taxol and PEGylated PTX without any loss of cancer cell destruction ability. A significant result was the 10-fold higher tumor uptake of PTX afforded by SWNT carriers, which is a key factor for the higher tumor suppression efficacy of SWNT–PTX than Taxol and PEG–PTX. Prolonged blood circulation and EPR effects are responsible for the significantly higher tumor uptake of PTX in the SWNT–PTX case (6.4% ID/g at 2 h after injection) than Taxol (0.6% ID/g) and PEG–PTX (1.1% ID/g). PTX in Taxol is cleared from the blood and taken up by various organs especially the kidney and liver for rapid renal and fecal excretion with very low tumor uptake. Taken together, the uptake of drug–nanomaterial complexes by RES could serve as a scavenger system to eliminate toxic drugs as well as carriers. The one-dimensional shape and length of nanotubes render easy tagging of targeting ligands, drugs, and multiple molecules for synergistic effects.

4.3.5 Nanofiber-Based Nanocarriers

Nanofibers are widely used in tissue engineering and drug delivery applications because of their structure and properties analogous to native extracellular matrix (ECM). Peptide amphiphiles (PAs) are a typical example of nanofibers, and they are peptide-based molecules that self-assemble into high-aspect-ratio nanofibers. PAs have been employed in breast cancer therapy for the past few years and have three regions: a hydrophobic tail, a region of β-sheet forming amino acids, and a peptide epitope designed to allow solubility of the molecule in water, which performs a biological function by interacting with living systems. The resultant nanostructures can be designed to display bioactive peptide epitopes at high density on their surfaces (Silva et al. 2004). PAs have been investigated in vivo as a vital component for therapy in regenerative medicine, including central nervous system repair, bone and cartilage regeneration, angiogenesis for hind limb ischemia, and myocardial infarction (Tysseling-Mattiace et al. 2008).

The use of PAs to form multifunctional nanostructures with tumoricidal activity has also been reported (Toft et al. 2012). The combination of a cationic, membrane-lytic PA co-assembled with a serum-protective, PEGylated PA was shown to self-assemble into nanofibers. Degradation of the cytolytic PA by the protease trypsin was limited by addition of the PEGylated PA to the nanostructure, which led to an eightfold increase in the amount of intact PA observed after digestion.

In contrast to the above study, Soukasene et al. (2011) employed self-assembling PA nanofibers to encapsulate camptothecin (CPT), a naturally occurring hydrophobic chemotherapy agent, using a solvent evaporation technique (Soukasene et al. 2011). Encapsulation by PA nanofibers improved the aqueous solubility of the CPT molecule by more than 50-fold. In vitro studies using human breast cancer cells showed an enhancement in antitumor activity of the CPT when encapsulated by the PA nanofibers. These data highlight the potential of this model system to be adapted for delivery of hydrophobic therapies to treat a variety of diseases including cancer.

4.3.6 NANOGEL-BASED NANOCARRIERS

Nanogels are nanoparticles composed of a hydrogel and are most often made of synthetic polymers or biopolymers that are chemically or physically cross-linked. Nanogels are usually in the range of 10–100 nm in diameter, and they mimic the hydrated form of native ECM. Nanogels are recently recognized as a potential carrier system for cancer therapeutics. Na et al. (2007) fabricated DOX-loaded self-organized nanogels composed of hydrophobized pullulan (PUL)-NR-Boc-L-histidine (bHis) conjugates (Na et al. 2007). The designed nanogel responses to tumor extracellular pH were determined, and their anticancer efficacy against MCF-7 was evaluated. For pH-dependent releasing kinetics, DOX-loaded nanogels were assessed. The release rate of DOX from the PUL-DO/bHis78 nanogels increased significantly with reductions in pH. This resulted in increased cytotoxicity (30% cell viability at a dose of 10 μg/ml DOX equivalent) against sensitive MCF-7 cells at a pH of 6.8 and low cytotoxicity at pH 7.4 (65% cell viability at an identical dose).

Galmarini et al. (2008) designed a strategy of nanoencapsulation of anticancer nucleoside analogs (NAs) for efficient delivery to tumors because active NATP cannot be directly administered owing to instability and the therapeutic efficiency of NAs strongly depends on their intracellular accumulation and conversion into 5′-triphosphates (Galmarini et al. 2008). Stable lyophilized formulations of 5-triphosphates of cytarabine (araCTP), gemcitabine (dFdCTP), and floxuridine (FdUTP) encapsulated in biodegradable PEG-cl-PEI or F127-cl-PEI nanogel networks (NGC and NGM, respectively) were prepared by a self-assembly procedure. Cellular penetration, in vitro cytotoxicity, and drug-induced cell cycle perturbations of these nanoformulations were analyzed in MCF-7. Nanoencapsulated araCTP, dFdCTP, and FdUTP showed cytotoxicity and cell cycle perturbations similar to those of NAs. Nanogels without drugs showed very low cytotoxicity, although NGM was more toxic than NGC.

4.3.7 QUANTUM DOTS

Quantum dots are semiconducting nanoparticles often used in breast cancer therapeutics having optical properties, which can overcome some limitations that exist in conventional molecular profiling. They have enhanced photostability and intensified fluorescence properties with unique fluorescence emission peaks, which mark the absence of photo-bleaching and high diagnostic sensitivity, respectively (Gao et al. 2004). Different types of quantum dots can be conjugated to various antibodies to target the protein biomarkers in breast tumor cells, and spectra obtained from this combination can be quantified simultaneously in a single breast tumor section

(Haq et al. 2009; Xing et al. 2007; Yezhelyev et al. 2007). Therefore, using quantum dots as nanoparticles offers added advantages over conventional molecular profiling, which involves quantification of several proteins simultaneously on small tumor specimens.

Weng et al. (2008) have carried out in vitro studies using quantum dot–labeled liposomes, which encapsulate DOX and conjugate with anti-HER-2 antibody to target HER-2-expressing receptor breast cancer cells (Weng et al. 2008). This study showed an example of targeted drug delivery systems that can be processed for simultaneous imaging and treatment of breast cancer. The results showed that the quantum dot–labeled liposome system had efficient antineoplastic activity compared to control MCF-7 cells (Weng et al. 2008).

Xiao et al. (2005) have reported that the quantitative detection of estrogen receptor (ER), progesterone receptor (PR), and HER-2 can be done by quantum dot–based assay in paraffin-embedded cultured breast cancer cell lines and clinical tissue sections (Xiao et al. 2005). The expression of the biomarkers has been quantitatively correlated to semiquantitative Western blotting conventional immunohistochemical analysis, and HER-2 overexpression can be assessed by fluorescence in situ hybridization (FISH) along with immunohistochemical staining (Jain 2005; Yezhelyev et al. 2005b).

Along with quantum dots of different sizes and emission spectra, the Raman probes of gold-containing nanoparticles will help in the simultaneous detection and quantification of several various proteins such as ER, PR, and HER-2 small tumor samples, which leads to the tailoring of specific anticancer treatment to an individual patient's specific tumor protein profile (Jain 2005).

The established method of bioconjugation involves the use of streptavidin and biotin as adapter molecules and labeling the sample with a primary and a biotinylated secondary antibody, followed by incubation with streptavidin-coated quantum dots for the treatment of breast cancer (Wu et al. 2003). This method is easy to use and highly effective for single staining of cell proteins, but it is not the optimum method for multiplex protein detection.

Yezhelyev et al. (2005a) conjugated antibodies to semiconductor, multicolor nanoparticles (quantum dots), allowing the quantification of ER, PR, and HER-2/neu on single breast cancer sections, which correlated with Western blotting and immunohistochemistry (Yezhelyev et al. 2005a). The use of QD-Abs allowed the detection of proteins such as ER, PR, HER-2/neu, mTOR (mammalian target of rapamycin), and EGFR simultaneously on a single section of breast cancer cell lines and breast tumors.

Quantum dots offer a simple and precise method to trace nodes, which is an important factor in breast cancer treatment, that is, without the use of a dye or radioactive tracer. Owing to the nano size ranges, the quantum dots do not flow past a sentinel lymph mode. Song et al. (2009) reported that after injection of semiconductor nanocrystals of quantum dots into the skin of a breast tumor–bearing animal, the lymphatic flow was followed to a sentinel lymph node and its location was easily identified (Song et al. 2009). This study enables more precise and sensitive imaging using the near-infrared light source of sentinel nodes over longer periods. In vivo imaging may in turn improve the precision and safety of sentinel node biopsies.

4.3.8 Protein Nanocarriers

Protein nanoparticles as nanocarriers can be used for the targeted delivery of drug for breast cancer treatment since the surface of the nanoparticle can be modified to impart new functional groups or immobilization of biomolecules, which helps in the prolonged circulation of therapeutic molecules to enhance drug localization that facilitates an increase in the efficacy of drug and also a decrease in the chance of multidrug resistance from occurring (Kommareddy and Amiji 2007). For example, thiolated gelatin nanoparticles, which are modified by the stealth molecule PEG, enhanced the circulation time of the nanoparticles to reach the targeted tumor site primarily because of their hydrophilicity (Kommareddy and Amiji 2007).

The function of protein nanoparticles is limited by the absence of specific chemical conjugation sites. To introduce new functional groups suitable for breast cancer treatment, a new strategy was introduced where the organic molecules loaded into the cavity of the protein nanoparticle through noncovalent interactions and the concept of drug delivery have been tested in MDA-MB-231 breast cancer cells (Ren et al. 2012). The authors have designed the biomimetic model with generalized binding sites by multiple phenylalanine incorporation and by redesigning the caged protein scaffold; the DOX as the antitumor agent was delivered. The addition of more phenylalanine leads to greater drug-loading capacity. Compared to conventional nanoparticle delivery systems, this model shows higher drug-loading levels. The DOX-loaded protein nanoparticles can be taken up by the breast cancer cells with subsequent intracellular drug release to induce cell death (Ren et al. 2012).

It has been noticed that the chelating agent linked to protein-based drug carriers can induce anticancer activity in breast cancer cells. Michaelis et al. (2004) revealed that the chelating agent diethylene triamine penta acetic acid (DTPA) inhibits human cytomegalovirus replication along with its potential to inhibit the activity of MCF-7 (Michaelis et al. 2004). To enhance cellular uptake, DTPA was coupled covalently to HSA molecules, HSA nanoparticles (HSA-NP), gelatin type B (GelB) molecules, and GelB nanoparticles (GelB-NP). This study showed that compared to the normal growth of cancer cells, a threefold reduced growth concentration was observed because of DTPA. This study concluded that coupling of DTPA to protein-based drug carrier systems increases its antiviral and anticancer activity probably by mediating cellular uptake (Michaelis et al. 2004).

Another interesting approach used in breast cancer treatment is the integration of nanocarriers with phage display techniques, which is used for targeted breast cancer therapy using MCF-7 breast cancer cells. In the landscape phage protein–based approach, the phage fusion proteins self-assemble with the liposomal drug carriers to create targeted nanoparticles with components coexisting in a compatible and synergistic form (Wang et al. 2011). The phage protein in the liposome does not affect the liposome morphology. It was found that liposomes are modified with MCF-7-specific phage fusion proteins (MCF-7 binding peptide, DMPGTVLP, fused to the phage PVIII coat protein), which offered strong bonding with target MCF-7 cancer cells but not with co-cultured, nontarget cells including C166-GFP and NIH3T3. The free binding peptide addition, DMPGTVLP, competitively inhibited the interaction of MCF-7-specific phage–liposome with target MCF-7 cells but showed no reduction of MCF-7-associated plain liposomes (Wang et al. 2011).

Otis et al. (2013) formulated peptide nanostructures from artificial crown such as ether amino acids made from L-3,4-dihydroxyphenylalanine that has been used for breast cancer treatment (Otis et al. 2013). Similar to the natural channel proteins, the design and development of peptide nanostructures help create ions or channels by aligning crown ethers in such a way that it forms alpha helical conformation. It has been said that the analogs of channel peptide nanostructures showed cytotoxicity against different cancer cells. The appropriate nanoscale length of the crown peptide has the ability to span the membrane to cause cytotoxicity in cells (Otis et al. 2013).

4.4 ALTERNATIVE THERAPEUTIC STRATEGIES

There are a few other techniques that are also being used in the treatment of breast cancer apart from the carrier systems discussed earlier. Hyperthermia and photo⁻dynamic therapy (PDT) are the most notable treatment strategies used for breast cancer treatment. Sadeghi-Aliabadi et al. (2013) reported that the minimal heat (42°C–45°C) used in hyperthermia is an effective cancer therapy treatment (Sadeghi-Aliabadi et al. 2013). The authors used magnetite nanoparticles to produce heat, which have been prepared via co-precipitation method. The cytotoxicity of nanoparticles has been evaluated by suspending the magnetite nanoparticles in liquid paraffin, DOX, and a mixture of both; they were then added to MDA-MB-468 cells in separate 15-ml tubes and were allowed to stand at room temperature or be subjected to magnetic field for 30 min. The results showed that at room temperature, magnetite nanoparticles alone were not cytotoxic, but when exposed to the magnetic field, more than 50% of cells were dead. Along with this, it has been observed that DOX in combination with magnetite helps kill more than 80% of the cells (Sadeghi-Aliabadi et al. 2013).

The ablation of cancer cells using radiofrequency heating techniques has been carried out in the past decades, accompanied by issues such as significant ablation of normal cells and inconsistent tumor ablation. This paves the way to develop a treatment via constant exposure to electric field using metallic nanoparticles that are more sensitive to breast cancer cells. The heating of functionalized antibody attached to the metallic nanoparticles induces necrosis in T47D breast cancer cells when exposed to nanosecond pulsed electric field. The electric field exposure between 60- and 300-ns pulses caused alterations in the cell viability and thermal ablation of cells in the range of 80% to 90%. These quantities of ablated cells were achieved using a cumulative exposure time 6 orders of magnitude less than most in vitro constant electric field studies (Burford et al. 2013).

PDT is used for the treatment of many cancers including breast cancer. Photosensitizers are light-sensitive elements, which are taken up by tumor cells more actively and are activated by light, and generate ROS, which causes cell death by necrosis or apoptosis. The general mechanism of PDT used to kill the tumorous cells is shown in Figure 4.7. Abo-Zeid et al. (2013) carried out a study where the efficacy of PDT was observed with the photosensitizer indocyanine green (ICG) through the investigation of TP53, HER-2, and TOP2A gene signals as breast cancer gene

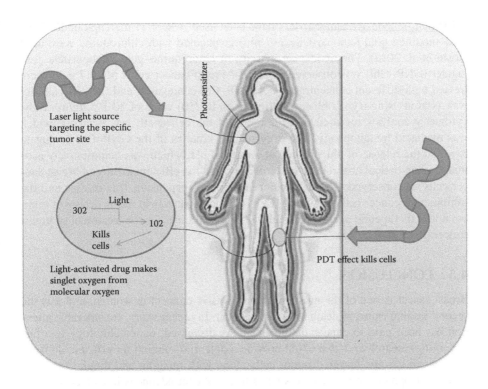

FIGURE 4.7   The general mechanism of PDT.

markers in MCF-7 breast cancer cells by interphase fluorescence in situ hybridization (nuc-FISH). The results showed that the viability of breast cancer cells was not reduced when they were treated with ICG followed by laser irradiation and incubation. The combination of ICG/PDT with laser irradiation exposure for 20 min reduced the cell viability after cell incubation in a time-dependent manner (12, 24, and 48 h) (Abo-Zeid et al. 2013).

In another study, Aggelidou et al. (2013) reported that the systemic or topical administration of 5-aminolevulinic acid (ALA) and its esters led to increased production and accumulation of protoporphyrin IX (PpIX) in cancerous lesions, which allows for effective application of PDT. In breast cancer treatment, the covalent bonding of PpIX with a drug carrier, β-cyclodextrin (βCD), was used to overcome the limitations that exist in the adjuvant chemotherapy of using large concentrations of exogenous ALA practically required to bypass the negative feedback control exerted by heme on enzymatic ALA synthesis and the strong dimerization propensity of ALA. The product is water soluble, because of which it was localized in the mitochondria and it can effectively solubilize the breast cancer drug tamoxifen metabolite *N*-desmethyl tamoxifen (NDMTAM) in water. The PpIX + βCD/NDMTAM complex was readily internalized by breast cells (Aggelidou et al. 2013).

Another interesting approach is the use of stimuli-responsive nanocarriers (which respond to various external and internal stimuli and act locally) that are being developed to improve the efficacy of current treatments. In this study, the pH stimuli-responsive nanocarriers have been used, where 11-mercaptoundecanoic acid–modified gold nanoparticles (~7 nm) conjugated with chloroquine were used (Joshi et al. 2012). The anticancer activity of chloroquine–gold nanoparticle conjugates (GNP–Chl) was observed in MCF-7 breast cancer cells. MCF-7 cells were treated with different concentrations of GNP–Chl conjugates, and the cell viability was assayed using trypan blue, resulting in an IC (50) value of 30 ± 5 µg/ml. Flow cytometry analysis revealed that the mode of the cell death was necrosis, which was mediated by autophagy. The drug release kinetics of the GNP–Chl conjugate revealed the release of chloroquine at an acidic pH, which was quantitatively estimated using optical absorbance spectroscopy, and the efficient killing of breast cancer cells was observed. Thus, the nature of stimuli-responsive drug release and the inhibition of cancer cell growth by GNP–Chl conjugates help in the design of combinatorial therapeutic agents, particularly nanomedicine, for the treatment of breast cancer (Joshi et al. 2012).

4.5 CONCLUSION

Breast cancer is one of the most common invasive cancers in women, and it is the second leading cause of death after lung cancer. In recent years, considerable attention has been paid to cancer therapeutics. As discussed, nanotechnology is a fast upcoming research area that could provide a potential solution for efficient delivery of drugs to specific targeted tumor cells along with imaging and diagnostics. The rapid development of nanocarriers leads to significant advances in cancer research and therapy that will help facilitate the noninvasive diagnostics and advancement in the analysis of tumor cells. The integration of nanotechnology into breast cancer therapy and diagnostics will have a great impact in improving breast cancer treatment in the near future where the ultrasensitive detection of metastasis with the help of contrast agents can be developed. The availability of nanocarriers for breast cancer treatment needs to be thoroughly analyzed with extensive safety testing such as toxicity and other side effects of the nanocarriers. Many nanocarrier-based drug formulations have already reached clinical trials. The success of these formulations and the materials to be developed keeping the above points in mind will decide the future of nanocarrier-based cancer therapy, with great challenges as well as great expectations ahead.

ACKNOWLEDGMENTS

This work was supported by the Centre for Stem Cell Research (CSCR). The authors would like to thank CSCR for the award of research fellowship.

REFERENCES

Abo-Zeid M.A.M., T. Liehr, S.M. El-Daly, A.M. Gamal-Eldeen, M. Glei, A. Shabaka, S. Bhatt, and A. Hamid, Molecular Cytogenetic Evaluation of the Efficacy of Photodynamic Therapy by Indocyanine Green in Breast Adenocarcinoma MCF-7 Cells, *Photodiagnosis Photodyn Ther*, 10, 194–202 (2013).

Aggelidou C., T.A. Theodossiou, and K. Yannakopoulou, Protoporphyrin IX-β-Cyclodextrin Bimodal Conjugate: Nanosized Drug Transporter and Potent Phototoxin, *Photochem Photobiol*, 89, 1011–1019 (2013).

Allen T.M., and F.J. Martin, Advantages of Liposomal Delivery Systems for Anthracyclines, *Semin Oncol*, 31, 5–15 (2004).

Artemov D., N. Mori, B. Okollie, and Z.M. Bhujwalla, MR Molecular Imaging of the HER-2/Neu Receptor in Breast Cancer Cells Using Targeted Iron Oxide Nanoparticles, *Magn Reson Med*, 49, 403–408 (2003).

Ashley C.E., E.C. Carnes, G.K. Phillips, D. Padilla, P.N. Durfee, P.A. Brown, T.N. Hanna, J. Liu, B. Phillips, M.B. Carter, N.J. Carroll, X. Jiang, D.R. Dunphy, C.L. Willman, D.N. Petsev, D.G. Evans, A.N. Parikh, B. Chackerian, W. Wharton, D.S. Peabody, and C.J. Brinker, The Targeted Delivery of Multicomponent Cargos to Cancer Cells by Nanoporous Particle-Supported Lipid Bilayers, *Nat Mater*, 10, 389–397 (2011).

Bassiouni Y., and L. Faddah, Nanocarrier-Based Drugs: The Future Promise for Treatment of Breast Cancer, *J Appl Pharm Sci*, 2, 225–232 (2012).

Bianco A., K. Kostarelos, and M. Prato, Applications of Carbon Nanotubes in Drug Delivery, *Curr Opin Chem Biol*, 9, 674–679 (2005).

Bickford L.R., R.J. Langsner, J. Chang, L.C. Kennedy, G.D. Agollah, and R. Drezek, Rapid Stereomicroscopic Imaging of HER2 Overexpression in Ex Vivo Breast Tissue Using Topically Applied Silica-Based Gold Nanoshells, *J Oncol*, 2012, 291898, 10 (2012).

Bleyer A., M. O'Leary, and R.R.L. Barr (eds.), *Cancer Epidemiology in Older Adolescents and Young Adults 15 to 29 Years of Age, Including SEER Incidence and Survival: 1975–2000*, National Cancer Institute, NIH Pub. No. 06-5767, Bethesda, MD (2006).

Boyle P., and B. Levin, *World Cancer Report 2008*, International Agency for Research on Cancer, Lyon (2008).

Brinton L.A., M.E. Sherman, J.D. Carreon, and W.F. Anderson, Recent Trends in Breast Cancer Among Younger Women in the United States, *J Natl Cancer Inst*, 100, 1643–1648 (2008).

Burford C.D., K.D. Bhattacharyya, N. Boriraksantikul, P.J.D. Whiteside, B.P. Robertson, S.M. Peth, N.E. Islam, and J.A. Viator, Nanoparticle Mediated Thermal Ablation of Breast Cancer Cells Using A Nanosecond Pulsed Electric Field, *IEEE Trans Nanobioscience*, 12, 112–118 (2013).

Canadian Cancer Statistics 2013, *Special Topic: Liver Cancer*, Canadian Cancer Society, Canada (2013).

Carmeliet P., and R.K. Jain, Angiogenesis in Cancer and Other Diseases, *Nature*, 407, 249–257 (2000).

Chen H., R. Ahn, J. Van den Bossche, D.H. Thompson, and T.V. O'Halloran, Folate-Mediated Intracellular Drug Delivery Increases the Anticancer Efficacy of Nanoparticulate Formulation of Arsenic Trioxide, *Mol Cancer Ther*, 8, 1955–1963 (2009).

Chen Z.G., Small-Molecule Delivery by Nanoparticles for Anticancer Therapy, *Trends Mol Med*, 16, 594–602 (2010).

Cho S.K., and Y.J. Kwon, Simultaneous Gene Transduction and Silencing Using Stimuli-Responsive Viral/Nonviral Chimeric Nanoparticles, *Biomaterials*, 33, 3316–3323 (2012).

Ciocca D.R., P. Frayssinet, and F.D. Cuello-Carrión, A Pilot Study with a Therapeutic Vaccine Based on Hydroxyapatite Ceramic Particles and Self-Antigens in Cancer Patients, *Cell Stress Chaperones*, 12, 33–43 (2007).

Desai N.P., V. Trieu, L.Y. Hwang, R. Wu, P. Soon-Shiong, and W.J. Gradishar, Improved Effectiveness of Nanoparticle Albumin-Bound (Nab) Paclitaxel Versus Polysorbate-Based Docetaxel in Multiple Xenografts as a Function of HER2 and SPARC Status, *Anticancer Drugs*, 19, 899–909 (2008).

Desai N., V. Trieu, Z. Yao, L. Louie, S. Ci, A. Yang, C. Tao, T. De, B. Beals, D. Dykes, P. Noker, R. Yao, E. Labao, M. Hawkins, and P. Soon-Shiong, Increased Antitumor Activity, Intratumor Paclitaxel Concentrations, and Endothelial Cell Transport of Cremophor-Free, Albumin-Bound Paclitaxel, ABI-007, Compared with Cremophor-Based Paclitaxel, *Clin Cancer Res*, 12, 1317–1324 (2006).

DeSantis C., R. Siegel, P. Bandi, and A. Jemal, Breast Cancer Statistics, 2011, *CA Cancer J Clin*, 61, 409–418 (2011).

Dhaheri Y.A., S. Attoub, K. Arafat, S. Abuqamar, J. Viallet, A. Saleh, H.A. Agha, A. Eid, and R. Iratni, Anti-Metastatic and Anti-Tumor Growth Effects of Origanum Majorana on Highly Metastatic Human Breast Cancer Cells: Inhibition of NFκB Signaling and Reduction of Nitric Oxide Production, *PLoS One*, 8, e68808 (2013).

Eghtedari M., A.V. Liopo, J.A. Copland, A.A. Oraevsky, and M. Motamedi, Engineering of Hetero-Functional Gold Nanorods for the In Vivo Molecular Targeting of Breast Cancer Cells, *Nano Lett*, 9, 287–291 (2009).

Elazar V., H. Adwan, T. Bäuerle, K. Rohekar, G. Golomb, and M.R. Berger, Sustained Delivery and Efficacy of Polymeric Nanoparticles Containing Osteopontin and Bone Sialoprotein Antisenses in Rats with Breast Cancer Bone Metastasis, *Int J Cancer*, 126, 1749–1760 (2010).

Elnemr A., T. Ohta, A. Yachie, M. Kayahara, H. Kitagawa, I. Ninomiya, S. Fushida, T. Fujimura, G. Nishimura, K. Shimizu, and K. Miwa, Human Pancreatic Cancer Cells Express Non-Functional Fas Receptors and Counterattack Lymphocytes by Expressing Fas Ligand; A Potential Mechanism for Immune Escape, *Int J Oncol*, 18, 33–39 (2001).

Ferrari M., Cancer Nanotechnology: Opportunities and Challenges, *Nat Rev Cancer*, 5, 161–171 (2005).

Gabizon A., and F. Martin, Polyethylene Glycol-Coated (Pegylated) Liposomal Doxorubicin. Rationale for Use in Solid Tumours, *Drugs*, 54 Suppl 4, 15–21 (1997).

Gabizon A., H. Shmeeda, and Y. Barenholz, Pharmacokinetics of Pegylated Liposomal Doxorubicin: Review of Animal and Human Studies, *Clin Pharmacokinet*, 42, 419–436 (2003).

Galmarini C.M., G. Warren, E. Kohli, A. Zeman, A. Mitin, and S.V. Vinogradov, Polymeric Nanogels Containing the Triphosphate Form of Cytotoxic Nucleoside Analogues Show Antitumor Activity Against Breast and Colorectal Cancer Cell Lines, *Mol Cancer Ther*, 7, 3373–3380 (2008).

Gao X., Y. Cui, R.M. Levenson, L.W.K. Chung, and S. Nie, In Vivo Cancer Targeting and Imaging with Semiconductor Quantum Dots, *Nat Biotechnol*, 22, 969–976 (2004).

García-Closas M., L.A. Brinton, J. Lissowska, N. Chatterjee, B. Peplonska, W.F. Anderson, N. Szeszenia-Dabrowska, A. Bardin-Mikolajczak, W. Zatonski, A. Blair, Z. Kalaylioglu, G. Rymkiewicz, D. Mazepa-Sikora, R. Kordek, S. Lukaszek, and M.E. Sherman, Established Breast Cancer Risk Factors by Clinically Important Tumour Characteristics, *Br J Cancer*, 95, 123–129 (2006).

Gradishar W.J., Albumin-Bound Paclitaxel: A Next-Generation Taxane, *Expert Opin Pharmacother*, 7, 1041–1053 (2006).

Gradishar W.J., S. Tjulandin, N. Davidson, H. Shaw, N. Desai, P. Bhar, M. Hawkins, and J. O'Shaughnessy, Phase III Trial of Nanoparticle Albumin-Bound Paclitaxel Compared with Polyethylated Castor Oil-Based Paclitaxel in Women with Breast Cancer, *J Clin Oncol*, 23, 7794–7803 (2005).

Hannun Y.A., Apoptosis and The Dilemma of Cancer Chemotherapy, *Blood*, 89, 1845–1853 (1997).

Haq A.I., C. Zabkiewicz, P. Grange, and M. Arya, Impact of Nanotechnology in Breast Cancer, *Expert Rev Anticancer Ther*, 9, 1021–1024 (2009).

Hu C.-M.J., S. Aryal, and L. Zhang, Nanoparticle-Assisted Combination Therapies for Effective Cancer Treatment, *Ther Deliv*, 1, 323–334 (2010).

Jain K.K., Personalised Medicine for Cancer: From Drug Development into Clinical Practice, *Expert Opin Pharmacother*, 6, 1463–1476 (2005).

Jemal A., R. Siegel, E. Ward, T. Murray, J. Xu, and M.J. Thun, Cancer Statistics, *CA Cancer J Clin*, 57, 43–66 (2007).

Jiang J., S.-J. Yang, J.-C. Wang, L.-J. Yang, Z.-Z. Xu, T. Yang, X.-Y. Liu, and Q. Zhang, Sequential Treatment of Drug-Resistant Tumors with RGD-Modified Liposomes Containing Sirna Or Doxorubicin, *Eur J Pharm Biopharm*, 76, 170–178 (2010).

Jiang W., B.Y.S. Kim, J.T. Rutka, and W.C.W. Chan, Nanoparticle-Mediated Cellular Response Is Size-Dependent, *Nat Nanotechnol*, 3, 145–150 (2008).

John T.A., S.M. Vogel, C. Tiruppathi, A.B. Malik, and R.D. Minshall, Quantitative Analysis of Albumin Uptake and Transport in the Rat Microvessel Endothelial Monolayer, *Am J Physiol Lung Cell Mol Physiol*, 284, L187–L196 (2003).

Johnston J., M. George, P.D. Karkos, R.C. Dwivedi, and S.C. Leong, Late Metastasis to Macroscopically Normal Paranasal Sinuses from Breast Cancer, *Ecancermedicalscience*, 7, 298 (2013).

Joshi P., S. Chakraborti, J.E. Ramirez-Vick, Z.A. Ansari, V. Shanker, P. Chakrabarti, and S.P. Singh, The Anticancer Activity of Chloroquine-Gold Nanoparticles Against MCF-7 Breast Cancer Cells, *Colloids Surf B Biointerfaces*, 95, 195–200 (2012).

Jun Y.-W., Y.-M. Huh, J.-S. Choi, J.-H. Lee, H.-T. Song, S. Kim, S. Yoon, K.-S. Kim, J.-S. Shin, J.-S. Suh, and J. Cheon, Nanoscale Size Effect of Magnetic Nanocrystals and Their Utilization for Cancer Diagnosis via Magnetic Resonance Imaging, *J Am Chem Soc*, 127, 5732–5733 (2005).

Karmali P.P., V.R. Kotamraju, M. Kastantin, M. Black, D. Missirlis, M. Tirrell, and E. Ruoslahti, Targeting of Albumin-Embedded Paclitaxel Nanoparticles to Tumors, *Nanomedicine*, 5, 73–82 (2009).

Kobayashi H., S. Kawamoto, Y. Sakai, P.L. Choyke, R. Star, M.W. Brechbiel, N. Sato, Y. Tagaya, J.C. Morris, and T. Waldmann, Lymphatic Drainage Imaging of Breast Cancer in Mice by Micro-Magnetic Resonance Lymphangiography Using a Nano-Size Paramagnetic Contrast Agent, *J Natl Cancer Inst*, 96, 703–708 (2004).

Kommareddy S., and M. Amiji, Biodistribution and Pharmacokinetic Analysis of Long-Circulating Thiolated Gelatin Nanoparticles Following Systemic Administration in Breast Cancer-Bearing Mice, *J Pharm Sci*, 96, 397–407 (2007).

Kumar M., M. Yigit, G. Dai, A. Moore, and Z. Medarova, Image-Guided Breast Tumor Therapy Using A Small Interfering RNA Nanodrug, *Cancer Res*, 70, 7553–7561 (2010).

Lee P.Y., and K.K. Wong, Nanomedicine: A New Frontier in Cancer Therapeutics, *Curr Drug Deliv*, 8, 245–253 (2011).

Lim Z.-Z.J., J.-E.J. Li, C.-T. Ng, L.-Y.L. Yung, and B.-H. Bay, Gold Nanoparticles in Cancer Therapy, *Acta Pharmacol Sin*, 32, 983–990 (2011).

Liu Z., K. Chen, C. Davis, S. Sherlock, Q. Cao, X. Chen, and H. Dai, Drug Delivery with Carbon Nanotubes for In Vivo Cancer Treatment, *Cancer Res*, 68, 6652–6660 (2008).

Mastrotto F., S. Salmaso, C. Alexander, G. Mantovani, and P. Caliceti, Novel pH-Responsive Nanovectors for Controlled Release of Ionisable Drugs, *J Mater Chem B*, 1, 5335–5346 (2013).

Mehlen P., and A. Puisieux, Metastasis: A Question of Life or Death, *Nat Rev Cancer*, 6, 449–458 (2006).

Michaelis M., K. Langer, S. Arnold, H.-W. Doerr, J. Kreuter, and J. Cinatl, Pharmacological Activity of DTPA Linked to Protein-Based Drug Carrier Systems, *Biochem Biophys Res Commun*, 323, 1236–1240 (2004).

Miele E., G.P. Spinelli, E. Miele, F. Tomao, and S. Tomao., Albumin-Bound Formulation of Paclitaxel (Abraxane ABI-007) in the Treatment of Breast Cancer, *Int J Nanomedicine*, 4, 99–105 (2009).

Min K.H., J.-H. Kim, S.M. Bae, H. Shin, M.S. Kim, S. Park, H. Lee, R.-W. Park, I.-S. Kim, K. Kim, I.C. Kwon, S.Y. Jeong, and D.S. Lee, Tumoral Acidic pH-Responsive MPEG-Poly(Beta-Amino Ester) Polymeric Micelles for Cancer Targeting Therapy, *J Control Release*, 144, 259–266 (2010).

Morawski A.M., G.A. Lanza, and S.A. Wickline, Targeted Contrast Agents for Magnetic Resonance Imaging and Ultrasound, *Curr Opin Biotechnol*, 16, 89–92 (2005).

Murphy E.A., B.K. Majeti, R. Mukthavaram, L.M. Acevedo, L.A. Barnes, and D.A. Cheresh, Targeted Nanogels: A Versatile Platform for Drug Delivery to Tumors, *Mol Cancer Ther*, 10, 972–982 (2011).

Na K., E.S. Lee, and Y.H. Bae, Self-Organized Nanogels Responding to Tumor Extracellular pH: pH-Dependent Drug Release and In Vitro Cytotoxicity Against MCF-7 Cells, *Bioconjugate Chem*, 18, 1568–1574 (2007).

Nelson H.D., L.H. Huffman, R. Fu, and E.L. Harris, Genetic Risk Assessment and BRCA Mutation Testing for Breast and Ovarian Cancer Susceptibility: Systematic Evidence Review for The U.S. Preventive Services Task Force, *Ann Intern Med*, 143, 362–379 (2005).

Nie S., Y. Xing, G.J. Kim, and J.W. Simons., Nanotechnology Applications in Cancer, *Annu Rev Biomed Eng*, 9, 257–288 (2007).

Noh J.M., D.H. Choi, S.J. Huh, W. Park, J.H. Yang, S.J. Nam, Y.H. Im, and J.S. Ahn, Patterns of Recurrence after Breast-Conserving Treatment for Early Stage Breast Cancer by Molecular Subtype, *J Breast Cancer*, 14, 46–51 (2011).

Otis F., M. Auger, and N. Voyer, Exploiting Peptide Nanostructures to Construct Functional Artificial Ion Channels, *Acc Chem Res*, 46, 2934–2943 (2013).

Peer D., J.M. Karp, S. Hong, O.C. Farokhzad, R. Margalit, and R. Langer, Nanocarriers as an Emerging Platform for Cancer Therapy, *Nat Nanotechnol*, 2, 751–760 (2007).

Rawat M., D. Singh, S. Saraf, and S. Saraf, Nanocarriers: Promising Vehicle for Bioactive Drugs, *Biol Pharm Bull*, 29, 1790–1798 (2006).

Ren D., M. Dalmau, A. Randall, M.M. Shindel, P. Baldi, and S.-W. Wang, Biomimetic Design of Protein Nanomaterials for Hydrophobic Molecular Transport, *Adv Funct Mater*, 22, 3170–3180 (2012).

Sadeghi-Aliabadi H., M. Mozaffari, B. Behdadfar, M. Raesizadeh, and H. Zarkesh-Esfahani, Preparation and Cytotoxic Evaluation of Magnetite (Fe3O4) Nanoparticles on Breast Cancer Cells and Its Combinatory Effects with Doxorubicin Used in Hyperthermia, *Avicenna J Med Biotechnol*, 5, 96–103 (2013).

Samuelson L.E., M.J. Dukes, C.R. Hunt, J.D. Casey, and D.J. Bornhop, TSPO Targeted Dendrimer Imaging Agent: Synthesis, Characterization, and Cellular Internalization, *Bioconjug Chem*, 20, 2082–2089 (2009).

Sethuraman V.A., K. Na, and Y.H. Bae, pH-Responsive Sulfonamide/PEI System for Tumor Specific Gene Delivery: An In Vitro Study, *Biomacromolecules*, 7, 64–70 (2006).

Shackleton M., E. Quintana, E.R. Fearon, and S.J. Morrison, Heterogeneity in Cancer: Cancer Stem Cells Versus Clonal Evolution, *Cell*, 138, 822–829 (2009).

Shao N., S. Lu, E. Wickstrom, and B. Panchapakesan, Integrated Molecular Targeting of IGF1R and HER2 Surface Receptors and Destruction of Breast Cancer Cells Using Single Wall Carbon Nanotubes, *Nanotechnology*, 18, 315101 (2007).

Sharma A., N. Jain, and R. Sareen, Nanocarriers for Diagnosis and Targeting of Breast Cancer, *Biomed Res Int*, 2013, 960821, 10 (2013).

Siddiqui M.A., M. Ahamed, J. Ahmad, M.A. Majeed Khan, J. Musarrat, A.A. Al-Khedhairy, and S.A. Alrokayan, Nickel Oxide Nanoparticles Induce Cytotoxicity, Oxidative Stress and Apoptosis in Cultured Human Cells That is Abrogated by the Dietary Antioxidant Curcumin, *Food Chem Toxicol*, 50, 641–647 (2012).

Silva G.A., C. Czeisler, K.L. Niece, E. Beniash, D.A. Harrington, J.A. Kessler, and S.I. Stupp, Selective Differentiation of Neural Progenitor Cells by High-Epitope Density Nanofibers, *Science*, 303, 1352–1355 (2004).

Song K.H., C. Kim, K. Maslov, and L.V. Wang, Noninvasive In Vivo Spectroscopic Nanorod-Contrast Photoacoustic Mapping of Sentinel Lymph Nodes, *Eur J Radiol*, 70, 227–231 (2009).

Soukasene S., D.J. Toft, T.J. Moyer, H. Lu, H.-K. Lee, S.M. Standley, V.L. Cryns, and S.I. Stupp, Antitumor Activity of Peptide Amphiphile Nanofiber Encapsulated Camptothecin, *ACS Nano*, 5, 9113–9121 (2011).

Tanaka T., P. Decuzzi, M. Cristofanilli, J.H. Sakamoto, E. Tasciotti, F.M. Robertson, and M. Ferrari, Nanotechnology for Breast Cancer Therapy, *Biomed Microdevices*, 11, 49–63 (2009).

Tang M.F., L. Lei, S.R. Guo, and W.L. Huang, Recent Progress in Nanotechnology for Cancer Therapy, *Chin J Cancer*, 29, 775–780 (2010).

Toft D.J., T.J. Moyer, S.M. Standley, Y. Ruff, A. Ugolkov, S.I. Stupp and V.L. Cryns, Co-Assembled Cytotoxic and Pegylated Peptide Amphiphiles Form Filamentous Nanostructures with Potent Anti-Tumor Activity in Models of Breast Cancer, *ACS Nano*, 6, 7956–7965 (2012).

Tysseling-Mattiace V.M., V. Sahni, K.L. Niece, D. Birch, C. Czeisler, M.G. Fehlings, S.I. Stupp, and J.A. Kessler, Self-Assembling Nanofibers Inhibit Glial Scar Formation and Promote Axon Elongation after Spinal Cord Injury, *J Neurosci*, 28, 3814–3823 (2008).

Vechasilp J., B. Tangtrakulwanich, K. Oungbho, and S. Yuenyongsawad, The Efficacy of Methotrexate-Impregnated Hydroxyapatite Composites on Human Mammary Carcinoma Cells, *J Orthop Surg (Hong Kong)*, 15, 56–61 (2007).

Wang H., P. Zhao, W. Su, S. Wang, Z. Liao, R. Niu, and J. Chang, PLGA/Polymeric Liposome for Targeted Drug and Gene Co-Delivery, *Biomaterials*, 31, 8741–8748 (2010a).

Wang P., X.-H. Zhao, Z.-Y. Wang, Z. Meng, X. Li, and Q. Ning, Generation 4 Polyamidoamine Dendrimers is a Novel Candidate of Nano-Carrier for Gene Delivery Agents in Breast Cancer Treatment, *Cancer Lett*, 298, 34–49 (2010b).

Wang T., N. Kulkarni, G.G.M. D'Souza, V.A. Petrenko, and V.P. Torchilin, On the Mechanism of Targeting of Phage Fusion Protein-Modified Nanocarriers: Only the Binding Peptide Sequence Matters, *Mol Pharm*, 8, 1720–1728 (2011).

Wang X., Y. Wang, Z.G. Chen, and D.M. Shin, Advances of Cancer Therapy by Nanotechnology, *Cancer Res Treat*, 41, 1–11 (2009).

Weng K.C., C.O. Noble, B. Papahadjopoulos-Sternberg, F.F. Chen, D.C. Drummond, D.B. Kirpotin, D. Wang, Y.K. Hom, B. Hann, and J.W. Park, Targeted Tumor Cell Internalization and Imaging of Multifunctional Quantum Dot-Conjugated Immunoliposomes In Vitro and In Vivo, *Nano Lett*, 8, 2851–2857 (2008).

Wooster R., and B.L. Weber, Breast and Ovarian Cancer, *N Engl J Med*, 348, 2339–2347 (2003).

Wu X., H. Liu, J. Liu, K.N. Haley, J.A. Treadway, J.P. Larson, N. Ge, F. Peale, and M.P. Bruchez, Immunofluorescent Labeling of Cancer Marker Her2 and Other Cellular Targets with Semiconductor Quantum Dots, *Nat Biotechnol*, 21, 41–46 (2003).

Xiao Y., W.G. Telford, J.C. Ball, L.E. Locascio, and P.E. Barker, Semiconductor Nanocrystal Conjugates, FISH and Ph, *Nat Methods*, 2, 723 (2005).

Xing Y., Q. Chaudry, C. Shen, K.Y. Kong, H.E. Zhau, L.W. Chung, J.A. Petros, R.M. O'Regan, M.V. Yezhelyev, J.W. Simons, M.D. Wang, and S. Nie, Bioconjugated Quantum Dots for Multiplexed and Quantitative Immunohistochemistry, *Nat Protoc*, 2, 1152–1165 (2007).

Xue Y., X. Tang, J. Huang, X. Zhang, J. Yu, Y. Zhang, and S. Gui, Anti-Tumor Efficacy of Polymer-Platinum(II) Complex Micelles Fabricated From Folate Conjugated PEG-Graft-A,B-Poly [(N-Amino Acidyl)-Aspartamide] and Cis-Dichlorodiammine Platinum(II) in Tumor-Bearing Mice, *Colloids Surf B Biointerfaces*, 85, 280–288 (2011).

Yezhelyev M., A. Al-Hajj, C. Morris, A. Marcus, T. Liu, M. Lewis, C. Cohen, P. Zrazhevskiy, J. Simons, A. Rogatko, S. Nie, X. Gao, and R. O'Regan, In Situ Molecular Profiling of Breast Cancer Biomarkers with Multicolor Quantum Dots, *Adv Mater*, 19, 3146–3151 (2007).

Yezhelyev M., C. Morris, X. Gao, A. Marcus, and R. M. O'Regan, Simultaneous and Quantitative Detection of Multiple Biomarkers in Human Breast Cancers Using Semiconductor Multicolor Quantum Dots Breast Cancer Research and Treatment, *Breast Cancer Res Treat*, 94 (Suppl. 1), S48 (Abstr. 1030) (2005a).

Yezhelyev M., C. Morris, X. Gao, S. Nie, M. Lewis, C. Cohen, and R.M. O'Regan, Multiplex Molecular Profiling of Breast Cancer Cell Lines with Quantum Dot-Antibody Conjugates, *AACR Meet Abstr*, 46, 510 (2005b).

Yezhelyev M., R. Yacoub, and R. O'Regan, Inorganic Nanoparticles for Predictive Oncology of Breast Cancer, *Nanomedicine (Lond)*, 4, 83–103 (2009).

Yezhelyev M.V., X. Gao, Y. Xing, A. Al-Hajj, S. Nie, and R.M. O'Regan, Emerging Use of Nanoparticles in Diagnosis and Treatment of Breast Cancer, *Lancet Oncol*, 7, 657–667 (2006).

Yoo K.-C., C.-H. Yoon, D. Kwon, K.-H. Hyun, S.J. Woo, R.-K. Kim, E.-J. Lim, Y. Suh, M.-J. Kim, T.H. Yoon, and S.-J. Lee, Titanium Dioxide Induces Apoptotic Cell Death through Reactive Oxygen Species-Mediated Fas Upregulation and Bax Activation, *Int J Nanomedicine*, 7, 1203–1214 (2012).

Zhang Y., H. Zhang, X. Wang, J. Wang, X. Zhang, and Q. Zhang, The Eradication of Breast Cancer and Cancer Stem Cells Using Octreotide Modified Paclitaxel Active Targeting Micelles and Salinomycin Passive Targeting Micelles, *Biomaterials*, 33, 679–691 (2012).

Zhou B.P., HER-2/Neu Blocks Tumor Necrosis Factor-Induced Apoptosis via the Akt/ NF-Kappa B Pathway, *J Biol Chem*, 275, 8027–8031 (2000).

5 Nanoparticles
A Promise for Host Defense Peptide Therapeutics

Carlos López-Abarrategui,
Anselmo J. Otero-González,
Annia Alba-Menéndez,
Edilso Reguera, and Octavio Luiz Franco

CONTENTS

ABSTRACT

Antibiotic resistance developed by bacterial and fungal pathogens is one of the current major health problems in the world; hence, the development of newer antimicrobial therapies based on novel antimicrobial molecules that diminish this resistance is urgently required. Antimicrobial peptides or, in a wider concept, host defense peptides (HDPs), a diverse set of peptides that are evolutionarily conserved to combat or enhance immunity to infections in all forms of life, could be a reassuring and complementary solution to this health emergency. Many antimicrobial peptides could combine antimicrobial activity with immunomodulatory and anti-inflammatory activities. Although bacteria and fungi have resistance mechanisms against these peptides, their multifunctionality can evade such resistance. HDPs exhibit a broad spectrum of activity against a wide range of microorganisms. Different mechanisms of action have been proposed for these molecules, which indicate that many of them could have more than one antimicrobial target at the cellular level. Many of them interact with plasma membrane (pore formation, physical and functional disorganization, or simply transit to localize intracellular targets). One of the main difficulties for the utilization of HDPs for microbial control is peptide inactivation by proteinases, which is a real resistance mechanism shared by multiple human pathogens. Also, inactivation in the presence of salts, serum, or microbial components is an additional cause of no *in vivo* activity. The preventive action of HDPs is controversial not only for its effectiveness itself but also from a cost–benefit point of view. The potential immunomodulatory effect of HDP is promising. The combination of new peptides with novel delivery techniques is another approach that could become effective for such peptides. Despite the success in preclinical models, the clinical results of these molecules have not been good enough to approve them for medical use. Alternatives to increase the stability, efficacy, and biodistribution of HDPs are required. Different nanosystems have been demonstrated to develop medical applications. Nanoparticles (1–100 nm) of different materials are characterized by large surface-to-volume ratio, with a large fraction of their atoms located at the surface with unsaturated coordination bonds. Nanoparticles basically are obtained by bottom-up procedures and by top-down routes. They can be functionalized by the incorporation, through acid–base reactions or coordination interactions, of molecular species to allow their conjugation to biomolecules or to provide functional properties. The antimicrobial activity of different types of nanoparticles has been demonstrated when metals exhibit antibacterial properties in their bulk. The antimicrobial effect of these metals increases at nanoscale dimensions. Conjugation of HDPs with nanoparticles could increase the antimicrobial activity of the combined parts. Nanoparticles could be a perfect carrier for HDPs because of their multifunctional activities.

Keywords: Nanoparticles, Antibiotics, Antimicrobial peptides, Host defense, Bacterial infection

5.1   INTRODUCTION

Nowadays, novel infectious diseases have emerged, many of which are responsible for life-threatening disorders (Snell 2003). A lack of new antibiotics for treatment of illnesses, combined with the appearance of multi–drug-resistant strains, has generated the imperative requirement for innovative strategies in the development of newer antimicrobial therapies (Arias and Murray 2009). Host defense peptides (HDPs) are an essential first line of defense against pathogenic infection, showing strictly correlated immunomodulatory and antimicrobial properties. They constitute a novel strategy for the development of antimicrobial therapies (Afacan et al. 2012). Since they mainly act over microbial membranes or host immune cells, HDPs have shown a wide spectrum of activity that included bacteria, virus, and fungi with an ability to cause infectious diseases (Mulder et al. 2013; Theberge et al. 2013). Furthermore, such compounds have also been the focus of attention because of their low risk of triggering microbial resistance owing to their multiple mechanism of action and, therefore, are also investigated as a novel class of antibiotics, additives, and vaccine adjuvants (Zhang and Sunkara 2014). Cathelicidins and β-defensins are among the most well-known classes of HDPs, which are commonly found in many different animal species (Silva et al. 2011).

Unfortunately, the preclinical success achieved with these molecules has not been translated to the clinic yet (Eckert 2011). The instability, efficacy, and biodistribution of HDPs in clinical trials have been the major drawbacks (Brogden and Brogden 2011). Development of nanoparticles for entrapment and delivery of HDPs could represent an alternative to bypass the abovementioned clinic obstacles (Brandelli 2012). Here, we provide an overview and discuss the potential application of nanoparticles conjugated to HDPs in overcoming infectious diseases.

5.2 HOST DEFENSE PEPTIDES

HDPs, formerly designed as host defense peptides, are widely spread in nature from prokaryotic organisms to vertebrates (Brown and Hancock 2006). These molecules are conserved elements of the natural immunity and have a broad-ranging activity against infectious agents (Jenssen et al. 2006). They can modulate cell functions such as chemoattraction, gene transcription, and cytokine production or release. Also, these peptides may be involved in wound healing and angiogenesis (Lai and Gallo 2009).

HDPs are generally small molecules currently containing approximately 12–50 amino acid residues (molecular weight generally <10 kDa), cationic (net charge of +2 to +7), and frequently quite hydrophobic (Brown and Hancock 2006; Jenssen et al. 2006; Yount et al. 2006). Many of these peptides suffer different posttranscriptional modifications, with disulfide bond formation and C-terminal amidation as the most common ones (Andreu and Rivas 1998). For example, defensins are a widely distributed family of HDPs characterized by specific rearrangements of disulfide bridges (Selsted and Ouellette 2005). The disulfide bridges improve proteolysis resistance and, in some cases, seem to be fundamental for microbial killing (Tanabe et al. 2007; Wanniarachchi et al. 2011), while in others, they do not appear to be a requirement for direct antimicrobial activity (Mandal et al. 2002; Schroeder et al. 2011). On the other hand, some antimicrobial peptides such as clavanins (Lee et al. 1997) present a C-terminal amidation that confers resistance to proteolysis by carboxypeptidases and increases the cationic charge of the molecule (Andreu and Rivas 1998).

Generally, HDPs are genetically encoded molecules included together in multigenic families such as defensins, cathelicidins, cecropins, and dermaseptins (Patrzykat and Douglas 2005). The expression of these molecules could be constitutive or inducible. In prokaryotes, the production of bacteriocins, which are bacterially produced antimicrobial peptides, is generally regulated by a quorum-sensing mechanism of autoinduction when arriving at a certain cell density (Turovskiy et al. 2007). On the other hand, in eukaryotes, the expression of several HDP genes is regulated in different physiological stages: infection (Diamond and Bevins 1994), injury or inflammation (Dorschner et al. 2001), and stress (Aberg et al. 2007). That situation depends on the stimulation and the cell type and it is controlled or synchronized with the expression of other elements of natural immunity and inflammation (Braff and Gallo 2006; Selsted and Ouellette 2005).

According to their secondary structure in solution, these molecules can be generally classified into one of four structural classes: (1) α-helix, (2) β-sheet stabilized by two or three disulfide bridges, (3) extended structures with one or more predominant residues (like tryptophan and proline rich), and (4) loop owing to the presence of a single disulfide bridge (Jenssen et al. 2006; Lai and Gallo 2009). Many of these peptides exist in a relatively unstructured conformation in solution and fold into their ultimate arrangement when interacting with the unique environment of biological membranes (Tossi et al. 2000). The capability to interact with lipid bilayers is essential for the diverse antimicrobial activities of HDPs, although complete membrane destabilization is not always required (Zasloff 2002). The enormous potential of HDPs to interact with biological membranes might bring some concerns on the possible toxicity of HDP-based therapy to host cells, and thus, the selectivity of these molecules constitutes an important issue.

5.3   MECHANISM OF ACTION OF HDPs

Regarding HDPs' mechanism of action, not only are they antibacterial molecules (even against strains resistant to conventional antibiotics) (Miyakawa et al. 1996; Saiman et al. 2001), they could also have antimicrobial activity against fungi (Silva et al. 2014), enveloped viruses like HIV and influenza (Chang et al. 2005; Salvatore et al. 2007), and protozoan parasites as important as *Plasmodium falciparum* (Gelhaus et al. 2008), *Trypanosoma cruzi*, and *Leishmania braziliensis* (Lofgren et al. 2007). Moreover, their toxicity toward cancerous cells has been documented (Do et al. 2014; Hsu et al. 2011). This antimicrobial activity could be by direct action against microbial cells or by an indirect activation of cells from the innate immune system at the site of infection (Alba et al. 2012; López-Abarrategui and Otero-Gonzalez 2013).

HDPs can deal with the lipid bilayer producing cellular death by different mechanisms: (1) changing membrane potential (Westerhoff et al. 1989), (2) transmembrane pore formation (Matsuzaki 1998), (3) modifying the current distribution of membrane lipids with destabilization of membrane structure (Matsuzaki et al. 1996), (4) triggering lethal processes such as the induction of autolytic enzymes (Bierbaum and Sahl 1985), and (5) striking crucial intracellular targets after membrane penetration (Cudic and Otvos 2002; De Brucker et al. 2011; Scocchi et al. 2011). All these different routes underlying the direct antimicrobial activity of HDPs require an initial interaction with biological bilayers, and therefore, the use of model membranes has been widely accepted for learning about this interaction (Hancock and Rozek 2002). The different models proposed can be divided into transmembrane pore models, which imply the formation of actual membrane pores or nonpore ones instead (Wimley and Hristova 2011).

Furthermore, even when the nonspecificity between the interaction of HDPs and membrane lipids has been widely accepted, recent data reveal a more complex scenario. The affinity of some defensins for some specific microbial lipids has been demonstrated (Wilmes et al. 2011). *In vitro*, the inhibition of cell wall synthesis combined with binding experiments and nuclear magnetic resonance spectroscopy demonstrated that Plectasin, a fungal defensin produced by *Pseudoplectania nigrella*, inhibits the growth of Gram-positive bacteria through the binding to the cell wall precursor Lipid II (Schneider et al. 2010). Also, the inhibition of *Staphylococcus aureus* growing by the interaction of the invertebrate defensins Cg-Defh1, Cg-Defh2, and Cg-Defm, from the oyster *Crassostrea gigas*, with Lipid II has been demonstrated (Schmitt et al. 2010). On the other hand, the binding of the plant defensins DmAMP1 and RsAFP2 to sphingolipids has been demonstrated (Aerts et al. 2007; Thevissen et al. 2003). All these data confirmed the existence of the specific interaction of HDPs with components of microbial membranes. This type of interaction was derived from a novel antimicrobial mechanism that could be conserved between different species.

As has been discussed, many of the mechanisms proposed for describing HDP–membrane interaction are derived from experimental data achieved with model membrane, and therefore, the conclusions might be limited. Also, the relevance of these considerations is limited in relation to *in vivo* infection experiments where the pharmacokinetic properties of peptides (Brinch et al. 2009), serum inhibition of peptide activity (Selsted and Ouellette 2005), and microbial resistance mechanisms (Kraus and Peschel 2006) could influence the active doses needed to eliminate the infection. For example, according to Selsted and Ouellette (2005), under physiological conditions, it is necessary for 1–10 mg/ml of defensin to be fungicidal, conditions only found locally in polymorphonuclear leukocytes, in phagolysosomes, and in the lumen of the crypts of Lieberkuhn. For this reason, it is not practical to consider a peptide-based therapy relying only on its direct antimicrobial activities. Instead, features like immunomodulation could complement and enhance the overall action of such peptides against infections. This balance could be critical in the success of peptide-based therapies.

5.4 HDP THERAPEUTICS

One of the main pitfalls for the utilization of HDPs for bacterial control is peptide inactivation by proteinases. HDP proteolytic inactivation is a real resistance mechanism shared by multiple human pathogens. In an interesting study using group A streptococci also known as GAS, the secretion of at least two factors, cysteine protease SpeB (Schmidtchen et al. 2002) and streptococcal inhibitor of complement (Frick et al. 2003), enabled *in vitro* inactivation of LL-37. Such hypothesis was also proven by Johansson et al. (2008) by using GAS *in vivo* models clearly showing SpeB-mediated LL-37 inactivation representing a bacterial resistance mechanism at severely infected tissue sites. Furthermore, as mentioned earlier, it is notable that HDPs' biological activities are frequently missing at physiologically significant concentrations of glycosaminoglycans, salt, and serum (Afacan et al. 2012). However, despite their enormous potential, are those peptides really effective at *in vivo* models? This is an important question to ask, since the *in vitro* activity does not reveal too much about the real activities of HDPs.

In this context, several *in vivo* trials using animal models have been performed in the last few years (Hilchie et al. 2013). Interestingly, the addition of HDP peptides before initiating infection in a mouse leads to infection reduction (Nijnik et al. 2010; Scott et al. 2007). Moreover, although an extremely weak antimicrobial activity, HNP-1 was able to protect mice from *S. aureus* and *Klebsiella pneumoniae* infections (Nizet et al. 2001). In principle, anti-infective HDPs' capability could be related to their ability to manipulate immune-cell functions (indirect activation of the innate immune system), direct antimicrobial activities, or a combination of both functions. Nevertheless, once bactericidal properties are mainly lost under physiological conditions (Afacan et al. 2012; Selsted and Ouellette 2005), it has been suggested that such peptides are anti-infective because of their immunomodulatory properties. This proposition was reinforced when the innate defense regulator peptide IDR-1, derived from bovine bactenecin, did not show *in vitro* antibacterial activities. However, such a peptide was extremely protective in several mouse models of bacterial infections (Scott et al. 2007). Surprisingly, such a peptide was protective when delivered topically or systemically through subcutaneous, intraperitoneal, and intravenous means and also effective when utilized after or before bacterial challenge. Undeniably, IDR-1 was capable of stimulating bacterial clearance by acting directly on the host innate immune response, decreasing tumor necrosis factor, and enhancing chemokine production including monocyte chemotactic protein-1.

Additionally, other IDR peptides including IDR-HH2, IDR-1002, and IDR-1018 were also effective in controlling *S. aureus* infections (Achtman et al. 2012; Rivas-Santiago et al. 2013). Moreover, IDR-1002 was also able to protect mice from invasive *Escherichia coli* infection but was unable to control *Mycobacterium tuberculosis* infections. Otherwise, IDR-HH2 and IDR-1018 were capable of reducing bacterial counts in mouse models of drug-sensitive and multidrug-resistant *M. tuberculosis* infections (Rivas-Santiago et al. 2013). Such data clearly suggest that structure and activity are clearly related, although it could be impossible to cross the specificity information for each bacterium. IDR-1018 was also evaluated in diabetic and nondiabetic wound-healing models (Steinstraesser et al. 2012). In such reports, IDR-1018 was compared to LL-37 and HDP-derived wound-healing peptide HB-107. IDR-1018 was suggestively less cytotoxic when compared to LL-37 or HB-107. Surprisingly, although there is complete inefficacy of IDR-1018 to control bacterial colonization, a significant improvement in wound healing in *S. aureus*–infected porcine and non-diabetic models was observed, improving the potential of IDRs and HDPs as pharmaceutical drugs.

Moreover, some studies have focused on polyalanine peptides. Among them is the multifunctional peptide Pa-MAP derived from the polar fish *Pleuronectes americanus* (Migliolo et al. 2012). Pa-MAP was evaluated in intraperitoneally infected mice with a sublethal concentration of *E. coli* (Teixeira et al. 2013), exhibiting the capability to prevent *E. coli* infection and the upsurge in mice survival, being as effective as ampicillin. In addition, mice treated with Pa-MAP have their weight loss reverted. Interestingly, despite other peptides having shown their main *in vivo* bactericidal activities related to immune response, no immunomodulatory activity was observed in such reports, suggesting that bacterial clearance activity obtained could be related to a direct bactericidal effect.

Another option is to discover not only novel peptides but also novel delivery techniques. For example, Ghali et al. (2009) established the viability of protein delivery via microvascular free flap gene therapy, challenging such approach for recalcitrant infections. In this context, authors investigated the LL37 production delivered by *ex vivo* transduction of the rodent superficial inferior epigastric free flap containing

Ad/CMV-LL37. A vascular permeabilizing agent, vascular endothelial growth factor, was also administered during transduction with adenoviral vectors in an effort to enhance transduction efficiency. Moreover, a rodent model of chronic wound infection sewn with bioluminescent *S. aureus* was utilized. Data obtained showed a significant reduction in bacterial loads from infected catheters owing to the expression of LL37 for 14 days, increasing bacterial clearance. Another option consists in the utilization of transgenic mice expressing HDPs. In this field, transgenic mice expressing human beta defensin 2 on different tissues including the intestine, trachea, lung, and skin were more resistant to *S. aureus* infection, despite not reaching complete protection (Zhang et al. 2006).

The pharmacological potentials are enormous and *in vivo* trials are just beginning. At the moment, the *in vivo* peptide activities are completely unpredictable and HDPs that show amazing *in vitro* activities could be extremely pharmacologically useless. Otherwise, peptides that show inconsiderable activities at bioassays could be amazing anti-infectives when challenged at *in vivo* models. The future of HDPs, as pharmaceutical drugs, is a complete open field and totally under construction.

Despite the success of HDPs in preclinical models, the clinical results of these molecules have not been good enough to approve them for medical use. There is no doubt that alternatives to augment the stability, efficacy, and biodistribution of HDPs are needed. Different nanosystems have emerged to develop biomedical applications (Kingsley et al. 2006; Seil and Webster 2012). In fact, some of them have been used to potentiate the activity of HDPs (Brandelli 2012; Urban et al. 2012).

5.5 NANOPARTICLES

Nanoparticles (metals, semiconductors, polymers, and magnets) have a size of between 1 and 100 nm and are characterized by large surface-to-volume ratio, and from this fact, a large fraction of their atoms are located at the surface with unsaturated coordination environments. These atoms are active species able to catalyze redox reactions and to form coordination bonds with surface guest molecules. These are probably the most attractive properties of nanoparticles for their application in biotechnology. For instance, the presence in transition metal oxide nanoparticles of partially naked surface metal sites explains their enzyme-like properties and microbial activity (Biju 2014; Ul-Islam et al. 2014). The coordination chemistry at the nanoparticle surface supports the possibility of their functionalization and conjugation to biomolecules to form programmable molecular engines with unique multifunctional properties, including molecular recognition, target-oriented biosensing, remote-guided nanodevices, and drug and gene transport and delivery, among others. The particles' core properties usually help in their interaction with external agents (e.g., they receive energy from an external source and liberate it in the form of heat into the biological environment). The hyperthermia treatment of cancer tumors using magnetic nanoparticles and a variable external magnetic field and the photodynamic therapy are good examples in that sense (Reddy et al. 2012; Vatansever et al. 2013). All these potential applications of nanoparticles in biomedical biotechnology will be briefly discussed below, with emphasis on the role of nanoparticles as antimicrobial agents conjugated or not with HDPs.

5.6   NANOPARTICLE PREPARATION, FUNCTIONALIZATION, AND BIOCONJUGATION

Nanoparticles, independently of their nature (metals, semiconductors, polymers, and magnets; inorganic, organic, and inorganic–organic hybrid), are obtained by two preparative routes: (1) bottom-up procedures, commonly using colloidal and coordination chemistry, molecular beam epitaxy, laser ablation, chemical vapor deposition, and so on; and (2) top-down routes, for example, milling or grinding (Faramarzi and Sadighi 2012; Sweet et al. 2012). Chemical routes, particularly those involving colloidal chemistry, allow appropriate control of particle size and shape, nanocrystal morphology, and surface active sites, which are structural features required for their biological applications, both *in vitro* and *in vivo*, including functionalization and bioconjugation. In this context, functionalization comprises the incorporation, through acid–base reactions or coordination interactions, of molecular species to the particles' surface to allow their conjugation to biomolecules or to provide functional properties for molecular recognition and separation, target modification and activation/inactivation, drug and gene delivery, bioimaging and sensing, and so forth (Schrofel et al. 2014). The chemical routes are also appropriate for tailoring the particles' composition, size, and shape, which determine their optical, electrical, thermal, and magnetic properties (Akbarzadeh et al. 2012).

The functionalization and bioconjugation of nanoparticles depend on their nature and surface composition. In this sense, silica nanoparticles illustrate the importance of the surface chemistry having an appropriate interface for the functionalization and bioconjugation processes. Silica is a hydrophilic and biocompatible material; it is transparent to the optical region of the electromagnetic spectral region and has a high physical and chemical stability. In addition, the preparative methods to obtain silica nanoparticles and mesoporous silica nanostructures from sol-gel and colloidal routes are well established, including the control of the pore size and shape (Trewyn et al. 2007). A wide diversity of reactive functional species (including carbonyl, primary and secondary amine, hydroxyl, azido, and alkyl halogen groups) can be incorporated into the silica surface during the preparative process through postsynthesis surface modification (Figure 5.1). Such reactive surface species, with both basic and acidic features, serve as anchoring sites for organic and biological molecules, including fluorescent markers, antibodies, nucleic acids, peptides, and proteins. Biological molecules have heteroatomic sites with basic and acidic characteristics able to form chemical bonds with the silica surface reactive groups. Practically all the available bioconjugation protocols are applicable for silica nanostructures (Trewyn et al. 2007).

The abovementioned features of silica support its incorporation to core@shell nanostructures, particularly when the core has limited chemical stability in biological environments or liberates toxic species (e.g., CdS luminescent quantum dots) or when the availability of an easily functionalizable shell is recommended. Quantum dots are semiconductor nanostructures (ZnS, ZnSe, ZnTe; CdS, CdSe, CdTe, ZnO, etc.) that absorb light in the UV-vis spectral region, promoting an electron from the valence band to the conduction band. Part of the energy of the resulting excited state is then transferred to the network solid as heat through the excitation of phonons

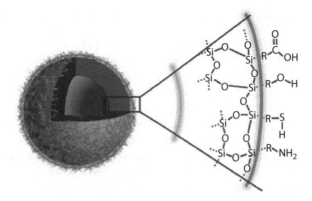

FIGURE 5.1 A nanoparticle (metallic, semiconducting, magnetic) with a surface layer (shell) of silica to facilitate its functionalization and bioconjugation. Indicated are four possible functional groups (R-NH$_2$, R-SH, R-OH, and R-CO$_2$H).

and that remaining is emitted as fluorescence, from trap states, in the visible and NIR spectral region. Both the spectral region where the quantum dot absorbs light and the region where it emits can be tuned, controlling its size and shape. The quantum efficiency for the emission process and the line width of the emitted light are controllable parameters through particle surface passivation incorporating a shell of appropriate molecular species (e.g., trioctylphosphine, trioctylphosphine oxide, etc.). The most important property of quantum dots, in the context of biomedical applications, is the tunable photoluminescence. This determines their application as fluorescent labels in analytical biochemistry, imaging, and sensing (Chinnathambi et al. 2014). Compared with organic fluorescent markers, quantum dots show a higher luminescence, with narrow emission lines, and are practically free of photo bleaching. The synthesis of high-quality quantum dots commonly involves the use of organic reagents, and the resulting nanoparticles are obtained with a surface layer of organic molecules with hydrophobic character. In consequence, their functionalization and bioconjugation must be preceded by an exchange of surface ligands. In order to prepare the surface for its further functionalization and bioconjugation, the ligand exchange reaction must produce a hydrophilic surface with available reactive species, for example, carboxyl, amine, and hydroxyl groups (Jiang et al. 2014; Kuzyniak et al. 2014). The degradation of quantum dots and the heavy metal liberation into the biological environment can be prevented, creating a thin surface coating of silica (Figure 5.1) and using the above-discussed benefits of this last material for the nanoparticles' functionalization and conjugation or growing a layer at the surface of a less toxic semiconductor, for instance, ZnX (X = O, S, Se, Te). In this last case, at the surface, an alloy or solid solution of the two semiconductors is formed, which also helps tune the emission spectra (Estévez-Hernández et al. 2012). Quantum dots have found applications in photodynamic therapy as well through their conjugation to photosensitizers. The energy of the excited state is transferred to the anchored sensitizer molecule and finally used for the singlet oxygen and reactive oxygen species (ROS) production (Biju et al. 2010).

Metallic nanoparticles have attracted considerable attention for biological applications not only because of their metal bioactivity but also because of their optical properties based on light absorption through surface plasmon resonance (Schrofel et al. 2014). Nanoparticles of silver and gold show a strong plasmon resonance effect in the UV-vis-NIR spectral region, which is tunable by modifying particle size and morphology and through the chemical species anchored to their surface. Plasmon resonance light absorption leads to a color change for the incident radiation, which is utilized for imaging the region where the nanoparticles are located. If the nanoparticles are functionalized with target-oriented groups, for example a monoclonal antibody, the optical spectra can be used for sensing purposes. The energy absorbed by the particle from the incident radiation is then partially liberated to the particle environment in the form of heat. This is exploited in photothermal cancer therapy. A fraction of the adsorbed light is reemitted as bright vis-NIR photoluminescence, which provides an image of the sites where the nanoparticles have been adsorbed (Schrofel et al. 2014). The surface plasmon resonance also supports surface-enhanced Raman spectroscopy, a technique with an ultrahigh sensitivity for adsorbed species on metallic surface. The adsorption of a molecule on a metal surface leads to an increase of approximately 10^{12} times in the Raman signal intensity. This technique allows the sensing of a single molecule when it is adsorbed on a metal nanoparticle, for instance, silver or gold. Such ultrahigh sensitivity makes possible the detection of quite a small amount of molecular pathological markers in biological fluids or tissues and for *in vitro* and *in vivo* marker-specific imaging (Schlücker 2010). Metals show strong x-ray absorption, and from this fact, the target-oriented biosensing and linking of metal nanoparticles to specific biological sites in tissues serve as contrast agent in x-ray imaging. Similar to quantum dots, as-synthesized metal nanoparticles usually require capping ligand exchange to allow their functionalization and bioconjugation. From such ligand exchange, nanoparticles with a wide diversity of reactive surface groups can be prepared, including carboxyl acids, amines, azides, maleimides, alcohols, amino acids, peptides, and proteins. These molecules have heteroatomic sites able to form a chemical bond with the surface metal sites. For instance, the conjugation of gold nanoparticles exchanged with thiolated carboxylic acids to peptides, proteins, amino acids, and antibodies is relatively simple (Shah et al. 2014).

Related to the large availability of carbon in nature, the wide diversity of carbon nanostructures (nanotubes, fullerenes, graphenes, nanodiamonds, and onions), and unique physical properties (strong absorption of light in the UV-vis-NIR spectral region, NIR photoluminescence, high photothermal response, tunable electrical behavior, etc.), the potential applications of carbon-based materials in biology and pharmacy are receiving increasing attention (Moon et al. 2009). Similar to silica, the surface of carbon nanostructures is functionalizable with a wide variety of reactive groups, among them, carboxylic acids, amides, phenols, alkyl halides, and alcohols. The conjugation to biomolecules and the incorporation in the surface of target-oriented molecules, for example antibodies, allow the conjugate sorption on specific molecular or tissue region for imaging, sensing, drug and gene delivery, or target modification. Target modification involves the therapy for cancer and microbial infections, through photothermal and oxidative stress effects. Carbon nanostructures show exceptional abilities for production of ROS, including singlet oxygen. The photothermal ablation of targeted cancer cells and tumors using NIR light or radiofrequency is an attractive research area currently in progress for the application of functionalized and bioconjugated carbon nanostructures (Moon et al. 2009).

Magnetic nanoparticles have additional attractive characteristics, compared with their metallic, semiconducting, silica- or carbon-based analogs, for biological and pharmaceutical applications. Magnetic nanoparticles are susceptible to remote guiding through an external magnetic field, and once they are located on the selected target, the application of an oscillating magnetic field permits local heating for target modification, including cellular death. This last possibility supports their potential application for cancer treatment. When magnetic nanoparticles are subjected to a time-varying magnetic field of low frequency (250 Hz), the particles receive energy from the applied magnetic field through orientation of their magnetic dipole moments, which is then liberated into the biological environment when they are disoriented (Figure 5.2). By this mechanism, the tumor is warmed to a temperature of 42°C–45°C, where the tumor cells are irreversibly damaged (Reddy et al. 2012). A heating time of approximately 30 min could be sufficient to destroy a tumor. Hyperthermia treatment of cancer is being intensively studied. It supposes that the magnetic nanoparticles are directed to and adsorbed by the target sites, by using an external magnetic field as well as through their functionalization with highly specific target-recognizing molecules, for example, monoclonal antibodies.

Nanoparticles of iron oxides, particularly of magnetite (Fe_3O_4), are the commonly used magnetic nanoparticles for biological and pharmaceutical applications. The preparation of this iron oxide is relatively simple; it can be obtained practically free of toxic by-products, and its tolerance for biological systems is high. The partially naked iron sites and the OH groups found at magnetite particles' surface are appropriate reactive species for their functionalization or bioconjugation. When a higher versatility for the functionalization is required or a higher chemical stability is recommended, a core–shell system with silica, $Fe_3O_4@SiO_2$, could be prepared (Figure 5.1). The applications of magnetic nanoparticles in biomedical sciences are diverse (Erathodiyil and Ying 2011; Lopez-Abarrategui et al. 2013; Reddy et al. 2012): analytical biochemistry for separation and concentration of analytes and

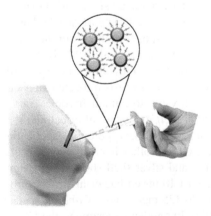

FIGURE 5.2 Localized drug delivery using magnetic nanoparticles and a magnetic tape.

molecular markers from biological fluids, drug and biomolecule transport and delivery in *in vivo* systems, chemoembolization for tumor vessel blockage in order to induce hypoxia, magnetically guided radioimmunotherapy, and as contrast agent for magnetic resonance imaging through the tuning of the transverse relaxation time.

5.7 ANTIMICROBIAL PROPERTIES OF NANOPARTICLES

The antimicrobial activity of different types of nanoparticles has been demonstrated. In fact, some metals like zinc, silver, and copper exhibit antibacterial properties in their bulk form. The antimicrobial effect of these metals increases at nanoscale dimensions (Seil and Webster 2012). The mechanism of action of these nanoparticles varies from one nanoparticle to another. Although these antimicrobial mechanisms are not fully understood, some are related to the damage caused by the physical structure of the nanoparticles, whereas others are associated with the release of metal ions from nanoparticle surfaces. For instance, the mode of action of silver nanoparticles is reliant on Ag+ ions, which interact with respiratory enzymes, the electron transport system, and DNA to inhibit microbial growth (Li et al. 2006).

The antibacterial activity against *S. aureus* of polysaccharide-reduced silver nanoparticles has been confirmed (Kemp et al. 2009). Furthermore, the inhibition (*in vitro* and *in vivo*) of different viruses by silver nanoparticles has also been established (Baram-Pinto et al. 2009; Rai et al. 2014; Xiang et al. 2013). Recently, an antimicrobial peptide (G3R6TAT) was conjugated to silver nanoparticles (Liu et al. 2013). The conjugated peptide showed enhanced antibacterial and antifungal activity compared with silver nanoparticles. These results suggest that silver nanoparticles have potential in antimicrobial therapeutic applications.

Antibacterial as well as antifungal activity has also been documented for ZnO nanoparticles (Jones et al. 2008; Siddique et al. 2013; Wahab et al. 2010). The mechanism of action of many of these ZnO nanoparticles involves the production of ROS (Dutta et al. 2012; Raghupathi et al. 2011).

Iron oxide is not antibacterial in its bulk form but may exhibit antibacterial properties as nanoparticles. For example, magnetite nanoparticles coated with quaternary ammonium were bactericidal against *E. coli* (Dong et al. 2011). Furthermore, bacitracin-conjugated iron oxide (Fe_3O_4) nanoparticles have shown higher antimicrobial activity against both Gram-positive and Gram-negative organisms, in comparison with the bacitracin peptide (Zhang et al. 2012). Because of this improved activity, conjugated magnetic nanoparticles allow lower dosages and collateral effects of the antibiotic. Moreover, cell cytotoxicity tests indicate that bacitracin magnetic nanoparticles show very low cytotoxicity to human fibroblast cells, even at relatively high concentrations. Because of their antibacterial effect and magnetism, the conjugated bacitracin magnetic nanoparticles have potential application in magnetic-targeting biomedical applications. On the other hand, the synthesis of multimodal nanoparticles with magnetic core and silver shell showed very significant antibacterial and antifungal activities against 10 tested bacterial strains (minimal inhibitory concentration [MIC] from 15.6 to 125 mg/l) and 4 *Candida* species (MIC from 1.9 to 31.3 mg/l) (Prucek et al. 2011). In another experiment, the HDP LL37 was conjugated to magnetic nickel nanoparticles coated with a nanolayer biofilm of polyacrylic acid. An

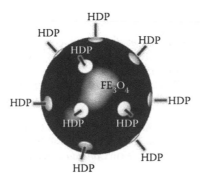

FIGURE 5.3 A possible conjugation route for HDPs to nanoparticles. The presence of gold islands or shell at the nanoparticles allows the peptide molecules to link to the nanoparticles' surface. This leads to the formation of multifunctional nanostructures.

effective bactericidal activity was demonstrated for the conjugated peptide (Chen et al. 2009). Similarly, citric acid–functionalized manganese ferrites were conjugated with the antifungal peptide Cmp5. The antimicrobial activity of the conjugated ferrites was higher than their bulk counterparts (Lopez-Abarrategui et al. 2013).

These results reinforce the importance of nanochemistry to fight different infectious diseases. On the other hand, the high affinity of gold for amino acids containing molecules can be used for HDP conjugation to magnetic and semiconductor nanoparticles, through the postsynthesis incorporation of a thin shell or islands of gold on the surface of magnetite or CdS, for instance (Odio et al. 2014). The adsorption of gold atoms on thiol-capped magnetite nanoparticles produces gold islands at their surface. The conjugation of peptides to such gold-containing nanostructures leads to the formation of multifunctional conjugates (Figure 5.3).

5.8 CONCLUSIONS

Despite the broad spectrum activity of HDPs and success in preclinical models, the clinical results of these molecules have not been good enough to approve them for medical use. Alternatives to reduce the toxicity and increase the stability, efficacy, and biodistribution of HDPs are urgently needed. Nanotechnology could provide a solution for these problems. Nanoparticles could be a perfect carrier for HDPs because of their multifunctional activities. Because the antimicrobial properties of both molecules have different mechanisms of action, the conjugated peptides (HDP–NP) could have an enhanced activity. The preparation and study of these multifunctional conjugates open unpredictable opportunities and result in biological and pharmacological applications to combating infectious diseases.

ACKNOWLEDGMENTS

We would like to thank the financial support of CNPq (project 490180-2011-6), Brazil, CAPES, FAPDF, FUNDECT, and the International Foundation of Science (IFS) (project IFS F 5199), Sweden.

REFERENCES

Aberg, K. M., K. A. Radek, E. H. Choi et al. 2007. Psychological stress downregulates epidermal antimicrobial peptide expression and increases severity of cutaneous infections in mice. *J. Clin. Invest.* 117 (11):3339–3349.

Achtman, A. H., S. Pilat, C. W. Law et al. 2012. Effective adjunctive therapy by an innate defense regulatory peptide in a preclinical model of severe malaria. *Sci. Transl. Med.* 4 (135):135–164.

Aerts, A. M., I. E. Francois, E. M. Meert, Q. T. Li, B. P. Cammue, and K. Thevissen. 2007. The antifungal activity of RsAFP2, a plant defensin from raphanus sativus, involves the induction of reactive oxygen species in *Candida albicans*. *J. Mol. Microbiol. Biotechnol.* 13 (4):243–247.

Afacan, N. J., A. T. Yeung, O. M. Pena, and R. E. Hancock. 2012. Therapeutic potential of host defense peptides in antibiotic-resistant infections. *Curr. Pharm. Des.* 18: 807–819.

Akbarzadeh, A., M. Samiei, and S. Davaran. 2012. Magnetic nanoparticles: Preparation, physical properties, and applications in biomedicine. *Nanoscale. Res. Lett.* 7 (1):144.

Alba, A., C. Lopez-Abarrategui, and A. J. Otero-Gonzalez. 2012. Host defense peptides: An alternative as antiinfective and immunomodulatory therapeutics. *Biopolymers* 98 (4):251–267.

Andreu, D., and L. Rivas. 1998. Animal antimicrobial peptides: An overview. *Biopolymers* 47 (6):415–433.

Arias, C. A., and B. E. Murray. 2009. Antibiotic-resistant bugs in the 21st century—A clinical super-challenge. *N. Engl. J. Med.* 360 (5):439–443.

Baram-Pinto, D., S. Shukla, N. Perkas, A. Gedanken, and R. Sarid. 2009. Inhibition of herpes simplex virus type 1 infection by silver nanoparticles capped with mercaptoethane sulfonate. *Bioconjug. Chem.* 20 (8):1497–1502.

Bierbaum, G., and H. G. Sahl. 1985. Induction of autolysis of staphylococci by the basic peptide antibiotics Pep 5 and nisin and their influence on the activity of autolytic enzymes. *Arch. Microbiol.* 141 (3):249–254.

Biju, V. 2014. Chemical modifications and bioconjugate reactions of nanomaterials for sensing, imaging, drug delivery and therapy. *Chem. Soc. Rev.* 43 (3):744–764.

Biju, V., S. Mundayoor, R. V. Omkumar, A. Anas, and M. Ishikawa. 2010. Bioconjugated quantum dots for cancer research: Present status, prospects and remaining issues. *Biotechnol. Adv.* 28 (2):199–213.

Braff, M. H., and R. L. Gallo. 2006. Antimicrobial peptides: An essential component of the skin defensive barrier. *Curr. Top. Microbiol. Immunol.* 306:91–110.

Brandelli, A. 2012. Nanostructures as promising tools for delivery of antimicrobial peptides. *Mini Rev. Med. Chem.* 12 (8):731–741.

Brinch, K. S., N. Frimodt-Moller, N. Hoiby, and H. H. Kristensen. 2009. Influence of antidrug antibodies on plectasin efficacy and pharmacokinetics. *Antimicrob. Agents Chemother.* 53 (11):4794–4800.

Brogden, N. K., and K. A. Brogden. 2011. Will new generations of modified antimicrobial peptides improve their potential as pharmaceuticals? *Int. J. Antimicrob. Agents* 38 (3):217–225.

Brown, K. L., and R. E. Hancock. 2006. Cationic host defense (antimicrobial) peptides. *Curr. Opin. Immunol.* 18 (1):24–30.

Chang, T. L., J. Vargas, Jr., A. DelPortillo, and M. E. Klotman. 2005. Dual role of alpha-defensin-1 in anti-HIV-1 innate immunity. *J. Clin. Invest.* 115 (3):765–773.

Chen, G., M. Zhou, S. Chen, G. Lv, and J. Yao. 2009. Nanolayer biofilm coated on magnetic nanoparticles by using a dielectric barrier discharge glow plasma fluidized bed for immobilizing an antimicrobial peptide. *Nanotechnology* 20 (46):465706.

Chinnathambi, S., S. Chen, S. Ganesan, and N. Hanagata. 2014. Silicon quantum dots for biological applications. *Adv. Healthcare Mater.* 3 (1):10–29.

Cudic, M., and L. Otvos, Jr. 2002. Intracellular targets of antibacterial peptides. *Curr. Drug Targets* 3 (2):101–106.

De Brucker, K., B. P. Cammue, and K. Thevissen. 2011. Apoptosis-inducing antifungal peptides and proteins. *Biochem. Soc. Trans.* 39 (5):1527–1532.

Diamond, G., and C. L. Bevins. 1994. Endotoxin upregulates expression of an antimicrobial peptide gene in mammalian airway epithelial cells. *Chest* 105 (3 Suppl):51S–52S.

Do, N., G. Weindl, L. Grohmann et al. 2014. Cationic membrane-active peptides—Anticancer and antifungal activity as well as penetration into human skin. *Exp. Dermatol.* 23 (5): 326–331.

Dong, H., J. Huang, R. R. Koepsel, P. Ye, A. J. Russell, and K. Matyjaszewski. 2011. Recyclable antibacterial magnetic nanoparticles grafted with quaternized poly(2-(dimethylamino) ethyl methacrylate) brushes. *Biomacromolecules* 12 (4):1305–1311.

Dorschner, R. A., V. K. Pestonjamasp, S. Tamakuwala et al. 2001. Cutaneous injury induces the release of cathelicidin anti-microbial peptides active against group A *Streptococcus*. *J. Invest. Dermatol.* 117 (1):91–97.

Dutta, R. K., B. P. Nenavathu, M. K. Gangishetty, and A. V. Reddy. 2012. Studies on antibacterial activity of ZnO nanoparticles by ROS induced lipid peroxidation. *Colloids Surf. B. Biointerfaces* 94:143–150.

Eckert, R. 2011. Road to clinical efficacy: Challenges and novel strategies for antimicrobial peptide development. *Future Microbiol.* 6 (6):635–651.

Erathodiyil, N., and J. Y. Ying. 2011. Functionalization of inorganic nanoparticles for bioimaging applications. *Acc. Chem. Res.* 44 (10):925–935.

Estévez-Hernández, O. L., J. González, J. Guzman et al. 2012. Mercaptopropionic acid capped CdS@ZnS nanocomposites: Interface structure and related optical properties. *Sci. Adv. Mater.* 4:771–779.

Faramarzi, M. A., and A. Sadighi. 2012. Insights into biogenic and chemical production of inorganic nanomaterials and nanostructures. *Adv. Colloid Interface Sci.* 1 (20):189–190.

Frick, I. M., P. Akesson, M. Rasmussen, A. Schmidtchen, and L. Bjorck. 2003. SIC, a secreted protein of Streptococcus pyogenes that inactivates antibacterial peptides. *J. Biol. Chem.* 278 (19):16561–16566.

Gelhaus, C., T. Jacobs, J. Andra, and M. Leippe. 2008. The antimicrobial peptide NK-2, the core region of mammalian NK-lysin, kills intraerythrocytic *Plasmodium falciparum*. *Antimicrob. Agents Chemother.* 52 (5):1713–1720.

Ghali, S., K. A. Bhatt, M. P. Dempsey et al. 2009. Treating chronic wound infections with genetically modified free flaps. *Plast. Reconstr. Surg.* 123 (4):1157–1168.

Hancock, R. E., and A. Rozek. 2002. Role of membranes in the activities of antimicrobial cationic peptides. *FEMS Microbiol. Lett.* 206:143–149.

Hilchie, A. L., K. Wuerth, and R. E. Hancock. 2013. Immune modulation by multifaceted cationic host defense (antimicrobial) peptides. *Nat. Chem. Biol.* 9 (12):761–768.

Hsu, J. C., L. C. Lin, J. T. Tzen, and J. Y. Chen. 2011. Pardaxin-induced apoptosis enhances antitumor activity in HeLa cells. *Peptides* 32 (6):1110–1116.

Jenssen, H., P. Hamill, and R. E. Hancock. 2006. Peptide antimicrobial agents. *Clin. Microbiol. Rev.* 19 (3):491–511.

Jiang, X., J. Bai, and T. Wang. 2014. Basics for the preparation of quantum dots and their interactions with living cells. *Methods Mol. Biol.* 1199:165–175.

Johansson, L., P. Thulin, P. Sendi et al. 2008. Cathelicidin LL-37 in severe Streptococcus pyogenes soft tissue infections in humans. *Infect. Immun.* 76 (8):3399–3404.

Jones, N., B. Ray, K. T. Ranjit, and A. C. Manna. 2008. Antibacterial activity of ZnO nanoparticle suspensions on a broad spectrum of microorganisms. *FEMS Microbiol. Lett.* 279 (1):71–76.

Kemp, M. M., A. Kumar, D. Clement, P. Ajayan, S. Mousa, and R. J. Linhardt. 2009. Hyaluronan- and heparin-reduced silver nanoparticles with antimicrobial properties. *Nanomedicine (Lond.)* 4 (4):421–429.

Kingsley, J. D., H. Dou, J. Morehead, B. Rabinow, H. E. Gendelman, and C. J. Destache. 2006. Nanotechnology: A focus on nanoparticles as a drug delivery system. *J. Neuroimmune Pharmacol.* 1 (3):340–350.

Kraus, D., and A. Peschel. 2006. Molecular mechanisms of bacterial resistance to antimicrobial peptides. *Curr. Top. Microbiol. Immunol.* 306:231–250.

Kuzyniak, W., O. Adegoke, K. Sekhosana et al. 2014. Synthesis and characterization of quantum dots designed for biomedical use. *Int. J. Pharm.* 466 (1–2):382–389.

Lai, Y., and R. L. Gallo. 2009. AMPed up immunity: How antimicrobial peptides have multiple roles in immune defense. *Trends Immunol.* 30 (3):131–141.

Lee, I. H., C. Zhao, Y. Cho, S. S. Harwig, E. L. Cooper, and R. I. Lehrer. 1997. Clavanins, alpha-helical antimicrobial peptides from tunicate hemocytes. *FEBS Lett.* 400 (2):158–162.

Li, Y., P. Leung, L. Yao, Q. W. Song, and E. Newton. 2006. Antimicrobial effect of surgical masks coated with nanoparticles. *J. Hosp. Infect.* 62 (1):58–63.

Liu, L., J. Yang, J. Xie et al. 2013. The potent antimicrobial properties of cell penetrating peptide-conjugated silver nanoparticles with excellent selectivity for Gram-positive bacteria over erythrocytes. *Nanoscale* 5:3834–3840.

Lofgren, S. E., L. C. Miletti, M. Steindel, E. Bachere, and M. A. Barracco. 2007. Trypanocidal and leishmanicidal activities of different antimicrobial peptides (AMPs) isolated from aquatic animals. *Exp. Parasitol.* 118:197–202.

Lopez-Abarrategui, C., V. Figueroa-Espi, O. Reyes-Acosta, E. Reguera, and A. J. Otero-Gonzalez. 2013. Magnetic nanoparticles: New players in antimicrobial peptide therapeutics. *Curr. Protein Pept. Sci.* 14 (7):595–606.

López-Abarrategui, C., and A. J. Otero-Gonzalez. 2013. Subcellular proteomics for understanding Host Defense Peptides mechanism of action. *Organelles Proteomics* 1:7–15.

Mandal, M., M. V. Jagannadham, and R. Nagaraj. 2002. Antibacterial activities and conformations of bovine beta-defensin BNBD-12 and analogs: Structural and disulfide bridge requirements for activity. *Peptides* 23 (3):413–418.

Matsuzaki, K. 1998. Magainins as paradigm for the mode of action of pore forming polypeptides. *Biochim. Biophys. Acta* 1376 (3):391–400.

Matsuzaki, K., O. Murase, N. Fujii, and K. Miyajima. 1996. An antimicrobial peptide, magainin 2, induced rapid flip-flop of phospholipids coupled with pore formation and peptide translocation. *Biochemistry* 35 (35):11361–11368.

Migliolo, L., O. N. Silva, P. A. Silva et al. 2012. Structural and functional characterization of a multifunctional alanine-rich peptide analogue from *Pleuronectes americanus*. *PLoS One* 7 (10):e47047.

Miyakawa, Y., P. Ratnakar, A. G. Rao et al. 1996. In vitro activity of the antimicrobial peptides human and rabbit defensins and porcine leukocyte protegrin against *Mycobacterium tuberculosis*. *Infect. Immun.* 64 (3):926–932.

Moon, H. K., S. H. Lee, and H. C. Choi. 2009. In vivo near-infrared mediated tumor destruction by photothermal effect of carbon nanotubes. *ACS Nano* 3 (11):3707–3713.

Mulder, K. C., L. A. Lima, V. J. Miranda, S. C. Dias, and O. L. Franco. 2013. Current scenario of peptide-based drugs: The key roles of cationic antitumor and antiviral peptides. *Front. Microbiol.* 4:321.

Nijnik, A., L. Madera, S. Ma et al. 2010. Synthetic cationic peptide IDR-1002 provides protection against bacterial infections through chemokine induction and enhanced leukocyte recruitment. *J. Immunol.* 184 (5):2539–2550.

Nizet, V., T. Ohtake, X. Lauth et al. 2001. Innate antimicrobial peptide protects the skin from invasive bacterial infection. *Nature* 414 (6862):454–457.

Odio, O. F., L. Lartundo-Rojas, P. Santiago-Jacinto, R. Martinez, and E. Reguera. 2014. Sorption of gold by naked and thiol-capped magnetite nanoparticles: An XPS approach. *J. Phys. Chem. C.* 118:2776–2791.

Patrzykat, A., and S. E. Douglas. 2005. Antimicrobial peptides: Cooperative approaches to protection. *Protein Pept. Lett.* 12 (1):19–25.

Prucek, R., J. Tucek, M. Kilianova et al. 2011. The targeted antibacterial and antifungal properties of magnetic nanocomposite of iron oxide and silver nanoparticles. *Biomaterials* 32 (21):4704–4713.

Raghupathi, K. R., R. T. Koodali, and A. C. Manna. 2011. Size-dependent bacterial growth inhibition and mechanism of antibacterial activity of zinc oxide nanoparticles. *Langmuir* 27 (7):4020–4028.

Rai, M., S. D. Deshmukh, A. P. Ingle, I. R. Gupta, M. Galdiero, and S. Galdiero. 2014. Metal nanoparticles: The protective nanoshield against virus infection. *Crit. Rev. Microbiol.* [epub ahead of print].

Reddy, L. H., J. L. Arias, J. Nicolas, and P. Couvreur. 2012. Magnetic nanoparticles: Design and characterization, toxicity and biocompatibility, pharmaceutical and biomedical applications. *Chem. Rev.* 112 (11):5818–5878.

Rivas-Santiago, B., J. E. Castaneda-Delgado, C. E. Rivas Santiago et al. 2013. Ability of innate defence regulator peptides IDR-1002, IDR-HH2 and IDR-1018 to protect against *Mycobacterium tuberculosis* infections in animal models. *PLoS One* 8 (3):e59119.

Saiman, L., S. Tabibi, T. D. Starner et al. 2001. Cathelicidin peptides inhibit multiply antibiotic-resistant pathogens from patients with cystic fibrosis. *Antimicrob. Agents Chemother.* 45 (10):2838–2844.

Salvatore, M., A. Garcia-Sastre, P. Ruchala, R. I. Lehrer, T. Chang, and M. E. Klotman. 2007. alpha-Defensin inhibits influenza virus replication by cell-mediated mechanism(s). *J. Infect. Dis.* 196 (6):835–843.

Schlücker, S. 2010. *Surface Enhanced Raman Spectroscopy: Analytical, Biophysical and Life Science Applications*. Weinheim, Germany: Wiley-VCH Verlag GmbH & Co. KGaA.

Schmidtchen, A., I. M. Frick, E. Andersson, H. Tapper, and L. Bjorck. 2002. Proteinases of common pathogenic bacteria degrade and inactivate the antibacterial peptide LL-37. *Mol. Microbiol.* 46 (1):157–168.

Schmitt, P., M. Wilmes, M. Pugniere et al. 2010. Insight into invertebrate defensin mechanism of action: Oyster defensins inhibit peptidoglycan biosynthesis by binding to lipid II. *J. Biol. Chem.* 285 (38):29208–29216.

Schneider, T., T. Kruse, R. Wimmer et al. 2010. Plectasin, a fungal defensin, targets the bacterial cell wall precursor Lipid II. *Science* 328 (5982):1168–1172.

Schroeder, B. O., Z. Wu, S. Nuding et al. 2011. Reduction of disulphide bonds unmasks potent antimicrobial activity of human beta-defensin 1. *Nature* 469 (7330):419–423.

Schrofel, A., G. Kratosova, I. Safarik, M. Safarikova, I. Raska, and L. M. Shor. 2014. Applications of biosynthesized metallic nanoparticles—A review. *Acta Biomater.* 10 (10): 4023–4042.

Scocchi, M., A. Tossi, and R. Gennaro. 2011. Proline-rich antimicrobial peptides: Converging to a non-lytic mechanism of action. *Cell Mol. Life Sci.* 68 (13):2317–2330.

Scott, M. G., E. Dullaghan, N. Mookherjee et al. 2007. An anti-infective peptide that selectively modulates the innate immune response. *Nat. Biotech.* 25 (4):465–472.

Seil, J. T., and T. J. Webster. 2012. Antimicrobial applications of nanotechnology: Methods and literature. *Int. J. Nanomedicine* 7:2767–2781.

Selsted, M. E., and A. J. Ouellette. 2005. Mammalian defensins in the antimicrobial immune response. *Nat. Immunol.* 6 (6):551–567.

Shah, M., V. D. Badwaik, and R. Dakshinamurthy. 2014. Biological applications of gold nanoparticles. *J. Nanosci. Nanotechnol.* 14 (1):344–362.

Siddique, S., Z. H. Shah, S. Shahid, and F. Yasmin. 2013. Preparation, characterization and antibacterial activity of ZnO nanoparticles on broad spectrum of microorganisms. *Acta Chim. Slov.* 60 (3):660–665.

Silva, O. N., K. C. Mulder, A. E. Barbosa et al. 2011. Exploring the pharmacological potential of promiscuous host-defense peptides: From natural screenings to biotechnological applications. *Front. Microbiol.* 2:232.

Silva, P. M., S. Goncalves, and N. C. Santos. 2014. Defensins: Antifungal lessons from eukaryotes. *Front. Microbiol.* 5:97.

Snell, N. J. 2003. Examining unmet needs in infectious disease. *Drug Discov. Today* 8 (1):22–30.

Steinstraesser, L., T. Hirsch, M. Schulte et al. 2012. Innate defense regulator peptide 1018 in wound healing and wound infection. *PLoS One* 7 (8):e39373.

Sweet, M. J., A. Chesser, and I. Singleton. 2012. Review: Metal-based nanoparticles; size, function, and areas for advancement in applied microbiology. *Adv. Appl. Microbiol.* 80:113–142.

Tanabe, H., T. Ayabe, A. Maemoto et al. 2007. Denatured human alpha-defensin attenuates the bactericidal activity and the stability against enzymatic digestion. *Biochem. Biophys. Res. Commun.* 358 (1):349–355.

Teixeira, L. D., O. N. Silva, L. Migliolo, I. C. Fensterseifer, and O. L. Franco. 2013. In vivo antimicrobial evaluation of an alanine-rich peptide derived from *Pleuronectes americanus*. *Peptides* 42:144–148.

Theberge, S., A. Semlali, A. Alamri, K. P. Leung, and M. Rouabhia. 2013. C. albicans growth, transition, biofilm formation, and gene expression modulation by antimicrobial decapeptide KSL-W. *BMC Microbiol.* 13 (1):246.

Thevissen, K., I. E. Francois, J. Y. Takemoto, K. K. Ferket, E. M. Meert, and B. P. Cammue. 2003. DmAMP1, an antifungal plant defensin from dahlia (*Dahlia merckii*), interacts with sphingolipids from Saccharomyces cerevisiae. *FEMS Microbiol. Lett.* 226 (1):169–173.

Tossi, A., L. Sandri, and A. Giangaspero. 2000. Amphipathic, alpha-helical antimicrobial peptides. *Biopolymers* 55 (1):4–30.

Trewyn, B. G., I. I. Slowing, S. Giri, H. T. Chen, and V. S. Lin. 2007. Synthesis and functionalization of a mesoporous silica nanoparticle based on the sol-gel process and applications in controlled release. *Acc. Chem. Res.* 40 (9):846–853.

Turovskiy, Y., D. Kashtanov, B. Paskhover, and M. L. Chikindas. 2007. Quorum sensing: Fact, fiction, and everything in between. *Adv. Appl. Microbiol.* 62:191–234.

Ul-Islam, M., A. Shehzad, S. Khan, W. A. Khattak, M. W. Ullah, and J. K. Park. 2014. Antimicrobial and biocompatible properties of nanomaterials. *J. Nanosci. Nanotechnol.* 14 (1):780–791.

Urban, P., J. J. Valle-Delgado, E. Moles, J. Marques, C. Diez, and X. Fernandez-Busquets. 2012. Nanotools for the delivery of antimicrobial peptides. *Curr. Drug Targets* 13 (9):1158–1172.

Vatansever, F., W. C. de Melo, P. Avci et al. 2013. Antimicrobial strategies centered around reactive oxygen species—Bactericidal antibiotics, photodynamic therapy, and beyond. *FEMS Microbiol. Rev.* 37 (6):955–989.

Wahab, R., A. Mishra, S. I. Yun, Y. S. Kim, and H. S. Shin. 2010. Antibacterial activity of ZnO nanoparticles prepared via non-hydrolytic solution route. *Appl. Microbiol. Biotechnol.* 87 (5):1917–1925.

Wanniarachchi, Y. A., P. Kaczmarek, A. Wan, and E. M. Nolan. 2011. Human defensin 5 disulfide array mutants: Disulfide bond deletion attenuates antibacterial activity against *Staphylococcus aureus*. *Biochemistry* 50 (37):8005–8017.

Westerhoff, H. V., D. Juretic, R. W. Hendler, and M. Zasloff. 1989. Magainins and the disruption of membrane-linked free-energy transduction. *Proc. Natl. Acad. Sci. U.S.A.* 86 (17):6597–6601.

Wilmes, M., B. P. Cammue, H. G. Sahl, and K. Thevissen. 2011. Antibiotic activities of host defense peptides: More to it than lipid bilayer perturbation. *Nat. Prod. Rep.* 28 (8):1350–1358.

Wimley, W. C., and K. Hristova. 2011. Antimicrobial peptides: Successes, challenges and unanswered questions. *J. Membr. Biol.* 239 (1–2):27–34.

Xiang, D., Y. Zheng, W. Duan et al. 2013. Inhibition of A/Human/Hubei/3/2005 (H3N2) influenza virus infection by silver nanoparticles in vitro and in vivo. *Int. J. Nanomedicine* 8:4103–4113.

Yount, N. Y., A. S. Bayer, Y. Q. Xiong, and M. R. Yeaman. 2006. Advances in antimicrobial peptide immunobiology. *Biopolymers* 84 (5):435–458.

Zasloff, M. 2002. Antimicrobial peptides of multicellular organisms. *Nature* 415 (6870): 389–395.

Zhang, G., and L. T. Sunkara. 2014. Avian antimicrobial host defense peptides: From biology to therapeutic applications. *Pharmaceuticals (Basel)* 7 (3):220–247.

Zhang, S., N. Huang, X. Zhao et al. 2006. [Construction and identification of HBD-2 transgenic mice]. *Sheng Wu Yi. Xue. Gong. Cheng Xue. Za Zhi.* 23 (2):396–399.

Zhang, W., X. Shi, J. Huang, Y. Zhang, Z. Wu, and Y. Xian. 2012. Bacitracin-conjugated superparamagnetic iron oxide nanoparticles: Synthesis, characterization and antibacterial activity. *Chem. Phys. Chem.* 13 (14):3388–3396.

6 Novel Nanostructured Bioactive Restorative Materials for Dental Applications

Mary Anne S. Melo, Lei Cheng, Ke Zhang,
Michael D. Weir, Xuedong Zhou, Yuxing Bai,
Lidiany K.A. Rodrigues, and Hockin H.K. Xu

CONTENTS

ABSTRACT

Dental restorative materials such as composites, glass ionomer cements, and adhesive systems are being widely used; however, they still have several drawbacks. Tooth restorations often fail and the replacement of failed restorations accounts for 50%–70% of all tooth cavity restorations performed. Nanotechnology has been applied to develop the next generation of dental restorative materials with desirable bioactive proprieties, to not only replace the missing tooth volume but also exert therapeutic effects to combat caries. Recurrent caries lesions around restorations have been the main reason for operative treatment failures. These lesions are related to oral biofilm accumulation and acid production. Nanomaterials with large surface-to-volume ratios and unique physical, chemical, and biological properties have demonstrated great potential to inhibit the formation of biofilms with improved caries inhibition efficacy. This chapter summarizes the ongoing advancement in studies of emerging functionalized nanoparticles as strategies for addressing dental restorative challenges. This includes new nanomaterials with potent antibacterial activity as well as remineralization capability, the combination of several bioactive agents together in resin for effective caries inhibition, and their promising *in vitro* properties and *in vivo* performance. Furthermore, research trends and future prospects in the area of resin-based dental materials with a wide range of applications in dental caries management are discussed. In addition, this chapter attempts to provide a glance into the potential future of these new nanomaterials to researchers in dental materials science, dental practitioners, and investigators in other related fields.

Keywords: Dental materials, Nanotechnology, Nanoparticles, Dental caries

6.1 INTRODUCTION

The micro-to-nano shift has provided tangible benefits in contemporary materials science.[1] In recent years, there has been an explosive growth in the application of nanotechnology in medicine and dentistry. Strategies based on nanotechnology are being developed to treat high-impact human diseases, such cancer and diabetes.[2] Despite much effort, dental caries still remain to be a widespread public health problem with significant medical and economic consequences.[3] The pathogenesis for dental caries is based on bacteria in dental plaques (biofilms) that metabolize dietary sugars to produce acids that then lead to tooth mineral loss.[4] The progressive dissolution of enamel and dentin could then lead to cavity formation. Resin composites and adhesives are increasingly popular in restorative procedures of cavities because of their esthetics and direct-filling capability.[5,6] The adoption of nanotechnology has improved the composite properties, especially in esthetics, and mechanical properties such as strength and fracture resistance.[7] For example, nanosized silica particles of diameters of approximately 40 nm were used in composites as reinforcement fillers.[8] Dental nanocomposites exhibited outstanding esthetics, had excellent polishability and surface finishing, and possessed an enhanced wear resistance.[9] The incorporation of nanoparticles into dental adhesive systems may also improve fracture toughness and adhesion to tooth tissues.

However, recurrent (secondary) caries lesions at the tooth-restoration interfaces still remain as the main challenge in restorative dentistry as represented in Figure 6.1 and are the primary reason for composite restoration failures; replacing the failed restorations accounts for 50%–70% of all tooth cavity restorations performed.[10,11] Dental resin composites tend to accumulate more biofilms and plaques *in vivo* than other restoratives.[12] The fact that resin composites accumulate more biofilms *in vivo* may also lead to the development of gingival inflammation.[13,14] Therefore, new restorative materials that are bioactive and can inhibit biofilm attachment and accumulation along with remineralizing tooth lesions need to be developed.

Nanotechnology is a promising approach for the development of the next generation of dental materials, not only to replace the missing tooth volume as traditional restorations but also to inhibit oral biofilms and remineralize tooth caries.[15] Recently,

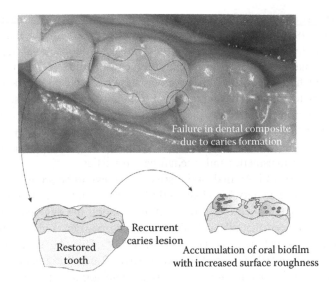

FIGURE 6.1 Schematic representation of a restored tooth showing the dental composite failure owing to oral biofilm accumulation and, consequently, formation of recurrent dental caries lesion, the primary reason for composite restoration failures.

nanotechnology was applied in developing functionalized nanoparticles for incorporation in dental materials.[16] This introduces opportunities for developing new strategies to prevent oral biofilm accumulation and repair the damage of mineral loss owing to bacterial acid attacks.[17] Based on nanotechnology, several agents with antimicrobial properties, such as silver, zinc oxide, and quaternary ammonium nanoparticles, were introduced into dental resins.[18] In addition, remineralizing agents such as calcium phosphates, calcium fluoride, and hydroxyapatite nanoparticles were also incorporated into dental resins. These agents imparted unique antimicrobial and remineralizing capabilities to dental restorations.[17] This chapter describes these and other new developments in nanostructured bioactive dental materials, as well as their antibacterial and caries-inhibiting properties.

6.2 ANTIBACTERIAL COMPOSITES AND BONDING AGENTS WITH SILVER NANOPARTICLES

The main cause of dental composite restoration failure is the occurrence of marginal leakage.[19] Detachment of the resin–tooth interface allows bacteria invasion into the gap with biofilm acid production, which eventually leads to marginal discoloration, secondary caries, and restoration failure.[20] A biofilm is a heterogeneous structure of bacteria consisting of clusters of various types of bacteria embedded in an extracellular matrix.[21]

Cariogenic bacteria such as *Streptococcus mutans* and lactobacilli in the dental plaque can metabolize carbohydrates to acids, causing demineralization of the tooth and the tooth-restoration margins beneath the biofilms.[22]

Nanoparticles of silver (NAg) were shown to possess effective antibacterial activity and require only a low concentration to be effective owing to their relatively large surface area-to-volume ratio.[23] The mechanism of antibacterial activity of Ag is based on the inactivation of bacterial enzymes, causing the DNA to lose its replication ability, which leads to cell death.[24] Ag was shown to have good biocompatibility and low toxicity to human cells and had long-term antibacterial effects.[25] Compared to traditional micrometer-sized Ag particles, the high surface area of nanoparticles potentially results in higher reactivity and stronger antibacterial activity.[26,27] For dental resin applications, a low filler level of NAg in resin is beneficial in order to not compromise the resin esthetics and mechanical properties.

The incorporation of NAg in dental resins was shown to be promising to achieve a strong antibacterial activity.[28,29] NAg could be formed in the resin *in situ*, without the need to mix nanoparticles with resin, thus avoiding the agglomeration issue.[30] A recent study showed that silver 2-ethylhexanoate powder could be dissolved in 2-(tert-butylamino)ethyl methacrylate (TBAEMA).[31] This Ag solution was then mixed into a resin at 0.05% mass fraction of silver 2-ethylhexanoate.[31] TBAEMA was selected since it contains reactive methacrylate groups and therefore can be chemically incorporated into a dental resin upon photopolymerization. This method produced NAg with a mean particle size of approximately 2.7 nm that were well dispersed in the cured resin matrix (Figure 6.2).[32]

Antibacterial dental nanocomposite was developed also by mixing filler particles into the resin containing NAg and then photopolymerizing the composite.[28,29] Using a dental plaque biofilm model, colony-forming unit (CFU) counts for total

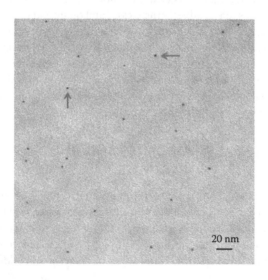

FIGURE 6.2 Representative transmission electron microscopy (TEM) images of nanoparticles of silver (NAg) in a dental resin. NAg were well dispersed in the resin matrix, without noticeable agglomeration. (Adapted from Cheng L et al., *J Dental Res* 2012; 91: 598–604. With permission.)

microorganisms, total streptococci, and *S. mutans* for nanocomposite with 0.042% mass fraction of NAg were approximately a quarter of those for commercial composite control (Figure 6.3).[31] Lactic acid production by biofilms on nanocomposite with 0.042% NAg was a third of that on commercial composite control. Metabolic activity of biofilms on nanocomposite with NAg was markedly reduced when compared to composite without NAg. In another study, different NAg mass fractions of 0.028%, 0.042%, 0.088%, and 0.175% were investigated and compared to controls (0%) to achieve antibacterial activity without reducing composite mechanical properties.[32] The composite containing 0.028% of NAg also showed great reductions in *S. mutans* biofilm CFU counts, metabolic activity, and lactic acid production, compared to two commercial control composites.[32] Furthermore, antibacterial composites containing NAg had strength and elastic modulus that matched those of a commercial composite control without antibacterial activity (Figure 6.4).[32]

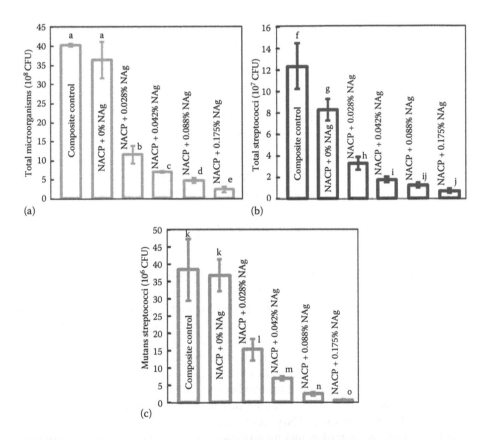

FIGURE 6.3 Dental plaque biofilm CFUs formed on the surface of composites containing different NAg mass fractions. (a) Total microorganisms, (b) total streptococci, and (c) mutans streptococci. Each value is (mean ± SD; $n = 6$). In each plot, values with dissimilar letters are significantly different ($p < 0.05$). The CFU counts on NACP nanocomposite with NAg were much lower than those without NAg and the commercial composite control. (Adapted from Cheng L et al., *J Biomed Mater Res B* 2012; 100: 1378–1386. With permission.)

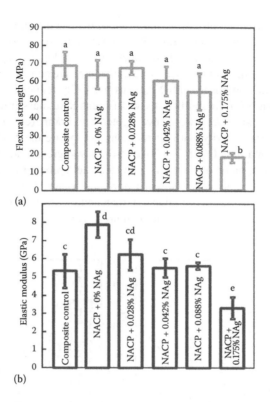

FIGURE 6.4 Mechanical properties of NACP nanocomposites containing NAg: (a) flexural strength and (b) elastic modulus. Each value is the mean of six measurements with the error bar showing one standard deviation (mean ± SD; $n = 6$). In each plot, values with dissimilar letters are significantly different from each other ($p < 0.05$). (Adapted from Cheng L et al., *J Biomed Mater Res B* 2012; 100: 1378–1386. With permission.)

Besides composites, NAg were also incorporated into dental bonding agents. Bonding agents are needed to adhere the composite restoration to the tooth structure. Antibacterial bonding agents have great potential to kill residual bacteria remaining in the prepared tooth cavity and inhibit subsequent bacteria invasion at the tooth-restoration interfaces during service. Dentin primers directly contact the tooth structure and could kill residual bacterial if rendered antibacterial.[17] Indeed, primer and adhesive with the addition of NAg achieved great antibacterial effects.[18,33] NAg presented additional benefits of inhibiting not only *S. mutans* on the resin surface but also *S. mutans* in culture medium away from the resin surface.[34] The incorporation of NAg into primer at a mass fraction of 0.05% indicated that this concentration had no adverse effect on the color of the primer.[23] The primer with 0.05% reduced biofilm CFU by an order of magnitude compared to control primer. Lactic acid production and metabolic activity from biofilms were also greatly reduced (Figures 6.5 and 6.6).[29] Furthermore, the dentin shear bond strength for primer containing 0.05% NAg was similar to control without

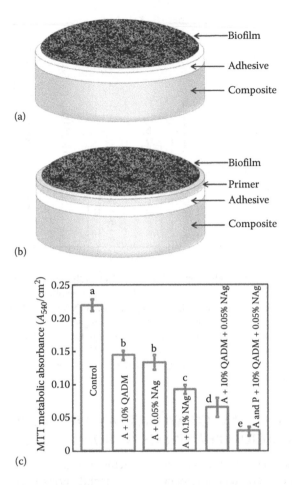

FIGURE 6.5 Schematic of dental plaque biofilm experiments and MTT metabolic activity of 2-day biofilms: (a) schematic of biofilm on adhesive surface covering the composite, (b) biofilm on the primer covering the adhesive and composite, and (c) MTT metabolic activity. Five adhesive groups were tested following schematic (a): Control, A + 10% QADM, A + 0.05% NAg, A + 0.1% NAg, A + 10% QADM + 0.05% NAg (A refers to adhesive). One group was tested following schematic (b) with a primer layer: A and P both contained 10% QADM and 0.05% NAg (A refers to adhesive, and P refers to primer). Each value is mean ± SD (*n* = 6). Values with dissimilar letters are different from each other (*p* < 0.05). (Adapted from Zhang K et al., *Dent Mater* 2012; 28: 842–852. With permission.)

NAg.[29] In the adhesive, NAg was added at a mass fraction of 0.10%, yet the dentin shear bond strength was comparable to that of control without NAg, ranging from approximately 32 to 35 MPa.[33] Therefore, strong anti-biofilm activity was achieved in dental bonding agents via NAg incorporation without compromising resin color and dentin bond strength.

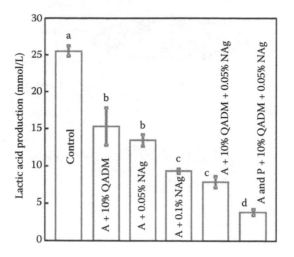

FIGURE 6.6 Lactic acid production by 2-day biofilms adherent on the six different types of disks. Five adhesive groups were tested following schematic described in Figure 6.5 (a): Control, A + 10% QADM, A + 0.05% NAg, A + 0.1% NAg, A + 10% QADM + 0.05% NAg (A refers to adhesive). One group was tested following schematic described in Figure 6.5 (b) with a primer layer: A and P both contained 10% QADM and 0.05% NAg (A refers to adhesive, and P refers to primer). Each value is mean ± SD (n = 6). Values with dissimilar letters are different from each other ($p < 0.05$). (Adapted from Zhang K et al., *Dent Mater* 2012; 28: 842–852. With permission.)

6.3 REMINERALIZING COMPOSITES AND BONDING AGENTS WITH CALCIUM PHOSPHATE NANOPARTICLES

Besides antibacterial restorations, nanostructured restorations with remineralization capability were also developed. Active dental caries occurs when the biofilm pH on the tooth surface decreases to below the dissolution threshold for the hydroxyapatite mineral in the dental tissues. Net mineral loss that characterizes the demineralization process is clinically evident as porosity, white-spot lesions, caries lesions, and cavitation.[35] A promising approach is to reverse this mineral loss through remineralization.[36] Previous remineralization strategies for dental hard tissues focused on the use of fluoride and calcium phosphates, including bioactive glass, fluoride-releasing materials, and amorphous calcium phosphate compounds.[36] A recent strategy, which is becoming the focus of much research in this field, is the use of remineralizing agents with nanoscale structures for increased surface area and bioactivity. Nanostructured calcium phosphates and fluoride-releasing materials could potentially be highly effective in remineralizing tooth lesions.[37,38] Calcium phosphate nanoparticles were synthesized via a spray-drying technique.[39–42] Typical nanoparticles of amorphous calcium phosphate (NACP) are shown in Figure 6.7a. To synthesize NACP, calcium carbonate ($CaCO_3$) and dicalcium phosphate anhydrous (Ca_2HPO_4) were dissolved into an acetic acid solution to obtain final calcium and phosphate ionic concentrations of 8 and 5.333 mmol/L, respectively. This solution

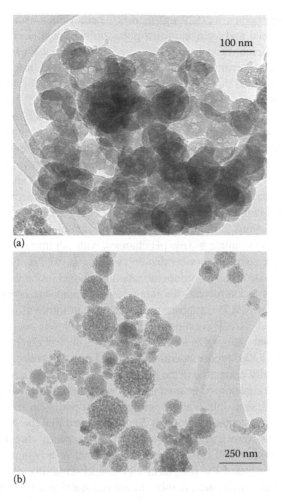

FIGURE 6.7 TEM images of (a) NACP. (Adapted from Xu et al., *Dent Mater* 2011; 27: 762–769. With permission.) (b) Nanoparticles of CaF_2 synthesized by using a spray-drying technique. (Adapted from Xu et al., *J Dent Res* 2010 Jan; 89(1): 19–28. With permission.)

was sprayed into a heated chamber to remove the liquid and volatile acids. Then, an electrostatic precipitator was used to collect the dried NACP powder, which had a mean particle size of approximately 116 nm (Figure 6.7a).[32,33]

In another study, a two-liquid nozzle was employed to allow two solutions to be mixed at the time of atomization, namely, a calcium solution and a fluoride solution.[43] This method produced CaF_2 nanoparticles that were trapped in the electrostatic precipitator and collected at the end of the process. The CaF_2 powder had a mean particle size of approximately 53 nm (Figure 6.7b).[43] Nanocomposite containing CaF_2 had a flexural strength of 110 MPa, matching the 108 MPa of a stress-bearing, nonreleasing commercial composite control.[43] The initial fluoride release rate from the nanocomposite was 2 μg/(h·cm²) and the sustained release rate after

10 weeks of immersion was $0.29\ \mu g/(h \cdot cm^2)$. These values exceeded the reported releases of traditional and resin-modified glass ionomer materials.[43]

The effect of calcium phosphate particle size on calcium and phosphate ion release from the composite was evaluated.[44] Using three different particle sizes (112 nm, 0.88 μm, and 12 μm), it was found that the ion release was inversely proportional to particle size and decreasing the particle size greatly increased the ion release.[45] Therefore, an advantage of using smaller particles was their higher surface area, which facilitated the release of cavity-fighting ions and resulted in higher ionic concentrations to promote remineralization.[38] Moreover, the NACP composite could greatly increase the ion release when the pH was lowered (e.g., at a cariogenic pH of 4) when these ions were most needed to inhibit caries (Figure 6.8).[46] In addition, the NACP composite possessed an acid neutralization ability and could quickly neutralize acid attacks to avoid enamel demineralization.[47]

Using extracted human teeth, NACP nanocomposite was shown to effectively remineralize enamel lesions.[41] In this study, a cyclic demineralization/remineralization regimen was used to simulate *in vivo* pH changes, with 1-h immersion in a pH 4 solution and 23-h immersion in a remineralization solution at pH 7 daily for 30 days.[41] The NACP nanocomposite achieved remineralization of enamel lesion that was fourfold the remineralization by a commercial fluoride-releasing composite control (Figure 6.9).[41] In another study, an NACP composite was tested in an intraoral *in situ* model in 25 human participants.[41] NACP composite produced much lower enamel mineral loss at the enamel-composite margins *in vivo*, compared to a control composite.[42] In addition, NACP composite yielded higher calcium and phosphorus ion concentrations in the biofilm plaque intraorally, compared to the plaque next to the control composite.[42]

Besides remineralization of enamel lesions and inhibition of secondary caries at composite-enamel lesions intraorally, load-bearing properties to resist chewing forces are also important for dental restorations. Studies showed that the flexural strengths of the nanocomposites were approximately 70–120 MPa, nearly threefold that of resin-modified glass ionomer, and matched or exceeded that of a commercial composite.[48] Another study investigated the long-term mechanical durability of nanocomposites.[49] In addition to physical resistance, another major requirement for the longevity of load-bearing restorations is resistance to occlusal wear. The three-body wear, a wear testing consisting of measurements of track, width, depth from multiple passes of a diamond tip under the abrasiveness of dentifrices/oral fluids, and other mechanical properties like flexural strength and elastic modulus after thermal cycling and water aging for 2 years of a nanocomposite, has shown comparable values to a commercial control composite.[49] These studies demonstrated that the new nanocomposites, while possessing desirable remineralization and caries-inhibiting capabilities, also possessed adequate load-bearing capability similar to the commercial control composites.

Besides being used in composites, the novel remineralizing agents can also be incorporated into bonding agents to help combat caries. NACP were incorporated into adhesives with different formulations to impart a remineralization capability without compromising the dentin bond strength.[49] Because of the small NACP size, NACP were able to flow with the bonding agent into dentinal tubules in the dentin so that they could release cavity-fighting ions and remineralize the remnants of lesions in the prepared tooth cavity.[50]

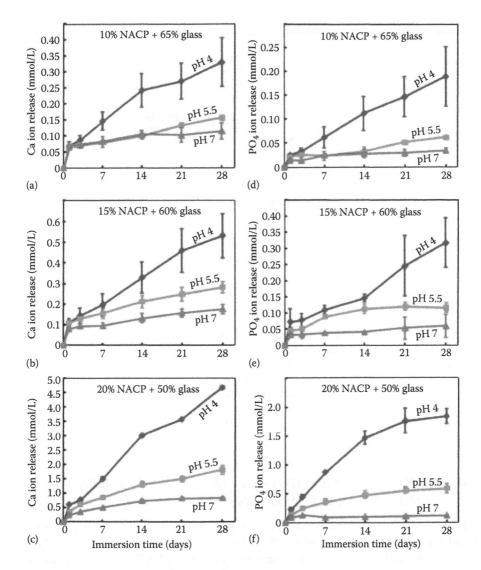

FIGURE 6.8 Calcium and phosphate ion release from the nanocomposite filled with 10% NACP and 65% glass (a and d), 15% NACP and 60% glass (b and e), or 20% NACP and 50% glass (c and f). Each value is the mean of three measurement, with the error bar showing one standard deviation (mean ± SD; $n = 3$). Calcium ion release increased with increasing the immersion time and the NACP filler level. Calcium ion release increased with decreasing the solution pH. The release of phosphate ions significantly increased with longer immersion time and higher NACP filler level, or with decreasing the solution pH. (Adapted from Xu et al., *Dent Mater* 2011; 27: 762–769. With permission.)

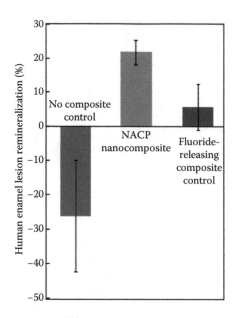

FIGURE 6.9 Remineralization of human enamel lesions in a demineralization/remineralization cyclic regimen for 30 days (mean ± SD; $n = 6$). Enamel lesions around NACP nanocomposite had the highest remineralization, 21.8% ± 3.7%. The fluoride-releasing commercial composite produced 5.7% ± 6.9% of enamel remineralization. Enamel sections without a composite had −26.1% ± 16.2%, which means further demineralization during the 30-day cyclic demineralization/remineralization treatment. These three values are significantly different from each other ($p < 0.05$). (Adapted from Weir MD et al., *J Dent Res* 2012; 91: 979–984. With permission.)

6.4 COMBINING NAg WITH QUATERNARY AMMONIUM AND NACP IN RESTORATIONS

It is beneficial for the restoration process to have the dual benefits of both antibacterial and remineralizing capabilities for caries prevention. Previous studies analyzed the mechanical properties of nanocomposite containing NACP, Nag, and antibacterial quaternary ammonium methacrylates (QAMs).[31,32] Antibacterial dental resins with QAMs were developed and 12-methacryloyloxydodecyl-pyridinium bromide (MDPB) was among the first antibacterial monomers.[51–53] MDPB has been extensively investigated and shown to possess potent antibacterial activities against various oral bacteria including facultative and obligate anaerobe in coronal lesions and other oral microorganism species isolated from root caries such as *Actinomyces* and *Candida albicans*.[54] An MDPB-containing primer was applied to cavities in teeth of dogs infected with *S. mutans* and exhibited *in vivo* antibacterial effects.[55] In addition, a composite restoration material containing MDPB was shown to inhibit the progression of artificial secondary root caries lesions using extracted human teeth with Class V cavities.[55] Other novel antibacterial formulations were also developed, including a methacryloxylethyl cetyl dimethyl ammonium chloride–containing adhesive,[56] antibacterial glass ionomer cements,[57] and antibacterial nanocomposites and bonding agents using a quaternary ammonium dimethacrylate (QADM).[31–33,58]

While these studies usually incorporated only one type of bioactive agent into a composite or bonding agent, recent studies sought to combine two or three bioactive agents into the same restoration material with the purpose of enhancing anti-caries efficacy. QADM and NAg were combined together in the NACP nanocomposite, while maintaining the flexural strength and elastic modulus to be similar to those of commercial composites without antibacterial activity.[32] Incorporation of both QADM and NAg together in the same composite significantly lowered the biofilm CFU counts, metabolic activity, and lactic acid production, compared to separately adding either QADM or NAg alone.[31]

Greater inhibition of oral biofilms was achieved when the primer and adhesive contained not only NAg but also a QAM. Antibacterial primer and adhesive containing both NAg and QAM were developed.[49,59] The results indicated that the addition of both NAg and QAM into the adhesive and primer did not compromise the dentin shear bond strength. With both NAg and QAM in the primer and adhesive, biofilm CFU, metabolic activity, and lactic acid production were all substantially reduced. Therefore, the method of incorporating dual agents (QAM + NAg) into adhesive and primer has the potential to more effectively combat residual bacteria in the tooth cavity and invade bacteria along the margins, compared to a single agent.[60,61] Furthermore, satisfactory bonding performance was achieved for the primer containing NAg or QAM and for the adhesive containing NACP with mass fractions ranging from 0% to 40%.[49,62] The antibacterial and remineralizing primer and adhesive were able to penetrate dentinal tubules and promote the mechanical interlock between dentin and composite (Figure 6.10). The viability of human saliva microcosm biofilms was substantially reduced when exposed to the cured

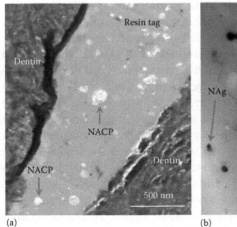 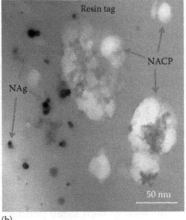

(a)   (b)

FIGURE 6.10 TEM images showing adhesive resin filling dentinal tubules in human dentin forming resin tags. (a) NACP successfully flowed with the adhesive into dentinal tubules. (b) Higher-magnification TEM revealed NAg as well as NACP in the resin tags in the dentinal tubules. The NAg appeared as black dots in TEM images with sizes of less than 10 nm. (Adapted from Melo MA et al., *J Biomed Mater Res B Appl Biomater* 2013; 101: 620–629. With permission.)

primer and adhesive disks containing NAg and QAM.[50,62] These novel materials containing NAg, quaternary ammonium, and NACP had the potential to kill residual bacteria in the tooth cavity and inhibit the invading bacteria along tooth-restoration margins with NACP to remineralize tooth lesions.

In vivo performance of these new materials was favorable in pilot studies.[58] The biocompatibility of composite and adhesive containing NACP and a new antibacterial quaternary ammonium dimethylaminododecyl methacrylate (DMADDM) was tested in a rat tooth cavity model.[58] The restorations containing 30% NACP, or 30% NACP plus 5% DMADDM, had significantly milder pulp inflammatory response than the control restoration.[58] Tertiary dentin formation was greatly enhanced for the NACP group and the NACP plus DMADDM group, compared to control.[58] Therefore, these novel nanocomposites and bonding agents with antibacterial and remineralizing capabilities are promising for dental clinical applications. Furthermore, NAg, QAM, and NACP are expected to have wide applicability to other dental composites, adhesives, sealants, and cements to inhibit biofilms and caries.

6.5   OTHER NANOSTRUCTURED ANTIBACTERIAL AND REMINERALIZING RESTORATIVES

For antibacterial activity, nanoparticles of quaternary ammonium polyethyleneimine (QA-PEI) were synthesized by cross-linking poly(ethylene imine) (PEI) that was *n*-alkylated with octyl halide, which was followed by quaternization of the amino groups with methyl iodide.[63] Dental composites containing 1% mass fraction of QA-PEI nanoparticles were tested for their antimicrobial activity.[63,64] The antibacterial properties of these composites were based on contact-killing mechanisms rather than on leaching of antibacterial agents; hence, the antibacterial effect was durable and not lost over time.[65] Although the detailed mechanism of the antibacterial effect of QAMs has not been fully determined, it was suggested that they cause lysis of the bacterial cells.[63] The QA-PEI composite showed strong antibacterial activity against *S. mutans*.[66] Furthermore, the anti-biofilm activity of the QA-PEI composite against oral biofilms *in vivo* was shown to be effective using a human *in situ* model.[64]

For remineralization, previous studies reported hydroxyapatite nanoparticle preparation in a solution environment, such as chemical precipitation, sol-gel, microemulsion, electrodeposition, and mechanochemical preparation methods followed by hydrothermal treatment.[66,67] A recent study[68] reported the synthesis of hydroxyapatite nanoparticles following a sol-gel technique similar to previous methods.[69,70] Hydroxyapatite nanoparticles of spherical shape and approximately 5 nm in size were obtained.[71] The remineralizing potential of hydroxyapatite nanoparticles was investigated.[68] Because of their small particle sizes, the hydroxyapatite nanoparticles had successful infiltration into the dentin matrix.[71] Hydroxyapatite nanoparticles were incorporated in dental composites, which increased the mechanical properties of these materials.[72] These findings support further investigation of the use of hydroxyapatite nanoparticles in dental materials for the remineralization of dental tissues.

Another class of materials that benefited from nanotechnology is resin-modified glass ionomer cements. This class of materials has the advantage of fluoride release;

however, the inferior mechanical properties of ionomer materials have limited their use. Recently, an improved glass ionomer material was developed, which contained fluoroaluminosilicate glass and nanofiller "clusters."[73] Resin-modified glass ionomer containing such nanoparticles showed suitable shear bond strength for clinical applications.[74] This was achieved without compromising the fluoride release rate.[75] Furthermore, the incorporation of nanohydroxyapatite into glass ionomer materials could also improve the mechanical properties.[69,76] The nanoparticles were shown to occupy the empty spaces between the glass-ionomer particles and acted as a reinforcement in the glass ionomer cement.[69] Therefore, nanotechnology is promising to yield a new generation of dental nanostructured materials with desirable properties to improve clinical efficacy and positively affect the field of restorative and preventive dentistry.

6.6 CONCLUSION

Nanotechnology is a promising approach to develop the next generation of dental materials to not only replace the missing tooth volume but also inhibit oral biofilms and remineralize tooth caries. These nanostructured and bioactive materials are able to provide therapeutic effects in dental tissues by deterring cariogenic bacteria adhesion and promoting tooth remineralization. Among them, NAg with a particle size of 2.7 nm were formed in dental resins, which greatly reduced oral biofilm CFU counts, metabolic activity, and lactic acid production, without negatively affecting the physical properties. NACP incorporation into dental resins yielded calcium and phosphate ion release, neutralized cariogenic acid attacks, remineralized tooth lesions, and inhibited secondary caries. Furthermore, the combination of two antibacterial agents into the same resin matrix substantially enhanced the antibacterial potency, compared to the use of a single agent. In addition, combining antibacterial and remineralizing agents into the same restoration imparted a higher capability of caries inhibition. These new nanostructured materials showed highly promising *in vivo* results in an animal model and in a human *in situ* model intraorally. Nanotechnology is yielding a new class of bioactive dental materials with the double benefits of antibacterial and remineralizing capabilities, which are promising to greatly enhance caries inhibition and improve future restorative and preventive dentistry.

ACKNOWLEDGMENTS

We thank Drs. Fang Li, Joseph M. Antonucci, Nancy J. Lin, and Sheng Lin-Gibson for discussions and help.

REFERENCES

1. Wilson M, Kannangara K, Smith G, Simmons M, Raguse B. *Nanotechnology: Basic Science and Emerging Technologies*. UNSW Press: Sidney, 2002.
2. Zhang M, Kataoka K. Nano-structured composites based on calcium phosphate for cellular delivery of therapeutic and diagnostic agents. *Nano Today*. 2009;4:508–517.

3. Rugg-Gunn A. Dental caries: Strategies to control this preventable disease. *Acta Med Acad.* 2013;42(2):117–130.

4. Pitts NB, Stamm JW. International Consensus Workshop on Caries Clinical Trials (ICW-CCT)—Final consensus statements: Agreeing where the evidence leads. *J Dental Res.* 2004;83(SPEC. ISS. C):C125–C128.

5. World Health Organization. Future use of materials for dental restoration: Report of the meeting convened at WHO HQ, Geneva, Switzerland, prepared by Dr. Poul Erik Petersen, 2009.

6. Arhun N, Celik C, Yamanel K. Clinical evaluation of resin-based composites in posterior restorations: Two-year results. *Oper Dent.* 2010;35(4):397–404.

7. Subramani K, Ahmed W. *Emerging Nanotechnologies in Dentistry: Processes, Materials and Applications.* Elsiever, Oxford, UK, 2012.

8. Jandt KD, Sigusch BW. Future perspectives of resin-based dental materials. *Dent Mater.* 2009;25(8):1001–1006.

9. Sarrett DC. Clinical challenges and the relevance of materials testing for posterior composite restorations. *Dent Mater.* 2005;21:9–20.

10. Demarco FF, Corrêa MB, Cenci MS, Moraes RR, Opdam NJ. Longevity of posterior composite restorations: Not only a matter of materials. *Dent Mater.* 2012;28(1):87–101.

11. Zalkind MM, Keisar O, Ever-Hadani P, Grinberg R, Sela MN. Accumulation of *Streptococcus mutans* on light-cured composites and amalgam: An in vitro study. *J Esthet Dent.* 1998;10:187–190.

12. Jung M, Sehr K, Klimek J. Surface texture of four nanofilled and one hybrid composite after finishing. *Oper Dent.* 2007;32(1):45–52.

13. Montanaro L, Campoccia D, Rizzi S, Donati ME, Breschi L, Prati C, Arciola CR. Evaluation of bacterial adhesion of *Streptococcus mutans* on dental restorative materials. *Biomaterials.* 2004;25:4457–4463.

14. De Fúcio SB, Puppin-Rontani RM, De Carvalho FG, Mattos-Graner RO, Correr-Sobrinho L, Garcia-Godoy F. Analyses of biofilms accumulated on dental restorative materials. *J Am Dent Assoc.* 2009;22(3):131–136.

15. Kanaparthy R, Kanaparthy A. The changing face of dentistry: Nanotechnology. *Int J Nanomed.* 2011;6(1):2799–2804.

16. Lainović T, Blažić L, Potran M. Nanotechnology in dentistry—Current state and future perspectives. *Serbian Dent J.* 2012;59(1):44–47.

17. Subramani K, Ahmed W. *Nanobiomaterials in Clinical Dentistry.* Elsevier, Oxford, UK, 2012.

18. Melo MA, Guedes SF, Xu HH, Rodrigues LK. Nanotechnology-based restorative materials for dental caries management. *Trends Biotechnol.* 2013;31(8):459–467.

19. Drummond JL. Degradation, fatigue, and failure of resin dental composite materials. *J Dent Res.* 2008;87(8):710–719.

20. Cramer NB, Stansbury JW, Bowman CN. Recent advances and developments in composite dental restorative materials. *J Dent Res.* 2011;90(4):402–416.

21. Bradshaw DJ, Lynch RJ. Diet and the microbial aetiology of dental caries: New paradigms. *Int Dent J.* 2013;63 Suppl 2:64–72.

22. Wang Z, Shen Y, Haapasalo M. Dental materials with antibiofilm properties. *Dent Mater.* 2014;30(2):e1–e16.

23. Hamouda IM. Current perspectives of nanoparticles in medical and dental biomaterials. *J Biomed Mater Res.* 2012;26:143–151.

24. Völker C, Oetken M, Oehlmann J. The biological effects and possible modes of action of nanosilver. *Rev Environ Contam Toxicol.* 2013;223:81–106.

25. Sotiriou GA, Pratsinis SE. Antibacterial activity of nanosilver ions and particles. *Environ Sci Technol.* 2010;44(14):5649–5654.

26. Lok CN, Ho CM, Chen R, He QY, Yu WY, Sun H, Tam PK, Chiu JF, Che CM. Proteomic analysis of the mode of antibacterial action of silver nanoparticles. *J Proteome Res.* 2006;5:916–924.
27. Lara HH, Ayala-Nunez NV, Turrent LDI, Padilla CR. Bactericidal effect of silver nanoparticles against multidrug-resistant bacteria. *World J Microbiol Biotechnol.* 2010;26:615–621.
28. Fan C, Chu L, Rawls HR, Norling BK, Cardenas HL, Whang K. Development of an antimicrobial resin—A pilot study. *Dent Mater.* 2011;27:322–328.
29. Cheng L, Zhang K, Melo MAS, Weir MD, Zhou X, Xu HHK. Anti-biofilm dentin primer with quaternary ammonium and silver nanoparticles. *J Dental Res.* 2012;91: 598–604.
30. Cheng YJ, Zeiger DN, Howarter JA, Zhang X, Lin NJ, Antonucci JM, Lin-Gibson S. In situ formation of silver nanoparticles in photocrosslinking polymers. *J Biomed Mater Res B Appl Biomater.* 2011;97:124–131.
31. Cheng L, Weir MD, Xu HK, Antonucci JM, Kraigsley AM, Lin NJ, Lin-Gibson S, Zhou X. Antibacterial amorphous calcium phosphate nanocomposites with a quaternary ammonium dimethacrylate and silver nanoparticles. *Dent Mater.* 2012;28:561–572.
32. Cheng L, Weir MD, Xu HHK, Antonucci JM, Lin NJ, Lin-Gibson S, Xu SM, Zhou X. Effect of amorphous calcium phosphate and silver nanocomposites on dental plaque microcosm biofilms. *J Biomed Mater Res B.* 2012;100:1378–1386.
33. Zhang K, Melo MAS, Cheng L, Weir MD, Bai Y, Xu HHK. Effect of quaternary ammonium and silver nanoparticle-containing adhesives on dentin bond strength and dental plaque microcosm biofilms. *Dent Mater.* 2012;28:842–852.
34. Li F, Weir MD, Chen J, Xu HH. Comparison of quaternary ammonium-containing with nano-silver-containing adhesive in antibacterial properties and cytotoxicity. *Dent Mater.* 2013;29:450–461.
35. Cury JA, Tenuta LM. Enamel remineralization: Controlling the caries disease or treating early caries lesions? *Braz Oral Res.* 2009;23:23–30.
36. Ten Cate JM. Novel anticaries and remineralizing agents: Prospects for the future. *J Dent Res.* 2012;91:813–815.
37. Xu HH, Moreau JL, Sun L, Chow LC. Nanocomposite containing amorphous calcium phosphate nanoparticles for caries inhibition. *Dent Mater.* 2011;27:762–769.
38. Xu HH, Weir MD, Sun L, Moreau JL, Takagi S, Chow LC, Antonucci JM. Strong nanocomposites with Ca, $PO_{(4)}$, and F release for caries inhibition. *J Dent Res.* 2010;89(1):19–28.
39. Chow LC, Sun L, Hockey B. Properties of nanostructured hydroxyapatite prepared by a spray drying technique. *J Res Natl Inst Stand Technol.* 2004;109:543–551.
40. Sun L, Chow LC, Frukhtbeyn SA, Bonevich JE. Preparation and properties of nanoparticles of calcium phosphates with various Ca/P ratios. *J Res Natl Inst Stand Technol.* 2010;115:243–255.
41. Weir MD, Chow LC, Xu HH. Remineralization of demineralized enamel via calcium phosphate nanocomposite. *J Dent Res.* 2012;91:979–984.
42. Melo MAS, Weir MD, Rodrigues LK, Xu HH. Novel calcium phosphate nanocomposite with caries-inhibition in a human in situ model. *Dent Mater.* 2013;29:231–240.
43. Xu HHK, Moreau JL, Sun L, Chow LC. Strength and fluoride release characteristics of a calcium fluoride based dental nanocomposite. *Biomaterials.* 2008;29:4261–4267.
44. Xu HH, Weir MD, Sun L, Ngai S, Takagi S, Chow LC. Effect of filler level and particle size on dental caries-inhibiting Ca-PO_4 composite. *J Mater Sci Mater Med.* 2009;20:1771–1779.
45. Xu HH, Weir MD, Sun L, Takagi S, Chow LC. Effects of calcium phosphate nanoparticles on Ca-PO_4 composite. *J Dent Res.* 2007;86:378–383.

46. Moreau JL, Sun L, Chow LC, Xu HH. Mechanical and acid neutralizing properties and bacteria inhibition of amorphous calcium phosphate dental nanocomposite. *J Biomed Mater Res B Appl Biomater.* 2011;98:80–88.
47. Xu HH, Weir MD, Sun L. Calcium and phosphate ion releasing composite: Effect of pH on release and mechanical properties. *Dent Mater.* 2009;25:535–542.
48. Xu HH, Moreau JL, Sun L, Chow LC. Novel CaF$_2$ nanocomposite with high strength and fluoride ion release. *J Dent Res.* 2010;89:739–745.
49. Weir MD, Moreau JL, Levine ED, Strassler HE, Chow LC, Xu HH. Nanocomposite containing CaF$_2$ nanoparticles: Thermal cycling, wear and long-term water-aging. *Dent Mater.* 2012;28:642–652.
50. Melo MA, Cheng L, Zhang K, Weir MD, Rodrigues LK, Xu HH. Novel dental adhesives containing nanoparticles of silver and amorphous calcium phosphate. *Dent Mater.* 2013;29:199–210.
51. Imazato S, Ehara A, Torii M, Ebisu S. Antibacterial activity of dentine primer containing MDPB after curing. *J Dent.* 1998;26:267–271.
52. Imazato S, Kuramoto A, Takahashi Y, Ebisu S, Peters MC. In vitro antibacterial effects of the dentin primer of Clearfil Protect Bond. *Dent Mater.* 2006;22:527–532.
53. Imazato S. Bio-active restorative materials with antibacterial effects: New dimension of innovation in restorative dentistry. *Dent Mater J.* 2009;28:11–19.
54. Imazato S, Kaneko T, Takahashi Y, Noiri Y, Ebisu S. In vivo antibacterial effects of dentin primer incorporating MDPB. *Oper Dent.* 2004;29:369–375.
55. Thome T, Mayer MP, Imazato S, Geraldo-Martins VR, Marques MM. In vitro analysis of inhibitory effects of the antibacterial monomer MDPB-containing restorations on the progression of secondary root caries. *J Dent.* 2009;37:705–711.
56. Li F, Chen J, Chai Z, Zhang L, Xiao Y, Fang M, Ma S. Effects of a dental adhesive incorporating antibacterial monomer on the growth, adherence and membrane integrity of *Streptococcus mutans. J Dent.* 2009;37:289–296.
57. Xie D, Weng Y, Guo X, Zhao J, Gregory RL, Zheng C. Preparation and evaluation of a novel glass-ionomer cement with antibacterial functions. *Dent Mater.* 2011;27:487–496.
58. Li F, Wang P, Weir MD, Fouad AF, Xu HH. Evaluation of antibacterial and remineralizing nanocomposite and adhesive in rat tooth cavity model. *Acta Biomater.* 2014;10(6):2804–2813.
59. Zhang K, Cheng L, Imazato S, Antonucci JM, Lin NJ, Lin-Gibson S, Bai Y, Xu HH. Effects of dual antibacterial agents MDPB and nano-silver in primer on microcosm biofilm, cytotoxicity and dentine bond properties. *J Dent.* 2013;41:464–474.
60. Cheng L, Weir MD, Zhang K, Arola DD, Zhou X, Xu HH. Dental primer and adhesive containing a new antibacterial quaternary ammonium monomer dimethylaminododecyl methacrylate. *J Dent.* 2013;41:345–355.
61. Cheng L, Zhang K, Weir MD, Liu H, Zhou X, Xu HH. Effects of antibacterial primers with quaternary ammonium and nano-silver on *Streptococcus mutans* impregnated in human dentin blocks. *Dent Mater.* 2013;29:462–472.
62. Melo MA, Cheng L, Weir MD, Hsia RC, Rodrigues LK, Xu HH. Novel dental adhesive containing antibacterial agents and calcium phosphate nanoparticles. *J Biomed Mater Res B Appl Biomater.* 2013;101:620–629.
63. Beyth N, Yudovin-Farber I, Bahir R, Domb AJ, Weiss EI. Antibacterial activity of dental composites containing quaternary ammonium polyethylenimine nanoparticles against *Streptococcus mutans. Biomaterials.* 2006;27:3995–4002.
64. Beyth N, Yudovin-Farber I, Perez-Davidi M, Domb AJ, Weiss EI. Polyethyleneimine nanoparticles incorporated into resin composite cause cell death and trigger biofilm stress in vivo. *Proc Natl Acad Sci U S A.* 2010;107:22038–22043.
65. Beyth N, Pilo R, Weiss EI. Antibacterial activity of dental cements containing quaternary ammonium polyethylenimine nanoparticles. *J Nanomater.* 2012;2012:814763.

66. Yudovin-Farber I, Beyth N, Nyska A, Weiss EI, Golenser J, Domb AJ. Surface characterization and biocompatibility of restorative resin containing nanoparticles. *Biomacromolecules*. 2008;9:3044–3050.
67. Sadat-Shojai M, Khorasani MT, Dinpanah-Khoshdargi E, Jamshidi A. Synthesis methods for nanosized hydroxyapatite with diverse structures. *Acta Biomater*. 2013;9:7591–7621.
68. Besinis A, van Noort R, Martin N. Remineralization potential of fully demineralized dentin infiltrated with silica and hydroxyapatite nanoparticles. *Dent Mater*. 2014;30(3):249–262.
69. Moshaverinia A, Ansari S, Movasaghi Z, Billington RW, Darr JA, Rehman IU. Modification of conventional glass-ionomer cements with N-vinylpyrrolidone containing polyacids, nano-hydroxy and fluoroapatite to improve mechanical properties. *Dent Mater*. 2008;24:1381–1390.
70. Lin J, Zhu J, Gu X, Wen W, Li Q, Fischer-Brandies H, Wang H, Mehl C. Effects of incorporation of nano-fluorapatite or nano-fluorohydroxyapatite on a resin-modified glass ionomer cement. *Acta Biomater*. 2011;7:1346–1353.
71. Besinis A, van Noort R, Martin N. Infiltration of demineralized dentin with silica and hydroxyapatite nanoparticles. *Dent Mater*. 2012;28:1012–1023.
72. Zakir M, Al Kheraif AA, Asif M, Wong FS, Rehman IU. A comparison of the mechanical properties of a modified silorane based dental composite with those of commercially available composite material. *Dent Mater*. 2013;29:e53–e59.
73. Neelakantan P, John S, Anand S, Sureshbabu N, Subbarao C. Fluoride release from a new glass-ionomer cement. *Oper Dent*. 2011;36:80–85.
74. Uysal T, Yagici A, Uysal B, Akdogan G. Are nano-composites and nano-ionomers suitable for orthodontic bracket bonding? *Eur J Orthod*. 2010;32:78–82.
75. Wadenya R, Smith J, Mante F. Microleakage of nano-particle-filled resin-modified glass ionomer using atraumatic restorative technique in primary molars. *N Y State Dent J*. 2010;76:36–39.
76. Mitra SB, Oxman JD, Falsafi A, Ton TT. Fluoride release and recharge behavior of a nano-filled resin-modified glass ionomer compared with that of other fluoride releasing materials. *J Am Dent Assoc*. 2011;24:372–378.

7 Redox-Triggered, Biocompatible, Inorganic Nanoplatforms for Cancer Theranostics

Xin-Chun Huang, Yun-Ling Luo, and Hsin-Yun Hsu

CONTENTS

ABSTRACT

Traditional chemotherapeutic agents do not discriminate between rapidly dividing normal cells and tumor cells. Here, a general discussion about the design of stimulus-responsive drug delivery, with special emphasis on the construction of redox-responsive, inorganic nanocarriers, based on the difference in extra- and intracellular glutathione levels is provided. The widely employed biocompatible inorganic nanomaterials including silica nanoparticle–, iron oxide nanoparticle–, and gold nanoparticle–based nanoplatforms have been reviewed.

Keywords: Silica nanoparticles, Gold nanoparticles, Iron oxide nanoparticles, Redox-responsive drug delivery, Cancer theranostics

7.1 INTRODUCTION

Cancer is a potentially fatal disease particularly when diagnosed in the late stages. Abnormal cells proliferate without control and can metastasize to various organs through the bloodstream and lymph systems. Traditional strategies for cancer intervention include hyperthermia, radiation therapy, surgery, chemotherapy, targeted therapy, and combinations of these strategies.[1] For metastasized carcinoma that cannot be treated locally, chemotherapy serves as a relatively efficient alternative. However, their poor selectivity leads to systemic side effects such as multidrug resistance.[2] As a result, therapeutic options can be further limited because of the insensitivity to the treatments, leading to the increase in drug dosage, costs, lengths of stay, and high mortality-to-incidence ratio.[3,4] This has been one of the critical challenges faced in providing effective chemotherapy to cancer patients. This chapter focuses on the delivery of drug through nanocarriers in the biological milieu with respect to their circulation and clearance from tissues and their uptake in cells. In addition, we aim to provide the insight into the rapid progress in developing redox-triggered smart nanomaterials for cancer theranostics.

7.1.1 NANOMATERIALS IN THE BIOLOGICAL MILIEU

The extremely small feature size is of the same scale as the critical size for physical phenomena. Fundamental electronic, magnetic, optical, chemical, and biological processes are different at these scales. Proteins (10–1000 nm in size) and cell walls (1–100 nm thick) may interact differently with nanomaterials than larger-scale bulk materials. To develop effective nanomaterials for biomedical applications, their behavior in biological systems must be considered. To enable efficient tumor targeting, it is essential to design materials that can escape renal filtration and prolong blood circulation time. Unlike conventional molecular drugs that generally diffuse throughout the tissue, nanomaterials show unique clearance profiles. Current studies suggest that multiple factors control the circulation and organ clearance of nanomaterials. The size, shape, surface characteristics, and the aspect ratio of nanomaterials play a key role in their biodistribution *in vivo*.[5]

7.1.2 NANOMATERIALS IN BLOOD CIRCULATION AND ORGAN CLEARANCE

Several modes have been employed to introduce drug carriers into the human body; these include oral administration,[6] inhalation,[7,8] and intravenous[9,10] and intraperitoneal injection.[11,12] Most of these *in vivo* studies have shown that nanomaterials circulating in the bloodstream mainly end up in the reticuloendothelial system (RES). Consequently, nanomaterials overaccumulate in organs such as the liver and spleen; the main reason for side effects and inefficient delivery to targeted tissue stems from nanomaterials that have slow degradation and excretion rates from the body.

In general, particle sizes smaller than 5 nm are removed from the bloodstream by rapid renal clearance, whereas 10- to 20-nm particles are mostly filtered by the liver. Particles larger than 200 nm are cleared by Kupffer cells or filtered in the sinusoidal spleen. In principle, synthesizing nanomaterials within the diameter range of

20–200 nm could prevent them from undergoing organ clearance and enhance the opportunity for correct targeting.[13] Additionally, the intrinsic surface properties of nanomaterials influence their biodistribution. Under biological milieu *in vivo*, protein adsorption occurs on many synthesized nanomaterials, resulting in their removal by macrophages.[14] Opsonins, molecules that can bind to foreign particles, enhance phagocytosis, thereby making nanomaterials more susceptible to the immune system. Optimization of surface chemistry will enable the inhibition of protein adsorption and prevention of hepatic and spleen filtration. Polyethylene glycol (PEG) is a biocompatible polymer that has been widely applied to prolong the circulation time of nanocarriers.

7.1.3　Accumulation of Nanomaterials in Tumor Tissue

Nanomaterials can either passively accumulate or actively target tumors. Matsumura and Maeda first described the enhanced permeability and retention (EPR) effect, which is the passive accumulation of nanomaterials.[15] The EPR effect is a unique phenomenon seen in solid tumors and is related to their anatomical and pathophysiological differences from normal tissues[16] (Figure 7.1). Tumor vessels have an irregular structure and larger endothelial pores compared to normal vessels, which enables the passage of small nanomaterials (400–600 nm). The vascular pore size is approximately 100–2000 nm in tumors and 2–6 nm in healthy tissue.[17] The defective vasculature is caused by rapid tumor cell growth, the lack of adequate nutrients, and poor waste removal via blood flow. During this process, tumors undergo rapid angiogenesis, but there is a lack of tight junctions between endothelial cells and mural cells.[18] Tumor vessels are poorly perfused with blood and are dysfunctional, which limits the delivery of blood-borne compounds to tumors.[19] Furthermore, tumors have a high interstitial pressure that is thought to result from dysfunctional lymphatics, which causes tissue fluid to flow out of the tumor, thereby inhibiting the diffusion of drugs from the blood vessels into the tumor.[20] The lack of functional lymphatic drainage in tumor regions extends the retention time of nanomaterials in cancer tissue. Research on approaches to exploit this alteration in tumor blood flow, the modulation of tumor vascular penetration, or targeting strategies to accumulate drug-loaded nanocarriers at tumor sites for a prolonged retention time (days to weeks) is thus of great importance.[21] In certain cases where tumors show no EPR effect, active targeting accumulation by using ligand–receptor interactions could be introduced.[22] Nanomaterials functionalized with tumor-specific ligands can be recognized by the receptors on the surface of the carcinoma, promoting active cellular uptake. By combining the active modes with the passive EPR effect, nanomaterials enable effective drug delivery and accumulation in targeted tumor tissue.

7.1.4　Uptake and Trafficking of Nanomaterials in Cells

Once nanomaterials have targeted the tumor lesions, the next barriers to overcome are cellular uptake, crossing the cytoplasm membrane, and lysosomal escape. Endocytosis is the most common uptake pathway for intracellular trafficking in mammalian cells. Several endocytotic mechanisms facilitate the internalization of

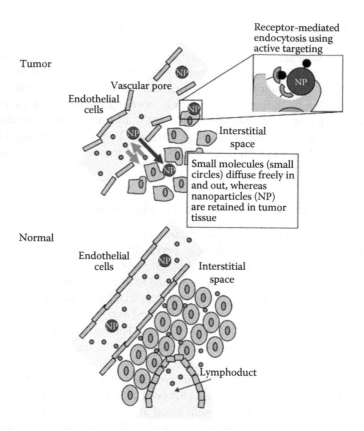

FIGURE 7.1 The EPR effect. Healthy tissue is characterized by a good flow in blood vessel, while in tumor, leaky vasculature and dysfunctional lymphatic network lead to the accumulation of nanoparticles in the tissue. (P.P. Adiseshaiah et al.: Nanomaterial standards for efficacy and toxicity assessment. *Wiley Interdisciplinary Reviews: Nanomedicine and Nanobiotechnology*. 2010. 2. 99–112. Copyright Wiley-VCH Verlag GmbH & Co. KGaA. Reproduced with permission.)

nanomaterials. Uptake of large particles (0.5–10 μm) can be through phagocytosis of specialized cells, such as macrophages and neutrophils, whereas smaller particles can be transported by different endocytosis modes, including macropinocytosis, micropinocytosis, clathrin-mediated endocytosis, caveola-mediated endocytosis, and clathrin- and caveola-independent endocytosis.[23,24] The mode of endocytosis determines the trafficking path of nanocarriers to various subcellular compartments. However, in most cases, they end up in lysosomes, which contain various digestive enzymes and have an acidic environment (pH 5–5.5), leading to the degradation of nanomaterials.[25]

7.2 STIMULUS-RESPONSIVE DELIVERY

Nanobiotechnology continues to be a rapidly developing field that offers new possibilities to improve the diagnosis and treatment of human diseases.[26–28] Various synthesized nanomaterials show potential benefits for diagnosing and treating metastatic cancer. These benefits include the ability to transport complex molecular cargos to the major sites of metastasis, such as the lungs, liver, and lymph nodes, and to target specific cell populations within these organs to enhance the EPR effect artificially in clinical settings. Nanocapsules and nanodevices may present new possibilities for drug delivery, gene therapy, and medical diagnostics. The anticancer nanoparticle drug, paclitaxel, which is albumin stabilized and hydrophobic, is one such drug delivery system (DDS) that has been approved by Food and Drug Administration (FDA).[29]

An optimal drug carrier typically consists of three key components:

1. Specific ligands to enhance tumor selectivity: Tumor targeting is usually achieved by immobilizing the ligands, which recognize the cancer-specific receptors to ensure effective cellular uptake.
2. Stimulus-responsive mechanisms for drug release: Drug unloading is usually designed to be triggered by specific mechanisms such as pH or redox potentials, which are known to be distinct between tumor and normal tissues.
3. Optical labeling or other detectable tracers: They allow direct visualization of the delivery.

Moreover, the biocompatibility and the ability to control the release of the drugs in a time- and site-specific manner are desired features for DDSs. With increase in interest regarding such targeted DDSs, significant effort[30–32] has been devoted during the last decade to improving drug efficacies and to minimizing nonspecific cytotoxicity based on the physical/chemical characteristics of tumors in various stimulus-responsive mechanisms.

The triggering stimuli could be classified as either internal or external[33] (Figure 7.2). External stimuli such as light,[34–40] temperature,[41–43] ultrasound,[44–46] or electromagnetic fields[47,48] have been used to specifically deliver drugs. For example,

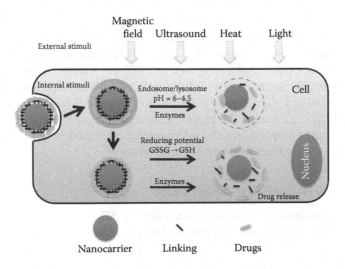

FIGURE 7.2 Stimulus-responsive drug delivery systems.

focused ultrasound has been applied to microbubbles to facilitate the delivery of therapeutic moieties across biologic barriers, including the blood–brain barrier,[49–51] extracranial endothelial layers,[52] and cellular membranes,[53,54] thereby enhancing local drug delivery. Sonoporation facilitates the delivery of standard drugs to target cells and shows significant potential for improving the delivery of plasmid DNA and small interfering RNAs[55,56] to enable genetic interventions.

Alternatively, depending on the cellular homeostasis, internal stimuli such as pH,[57–59] redox status,[60–62] or enzyme activities[50,63] can be used for this purpose. However, release mechanisms based on specific changes in the surrounding medium may cause unpredictable drug release before reaching the targeted sites. A sensitive stimuli-responsive drug carrier that is tunable in response to subtle environmental variations remains a major challenge.[64]

7.2.1 REDOX-RESPONSIVE DELIVERY SYSTEM

Among different stimulus-responsive drug carriers, redox-triggered delivery systems have been highlighted. The large difference of the redox potential inside and outside the cell could provide an advantageous niche for the design of intracellular DDSs.[65,66] Glutathione (GSH) is probably the most abundant redox-active compound in the cell. It is a tripeptide thiol composed of cysteine, glycine, and glutamic acid and is often found in the millimolar range in the cytoplasm of living cells. The GSH level in the cytosol (approximately 2–10 mM) is approximately two to three orders of magnitude higher than the level in extracellular fluids (approximately 2–20 μM).[67] GSH is recognized as an ideal internal stimulus for the destabilization of redox-responsive nanomaterials to accomplish efficient intracellular release. GSH disulfide is maintained at a reduced status by enzymes such as GSH reductase, and the intracellular GSH level has been tightly regulated by NADH/NAD$^+$, NADPH/NADP$^+$, and thioredoxin$_{red}$/thioredoxin$_{ox}$ levels.[65] A reduced microenvironment is also found in the endocytic pathway. The enzyme gamma interferon–inducible lysosomal thiol-reductase and the excess level of cysteine in a lysosome favor the reduction of disulfide bonds. In cancer cells, sustained oxidative stress followed by a high level of generated reactive oxygen species often induces redox adaptation leading to the up-regulation of antioxidant molecules, such as GSH. As a result, the redox potential gradient existing between the extracellular and intracellular environments has been widely exploited as a physiological stimulus in subcellular therapeutics delivery.[68]

Sections 7.2.2, 7.2.3, and 7.2.4 provide a summarized overview of silica nanoparticle–, iron oxide nanoparticle–, and gold nanoparticle–based, redox-responsive systems developed for cancer therapeutics, respectively.

7.2.2 SILICA NANOPARTICLE–BASED DDSs

During the past decades, solid silica nanoparticles (SiNPs) and mesoporous SiNPs (MSNs) have been extensively characterized for use in diverse applications. Although the SiNPs have been widely applied in DDS and as optical contrast agents for imaging, their functionalization is often limited by the surface of the SiNPs. MSNs exhibit higher surface areas and tunable pore volumes that allow for higher loading capacities of therapeutic drugs. Recently, enzyme immobilization on silica materials has been extensively explored. A comparative study of enzyme immobilization on SiNPs and hollow SiNPs has demonstrated that the protein-loading capacity of hollow silica nanospheres can be more than twice the capacity of SiNPs. Silica materials with hollow structures and tunable pore sizes can be adapted with diverse chemical conjugations to facilitate the immobilization of therapeutic proteins or drugs. Hence, MSNs currently have become prevalent nanoplatforms to design smart DDS for biomedical applications.

Various methods have been established to prepare MSNs.[69–72] In the late 1960s, Stöber and coworkers were the first to report the synthesis of monodispersed and spherical SiNPs by introducing a high concentration of surfactants to the traditional sol-gel method. Mobil Composition of Matter No. 41 (MCM-41), fabricated by Mobil's researchers, is one of the most well-known MSN structures. Although the silica wall is amorphous, its interior possesses an extremely ordered framework with uniform mesopores. It was proposed that the cationic surfactant molecules self-organize into a hexagonal structure and that the silica precursors co-condense with the cylindrical micelles to form MSNs with porosities of 2–50 nm.[70] Some studies have further found that the pore structure of MSNs can be tuned by controlling the relative amounts of silica and surfactant molecules in the reaction[73] or switching the length of carbon chain of surfactants.[74] Synthesis of smaller MSNs (<100 nm) can be achieved by diluting the surfactant or using a double surfactant system. A significant number of studies have demonstrated successful control of particle size, morphology, and surface functionalization of the MSNs for diverse applications.

MSN-based stimulus-responsive nanosystems for drug release in cancer theranostics include various triggers such as pH, redox gradient, light irradiation, and magnetic field. In recent years, the design of novel redox-responsive drug nanocarriers for achieving therapeutic selectivity in cancer theranostics by using the response to the redox gradient in the intracellular milieu of carcinomas has received considerable attention. Most of the current MSN-based, GSH-mediated controlled release systems share a setup similar to that of pH-responsive DDS. Cap or gatekeeper molecules, such as collagen, PEG, or cyclodextrin, have been functionalized on the surface of MSNs using disulfide bonds to prevent drug leakage during delivery until the drugs are released under reduced conditions. For example, the stimulus-responsive nanocarrier based on MSNs shown in Figure 7.3 is end capped with collagen and uses lactobionic acid as the target ligand. The hydrophobic dye, fluorescein isothiocyanate (FITC), serves as both a model drug and an optical probe for intracellular tracing of MSNs to demonstrate the cell-specific targeting and redox-responsive controlled drug release.[75]

Anticancer drugs, such as doxorubicin (DOX) or dye molecules, could also be covalently linked to the inner channels of MSNs via disulfide bonds to minimize the potential degradation triggered by the chaotic milieu of biological systems. The redox-sensitive delivery system functionalized with cysteine-labeled ATTO633 by disulfide formation at the inner core of MSNs has been demonstrated.[76] This study indicated that endosomal escape is a limiting factor for the redox-triggered intracellular release of disulfide-bound cysteine from core–shell functionalized colloidal

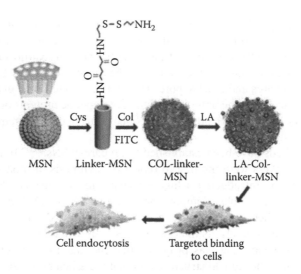

FIGURE 7.3 Scheme of redox-responsive MSNs with a collagen cap for targeted drug delivery. (Z. Luo et al.: Mesoporous silica nanoparticles end-capped with collagen: Redox-responsive nanoreservoirs for targeted drug delivery. *Angewandte Chemie International Edition*. 2011. 50. 640–643. Copyright Wiley-VCH Verlag GmbH & Co. KGaA. Reproduced with permission.)

mesoporous silica. In our recent work (Figure 7.4), we have demonstrated a self-destructive silica-based nanosystem in which the degradation was induced by the concentration gradient of dithiothreitol (DTT). This is attributed to the disulfide-linked structure in the synthesized silica nanobeads (ReSiN: redox-responsive silica nanobeads). An *in vitro* cytotoxicity assay indicated that ReSiN had insignificant

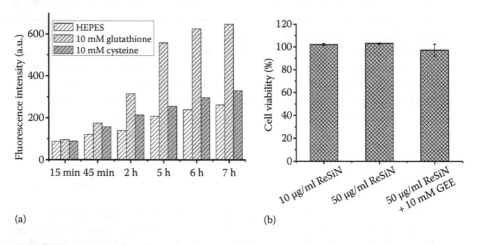

FIGURE 7.4 *In vitro* studies of ReSiN degradation in the presence of cysteine and GSH (a). MTT assays were performed to evaluate the *in vitro* cytotoxicity of ReSiN (b). HeLa cells showed no significant cytotoxicity after 24-h incubation with 10 and 50 μg/ml ReSiNs. The unaffected viability of glutathione ethyl ester (GEE)–treated cells indicated that the degraded by-products were not hazardous. (Courtesy of Huang et al., unpublished data.)

effects on HeLa cells. Our current results indicate that this novel nanocarrier may potentially be responsive to redox stimuli and has great biocompatibility for *in vivo* applications.

7.2.3 Magnetic Iron Oxide Nanoparticle–Based DDSs

The magnetic iron oxide nanoparticle has been an alternative material widely employed in biological applications, including microorganism detection, diagnostic magnetic resonance imaging (MRI), and magnetic fluid hyperthermia therapy. Their magnetic properties enable the accumulation of drug nanocarriers at a target region by switching on a local magnetic field. However, the synthesis of magnetic nanoparticles is challenging because of the high reactivity of bare iron oxide nanoparticles, which makes them easily oxidizable in air, thus resulting in loss of their magnetism and dispersibility. Consequently, surface modifications are often introduced to passivate the surface of these particles to avoid aggregation during or after the synthesis procedures. In order to increase stability and biocompatibility, iron oxide nanoparticles have been chemically functionalized with various compounds, including polymers, surfactants, biomolecules, and inorganic layers. Moreover, these protecting shells also provide functional groups for further ligand conjugation and drug loading via covalent bonding or physical adsorption. Similar to most designs, the development of iron oxide-based, redox-responsive nanocarriers has incorporated the disulfide linkage at the surface of the nanoparticles to enable thiol-triggered drug delivery. The hydrophobic anticancer drugs can be encapsulated in nanoreservoirs via a disulfide linker, and the intracellular drug delivery can be monitored by conjugation with imaging probes. It has been reported that polyethylenimine (PEI)- and β-cyclodextrin (β-CD)-functionalized magnetic nanoparticle MNP–S–S–PEI/β-CD@CAMP could deliver the anticancer drug camptothecin (CAMP) into the cells and induce cell apoptosis *in situ*. PEI and β-CD were conjugated to MNP via disulfide bonds, and CAMP was encapsulated in the PEI/β-CD nanostructure through hydrophobic interaction.[77] The results indicated that surface modification with PEI and β-CD improved internalization efficiency through physical adsorption and interaction between β-CD, cholesterols, and phospholipids. Moreover, PEI provides a relatively high density of positive charge and induces endosomal escape (Figure 7.5).

An alternative strategy combined superparamagnetic iron oxide nanoparticles (SPIONs) with mesoporous silica nanorods.[78] SPIONs served as a gatekeeper here. The chemically labile disulfide linkage between SPIONs and MSNs can react with cellular antioxidants (e.g., dihydrolipoic acid [DHLA]) or thiols. The release of the gatekeeper was regulated by the concentration of reducing agents. The results revealed that SPIONs efficiently prevented the fluorescent dyes from leaking out of the nanoconjugate and a rapid release could only be observed on treatment with reducing agents. Significant fluorescence was found in HeLa cells, indicating the cleavage of the disulfide linkers in the nanoconjugates on exposure to redox stimuli in cancer cells (Figure 7.6). The feasibility of iron oxide–based DDSs as redox-responsive anticancer drug carriers has been demonstrated; these DDSs have the potential to be manipulated by external magnetic fields for site-specific drug release and MRI.[78]

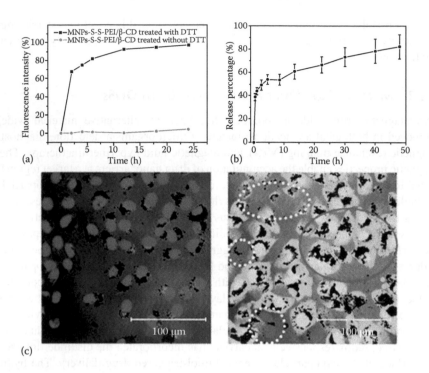

FIGURE 7.5 (a) Redox-responsive MNP–S–S–PEI/β-CD nanoconjugate upon DTT stimulus and (b) the cumulative FITC release. (c) The confocal images of HepaG2 cell cultured with MNPs-FITC (left) and MNP–S–S–PEI/β-CD@FITC (right) for 48 h. Note: green, FITC; black particulates, MNPs and MNP–S–S–PEI/β-CD; red, lysosome; blue, nuclei. (Z. Luo et al.: Redox-responsive molecular nanoreservoirs for controlled intracellular anticancer drug delivery based on magnetic nanoparticles. *Advanced Materials*. 2012. 24. 431–435. Copyright Wiley-VCH Verlag GmbH & Co. KGaA. Reproduced with permission.)

7.2.4 Gold Nanoparticle–Based DDSs

Gold nanoparticles have emerged as an attractive nanomaterial for biological and biomedical applications because of their reproducible synthesis with atomic-level precision, unique physical and chemical properties, versatile morphologies, flexibility in functionalization, ease of targeting, efficiency in drug delivery, and opportunities for multimodal therapy.[79,80] The intriguing optical properties of these nanoparticles reflected by their characteristic extinction spectra are attributed to their unique interaction with incident light. When a metal nanoparticle is exposed to electromagnetic radiation with a frequency matching the material's characteristic resonant frequency, all the "free" electrons within the conduction band of the particle will undergo an in-phase oscillation with the frequency of radiation. This is generally called surface plasmon resonance (SPR).[81]

The dipolar oscillation is resonant with the incoming light at a specific frequency, which is influenced by the particle's size, shape, structure, dielectric properties, and the surrounding medium, resulting in an altered distribution of electron charge

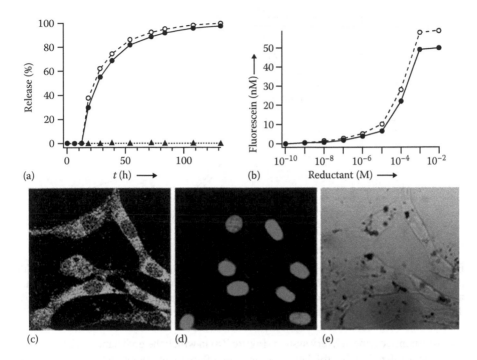

FIGURE 7.6   (a) Controlled release of fluorescein from magnetic Fe_3O_4-capped fluorescein-loaded MSNs triggered by DHLA (●) or DTT (○). No noticeable release was observed in the absence of a reductant (▲). (b) The dependency of fluorescein release from magnetic MSNs on the reductant concentration was measured 72 h after the addition of DHLA (●) or DTT (○). (c through e) Confocal images of HeLa cells after 10-h incubation with magnetic MSNs. The results showed the release of FITC (excited at 494 nm) and the aggregation of dark magnetic MSNs. Note: green, FITC; blue, DAPI; black particulates, Fe_3O_4. (S. Giri et al.: Stimuli-responsive controlled-release delivery system based on mesoporous silica nanorods capped with magnetic nanoparticles. *Angewandte Chemie International Edition.* 2005. 44. 5038–5044. Copyright Wiley-VCH Verlag GmbH & Co. KGaA. Reproduced with permission.)

density on the particle's surface. The absorption and scattering properties of gold nanoparticles can be tuned by controlling the particle size and the local refractive index near the particle surface. The monodispersed nanoparticles with diameters ranging from 9 to 99 nm can be synthesized to tune the plasmon resonance band over a wide spectral range. The absorption maximum of gold nanoparticle results in a red shift with increase in size (Figure 7.7).[82,83] The biocompatibility of gold nanoparticles and their simple functionalization by thiolated guest molecules allow the nanomaterial to serve as excellent drug delivery nanocarriers. Moreover, the geometrically tunable optical characteristics, the surface-enhanced Raman spectra, and the high-fluorescence quenching efficiency also indicate their great potential to serve as optical tracers and for biosensing applications.[84]

The characteristic GSH difference led scientists to design diverse disulfide-linked nanomaterials for smart drug delivery applications. Hong et al. developed a

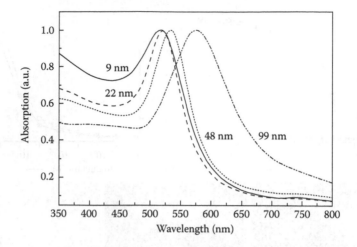

FIGURE 7.7 The absorption spectra of differently sized gold nanoparticles. (Reprinted with permission from S. Link and M.A. El-Sayed, Size and temperature dependence of the plasmon absorption of colloidal gold nanoparticles. *The Journal of Physical Chemistry B*, 103, 4212–4217. Copyright 1999 American Chemical Society.)

redox-responsive gene delivery system (Figure 7.8) in which the gold nanoparticle surface was functionalized with a thiolated, cationic, and fluorogenic ligand-labeled monolayer. GSH triggered the drug release from nanocarrier *in vitro* and *in vivo*.[60] Redox-sensitive systems have also been constructed by employing the thiol-cleavable bonds in the drug conjugates. For instance, the polyethylene glycosylated (PEGylated) gold nanoparticles were grafted with the anticancer drug, DOX, via a cleavable disulfide linkage (Au-PEG-SS-DOX). Upon endocytotic entry, the disulfide-containing Au-PEG-SS-DOX nano-conjugates were degraded by thiol-reducing enzymes in the lysosomes. The released molecules could escape from lysosomal vesicles and accumulate in the cytoplasm, inducing significant cell death of the multidrug-resistant cells.[11]

A new gold nanoparticle–based nanocarrier consisting of an extra-thin-layer disulfide network for improving the sensitivity of redox-responsive DDSs has been recently developed in our laboratory (Figure 7.9). ReSiN, a silica-based, disulfide bond–linked structure, is employed as a redox-sensitive material to modify the surface of gold nanoparticles. In addition, the transferrin serves as a cancer-specific ligand. The FITC dye is used as a model drug to facilitate the intracellular monitoring of the nanoconjugate. Under high concentrations of GSH in the cell, we expect that the rapid destruction of the thin-layer disulfide network can lead to the release of encapsulated FITC and the aggregation of the gold nanoparticles. This multimodality optical detection may also be feasible for further *in vivo* studies.

Additionally, by taking advantage of the gold nanoparticles that absorb near-infrared (NIR) light, intensive investigation of their potential in combination with hyperthermia therapy has been performed. Although the SPR of the conventional spherical gold nanoparticles is at the visible wavelength region, the resonance peak can be shifted to the NIR range (800–1200 nm) by modulating their shapes, for example, as gold nanorods,[85] gold nanocages,[34,35,44] and many multifunctional nanocomposites.[86]

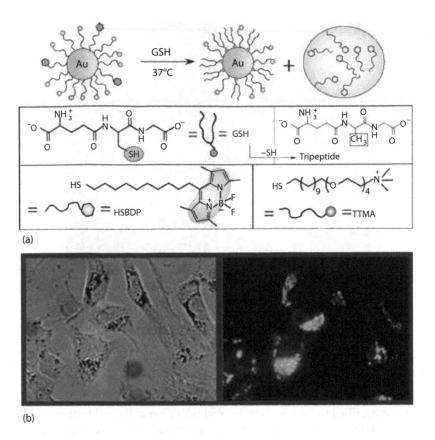

(a)

(b)

FIGURE 7.8 (a) GSH-triggered drug release of mixed TTMA/HSBDP monolayer–functionalized gold nanoparticles. (b) The fluorescence recovery in human liver carcinoma (Hep G2). (Reprinted with permission from R. Hong et al., Glutathione-mediated delivery and release using monolayer protected nanoparticle carriers. *Journal of the American Chemical Society*, 128, 1078–1079. Copyright 2006 American Chemical Society.)

The photothermal effect of gold nanoparticles leads to the rapid dissipation of heat to the surroundings by laser illumination exposure, and thus the cancer cells can be killed without damaging normal cells.[34,35,86]

A promising strategy to construct a stimuli-responsive nanocarrier is to modify the nanoparticle solid phase with polymers. The polymer chains change conformation in response to temperature at a point known as low critical solution temperature (LCST). By modulating the temperature, the properties of the polymer can be altered significantly. A smart copolymer based on poly-(*N*-isopropylacrylamide) (pNIPAAm)-co-poly-(acrylamide) (pAAm) with 39°C LCST was functionalized at a gold–silver nanocage to enable controlled drug release via structural changes in the polymers owing to absorption of NIR light. Without light exposure, the polymer returned to the extended conformation and drug release was terminated.[36] Another light-responsive drug delivery platform has been fabricated by coating a dense monolayer of drug-loading DNA at the gold nanoparticle surface. The light-induced drug

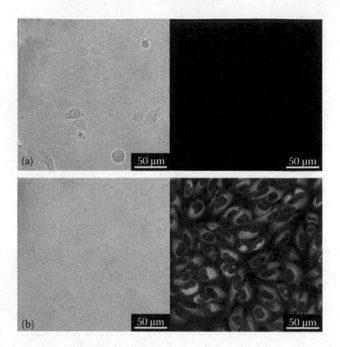

FIGURE 7.9 (a) Confocal images of control HeLa cells and (b) cells treated with redox-responsive silica–Au nanoconjugates. (Courtesy of Luo, Y.-L. et al., unpublished data.)

release was ascribed to the rapid DNA dehybridization at the gold nanoparticle surface under illumination, thereby triggering the release of encapsulated molecules.[38]

Chemical functionalization in conjunction with photothermal or photodynamic therapy is a new therapeutic strategy for cancer treatment. As the development of redox-responsive drug nanocarriers continues to evolve by various disulfide linkage incorporation strategies, a lot of effort has been devoted to the mechanisms of disulfide cleavage and the time- and spatial-resolved thiol levels in different cells and tissues.[76,87,88] The DDSs can be designed to respond to specific internal redox or pH stimuli with external light illumination to achieve synergistic efficacy in disease management.

7.3   FUTURE PERSPECTIVES

As more knowledge is gained regarding disease mechanisms, including ever-evolving understanding of the cancer microenvironment and new treatments resulting from discoveries of bioactive molecules and gene therapies, researchers can develop more effective DDSs for cancer management.[89–92] In the past decades, various inorganic nanomaterials have been successfully fabricated and applied in DDSs. The dye-doped SiNPs (called Cornell dots) were the first investigational new drug to receive FDA approval for targeted cancer imaging. Drugs based on gold nanoparticles have been used in phase I/II clinical trials for solid tumor treatment. Furthermore, studies of Feridex (iron oxide nanoparticles) have been employed as magnetic resonance contrast agents at very low dosages to label human cancer and stem cells. All these nanoconjugates have shown potential for their clinical relevance in transitioning their application from bench to bedside. Despite this promising progress, most of the other nanomaterials are still under *in vitro* optimization or withdrawn from the market. Mylotarg, a calicheamicin disulfide-linked anti-CD33 antibody commercialized by Pfizer, which was approved by FDA for acute myeloid leukemia, failed to confirm its benefit to patients and voluntary withdrawal of the drug was announced in 2010.

The current DDSs exhibit several issues that scientists are still attempting to address. The improvement in theranostics of malignancies is of great necessity. Although the EPR effect permits passive accumulation of nanoparticles in the tumor interstitium, only suboptimal delivery is achieved with most nanoparticles because of heterogeneities in vascular permeability. Furthermore, slow drug release limits bioavailability. Many drug potencies and therapeutic effects are limited or reduced because of the partial degradation that occurs before they reach a desired target in the body. In most cases, once ingested, the release of medications traditionally has been diffusion controlled. Time-dependent drug release delivers treatment continuously rather than providing instant relief from symptoms and protection from adverse events. The adoption of formulations that control the rate and period of drug delivery and target specific areas of the body for treatment has become a well-accepted trend. Evidently, to prepare such smart multifunctional pharmaceutical nanocarriers, chemical moieties providing certain required individual properties have to be simultaneously assembled either on the surface or within the structure of the same nanoconstructs. To achieve maximum therapeutic efficacy at the nano/bio interface, extensive pharmacokinetic studies and studies on the biocompatibility of therapeutic nanocarriers must be performed. The development of multifunctional nanoscale systems for combined sensing, imaging, and therapy continues to be an active subject of pharmaceutical research.

ACKNOWLEDGMENTS

This work was supported by the National Science Council of Taiwan (Grant No. NSC101-2113-M-009-006-MY2) and the Ministry of Education, Taiwan ("Aim for the Top University Plan" of National Chiao Tung University).

REFERENCES

1. A. B. Miller; B. Hoogstraten; M. Staquet; A. Winkler, Reporting results of cancer treatment. *Cancer*, 47, 207–214 (1981).
2. M. Dean; T. Fojo; S. Bates, Tumour stem cells and drug resistance. *Nature Reviews Cancer*, 5, 275–284 (2005).
3. A. Persidis, Cancer multidrug resistance. *Nature Biotechnology*, 17, 94–95 (1999).
4. M. Saraswathy; S. Gong, Different strategies to overcome multidrug resistance in cancer. *Biotechnology Advances*, 31, 1397–1407 (2013).
5. A. Albanese; P. S. Tang; W. C. Chan, The effect of nanoparticle size, shape, and surface chemistry on biological systems. *Annual Review of Biomedical Engineering*, 14, 1–16 (2012).
6. M. van der Zande; R. J. Vandebriel; E. Van Doren; E. Kramer; Z. Herrera Rivera; C. S. Serrano-Rojero; E. R. Gremmer; J. Mast; R. J. Peters; P. C. Hollman, Distribution,

elimination, and toxicity of silver nanoparticles and silver ions in rats after 28-day oral exposure. *ACS Nano*, 6, 7427–7442 (2012).

7. H. Xiao; Z. Haifeng; M. Yuhui; B. Wei; Z. Zhiyong; L. Kai; D. Yayun; Z. Yuliang; C. Zhifang, Lung deposition and extrapulmonary translocation of nano-ceria after intratracheal instillation. *Nanotechnology*, 21, 285103 (2010).

8. M.-T. Zhu; W.-Y. Feng; Y. Wang; B. Wang; M. Wang; H. Ouyang; Y.-L. Zhao; Z.-F. Chai, Particokinetics and extrapulmonary translocation of intratracheally instilled ferric oxide nanoparticles in rats and the potential health risk assessment. *Toxicological Sciences*, 107, 342–351 (2009).

9. W. H. De Jong; W. I. Hagens; P. Krystek; M. C. Burger; A. J. A. M. Sips; R. E. Geertsma, Particle size-dependent organ distribution of gold nanoparticles after intravenous administration. *Biomaterials*, 29, 1912–1919 (2008).

10. R. Kumar; I. Roy; T. Y. Ohulchanskky; L. A. Vathy; E. J. Bergey; M. Sajjad; P. N. Prasad, In vivo biodistribution and clearance studies using multimodal organically modified silica nanoparticles. *ACS Nano*, 4, 699–708 (2010).

11. Y.-J. Gu; J. Cheng; C. W.-Y. Man; W.-T. Wong; S. H. Cheng, Gold-doxorubicin nanoconjugates for overcoming multidrug resistance. *Nanomedicine: Nanotechnology, Biology and Medicine*, 8, 204–211 (2012).

12. J. S. Kim; T.-J. Yoon; K. N. Yu; B. G. Kim; S. J. Park; H. W. Kim; K. H. Lee; S. B. Park; J.-K. Lee; M. H. Cho, Toxicity and tissue distribution of magnetic nanoparticles in mice. *Toxicological Sciences*, 89, 338–347 (2006).

13. B. Wang; X. He; Z. Zhang; Y. Zhao; W. Feng, Metabolism of nanomaterials in vivo: Blood circulation and organ clearance. *Accounts of Chemical Research*, 46, 761–769 (2012).

14. P. Opanasopit; M. Nishikawa; M. Hashida, Factors affecting drug and gene delivery: Effects of interaction with blood components. *Critical Reviews in Therapeutic Drug Carrier Systems*, 19, 191–233 (2002).

15. Y. Matsumura; H. Maeda, A new concept for macromolecular therapeutics in cancer chemotherapy: Mechanism of tumoritropic accumulation of proteins and the antitumor agent smancs. *Cancer Research*, 46, 6387–6392 (1986).

16. F. Yuan; M. Dellian; D. Fukumura; M. Leunig; D. A. Berk; V. P. Torchilin; R. K. Jain, Vascular permeability in a human tumor xenograft: Molecular size dependence and cutoff size. *Cancer Research*, 55, 3752–3756 (1995).

17. M. R. Dreher; A. Chilkoti, Toward a systems engineering approach to cancer drug delivery. *Journal of the National Cancer Institute*, 99, 983–985 (2007).

18. R. A. Petros; J. M. DeSimone, Strategies in the design of nanoparticles for therapeutic applications. *Nature Reviews Drug Discovery*, 9, 615–627 (2010).

19. P. P. Adiseshaiah; J. B. Hall; S. E. McNeil, Nanomaterial standards for efficacy and toxicity assessment. *Wiley Interdisciplinary Reviews: Nanomedicine and Nanobiotechnology*, 2, 99–112 (2010).

20. P. Carmeliet; R. K. Jain, Angiogenesis in cancer and other diseases. *Nature*, 407, 249–257 (2000).

21. K. Greish; T. Sawa; J. Fang; T. Akaike; H. Maeda, SMA–doxorubicin, a new polymeric micellar drug for effective targeting to solid tumours. *Journal of Controlled Release*, 97, 219–230 (2004).

22. R. K. Jain, Barriers to drug-delivery in solid tumors. *Scientific American*, 271, 58–65 (1994).

23. N. Oh; J.-H. Park, Endocytosis and exocytosis of nanoparticles in mammalian cells. *International Journal of Nanomedicine*, 9, 51 (2014).

24. K. Makino; N. Yamamoto; K. Higuchi; N. Harada; H. Ohshima; H. Terada, Phagocytic uptake of polystyrene microspheres by alveolar macrophages: Effects of the size and surface properties of the microspheres. *Colloids and Surfaces B: Biointerfaces*, 27, 33–39 (2003).

25. T.-G. Iversen; T. Skotland; K. Sandvig, Endocytosis and intracellular transport of nanoparticles: Present knowledge and need for future studies. *Nano Today*, 6, 176–185 (2011).
26. J. Gallo; N. J. Long; E. O. Aboagye, Magnetic nanoparticles as contrast agents in the diagnosis and treatment of cancer. *Chemical Society Reviews*, 42, 7816–7833 (2013).
27. Y.-C. Chen; X.-C. Huang; Y.-L. Luo; Y.-C. Chang; Y.-Z. Hsieh; H.-Y. Hsu, Non-metallic nanomaterials in cancer theranostics: A review of silica- and carbon-based drug delivery systems. *Science and Technology of Advanced Materials*, 14, 044407 (2013).
28. A. J. Mieszawska; W. J. M. Mulder; Z. A. Fayad; D. P. Cormode, Multifunctional gold nanoparticles for diagnosis and therapy of disease. *Molecular Pharmaceutics*, 10, 831–847 (2013).
29. E. Miele; G. P. Spinelli; E. Miele; F. Tomao; S. Tomao, Albumin-bound formulation of paclitaxel (Abraxane® ABI-007) in the treatment of breast cancer. *International Journal of Nanomedicine*, 4, 99 (2009).
30. J. Kost; R. Langer, Responsive polymeric delivery systems. *Advanced Drug Delivery Reviews*, 64 Suppl., 327–341 (2012).
31. S. Mura; J. Nicolas; P. Couvreur, Stimuli-responsive nanocarriers for drug delivery. *Nature Materials*, 12, 991–1003 (2013).
32. V. P. Torchilin, Multifunctional nanocarriers. *Advanced Drug Delivery Reviews*, 64 Suppl., 302–315 (2012).
33. E. Fleige; M. A. Quadir; R. Haag, Stimuli-responsive polymeric nanocarriers for the controlled transport of active compounds: Concepts and applications. *Advanced Drug Delivery Reviews*, 64, 866–884 (2012).
34. J. Chen; C. Glaus; R. Laforest; Q. Zhang; M. Yang; M. Gidding; M. J. Welch; Y. Xia, Gold nanocages as photothermal transducers for cancer treatment. *Small*, 6, 811–817 (2010).
35. C. M. Cobley; L. Au; J. Chen; Y. Xia, Targeting gold nanocages to cancer cells for photothermal destruction and drug delivery. *Expert Opinion on Drug Delivery*, 7, 577–587 (2010).
36. M. S. Yavuz; Y. Cheng; J. Chen; C. M. Cobley; Q. Zhang; M. Rycenga; J. Xie; C. Kim; K. H. Song; A. G. Schwartz; L. V. Wang; Y. Xia, Gold nanocages covered by smart polymers for controlled release with near-infrared light. *Nature Materials*, 8, 935–939 (2009).
37. S. S. Agasti; A. Chompoosor; C.-C. You; P. Ghosh; C. K. Kim; V. M. Rotello, Photoregulated release of caged anticancer drugs from gold nanoparticles. *Journal of the American Chemical Society*, 131, 5728–5729 (2009).
38. Y.-L. Luo; Y.-S. Shiao; Y.-F. Huang, Release of photoactivatable drugs from plasmonic nanoparticles for targeted cancer therapy. *ACS Nano*, 5, 7796–7804 (2011).
39. I. H. El-Sayed; X. Huang; M. A. El-Sayed, Selective laser photo-thermal therapy of epithelial carcinoma using anti-EGFR antibody conjugated gold nanoparticles. *Cancer Letters*, 239, 129–135 (2006).
40. X. Huang; P. K. Jain; I. H. El-Sayed; M. A. El-Sayed, Determination of the minimum temperature required for selective photothermal destruction of cancer cells with the use of immunotargeted gold nanoparticles. *Photochemistry and Photobiology*, 82, 412–417 (2006).
41. L. A. Lyon; Z. Meng; N. Singh; C. D. Sorrell; A. St. John, Thermoresponsive microgel-based materials. *Chemical Society Reviews*, 38, 865–874 (2009).
42. D. M. Nelson; Z. Ma; C. E. Leeson; W. R. Wagner, Extended and sequential delivery of protein from injectable thermoresponsive hydrogels. *Journal of Biomedical Materials Research Part A*, 100A, 776–785 (2012).
43. M. Nakayama; T. Okano; T. Miyazaki; F. Kohori; K. Sakai; M. Yokoyama, Molecular design of biodegradable polymeric micelles for temperature-responsive drug release. *Journal of Controlled Release*, 115, 46–56 (2006).

44. W. Li; X. Cai; C. Kim; G. Sun; Y. Zhang; R. Deng; M. Yang; J. Chen; S. Achilefu; L. V. Wang, Gold nanocages covered with thermally-responsive polymers for controlled release by high-intensity focused ultrasound. *Nanoscale*, 3, 1724–1730 (2011).

45. C.-H. Wang; S.-T. Kang; Y.-H. Lee; Y.-L. Luo; Y.-F. Huang; C.-K. Yeh, Aptamer-conjugated and drug-loaded acoustic droplets for ultrasound theranosis. *Biomaterials*, 33, 1939–1947 (2012).

46. G. D. Moon; S.-W. Choi; X. Cai; W. Li; E. C. Cho; U. Jeong; L. V. Wang; Y. Xia, A new theranostic system based on gold nanocages and phase-change materials with unique features for photoacoustic imaging and controlled release. *Journal of the American Chemical Society*, 133, 4762–4765 (2011).

47. C. S. S. R. Kumar; F. Mohammad, Magnetic nanomaterials for hyperthermia-based therapy and controlled drug delivery. *Advanced Drug Delivery Reviews*, 63, 789–808 (2011).

48. J. Klostergaard; C. E. Seeney, Magnetic nanovectors for drug delivery. *Maturitas*, 73, 33–44 (2012).

49. M. Kinoshita; N. McDannold; F. A. Jolesz; K. Hynynen, Noninvasive localized delivery of Herceptin to the mouse brain by MRI-guided focused ultrasound-induced blood–brain barrier disruption. *Proceedings of the National Academy of Sciences of the United States of America*, 103, 11719–11723 (2006).

50. C.-Y. Ting; C.-H. Fan; H.-L. Liu; C.-Y. Huang; H.-Y. Hsieh; T.-C. Yen; K.-C. Wei; C.-K. Yeh, Concurrent blood–brain barrier opening and local drug delivery using drug-carrying microbubbles and focused ultrasound for brain glioma treatment. *Biomaterials*, 33, 704–712 (2012).

51. H.-L. Liu; M.-Y. Hua; P.-Y. Chen; P.-C. Chu; C.-H. Pan; H.-W. Yang; C.-Y. Huang; J.-J. Wang; T.-C. Yen; K.-C. Wei, Blood-brain barrier disruption with focused ultrasound enhances delivery of chemotherapeutic drugs for glioblastoma treatment. *Radiology*, 255, 415–425 (2010).

52. F. Kiessling; S. Fokong; P. Koczera; W. Lederle; T. Lammers, Ultrasound microbubbles for molecular diagnosis, therapy, and theranostics. *Journal of Nuclear Medicine*, 53, 345–348 (2012).

53. H. R. Guzmán; D. X. Nguyen; S. Khan; M. R. Prausnitz, Ultrasound-mediated disruption of cell membranes. I. Quantification of molecular uptake and cell viability. *The Journal of the Acoustical Society of America*, 110, 588–596 (2001).

54. J. Sundaram; B. R. Mellein; S. Mitragotri, An experimental and theoretical analysis of ultrasound-induced permeabilization of cell membranes. *Biophysical Journal*, 84, 3087–3101 (2003).

55. M. Kinoshita; K. Hynynen, A novel method for the intracellular delivery of siRNA using microbubble-enhanced focused ultrasound. *Biochemical and Biophysical Research Communications*, 335, 393–399 (2005).

56. Y. Negishi; Y. Endo; T. Fukuyama; R. Suzuki; T. Takizawa; D. Omata; K. Maruyama; Y. Aramaki, Delivery of siRNA into the cytoplasm by liposomal bubbles and ultrasound. *Journal of Controlled Release*, 132, 124–130 (2008).

57. F. Wang; Y.-C. Wang; S. Dou; M.-H. Xiong; T.-M. Sun; J. Wang, Doxorubicin-tethered responsive gold nanoparticles facilitate intracellular drug delivery for overcoming multidrug resistance in cancer cells. *ACS Nano*, 5, 3679–3692 (2011).

58. R. Liu; Y. Zhang; X. Zhao; A. Agarwal; L. J. Mueller; P. Feng, pH-responsive nanogated ensemble based on gold-capped mesoporous silica through an acid-labile acetal linker. *Journal of the American Chemical Society*, 132, 1500–1501 (2010).

59. S. Aryal; J. J. Grailer; S. Pilla; D. A. Steeber; S. Gong, Doxorubicin conjugated gold nanoparticles as water-soluble and pH-responsive anticancer drug nanocarriers. *Journal of Materials Chemistry*, 19, 7879–7884 (2009).

60. R. Hong; G. Han; J. M. Fernández; B.-J. Kim; N. S. Forbes; V. M. Rotello, Glutathione-mediated delivery and release using monolayer protected nanoparticle carriers. *Journal of the American Chemical Society*, 128, 1078–1079 (2006).
61. N. Graf; S. J. Lippard, Redox activation of metal-based prodrugs as a strategy for drug delivery. *Advanced Drug Delivery Reviews*, 64, 993–1004 (2012).
62. J. Liu; Y. Pang; W. Huang; Z. Zhu; X. Zhu; Y. Zhou; D. Yan, Redox-responsive polyphosphate nanosized assemblies: A smart drug delivery platform for cancer therapy. *Biomacromolecules*, 12, 2407–2415 (2011).
63. R. de la Rica; D. Aili; M. M. Stevens, Enzyme-responsive nanoparticles for drug release and diagnostics. *Advanced Drug Delivery Reviews*, 64, 967–978 (2012).
64. Q. He; J. Shi, Mesoporous silica nanoparticle based nano drug delivery systems: Synthesis, controlled drug release and delivery, pharmacokinetics and biocompatibility. *Journal of Materials Chemistry*, 21, 5845–5855 (2011).
65. R. Cheng; F. Feng; F. Meng; C. Deng; J. Feijen; Z. Zhong, Glutathione-responsive nano-vehicles as a promising platform for targeted intracellular drug and gene delivery. *Journal of Controlled Release*, 152, 2–12 (2011).
66. A. N. Koo; H. J. Lee; S. E. Kim; J. H. Chang; C. Park; C. Kim; J. H. Park; S. C. Lee, Disulfide-cross-linked PEG-poly(amino acid)s copolymer micelles for glutathione-mediated intracellular drug delivery. *Chemical Communications*, 48, 6570–6572 (2008).
67. D. P. Jones; J. L. Carlson; P. S. Samiec; P. Sternberg Jr; V. C. Mody Jr; R. L. Reed; L. A. S. Brown, Glutathione measurement in human plasma: Evaluation of sample collection, storage and derivatization conditions for analysis of dansyl derivatives by HPLC. *Clinica Chimica Acta*, 275, 175–184 (1998).
68. S. Ganta; H. Devalapally; A. Shahiwala; M. Amiji, A review of stimuli-responsive nanocarriers for drug and gene delivery. *Journal of Controlled Release*, 126, 187–204 (2008).
69. J. Jansen; Z. Shan; L. Marchese; W. Zhou; N. van der Puil; T. Maschmeyer, A new templating method for three-dimensional mesopore networks. *Chemical Communications*, 8, 713–714 (2001).
70. J. S. Beck; J. C. Vartuli; W. J. Roth; M. E. Leonowicz; C. T. Kresge; K. D. Schmitt; C. T. W. Chu; D. H. Olson; E. W. Sheppard, A new family of mesoporous molecular sieves prepared with liquid crystal templates. *Journal of the American Chemical Society*, 114, 10834–10843 (1992).
71. C. Kresge; M. Leonowicz; W. Roth; J. Vartuli; J. Beck, Ordered mesoporous molecular sieves synthesized by a liquid-crystal template mechanism. *Nature*, 359, 710–712 (1992).
72. S. Inagaki; Y. Fukushima; K. Kuroda, Synthesis of highly ordered mesoporous materials from a layered polysilicate. *Journal of the Chemical Society, Chemical Communications*, 8, 680–682 (1993).
73. A. Corma; Q. Kan; M. T. Navarro; J. Pérez-Pariente; F. Rey, Synthesis of MCM-41 with different pore diameters without addition of auxiliary organics. *Chemistry of Materials*, 9, 2123–2126 (1997).
74. S. Namba; A. Mochizuki; M. Kito, Preparation of highly ordered MCM-41 with docosyltrimethylammonium chloride (C_{22} TMAC1) as a template and fine control of its pore size. *Studies in Surface Science and Catalysis*, 117, 257–264 (1998).
75. Z. Luo; K. Cai; Y. Hu; L. Zhao; P. Liu; L. Duan; W. Yang, Mesoporous silica nanoparticles end-capped with collagen: Redox-responsive nanoreservoirs for targeted drug delivery. *Angewandte Chemie International Edition*, 50, 640–643 (2011).
76. A. M. Sauer; A. Schlossbauer; N. Ruthardt; V. Cauda; T. Bein; C. Bräuchle, Role of endosomal escape for disulfide-based drug delivery from colloidal mesoporous silica evaluated by live-cell imaging. *Nano Letters*, 10, 3684–3691 (2010).

77. Z. Luo; K. Cai; Y. Hu; J. Li; X. Ding; B. Zhang; D. Xu; W. Yang; P. Liu, Redox-responsive molecular nanoreservoirs for controlled intracellular anticancer drug delivery based on magnetic nanoparticles. *Advanced Materials*, 24, 431–435 (2012).

78. S. Giri; B. G. Trewyn; M. P. Stellmaker; V. S. Y. Lin, Stimuli-responsive controlled-release delivery system based on mesoporous silica nanorods capped with magnetic nanoparticles. *Angewandte Chemie International Edition*, 44, 5038–5044 (2005).

79. D. A. Giljohann; D. S. Seferos; W. L. Daniel; M. D. Massich; P. C. Patel; C. A. Mirkin, Gold nanoparticles for biology and medicine. *Angewandte Chemie International Edition*, 49, 3280–3294 (2010).

80. S. Eustis; M. A. El-Sayed, Why gold nanoparticles are more precious than pretty gold: Noble metal surface plasmon resonance and its enhancement of the radiative and non-radiative properties of nanocrystals of different shapes. *Chemical Society Reviews*, 35, 209–217 (2006).

81. C. F. Bohren; D. R. Huffman, *Absorption and Scattering of Light by Small Particles*. Wiley-VCH Verlag, Weinheim, Germany: 2008.

82. S. Link; M. A. El-Sayed, Size and temperature dependence of the plasmon absorption of colloidal gold nanoparticles. *The Journal of Physical Chemistry B*, 103, 4212–4217 (1999).

83. K.-S. Lee; M. A. El-Sayed, Gold and silver nanoparticles in sensing and imaging: Sensitivity of plasmon response to size, shape, and metal composition. *The Journal of Physical Chemistry B*, 110, 19220–19225 (2006).

84. K. Saha; S. S. Agasti; C. Kim; X. Li; V. M. Rotello, Gold nanoparticles in chemical and biological sensing. *Chemical Reviews*, 112, 2739–2779 (2012).

85. V. Biju, Chemical modifications and bioconjugate reactions of nanomaterials for sensing, imaging, drug delivery and therapy. *Chemical Society Reviews*, 43, 744–764 (2014).

86. H. Liu; T. Liu; X. Wu; L. Li; L. Tan; D. Chen; F. Tang, Targeting gold nanoshells on silica nanorattles: A drug cocktail to fight breast tumors via a single irradiation with near-infrared laser light. *Advanced Materials*, 24, 755–761 (2012).

87. K. Ock; W. I. Jeon; E. O. Ganbold; M. Kim; J. Park; J. H. Seo; K. Cho; S.-W. Joo; S. Y. Lee, Real-time monitoring of glutathione-triggered thiopurine anticancer drug release in live cells investigated by surface-enhanced Raman scattering. *Analytical Chemistry*, 84, 2172–2178 (2012).

88. G. Saito; J. A. Swanson; K.-D. Lee, Drug delivery strategy utilizing conjugation via reversible disulfide linkages: Role and site of cellular reducing activities. *Advanced Drug Delivery Reviews*, 55, 199–215 (2003).

89. P. P. Shanbhag; S. V. Jog; M. M. Chogale; S. S. Gaikwad, Theranostics for cancer therapy. *Current Drug Delivery*, 10, 357–362 (2013).

90. S. P. Povoski; I. S. Hatzaras; C. M. Mojzisik; E. W. Martin, Jr., Oncologic theranostics: Recognition of this concept in antigen-directed cancer therapy for colorectal cancer with anti-TAG-72 monoclonal antibodies. *Expert Review of Molecular Diagnostics*, 11, 667–670 (2011).

91. Y. Omidi, Smart multifunctional theranostics: Simultaneous diagnosis and therapy of cancer. *BioImpacts: BI*, 1, 145–147 (2011).

92. W. Chen; N. Xu; L. Xu; L. Wang; Z. Li; W. Ma; Y. Zhu; C. Xu; N. A. Kotov, Multifunctional magnetoplasmonic nanoparticle assemblies for cancer therapy and diagnostics (theranostics). *Macromolecular Rapid Communications*, 31, 228–236 (2010).

Section II

Antimicrobial Nanomaterials

Section II

Antimicrobial Nanomaterials

8 Surface Characteristics Dictate Microbial Adhesion Ability

*Klemen Bohinc, Mojca Jevšnik, Rok Fink,
Goran Dražić, and Peter Raspor*

CONTENTS

ABSTRACT

Bacterial adhesion can be inhibited or promoted by different material surface characteristics. In this review, we give a short overview of bacterial and material characteristics as well as conditions for microbial adhesion to contact surfaces. Bacterial adhesion is related to food safety and its implications for human health. One of the surface characteristics is its roughness, which we will concentrate on in this review. In our experiment, we prepared four different glass surfaces by polishing the glass plates with different gradations. The surface roughness was controlled by profilometry and atomic force microscopy. We used three different bacteria (*Staphylococcus aureus*, *Pseudomonas aeruginosa*, and *Escherichia coli*). The rate of adhered bacteria on glass surfaces was determined spectrophotometrically. The results showed that the rate of adhered bacteria increases with increasing surface roughness. The increased adhesion of bacteria on rougher surfaces is the interplay between the increasing effective surface and increasing number of defects on the surface.

Keywords: Bacterial adhesion, Material surfaces, Roughness

8.1   INTRODUCTION

8.1.1   GENERAL

The phenomenon of adherence of microorganisms on different surfaces is widespread in the food industry, medical equipment (prostheses, implants), natural environments, and water supply systems. Otto (2008) described how microorganisms can live and proliferate as individual cells or they can attach to surfaces, where they grow as highly organized multicellular communities that are referred to as biofilms and are now regarded as the predominant mode of microbial life in nature and disease.

8.1.2   BIOFILM FORMATION

Bacteria can be considered as either planktonic cells freely flowing in a solution or as biofilms where the bacteria are attached to a material surface. Vickery et al. (2004) state that bacteria readily adhere to wet surfaces and form organized colonies of cells enclosed in a self-excreted matrix composed principally of polysaccharide (EPS) that facilitates adhesion to the surface and each other. This type of bacterial organization is termed biofilm and was originally noted in 1936 (Vickery et al. 2004; Zobell and Anderson 1936). The adhesion process is governed by physical and chemical interactions between microorganisms and surface and represents the first step, by attachment, followed by survival, and if the nutrients at the surface allow, microbes can multiply, colonize the surface, and finally form biofilm, which is an essential source of further contamination (Hori and Matsumoto 2010; Zupan et al. 2009). The theory of biofilms was first described by J.W. Costerton in 1978 (Costerton et al. 1978). A biofilm is defined as a microbial-derived sessile community that is characterized by cells that are irreversibly attached to a substratum, to an interface, or to each other. The biofilm is irreversibly attached to the surface and rinsing cannot remove it. These cells are embedded in an extracellular polymeric matrix. Cells in a biofilm exhibit altered growth and gene transcription compared to unattached cells (Agle 2007; Donlan and Costerton 2002). Biofilms are the preferential mode of growth for many types of organisms (Agle 2007). Understanding of bacterial accumulation at interfaces is of biological, medical, technological, and sanitary importance.

The extensive and pervasive role of biofilms in the environment, industry, and medicine is well established thanks to the pioneering efforts of many important authors (Costerton et al. 1987; Fletcher and Loeb 1979; Fletcher and Marshall 1982; Geesey et al. 1977; Marshall and Cruickshank 1973; Marshall et al. 1971; Zobell 1943), among a host of others, yet our understanding of the molecular basis for biofilm formation remains limited. A number of studies have demonstrated that biofilm formation depends on the deposition of a conditioning layer, which adsorbs onto the surface, rather than through a direct interaction with the surface, and that one needs to modulate conditioning film formation and/or bacterial binding to adsorbed organic material to control biofilm formation (Pringle and Fletcher 1986; Renner and Weibel 2011).

Bacteria can adhere to various natural and synthetic surfaces, a phenomenon with widely different fields of application ranging from marine fouling, soil remediation, and food and drinking water processing to medicine and dentistry (Chen et al. 2011; Cunliffe et al. 1999; Stenström 1989). Bacterial adhesion to surfaces can be approached by biochemical methods, by which the molecular structures mediating adhesion are unraveled, or by physicochemical methods. Adhesion of viable bacteria to material surfaces is a necessary condition for biofilm formation in both hygienic and industrial contexts. The adhesion process is sufficiently complex that engineered prevention and promotion of bacterial adhesion remains an elusive goal (Lichter et al. 2009).

Bacteria seem to initiate biofilm formation in response to specific environmental cues, such as nutrient and oxygen availability, pH values, and water activity. These external conditions trigger alterations in the expression of a subset of genes required for biofilm formation. Strictly aerobic bacteria (i.e., *Bacillus subtilis*) form rough biofilms at the air–liquid interface rather than on the surface of a solid phase in a liquid, owing to the aerotaxis of the cells. This observation indicates that the depletion of dissolving oxygen triggers the formation of floating biofilms. It has been reported that glucose inhibits biofilm formation by *B. subtilis* through the catabolite control protein. The rapid metabolism of carbon under carbon-rich conditions does not seem to induce *B. subtilis* to undergo biofilm formation but allows cells to grow as free-living organisms. It was reported that exopolysaccharide expression and biofilm elaboration are markedly enhanced in certain bacteria, including *Pseudomonas*, *Escherichia coli*, *Staphylococcus*, and *Streptococcus*, when glucose or another utilizable carbon source is abundant. When nutrient sources are depleted, the bacteria detach and become planktonic, suggesting that nutrient deprivation is a trigger to move on, in search of a better habitat. The lower number of attached bacterial cells was found at lower pH values and higher concentrations of NaCl.

Vickery et al. (2004) pointed out that removal of biofilm poses considerable difficulties in the hospital environment. Although physical methods such as ultrasonication and mechanical cleaning or scraping are generally effective if carried out efficiently, chemical methods are often ineffective because of the resistance of biofilms to antibiotics, disinfectants, and biocides. Bacteria within biofilms are up to 1000 times more resistant to antimicrobials than the same bacteria in suspension (Vickery et al. 2004). Chmielewski and Frank (2003) stressed that poor sanitation of food contact surfaces, equipment, and processing environments has been a contributing factor in food-borne disease outbreaks, especially those involving *Listeria monocytogenes* and *Salmonella*. Elhariry (2008) pointed out that evaluating and understanding the formation of microbial biofilm are essential components of the Hazard Analysis and Critical Control Point system for food and processing industry because closed systems (e.g., pipes, valves, pumps) or open systems (e.g., conveyors) are regularly found to be contaminated by microorganisms such as *Bacillus* spp., *E. coli*, or *L. monocytogenes*. Hamadi and Yousif (2014) warn that *Staphylococcus aureus* are being occasionally found in food processing plants and have the ability to adhere to inert surfaces such as stainless steel commonly used in the food industry and consequently form biofilms.

8.1.3 CONTACT MATERIALS

The majority of bacteria can adhere to most surfaces and form biofilms (Bos et al. 1999). Different contact materials (e.g., stainless steel, glass and metal oxide surfaces, polymeric materials, surfaces with nanocoating, and many others related to ecology, food, and medical areas) are in contact with different types of microorganisms and their forms, which can cause harm to consumers' health because of their pathogenic properties (Raspor 2008) or great economic losses owing to food spoilage and reduced quality of products (Frank 2001). Materials have different characteristics for adhering and loading for various contaminants like bacteria, yeasts, fungal and bacterial spores, and viruses. Because of their characteristic attachment/adhesion, they serve as vehicles to transfer contamination vectors from place to place. If the contact materials allow microbes to survive, then the probability of contaminating the next recipient is very high, which has a strong impact on the safety and quality of the final product or service (Vesterlund et al. 2005). Current contact surfaces in the process and service industry are not strictly designed in that direction. For this reason, this issue has direct and indirect influence on the economic efficiency of production as well as on human health and the environment.

Interactions between microorganisms and contact material surfaces play an important role in biology and in different technologies like the food, pharmaceutical, and service industry (Raspor and Jevšnik 2008).

The adhesion process is governed by physical and chemical interactions between microorganisms and surface and represents the first step, by attachment, followed by survival, and if the nutrients at the surface allow, microbes can multiply, colonize the surface, and finally form biofilm, which is an essential source of further contamination (Hori and Matsumoto 2010; Zupan et al. 2009). Current comprehension of microbial adhesion and colonization of contact materials is limited to partial understanding of various model microbial cells from different genera and their biology (i.e., active growing cells, viable but nonculturable [VBNC], spores) (Henriques and Moran 2007), microbial morphology (shape, size, biofilm formation), physiology and biochemistry (i.e., polysaccharide secretion, acid production), and properties and surface chemistry of contact materials (i.e., stainless steel). However, it remains to be clarified for many contaminants how strong the influence is of various parameters such as properties of microbial cell like surface hydrophobicity (van der Mei et al. 1989) and charge (Wilson et al. 2001), extracellular appendages (Davey and O'Toole 2000), extracellular polymeric substances (Christensen 1989), signaling molecules and contact fluids in process (polarity, flow velocity, pH, ionic strength, temperature, presence of salts, antimicrobials, nutrient availability), and surface chemistry of contact materials (hydrophobicity, electric charge, surface roughness).

During processing, workers with their activities or products can injure material surfaces and transfer microbial contaminants to the contact surfaces if they have characteristics to adhere to microparticles. Since contact materials are in regular and permanent contact with substrates or final foods or drugs in the production process (food, pharmaceutical, and medical industry), there is a high probability of acquiring and loading surface contaminants from contact materials into products. Consequently, there is an evident need to determine the potential influence of various parameters such as properties of microbial cells (cell surface hydrophobicity and charge, extracellular appendages, extracellular polymeric substances, and signaling molecules), fluid characteristics (polarity, flow velocity, pH, ionic strength, temperature, presence of salts, antimicrobials, and nutrient availability), and the surface chemistry of contact materials (hydrophobicity, electric charge, and surface roughness). Understanding all these processes and their impact, it would be possible to foresee possible outcomes and thus prevent negative impact on food/drug product safety and quality.

Available methods for studying bacterial adhesion have been developed based on three vital steps: bacterial contact with surface, removal of unattached bacteria, and bacterial counting. One of the major concerns of positioning a sample surface in bacteria suspension is the surface's consistent contact with the suspension, which can be static (Murga et al. 2001). Rinsing is a very important part of a bacterial adhesion study. Attention should be paid to the force, direction, and content of the rinsing fluid. Liquids commonly used for rinsing include sterile water, normal saline, and phosphate buffered saline. A fundamental aspect of the study of bacterial adhesion and attachment to surfaces is the need for reliable quantification of the microbiological population that attaches to the surface. Few methods for bacteria counting have been introduced including direct counting methods, such as scanning electron microscopy (SEM), and indirect counting methods, such as colony-forming units, plate count, and staining methods (An and Friedman 1997; Jaryszak et al. 2009).

The results of the Bohinc et al. (2014) study showed that the rate of adhered bacteria increases with increasing surface roughness. The increased adhesion of bacteria on rougher surfaces is attributed to the interplay between the increasing effective surface and the increasing number of defects on the surface where bacteria preferentially adhere. The effect of surface roughness on bacterial adhesion is still far from being fully understood. Besides the polishing of the surface, other mechanisms that can change the roughness also exist (Quirynen et al. 1993). Truong et al. (2010) have shown that the adhesion of bacterial cells of *Pseudomonas aeruginosa* and *S. aureus* on titanium surfaces is enhanced by the presence of nanoscale topographical features. Similar trends have been reported by Bakker et al. (2004) for polymer surfaces with nanometer-scale roughness. Taylor et al. (1998) found that a small increase in surface roughness (Ra = 0.04–1.24 µm) resulted in a significant increase in bacterial adhesion, while a large increase in surface roughness (Ra = 1.86–7.89 µm) did not result in a very significant increase in adhesion, although the adhesion was still higher than to the smooth surface. On the other hand, Díaz et al. (2007, 2009) have proven that submicroscaled materials decrease microbial adhesion, whereas microscaled materials promote microbial adhesion (Whitehead et al. 2005). Xu and Siedlecki (2012) have confirmed the results obtained by Díaz et al. (2007, 2009) and, in addition, explained their reasons. In submicroscaled materials, the contact surface for adhesion is decreased owing to a small gap to fit in. Some research on eye lens showed stronger adhesion of bacteria to the materials with higher surface roughness (Giraldez et al. 2010; Tang et al. 2008). Results of Singh et al. (2011) on *E. coli* and *S. aureus* show that the increase in surface pore aspect ratio and volume, related to the increase of surface roughness, improves protein adsorption, which in turn downplays bacterial adhesion and biofilm formation. Giraldez et al. (2010) reported that greater surface roughness determines a greater specific surface area, thus creating more available surface active sites for thermodynamic reactions. Terada et al. (2006) estimated that the bacterial adhesion rate constant of *E. coli* markedly increased at a membrane potential higher than −7.8 mV, whereas that of *B. subtilis* increased at a membrane potential higher than −8.3 mV, at which the dominant effect on bacterial adhesion is expected to change.

Quirynen et al. (1993) have studied the influence of the surface roughness of implants on microbial adhesion. They showed that rough surfaces harbored more bacteria. Zhao et al. (2007) evaluated bacterial adhesion to Si-doped DLC films with *P. aeruginosa, Staphylococcus epidermidis*, and *S. aureus*, which frequently cause medical device–associated infections. Their results showed that bacterial adhesion decreased with increasing the silicon content in the films. They found out that all the Si-doped DLC films performed much better than stainless steel 316L on reducing bacterial attachment.

There are also some studies that showed that surface roughness has no effect on bacterial adhesion. Li and Logan (2004) reported that there was no significant effect of surface roughness (glass and metal oxide) on bacterial (*P. aeruginosa* and *E. coli*) adhesion. Hahnel et al. (2009) showed that the surface roughness of different ceramic materials has no significant influence on bacterial adhesion. Also, Flint et al. (2000) showed that bacterial adhesion to stainless steel with a range of surface roughness values (Ra = 0.5–3.3 μm) was largely independent on substrate topography.

Bohinc et al. (2014) pointed out that taking into account all available findings documented in the literature, this field of microbial adhesion to various material surfaces is not yet clear enough to enable prediction of when and how strongly one particular strain with defined surface hydrophobicity will adhere.

8.1.4 MICROBIAL ADHESION AND MICROORGANISM CHARACTERISTICS

By understanding the relationship between surface conditions and microbial adhesion, strategies can be developed that when realized would greatly inhibit, if not prevent, the attachment of bacteria and spores (Bower et al. 1996; Foschino et al. 2003).

The physicochemical properties of cell surfaces are an important aspect in active bacterial adhesion to different material surfaces. All bacterial cells are surrounded by a porous, three-dimensional macromolecular network, which is generally known as the bacterial cell wall. An important cell wall polymer is peptidoglycan. Gram-positive cell walls generally contain high peptidoglycan concentrations, whereas in the case of the more complex envelopes of Gram-negative cells, it is restricted to a thin layer between the cytoplasmic and the outer membrane. Besides peptidoglycan, many other macromolecules may be present in the cell wall, including teichuronic acid, lipoteichoic acid, lipopolysaccharides (LPSs), lipoproteins, enzymes, and mycolic acids. Most of these macromolecules are polyelectrolytes, because they carry charged groups such as carboxyl, phosphate, or amino groups. The presence of anionic and cationic groups gives the bacterial wall amphoteric properties, which implies that, depending on the pH, the net charge in the wall can be either positive, negative, or zero (Madigan et al. 2009; Van der Wal et al. 1997). The surfaces of most bacterial cells are at physiological pH values, that is, between 5 and 7 negatively charged, and the extent of the negative charge varies with growth environments. The net negative charge of the cell surface is adverse to bacterial adhesion owing to electrostatic repulsive force. This keeps cells a short distance away from the surface. However, the bacterial cell surface possesses hydrophobicity owing to fimbriae, flagella, and LPS. Fimbriae are cell appendages that possess hydrophobic amino acid residues (Rosenberg and Kjelleberg 1986). The main function of fimbriae is to overcome the initial electrostatic repulsion barrier that exists between the cell and the substratum (Corpe 1980). LPS is a part of the outer membrane of Gram-negative bacteria and reduces the cell's ability to interact with hydrophilic surfaces (Makin and Beveridge 1996). Adhesion of bacteria is greatly dependent on surface characteristics. The basic stages of bacterial adhesion are generally described by a two-stage kinetic binding model. In the first stage, there is an initial, rapid, and easily reversible interaction between the bacteria cell surface and the material surface. The adhesion of bacteria onto the interface is mainly governed by electrostatic, van der Waals, hydrophobic effects and contact interactions (Boks et al. 2008; Van Loosdrecht et al. 1989). Generally, the interaction free energy of the adhesion process shows two minima. The first minimum appears at a separation of 10 nm (a few kiloteslas). In this minimum, the microorganism is weakly and reversibly bound. The second stage includes specific and nonspecific interactions between so-called adhesion proteins expressed on bacterial surface structures (fimbriae or pili) and binding molecules on the material surfaces. The second minimum in the interaction free energy appears at a contact distance of 1 nm. Here, the microorganism is strongly and irreversibly adhered. The microorganism has to surpass a large energy barrier of a few kiloteslas to move on from the first to the second minimum at contact.

Numerous studies have shown that *L. monocytogenes* is capable of adhering to and forming biofilm on food contact surfaces (Blackman and Frank 1996) such as polystyrene, glass, and stainless steel (Mafu et al. 1990). Di Bonaventura et al. (2008) determined that by *L. monocytogenes*, biofilm formation is significantly influenced by temperature, which probably modifies cell surface hydrophobicity.

The behavior of the microorganisms used in the study of Foschino et al. (2003) turns out to be quite different. Particularly, *E. coli, Listeria innocua*, and *P. aeruginosa* do not have the capability to adhere to any surface since the shearing action generated by distilled water is sufficient to detach cells from the specimens. In contrast, the spores of *Aspergillus niger* show an evident adhesive ability; as a result, the removal from the surface becomes efficient only by means of an alkaline solution. *S. aureus* demonstrates an intermediate behavior with a clear improvement in the detachment when the detergent solution is used. Boulané-Petermann (1996) presents two physicochemical theories that can be applied to predict simple cases of bacterial adhesion. However, these models are limited in their applicability owing to the complexity of bacterial surfaces and the surrounding medium. Various factors that can affect the bacterial adhesion process have been listed, all directly linked to the solid substratum, the suspension liquid, or the microorganism. For stainless steel surfaces, it is important to take into account the grade of steel, the type of finish, surface roughness, the cleaning procedures used, and the age of the steel. Regarding the suspension fluid within which adhesion takes place, pH, ionic composition, and the presence of macromolecules are important variables. In addition, the adhering microorganisms have extremely complex surfaces and many factors must be taken into account when conducting adhesion tests, such as the presence of cell append-ages, the method of culture, the contact time between the microorganism and the surface, and exopolymer synthesis. Research on biofilms growing on stainless steel has confirmed results obtained with other materials, regarding resistance to disin-fectants, the role of the extracellular matrix, and the process by which the biofilm forms. However, it appears that the bactericidal activity of disinfectants on biofilms differs according to the type of surface on which they are growing. The main clean-ers and disinfectants used in the food industry are alkaline and acid detergents, per-acetic acid, quaternary ammonium chlorides, and iodophors. The cleanability and disinfectability of stainless steel surfaces have been compared with those of other materials. According to the published research findings, stainless steel is compa-rable in its biological cleanability to glass and significantly better than polymers, aluminum, or copper. Moreover, microorganisms in a biofilm developing on a stain-less steel surface can be killed with lower concentrations of disinfectant than those on polymer surfaces. Bower et al. (1996) warn that bacteria within a biofilm are more resistant to disinfectants, which may assist the survival of *Listeria* spp. and other food-borne pathogens in the food processing environment. Direct evidence that pathogen-containing biofilms play a role in the spread of food-borne illness is lacking, as identification and characterization of biofilms have not been included in food-borne illness investigations (Chmielewski and Frank 2003).

Since contact materials are in regular and permanent contact with substrates or final foods or drugs in the production process (food, pharmaceutical, and medical industry), there is high probability to acquire and load surface contaminants from contact materials into/onto products. Clean surfaces are acquired owing to sanitary hygiene conditions. Removal of biofilm poses considerable difficulties in the food industry and the hospital environment. Vickery et al. (2004) state that although physical methods such as ultrasonication and mechanical cleaning or scraping are generally effective if carried out efficiently, chemical methods are often ineffective because of the resistance of biofilms to antibiotics, disinfectants, and biocides. They also indicate that bacteria within biofilms are up to 1000 times more resistant to anti-microbials than the same bacteria in suspension (Gilbert and McBain 2001; Ntsama-Essomba et al. 1997; Vickery et al. 2004). By understanding all these processes and their impact, it would be possible to foresee possible outcomes and thus prevent negative impact on food/drug product safety and quality (Raspor 2008; Raspor and Jevšnik 2008).

8.2 CONTACT SURFACES AND FOOD SAFETY

Food contact materials have an important impact on bacterial attachment and bio-film formation. Recent food-borne outbreaks have focused on biofilms in food con-tact materials, searching the sources of food contamination (Al-Ahmad et al. 2010; Janssens et al. 2008; Wang et al. 2013). Commonly used materials in the food industry include stainless steel, glass, rubber, polyurethane (Cappitelli et al. 2014;

Chia et al. 2009; Faille and Carpentier 2009; Jun et al. 2010), Teflon, nitrile butyl rubber (Storgårds et al. 1999), and wood (Filip et al. 2012; Mariani et al. 2011), among others.

Adetunji and Isola (2011) analyzed biofilm formation on various materials such as wood, stainless steel, and glass and found the highest biofilm formation on wood surfaces and the lowest on the glass, while stainless steel can prevent the colonization, but it is vulnerable to corrosion. They found that *Salmonella* spp. can be attached to different surfaces, but it seems that more cells are attached to the Teflon surface and stainless steel than to polyurethane. This indicates that material properties have a large impact on initial adhesion and biofilm formation (Chia et al. 2009). As reported by Stepanović et al. (2004), *Salmonella* spp. and *L. monocytogenes* form biofilms on plastic material. In another study, Bernardes et al. (2013) studied adhesion of *Bacillus cereus* on stainless steel and found temperature and time to be the most important factors promoting the attachment. In the study of Arnold et al. (2004), fewer bacterial cells were attached to the electropolished stainless steel food contact surface than on the untreated one. Meanwhile, Guobjörnsdóttir et al. (2005) pointed out that not only the material properties but also the hygienic design such as welding, joints, corners, and equipment design could have an important impact on bacterial adhesion. One of the critical control points in the process of producing fresh products is packing, which should prevent cross-contamination. For produce that are generally consumed raw, packing as the last step of processing is considered as one of the critical control points. This last step should be controlled attentively and regularly to avoid recontamination. Carron (2011) reported an outbreak of *L. monocytogenes* that was connected to the unhygienic packing of melons. Keskinen et al. (2008) studied *Listeria* spp. biofilm on stainless steel knives for ready-to-eat food and found a significantly higher amount of transfer of strongly adhered biofilm than weakly adhered biofilm to turkey. In another study, Somers and Lee Wong (2004) found that the *L. monocytogenes* biofilm was the most resistant on brick and conveyor material in ready-to-eat production. Silagyi et al. (2009) reported that *E. coli* is considered to be very important in the ready-to-eat industry since it can form biofilms on food contact surfaces during food processing. Some of the studies reported colonization of bacteria on the conveyor belt, drying area, and floor drain (Filip et al. 2012; Neuman 2011). Bacteria can adhere to several surfaces. When the cells are irreversibly attached to the surface, they form the biofilm that can contaminate the whole process line or even the whole production (Sapers 2001). Regular sanitation can damage surfaces, causing cracks and scratches. Organic material with microorganisms can gather on these sites, forming biofilms that are protected against antimicrobial agents. In their study, Latorre et al. (2010) analyzed the sources of *L. monocytogenes* in dairy farms and found biofilms in the scratched surfaces. Boyd et al. (2001) studied the different types of stainless steel cleaning methods such as spraying and brushing and found that brushing is more efficient than spraying. The retention of organic matter was greater on rough samples. Guobjörnsdóttir et al. (2005) reported that adhered bacteria cells were found in the fish processing industry even if sanitation and disinfection measures were provided correctly. From shrimp processing plant surfaces, bacteria like *Pseudomonas* spp., *Aeromonas* spp., and *Enterobacteriaceae*, as well as yeast, were isolated (Gram and Huss 1996). In their study, Guobjörnsdóttir et al. demonstrated that *Pseudomonas* spp. promote the adhesion of *L. monocytogenes* on stainless steel (Guobjörnsdóttir et al. 2005). The research by Chia et al. (2009) has shown that *Salmonella typhimurium* seem to adhere more efficiently to stainless steel than to rubber. Abdallah et al. (2009) reported that *Salmonella* spp. isolated from Tunisian poultry produced moderate amounts of biofilm on PVC in more than 50% of samples. Hansson et al. (2012) studied adhesion of bacteria to dairy packing materials and found that adhesion is dependent on the product's contact time and surface.

Bacteria can colonize all food contact materials, although the rate of adhesion is strongly influenced by food and surface characteristics (Ismaïl et al. 2013; Olszewska 2013). Nevertheless, proper cleaning and disinfection should prevent bacterial adhesion and biofilm growth. Also, proper equipment, based on good hygiene practice, will reduce the risk of food contamination. Above all, the surfaces that are already in use can be changed by antifouling coating.

8.2.1 IMPLICATIONS FOR HUMAN HEALTH

Bacterial adhesion has implications for human health and the environment. Namely, many infections in hospitals are caused by attachment of bacteria to medical devices and implants. Vickery et al. (2004) described that fouling and corrosion of plant and pipework by biofilms has been a major problem in the industry. In the field of medicine and in the food industry, control of biofilm formation has a major impact on infection control. Bacterial adhesion to medical devices is the first step in the development of such infection (Zhao et al. 2007). Adhesion is an important aspect of many bacterial diseases, including native valve endocarditis, osteomyelitis, dental caries, middle ear infections, and ocular implant infections. Most pathogen microorganisms adhere themselves to the host cells of mucous membranes, tissues, and fluids of a human organism and cause the cells' degradation or toxication. The ability to grow as part of a sessile, exopolymer-enshrouded community referred to as biofilm is an important and clinically relevant example of bacterial adaptation through systematized gene expression, which is in most cases resulted as an adaptation to environments with rapidly changing conditions. The removal of infected devices and the additional treatment greatly increase patients' discomfort, treatment costs, and mortality (Weinstein 2001). Flock and Brennan (1999) stressed that in the United Kingdom, implant-associated infections are estimated to cost 7–11 million pounds per year. Approximately half of the two million cases of nosocomial infections per year in the United States are associated with indwelling devices (Darouiche 2004).

An effective but costly and stressful procedure in treating biofilm infections involves removing the implant, fighting the infection with antibiotics, and replacing the implant (Carmen et al. 2005). An and Friedman (1997) described a prosthetic infection and emphasized that the biofilm makes the embedded bacteria less accessible to the human defense system and significantly decreases antibiotic susceptibility.

Zhao et al. (2007) analyzed the many surface properties of the implanted surfaces. They evaluated, under static and laminar flow conditions, bacterial adhesion of *P. aeruginosa*, *S. epidermidis*, and *S. aureus*, which frequently cause medical device–associated infections. Their results showed that SiF_3^+-implanted stainless steel performed much better than N^+-implanted steel, O^+-implanted steel, and untreated steel control in reducing bacterial attachment under identical experimental conditions.

8.3   SURFACE CHARACTERIZATION

Characterization of glass surfaces was carried out using atomic force microscopy (AFM) and profilometry. The characterization of the surfaces resulted in determining roughness parameters. Surface hydrophobicity was determined by contact angle measurement.

For surface topography imaging and to ascertain the distribution and location of preferential adhesion of microorganisms on the surface, SEM was used. The FEI Helios Nanolab 650 dual-beam system was used for SEM investigation. The samples were coated with carbon film (a few nanometers thick) to prevent charging. On surfaces with low roughness, the microbes are preferentially adhered to pits, cavities, and other defects, and they grow more or less laterally in one layer. On surfaces with higher roughness, the microbes are concentrated in pores and scratches (Figure 8.1) and could grow in multilayers. Bacterial surface characterization was determined by measuring zeta potential, which is an indirect measure of the net cell surface charge on bacteria. Zeta potential was measured using a Zetasizer Nano ZS equipped with a universal dip cell. In this study, zeta potential was approximated from the

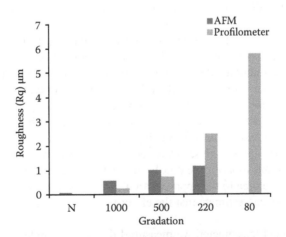

FIGURE 8.1   Roughness measurements (Rq) as a function of abrasion achieved by abrasive particles of different sizes measured with AFM and profilometer (gradation). (Reprinted with permission from Bohinc, K. et al. 2014. *Int J Adhes Adhes* 5: 265–272.)

electrophoretic mobility according to the Helmholtz–von Smoluchowski equation. Surface hydrophobicity was determined by contact angle measurement. The hydrophobicity of bacteria was determined by the procedure described by Rosenberg et al. (1980) and Tahmourespour et al. (2008) with some modifications. In this method, the nonpolar liquid xylene is added to the suspension. In this way, the polar and apolar phase are produced. The hydrophobicity rate h was calculated as the ratio between the absorbance of the initial bacterial suspension Ai and the absorbance of the aqueous phase after mixing with xylene.

8.4 BACTERIAL ADHESION TO GLASS SURFACES

We consider the influence of bacterial adhesion to surfaces with different roughness. The glass surfaces were prepared by abrasion to achieve different gradations. Roughness was determined by profilometry and AFM. The electrostatic surface potential and hydrophobicity of glass and bacteria were kept under standard conditions.

In this study, we used TEMPAX sheet glass from Schott (borosilicate glass). Two-millimeter-thick pieces were cut from the 2 cm × 2 cm glass rods, and the surfaces of glass pieces were fused using a gas burner. To achieve different surface roughness, sets of glass samples were ground to specific gradation using abrasive particles with different sizes. Gradation P80, P220, and P500 were used where abrasive particles with a size of 201, 68, and 30 μm, respectively, were used.

We made experiments with three different strains of bacteria: *E. coli*, *P. aeruginosa*, and *S. aureus*. They differ in their adhesive and surface properties. *E. coli* is a Gram-negative rod; *P. aeruginosa* is a Gram-negative, straight or slightly curved rod with several polar flagella, whereas *S. aureus* is spherical and nonmotile and occurs in irregular clusters.

To monitor the adhesion level of the strains, we used the method of O'Toole et al. (1999) and Kubota et al. (2008) with modifications. The supernatant was poured off three times with phosphate buffered saline buffer, and the biofilms were stained with crystal violet suspension. The dye in the cells was remobilized in 96% ethanol. The absorbance of the solution, OD_{620}, at a wavelength of 620 nm was determined using the microplate reader Infinite 200 PRO (Tecan Austria GmbH).

Surface roughness was estimated by AFM and profilometry. Samples with P220 gradation could be measured using AFM, while samples with P80 gradation were too rough to obtain reasonable results using AFM. Consequently, we showed that, at low roughness, AFM is a more sensitive tool, while at high roughness, the profilometer is a more suitable tool (Figure 8.1). From AFM images and profilometer profiles, the ratio of the true area to the apparent area (Wenzel's ratio) was calculated. From Wenzel's ratio, we can estimate that the effective area increased up to 30% because of grinding.

Using an optical tensiometer, we measured the contact angles of a water drop at the glass surface as a function of roughness. Several measurements were performed on each sample, and standard deviation was calculated. The lowest contact angle (28°) was measured at the untreated sample surface (plane fused glass). After grinding, the contact angles rose to values above 40°. A slight decrease in contact angles with an increase in roughness was observed.

The zeta potential of bacterial cells is the negative surface charge of all tested bacteria. We found that *E. coli* has the most negative charge, followed by *S. aureus* and *P. aeruginosa*. Measurements were provided in phosphate buffer solution at two ionic strengths: 1 and 100 mmol/L. The results show that a concentration of 1 mmol/L is more suitable for the zeta potential study than 100 mmol/L, owing to larger standard deviations. The zeta potential increases with increasing ionic strength. Namely, the counterions neutralize the cell surface. With the increasing ionic strength, the screening of the bacterial surface charge is increased. For very large ionic strengths, the zeta potential converges to zero. The results are given in Table 8.1.

Nostro et al. (2004) reported that isolates with *h* greater than 0.7 are arbitrarily classified as highly hydrophobic. Isolates with hydrophobicity rate *h* between 0.5 and 0.7 are classified as moderate, and isolates with *h* lower than 0.5 are classified as hydrophilic. Our results show that *E. coli* cells were hydrophilic ($h \approx 0.23$), *P. aeruginosa* cells were also hydrophilic ($h \approx 0.35$), whereas *S. aureus* cells were highly hydrophobic ($h \approx 0.92$). The results are given in Table 8.2.

The measured OD_{620} as a function of adhered cells to glass plate shows that adhesion of bacteria greatly depends on surface characteristics and type of bacteria. The measured OD_{620} shows that the adhesion of *P. aeruginosa* ATCC 27853, *S. aureus* ATCC 25923, and *E. coli* ATCC 35218 to untreated glass plates (type N) was the poorest, whereas adhesion of cells to most rough glass plates (type 80) was the greatest. The adhesion of all three bacteria increased with increasing roughness (Figure 8.2 and Table 8.3).

TABLE 8.1
Zeta Potential for Three Different Bacteria and Two Different Concentrations

	1 mmol/L	σ	100 mmol/L	σ
S. aureus	−31.87	4.84	−18.56	2.15
E. coli	−36.61	1.7	−21.7	6.8
P. aeruginosa	−16.92	2.42	−7.85	12.83

Note: The experimental error is added.

TABLE 8.2
Hydrophobicity of Investigated Bacteria

Bacteria	Hydrophobicity (*h*)
E. coli	0.23 ± 0.01
S. aureus	0.92 ± 0.10
P. aeruginosa	0.35 ± 0.04

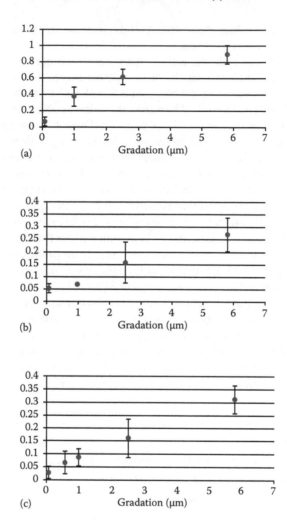

FIGURE 8.2 Available surface as a function of roughness dictates microbial adhesion capacity. The adhered cells were stained with crystal violet after 18 h, and the optical density at 620 nm (OD_{620}) was measured. (a) *P. aeruginosa* ATCC 27853, (b) *S. aureus* ATCC 25923, and (c) *E. coli* ATCC 35218. (Reprinted with permission from Bohinc, K. et al. 2014. *Int J Adhes Adhes* 5: 265–272.)

Optical density OD_{620} with SD of *P. aeruginosa* ATCC 27853 shows significantly greater adhesion to rough glass plates compared to *S. aureus* ATCC 25923 and *E. coli* ATCC 35218.

SEM was used to image the surfaces of the samples and to determine where the microbes are adhered. A SEM micrograph of the surface (P220) with bacteria at the beginning of the experiments showed that most of the bacteria are adhered to some defects, like cracks, voids, and gaps. Flat surfaces were more or less clear. After 8 h, the number of microbes increased substantially and they cover also flat areas (Figure 8.3).

TABLE 8.3
Crystal Violet Optical Density at 620 nm (OD$_{620}$) after 18-h Bacteria Incubation on Different Glass Plates

	P. aeruginosa ATCC 27853	S. aureus ATCC 25923	E. coli ATCC 35218
Control	0.051 ± 0.072	0.053 ± 0.019	0.026 ± 0.024
500	0.437 ± 0.023	0.069 ± 0.006	0.086 ± 0.033
220	0.661 ± 0.073	0.156 ± 0.082	0.160 ± 0.074
80	0.941 ± 0.113	0.269 ± 0.068	0.311 ± 0.054

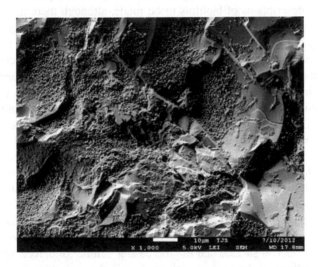

FIGURE 8.3 SEM image of the bacteria *S. aureus* after 8 h. Besides gaps, flat surfaces are also covered with microorganisms. (Reprinted with permission from Bohinc, K. et al. 2014. *Int J Adhes Adhes* 5: 265–272.)

8.5 CONCLUSIONS

Although descriptions of biofilms have varied over the years since 1674, when Antonie van Leuwenhoek used his primitive but effective microscope to describe aggregates of "animalcules" that he scraped from various surfaces, the fundamental characteristics of film formers are maintained, although we tried to explain them with different methods and different concepts in the last century when methods in biology, chemistry, and physics gradually improved and went from macro- to microscale and entered nanoscale levels in the last decades. But despite this methodological development, or because of it, a biofilm attached to a contact surface of technological, environmental, or medical importance can be observed and monitored as well as mechanistically explained in positive, negative, or even pathogenic functions. Research and development is far from reaching its end because we are implementing new materials, new technologies and processes, and new applications (from very traditional to very modern) in various industries (e.g., environmental, food, pharmaceutical, automotive, and space), not to mention added industrialized approaches in medical care. Consequently, microbes are under selection pressure and generate new strains with modified characteristics regarding film forming, on one hand, and accumulating a selection of characteristics, on the other, which might be beneficial in wastewater processing, such as xenodegradation, or in the food and medical industry, such as antibiotic and disinfectant resistance.

The essential requirements for biofilm growth are the microbes themselves, a substrate, and contact surface. When we expose them to new (or at least novel) niches that are unique to the microbial community, we expected to solve the problem of biofilm forming. Actually, it is just question of when will microbes overcome this obstacle. However, many advances in technology and laboratory working practices have allowed more accurate descriptions of biofilms to be made, although there is still ambiguity today: A biofilm consists of cells immobilized at a substratum and frequently embedded in an organic polymer matrix of microbial origin, which makes research more challenging and practice more complex. Biofilms are a biologically active matrix of cells and extracellular substances in association with a solid surface, and this can be good or bad, depending on point of view and application. Clean surfaces are acquired because of sanitary hygiene conditions, and removal of biofilm poses considerable difficulties in the food industry and the hospital environment. On the other hand, where biofilms represent the biologically active part of bioreactors, we need it to be stable and persistent. Hence, contact materials and bacterial adhesion potential are and will remain a focal point owing to their unique characteristics, which can be inhibited or enhanced by different surfaces. One of which is surface roughness, which we focused on in our study and can be designed and reproduced identically. Undoubtedly, results showed that the rate of adhered bacteria increases with increasing surface roughness. The increased adhesion of bacteria to rougher surfaces involves the interplay between the increasing effective surface and the increasing number of defects where bacteria preferentially adhere to the contact surface. Is this the case with microbial surface material or microbial substrate matrix, which already creates slightly different matrices from time to time? Is this the real issue? It is clear that this complexity dictates research and development in all areas where biofilms can be a friend or foe.

ACKNOWLEDGMENTS

The authors thank the Slovenian Research Agency for support through grant L1-4067 and Iskra Pio d.o.o. Collaborators from the Faculty of Health Studies, University of Ljubljana, are also acknowledged.

REFERENCES

Abdallah, F. B., Chaieb, K., Zmantar, T., Kallel, H., Bakhrouf, A. 2009. Adherence assays and slime production of *Vibrio alginolyticus* and *Vibrio parahaemolyticus*. *Braz J Microbiol* 40:394–398.
Adetunji, V. O., Isola, T. O. 2011. Crystal violet binding assay for assessment of biofilm formation by *Listeria monocytogenes* and *Listeria* spp. on wood, steel and glass surfaces. *Global Vet* 6:6–10.

Agle, M. E. 2007. Biofilms in the food industry. In: Blaschek, H. P., Wang, H. H., Agle, M. E. (eds.), *Biofilms in the Food Environment*. Iowa, Blackwell Publishing and the Institute of Food Technologists; pp. 3–17.

Al-Ahmad, A., Maier, J., Follo, M., Spitzmüller, B., Wittmer, A., Hellwig, E., Hübner, J., Jonas, D. 2010. Food-borne *Enterococci* integrate into oral biofilm: An in vivo study. *J Endod* 36:1812–1819.

An, Y. H., Friedman, R. J. 1997. Laboratory methods for studies of bacterial adhesion. *J Microbiol Methods* 30:141–152.

Arnold, J. W., Boothe, D. H., Suzuki, O., Bailey, G. W. 2004. Multiple imaging techniques demonstrate the manipulation of surfaces to reduce bacterial contamination and corrosion. *J Microsc* 216:215–221.

Bakker, D. P., Busscher, H. J., van Zanten, J., de Vries, J., Klijnstra, J. W. 2004. Multiple linear regression analysis of bacterial deposition to polyurethane coatings after conditioning film formation in the marine environment. *Microbiology* 150:1779–1784.

Bernardes, P. C., Andrade, N. J. D., Penã, W. E. L., Minim, L. A., Sá, J. P. N., Fernandes, P. E., Colombari, D. D. S. 2013. Modeling of the adhesion of *Bacillus cereus* isolated from a dairy plant as a function of time and temperature. *J Food Process Eng* 36:187–191.

Blackman, I. C., Frank, J. F. 1996. Growth of Listeria monocytogenes as a biofilm on various food-processing surfaces. *J Food Prot* 59:827–831.

Bohinc, K., Dražić, G., Fink, R., Oder, M., Jevšnik, M., Nipič, D., Godič-Torkar, K., Raspor, P. 2014. Available surface dictates microbial adhesion capacity. *Int J Adhes Adhes* 5:265–272.

Boks, N. P., Norde, W., Van der Mei, H. C., Busscher, H. J. 2008. Forces involved in bacterial adhesion to hydrophilic and hydrophobic surfaces. *Microbiology* 154:3122–3133.

Bos, R., van der Mei, H. C., Busscher, H. J. 1999. Physico-chemistry of initial microbial adhesive interactions its mechanisms and methods for study. *FEMS Microbiol Rev* 23:179–230.

Boulané-Petermann, L. 1996. Processes of bioadhesion on stainless steel surfaces and cleanability: A review with special reference to the food industry. *Biofouling* 10(4):275–300.

Bower, C. K., McGuire, J., Daeschel, M. 1996. The adhesion and detachment of bacteria and spores on food-contact surfaces. *Trends Food* 7:162–167.

Boyd, R. D., Cole, D., Rowe, D., Verran, J., Paul, A. J., West, R. H. 2001. Cleanability of soiled stainless steel as studied by atomic force microscopy and time of flight secondary ion mass spectrometry. *J Food Prot* 64:87–93.

Cappitelli, F., Polo, A., Villa, F. 2014. Biofilm formation in food processing environments is still poorly understood and controlled. *Food Eng Rev* 6:29–42.

Carmen, J. C., Roeder, B. L., Nelson, J. L., Robison Ogilvie, R. L., Robison, R. A., Schaalje, G. B., Pitt, W. G. 2005. Treatment of biofilm detection on implants with low-frequency ultrasound and antibiotics. *Am J Infect Control* 33:78–82.

Caron, C. 2011. CDC: Cantaloupe listeria outbreak deadliest in a decade—ABC news. Retrieved November 21, 2012, from http://abcnews.go.com/Health/cdc-cantaloupe listeria-outbreak-deadliest-decade/story?id¼14622507#.UKx7K-SE3pw.

Chen, Y., Busscher, H. J., van der Mei, H. C., Norde, W. 2011. Statistical analysis of long and short range forces involved in bacterial adhesion to substratum surfaces as measured using atomic force microscopy. *Appl Environ Microbiol* 77:5065–5070.

Chia, T. W. R., Goultera, R. M., McMeekinb, T., Dykesa, G. A., Fegana, N. 2009. Attachment of different Salmonella serovars to materials commonly used in a poultry processing plant. *Food Microbiol* 26:853–859.

Chmielewski, R. A. N., Frank, J. F. 2003. Biofilm formation and control in food processing facilities. *Comp Rev Food Sci Food Saf* 2:22–32.

Christensen, B. E. 1989. The role of extracellular polysaccharides in biofilms. *J. Biotechnol.* 10:181–202.

Corpe, W. 1980. *Adsorption of Microorganisms to Surfaces*. New York: John Wiley & Sons; pp. 105–144.

Costerton, J. W., Cheng, K. J., Geesey, G. G., Ladd, T. I., Nickel, J. C., Dasgupta, M. 1987. Bacterial biofilms in nature and disease. *Annu Rev Microbiol* 41:435–464.

Costerton, J. W., Geesey, G. G., Cheng, K. J. 1978. How bacteria stick. *Sci Am* 238:86–95.

Cunliffe, D., Smart, C. A., Alexander, C., Vulfson, E. N. 1999. Bacterial adhesion of synthetic surfaces. *Appl Environ Microbiol* 65:4995–5002.

Darouiche, R. O. 2004. Treatment of infections associated with surgical implants. *N Engl J Med* 350:1422–1429.

Davey, M. E., O'Toole, G. A. 2000. Microbial biofilms: From ecology to molecular genetics. *Microbiol Mol Biol Rev* 64:847–867.

Di Bonaventura, G., Piccolomini, R., Paludi, D., D'Orio, V. J. 2008. Influence of temperature on biofilm formation by Listeria monocytogenes on various food contact surfaces. *Appl Microbiol* 104:1552–1561.

Díaz, C., Schilardi, P. L., Salvarezza, R. C., Fernandez Lorenzo de Mele, M. 2007. AFM study using patterned substrates. *Langmuir* 23:11206–11210.

Díaz, C., Schilardi, P. L., dos Santos Claro, P. C., Salvarezza, R. C., Fernández Lorenzo de Mele, M. A. 2009. Submicron trenches reduce the *Pseudomonas fluorescens* colonization rate on solid surfaces. *Appl Mater Interfaces* 1:136–143.

Donlan, R. M., Costerton, J. W. 2002. Biofilms: Survival mechanisms of clinically relevant microorganisms. *Clin Microbiol Rev* 15:167–193.

Elhariry, H. M. 2008. Biofilm formation by endospore-forming *Bacilli* on plastic surface under some food-related and environmental stress conditions. *Global J Biotechnol Biochem* 3(2):69–78.

Faille, C., Carpentier, B. 2009. Food contact surfaces, surface soiling and biofilm formation. In: Fratamico, P. M., Annous, B. A., Guenther, N. W. (eds.), *Biofilms in the Food and Beverage Industries*. Cambridge, UK: Woodhead Publishing; pp. 303–330.

Filip, S., Fink, R., Oder, M., Jevšnik, M. 2012. Hygienic acceptance of wood in food industry. *Wood Sci Technol* 46:657–665.

Fletcher, M., Loeb, G. I. 1979. Influence of substratum characteristics on the attachment of a marine *Pseudomonas* to solid surfaces. *Appl Environ Microbiol* 37:67–72.

Fletcher, M., Marshall, K. C. 1982. Bubble contact angle method for evaluating substratum interfacial characteristics and its relevance to bacterial attachment. *Appl Environ Microbiol* 44:184–192.

Flint, S. H., Brooks, J. D., Bremer, P. J. 2000. Properties of stainless steel substrate, influencing the adhesion of thermo-resistant *Streptococci*. *J Food Eng* 43:235–242.

Flock, J. I., Brennan, F. 1999. Antibodies that block adherence of *Staphylococcus aureus* fibronectin. *Trends Microbiol* 7:140–141.

Foschino, R., Picozzi, C., Giorgi, E., Bontempi, A. 2003. Cleanability of floor surface materials in terms of removal of microorganisms at a low contamination level. *Ann Microbiol* 53:253–265.

Frank, J. F. 2001. Microbial attachment to food and food contact surfaces. *Adv Food Nutr Res* 43:319–370.

Geesey, G. G., Richardson, W. T., Yeomans, H. G., Irvin, R. T., Costerton, J. W. 1977. Microscopic examination of natural sessile bacterial populations from an alpine stream. *Can J Microbiol* 23:1733–1736.

Gilbert, P., McBain, A. J. 2001. Biofilms: Their impact on health and their recalcitrance toward biocides. *Am J Infect Control* 29:252–255.

Giraldez, M. J., Resua, C. G., Lira, M., Oliveira, M. E., Magarinos, B., Toranzo, A. E., Yebra-Pimentel, E. 2010. Soft contact lens surface profile by atomic force microscopy. *Optom Vis Sci* 87:426–431.

Gram, L., Huss, H. H. 1996. Microbiological spoilage of fish and fish products. *Int J Food Microbiol* 33:121–137.

Guobjörnsdóttir, B., Einarsson, H., Thorkelsson, G. 2005. Microbial adhesion to processing lines for fish fillets and cooked shrimp: Influence of stainless steel surface finish and presence of gram-negative bacteria on the attachment of *Listeria monocytogenes*. *Food Technol Biotech* 43:55–61.

Hahnel, S., Rosentritt, M., Handel, G., Bürgers, R. 2009. Surface characterization of dental ceramics and initial *streptococcal* adhesion in vitro. *Dent Mater* 25:969–975.

Hamadi, K. M., Yousif, A. A. 2014. Detection of slime material in *Staphylococcus aureus* bacteria from ovine mastitis by transmission electron microscope and Congo red agar method. *Int J Curr Microbiol App Sci* 3(4):304–309.

Hansson, K., Andersson, T., Skepö, M. 2012. Adhesion of fermented diary products to packaging materials. Effect of material functionality, storage time, and fat content of the product. An empirical study. *J Food Eng* 111:318–325.

Henriques, A. O., Moran, C. P. 2007. Structure, assembly, and function of the spore surface layers. *Annu Rev Microbiol* 61:555–588.

Hori, K., Matsumoto, S. 2010. Bacterial adhesion: From mechanisms to control. *Biochem Eng J* 48:424–434.

Ismaïl, R., Aviat, F., Michel, V., Le Bayon, I., Gay-Perret, P., Kutnik, M., Fédérighiet, M. 2013. Methods for recovering microorganisms from solid surfaces used in the food industry: A review of the literature. *Int J Environ Res Public Health* 10:6169–6183.

Janssens, J. C. A., Steenackers, H., Robijns, S., Gellens, E., Levin, J., Zhao, H., Hermans, K., De Coster, D., Verhoeven, T. L., Marchal, K., Vanderleyden, J., De Vos, D. E., De Keersmaecker, S. C. J. 2008. Brominated furanones inhibit biofilm formation by *Salmonella enterica* serovar *Typhimurium*. *Appl Environ Microbiol* 74:6639–6648.

Jaryszak, E. M., Sampson, E. M., Antonelli, P. J. 2009. Biofilm formation by *Pseudomonas aeruginosa* on ossicular reconstruction prostheses. *Curr Opin Otolaryngol Head Neck Surg* 30:367–370.

Jun, W., Kim, M. S., Cho, B. K., Millner, P. D., Chao, K., Chan, D. E. 2010. Microbial biofilm detection on food contact surfaces by macro-scale fluorescence imaging. *J Food Eng* 99:314–322.

Keskinen, L. A., Todd, E. C. D., Ryser, E. T. 2008. Transfer of surface-dried *Listeria monocytogenes* from stainless steel knife blades to roast Turkey breast. *J Food Prot* 71:176–181.

Kubota, H., Senda, S., Nomura, N., Tokuda, H., Uchiyama, H. J. 2008. Biofilm formation by lactic acid bacteria and resistance to environmental stress. *J Biosci Bioeng* 106:381–386.

Latorre, A. A., Van Kessel, J. S., Karns, J. S., Zurakowski, M. J., Pradhan, A. K., Boor, K. J., Jayarao, B. M., Houser, B. A., Daugherty, C. S., Schukken, Y. H. 2010. Biofilm in milking equipment on a dairy farm as a potential source of bulk tank milk contamination with *Listeria monocytogenes*. *J Dairy Sci* 93:2792–2802.

Li, B., Logan, B. E. 2004. Bacterial adhesion to glass and metal-oxide surfaces. *Biointerfaces* 36:81–90.

Lichter, J. A., J. Van Vliet, K., Rubner, M. F. 2009. Design of antibacterial surfaces and interfaces: Polyelectrolyte multilayers as a multifunctional platform. *Macromoleculs* 42:8573–8586.

Madigan, M. T., Martinko, J. M., Dunlap, P. V., Clark, D. P. 2009. *Brock Biology of Microorganisms*, 12th ed. San Francisco: Pearson International; p. 68.

Mafu, A. A., Roy, D., Goulet, J., Magny, P. 1990. Attachment of Listeria monocytogenes to stainless steel, glass, polypropylene and rubber surfaces after short contact time. *J Food Prot* 53:742–746.

Makin, S. A., Beveridge, T. J. 1996. The influence of A-band and B-band lipopolysaccharide on the surface characteristics and adhesion of *Pseudomonas aeruginosa* to surfaces. *Microbiology* 142:299–307.

Mariani, C., Oulahal, N., Chamba, J. F., Dubois Brissonnet, F., Notz, E., Briandet, R. 2011. Inhibition of *Listeria monocytogenes* by resident biofilms present on wooden shelves used for cheese ripening. *Food Control* 22:1357–1362.

Marshall, K. C., Cruickshank, R. H. 1973. Cell surface hydrophobicity and the orientation of certain bacteria at interfaces. *Arch Mikrobiol* 91:29–40.

Marshall, K. C., Stout, R., Mitchell, R. 1971. Selective sorption of bacteria from seawater. *Can J Microbiol* 17:1413–1416.

Murga, R., Forster, T. S., Brown, E., Pruckler, J. M., Fields, B. S., Donlan, R. M. 2001. Role of biofilms in the survival of *Legionella pneumophila* in a model potable-water system. *Microbiology* 147:3121–3126.

Neuman, W. 2011. Listeria outbreak traced to Colorado cantaloupe packing shed. *NY Times,* B1.

Nostro, A., Cannatelli, M. A., Crisafi, G., Musolino, A. D., Procopio, F., Alonzo, V. 2004. Modification of hydrophobicity in vitro adherence and cellular aggregation. *Lett Appl Microbiol* 38:423–427.

Ntsama-Essomba, C., Bouttier, S., Ramaldes, M., Dubois-Brissonnet, F., Fourniat, J. 1997. Resistance of *Escherichia coli* growing as biofilms to disinfectants. *Vet Res* 28: 353–363.

Olszewska, M. A. 2013. Microscopic findings for the study of biofilms in food environments. *Acta Biochim Pol* 60:531–537.

O'Toole, G. A., Pratt, L. A., Watnick, P. I., Newman, D. K., Weaver, V. B., Kolter, R. 1999. Genetic approaches to study of biofilms. *Methods Enzymol* 310:91–109.

Otto, K. 2008. Biophysical approaches to study the dynamic process of bacterial adhesion. *Res Microbiol* 159:415–422.

Pringle, J. H., Fletcher, M. 1986. Influence of substratum hydration and adsorbed macromolecules on bacterial attachment to surfaces. *Appl Environ Microbiol* 51:1321–1325.

Quirynen, M., Vandermei, H. C., Bollen, C. M. L., Schotte, A., Marechal, M., Doornbusch, G. I., Naert, I., Busscher, H. J., Vansteenberghe, D. J. 1993. An in vivo study of the influence of the surface roughness of implants on the microbiology of supra- and subgingival plaque. *Dent Res* 72:1304–1309.

Raspor, P. 2008. Total food chain safety: How good practices can contribute? *Trends Food Sci Technol* 19:405–412.

Raspor, P., Jevšnik, M. 2008. Good nutritional practice from producer to consumer. *Crit Rev Food Sci Nutr* 48:276–292.

Renner, L. D., Weibel, D. B. 2011. Physicochemical regulation of biofilm formation. *MRS Bull* 36:347–355.

Rosenberg, M., Gutniek, D., Rosenberg, E. 1980. Adherence of bacteria to hydrocarbons: A simple method for measuring cell-surface hydrophobicity. *FEMS Micro Lett* 9:29–33.

Rosenberg, M., Kjelleberg, S. 1986. Hydrophobic interactions: Role in bacterial adhesion. *Adv Microb Ecol* 9:353–396.

Sapers, G. M. 2001. Efficacy of washing and sanitizing methods for disinfection of fresh fruit and vegetable products. *Food Technol Biotechnol* 39:305–311.

Silagyi, K., Kim, S. H., Martin Lo, Y., Wei, C. 2009. Production of biofilm and quorum sensing by *Escherichia coli* O157:H7 and its transfer from contact surfaces to meat, poultry, ready-to-eat deli, and produce products. *Food Microbiol* 26:514–519.

Singh, A. V., Vyas, V., Patil, R., Sharma, V., Scopelliti, P. E., Bongiorno, G., Podesta, A., Lenardi, C., Gade, W. M., Milani, P. 2011. Quantitative characterization of the influence of the nanoscale morphology of nanostructured surfaces on bacterial adhesion and biofilm formation. *PLoS One*, 6:e25029.

Somers, E. B., Lee Wong, A. C. 2004. Efficacy of two cleaning and sanitizing combinations on *Listeria monocytogenes* biofilms formed at low temperature on a variety of materials in the presence of ready-to-eat meat residue. *J Food Prot* 67:2218–2229.

Stenström, T. A. 1989. Bacterial hydrophobicity, an overall parameter for the measurement of adhesion potential to soil particles. *Appl Environ Microbiol* 55:142–147.

Stepanović, S., Ćirković, I., Ranin, L., Švabić-Vlahović, M. 2004. Biofilm formation by *Salmonella* spp. and *Listeria monocytogenes* on plastic surface. *Lett Appl Microbiol* 38:428–432.

Storgårds, E., Simola, H., Sjöberg, A. M., Wirtanen, G. 1999. Hygiene of gasket materials used in food processing equipment part 1: New materials. *Food Bioprod Process: Trans Inst Chem Eng C* 77:137–145.

Tahmourespour, A., Kermanshahi, R. K., Salehi, R., Nabinejad, A. 2008. The relationship between cell surface hydrophobicity and antibiotic resistance of streptococcal strains isolated from dental plaque and caries. *Iranian J Basic Med Sci* 10:251–255.

Tang, H., Cao, T., Liang, X., Wang, A., Salley, S. O., McAllister, J., Ng, K. Y. 2008. Influence of silicone surface roughness and hydrophobicity on adhesion and colonization of *Staphylococcus epidermidis*. *J Biomed Mater Res A* 88:454–463.

Taylor, R. L., Verran, J., Lees, G. C., Ward, A. J. P. 1998. The influence of substratum topography on bacterial adhesion to polymethyl methacrylate. *J Mater Sci-Mater Med* 9:17–22.

Terada, A., Yuasa, A., Kushimoto, T., Tsuneda, S., Katakai, A., Tamada, M. 2006. Bacterial adhesion to and viability on positively charged polymer surfaces. *Microbiology* 152:3575–3583.

Truong, V. K., Lapovok, R., Estrin, Y. S., Rundell, S., Wang, J. Y. 2010. The influence of nanoscale surface roughness on bacterial adhesion to ultrafine-grained titanium. *Biomaterials* 31:3674–3683.

van der Mei, H. C., Brokke, P., Dankert, J., Feyen, J., Rouxhet, P. G., Busscher, H. J. 1989. Physicochemical surface properties of nonencapsulated and encapsulated coagulase-negative staphylococci. *Appl Environ Microbiol* 55:2806–2814.

Van der Wal, A., Norde, W., Zehnder, A. J. B., Lyklema, J. 1997. Conductivity and dielectric dispersion of gram-positive bacterial cells. *Biointerfaces* 9:81–100.

Van Loosdrecht, M. C. M., Lyklema, J., Norde, W., Zehnder, A. J. B. 1989. Bacterial adhesion: A physicochemical approach. *Microb Ecol* 17:1–15.

Vesterlund, S., Paltta, J., Karp, M., Ouwehand, A. C. 2005. Measurement of bacterial adhesion— In vitro evaluation of different methods. *J Microbiol Methods* 60:225–233.

Vickery, K., Pajkos, A., Cossart, Y. 2004. Removal of biofilm from endoscopes: Evaluation of detergent efficiency. *Am J Infect Control* 32:170–176.

Wang, H.-H., Ye, K. P., Zhang, Q. Q., Dong, Y., Xu, X. L., Zhou, G. H. 2013. Biofilm formation of meat-borne Salmonella enterica and inhibition by the cell-free supernatant from *Pseudomonas aeruginosa*. *Food Control* 32:650–658.

Weinstein, R. A. 2001. Device-related infections. *Clin Infect Dis* 33:1386.

Whitehead, K. A., Colligon, J., Verran, J. 2005. Retention of microbial cells in substratum surface features of micrometer and sub-micrometer dimensions. *Colloids Surf B Biointerfaces* 41:129–138.

Wilson, W. W., Wade, M. M., Holman, S. C., Champlin, F. R. 2001. Status of methods for assessing bacterial cell surface charge properties based on zeta potential measurements. *J Microbiol Methods* 43:153–164.

Xu, L. C., Siedlecki, C. A. 2012. Submicron-textured biomaterial surface reduces staphylococcal bacterial adhesion and biofilm formation. *Acta Biomater* 8:72–81.

Zhao, Q., Liu, Y., Wang, C., Wang, S. 2007. Bacterial adhesion on silicon-doped diamond-like carbon films. *Diamond Relat Mater* 16:1682–1687.

Zobell, C. E. 1943. The effect of solid surfaces upon bacterial activity. *J Bacteriol* 46:39–56.

Zobell, C. E., Anderson, D. Q. 1936. Observations on the multiplication of bacteria in different volumes of stored seawater and the influence of oxygen tension and solid surfaces. *Biol Bull Woods Hole* 71:324–342.

Zupan, J., Mavri, J., Raspor, P. 2009. Quantitative cell wall protein profiling of invasive and non-invasive *Saccharomyces cerevisiae* strains. *J Microbiol Methods* 79:260–265.

9 Antimicrobial Polymers Based on Nanostructures
A New Generation of Materials with Medical Applications

María Isabel González-Sánchez,
Stefano Perni, and Polina Prokopovich

CONTENTS

ABSTRACT

Contamination by microorganisms is a major problem that affects different areas such as medicine, health care, or industry. For example, infections associated with biofilm formation in medical implants are becoming very common in hospitals. Very frequently, biofilms have high resistance to antibacterial drugs and are very difficult to remove. Therefore, the development of new materials with antimicrobial properties is highly required. In recent years, antimicrobial polymers represent a class of biocides that has become increasingly important as an alternative to existing biocides. In addition, formulating these polymers into nanostructures can be very convenient to enhance their antibacterial activity. Different structures such as nanoparticles, core–shell nanoparticles, one-dimensional polymer nanostructures, and thin films can be prepared to inhibit the growth of microorganisms such as bacteria, fungi, or protozoa. These structures have unique physicochemical properties that make them suited for medical purpose.

The present chapter provides an overview of the latest innovations in antimicrobial polymers based on nanostructures. It is organized into sections that discuss their basic properties, the factors affecting their antimicrobial activity, the different natural and synthetic types, their major medical applications, the environmental impact, and their possible cytotoxicity in humans.

Keywords: Antimicrobial, Biofilm, Biomaterials, Microorganisms, Nanostructures, Polymers

9.1   INTRODUCTION

Contamination by microorganisms is a major problem in different areas such as medical devices, drugs, health care, water purification systems, hospital and dental surgery equipment, textiles, food packaging, and food storage [1]. The use of antibiotics entails some problems because sometimes microorganisms have developed resistance to these drugs. Some microbes are able to mutate their genes rapidly and easily, which makes their elimination difficult. For example, some *Staphylococcus aureus* are resistant to the antibiotic methicillin, methicillin-resistant *S. aureus* (MRSA), and different antibiotic types are often required to treat them [2]. Almost 70% of present-day infections are suspected to be attributed to drug-resistant bacteria [3]. For this reason, alternatives to treat infections are required.

While new biomaterials have been developed, a growing need for materials with antimicrobial properties to prevent infections has emerged. Antimicrobial refers to a substance that kills or inhibits the growth of microorganisms. Numerous substances are known to possess antimicrobial properties, among them several metals such as silver, zinc, and copper. Silver is certainly the most commonly used metal to confer anti-infective properties to biomedical devices [4]. The antimicrobial activity of silver is well known; hence, silver-coated orthopedic implants have become the subject of extensive research works [5–7]. Controversially, however, a long-standing debate about possible cytotoxicity in living organisms still persists. Other antimicrobial agents are bioactive glasses, cationic surfactants, lipids, peptides, and natural or synthetic polymers, which have been intensively investigated as antimicrobial agents themselves or in formulations [8,9].

Chen et al. [10] compared the antimicrobial properties of small biocides, dendrimer biocides, and antimicrobial polymers taking into account the different bactericidal mechanisms. The authors found that polymer biocides display stronger initial adsorption onto the bacteria cell surface than small-molecule biocides but that they exhibit less diffusion to the cytoplasmic membrane.

This chapter focuses on antimicrobial polymers, also known as polymeric biocides that can inhibit the growth of microorganisms such as bacteria, fungi, or protozoa. Anti-infective polymers have progressively become a primary strategy to prevent medical device–associated infection [8]. Polymers containing quaternary ammonium groups, polycations with phosphonium, tertiary sulfonium, rhodamine derivatives, polymeric N-halamines, peptides, and chitosan are some examples of this class of polymers. These macromolecular compounds damage microorganism membranes and proved to be more effective against antibiotic-resistant bacteria than antibiotics. In addition, these compounds are generally not toxic since the vast majority of them are not volatile, but chemically stable, and nonpermeable through skin [1] as compared to other chemical disinfectants. Although this chapter focuses more on the use of antimicrobial polymers in medicine, several other applications exist, like water disinfection [11], food packaging [12], health care products [13], and textile products [14].

Polymer nanotechnology is a broad interdisciplinary area of research that involves the design, manufacture, processing, and application of polymer materials that are capable of self-organizing into a variety of periodic or nonperiodic morphologies and are filled with particles, and have at least one length scale dimension in the order of 100 nm or less [12,15]. Nanosized antimicrobial polymers have been reported to be better antimicrobial agents than macromolecular polymers [16]. Therefore, processing polymers into nanostructures can be a very convenient way to enhance their antibacterial activity. Different structures such as nanoparticles, core–shell nanoparticles, one-dimensional polymer nanostructures, and thin films can be synthesized [17]. Nanostructural features of material surfaces have been found to be capable of altering the three-dimensional conformation of adsorbed proteins, which can also have a potential effect on biofilms [8]. Moreover, nanomaterials are excellent adsorbents and catalysts thanks to their large specific surface area and high reactivity [11]. This extremely large relative surface area is the cause of the improvement of the antibacterial properties of antimicrobial polymers.

Despite several different biocide polymeric material classifications being available, a classification that basically divides these natural and synthetic polymers is shown here. In addition, belonging to synthetic polymers, a classification based on the review published by Muñoz-Bonilla and Fernandez-García [2] has been made: polymers that exhibit antimicrobial activity themselves and those whose biocidal activity is conferred by incorporating antimicrobial organic and inorganic compounds.

The present chapter provides an overview of the latest innovations in antimicrobial polymers based on nanostructures. It is organized into sections that discuss their basic properties, the factors affecting their antimicrobial activity, the different natural and synthetic types, and their major medical applications.

9.2 BACTERIA ADHESION AND BIOCIDE MECHANISM OF ANTIMICROBIAL POLYMERS

The earliest step in the pathogenesis of foreign body–related infections is bacterial adhesion. When bacteria attach to a material surface and their cell number increases, they start to form a biofilm that consists of cells being attached to a surface. Microbial infection resulting from bacteria adhesion to biomaterial surfaces has been observed on almost all medical devices [18]. This process is driven by mass transport, electrostatic interactions, van der Waals forces, hydrophobic interactions, and hydrogen bonding [8]. After developing on a surface, biofilms are extremely difficult to remove, which allows microbial cells to survive, even under severe conditions. Bacterial adhesion and biofilm formation are very important concepts in bacterial diseases and control [19]. Not only do they help colonization, but they often provide a degree of protection against outside stresses [20]. The formation and structure of biofilm communities depend on a wide variety of parameters, including species, temperature, pH, and presence of salts [21]. In addition, adhesion to material surfaces is critically influenced by the pathogen type and the nature of the physiological fluids that come into contact [8].

Biofilm inhibition can be achieved in early bacterial adhesion stages by means of two main processes:

1. Killing bacteria before adhesion using low-molecular-weight compounds such as antibiotics
2. Modifying surface properties to prevent bacteria adhesion

In the first case, the problem lies in the fact that the pathogen population can exhibit resistance properties against these compounds, and bacteria often require different types of antibiotics to be treated. Regarding the second case, the polymer-based antimicrobial design will provide a new versatile strategy to create a diversity of antimicrobial agents to fight against resistant bacteria. On the surfaces based on positively charged polymers, such as quaternary ammonium compounds, high electrostatic forces are responsible for disrupting bacterial cell membranes by allowing the removal of anionic lipids [22].

In general terms, Carmona-Ribeiro and Carrasco [9] summarized the biocide mechanism of contact-active polymers by means of specific events:

1. Adsorption and penetration of the agent into the cell wall
2. Reaction with the cytoplasmic membrane followed by membrane disorganization
3. Leakage of intracellular low-molecular-weight material
4. Degradation of proteins and nucleic acids
5. Wall lysis caused by autolytic enzymes

All these processes lead to loss of structural organization and the integrity of the cytoplasmic membrane in bacteria, and to other damaging effects on bacteria cells [9,23]. Depending on the bacteria type, the mechanism might differ since bacteria can be classified into two types: Gram+ and Gram−. Between them, the most important difference is that the cell wall can be easily lost in the former, whereas the latter has an outer membrane structure that makes it more resistant. Regarding nanostructures, different mechanisms have been identified depending on the specific chemistry of the nanoparticle.

9.3 FACTORS AFFECTING ANTIMICROBIAL ACTIVITY OF POLYMERS

Before we go on to introduce several examples of nanostructured polymers in the bibliography, it is important to be aware of some general concerns about the factors affecting antimicrobial activity in polymers. Some of them are molecular weight, hydrophobicity, type of counterions, and spacer length of the alkyl chain on the bactericide [1]. Bearing in mind that this chapter focuses on nanostructure polymers, nanostructure size must also be added to this classification.

9.3.1 EFFECT OF MOLECULAR WEIGHT

Molecular weight dependence has been studied by several research groups [1]. Some years ago, Ikeda and Tazuke [24] investigated the molecular weight dependence of poly(trialkylvinylbenzylammonium chloride) against *S. aureus* and found that up to 7.7×10^4 Da, the antimicrobial activity was monotonically increasing: however, higher Mw were tested. On the contrary, bacteriostatic activities against *S. aureus*, *Bacillus subtilis*, *Escherichia coli*, *Aerobacter aerogenes*, and *Pseudomonas aeruginosa* had have little dependence on the molecular weight of polymeric quaternary ammonium salts. In addition, they also evaluated the antimicrobial activity of homopolymers of polyacrylates and polymethyl acrylates with side-chain biguanide groups and their copolymers with acrylamide [25]. These authors showed that a strong dependence existed between the molecular weight of the polymers and their biocidal action against *S. aureus*. They obtained an optimal molecular weight region (5×10^4 and 1.2×10^5 Da) for bactericide activity, which they explained on the basis of permeability through the cell wall. Similarly, the optimum Mw of poly(tributyl 4-vinylbenzyl)phosphonium chloride against *S. aureus* was in the range 1.6×10^4 to 9.4×10^4 Da [26].

The antibacterial activity of chitosan also depends on molecular weight [27]. They used three different molecular weight chitosan samples to prepare water-soluble quaternary ammonium salts and to determine the minimum inhibitory concentration and the minimum bactericidal concentration against *E. coli*. The results showed that antibacterial activity was greater using the polymer with a viscosity average molecular weight (Mv) of 2.14×10^5.

9.3.2 NANOSTRUCTURE SIZE

On occasion, antimicrobial macromolecules are very large; hence, they may not act as quickly as small-molecular biocides. This is when polymeric nanoparticles may be an alternative. The bactericide activity of nanoparticles is very closely related to their size. The size of antimicrobial agent–based nanostructures has been demonstrated to be a key factor in biocide efficacy because antimicrobial activity depends on the particle's exposed active area [17].

Riaz et al. [28] studied the antibacterial properties of nanostructured poly(1-naphthylamine) (PNA) and its composites and demonstrated that particle size and the morphology play a significant role in antimicrobial efficiency. Nanostructures with smaller particle size and higher charged surface area-to-volume ratio displayed better antimicrobial activity as they prevent the nutrient transport and energy transduction of the cell wall through interactions of amino groups. Song et al. [29] published the synthesis and the bactericide properties of the silica nanoparticles modified on the surface by the poly[2-(tert-butylaminoethyl)methacrylate-co-ethyleneglycol dimethacrylate] copolymer (Figure 9.1).

These authors discovered that the smaller the size of the core–shell nanoparticles, the greater the antimicrobial efficacy shown against Gram− and Gram+ bacteria. The same authors later [30] evaluated the relationship between the size of silica/polyrhodanine core–shell nanoparticles (Figure 9.2) and their bactericidal activity using a kinetic bactericidal test. Once again, they found the same dependence.

In conclusion, diminished nanostructure size usually leads to enhanced effectiveness against pathogens as the active surface is larger. This is a major observation because the size of synthesized nanoparticles is controllable on occasion.

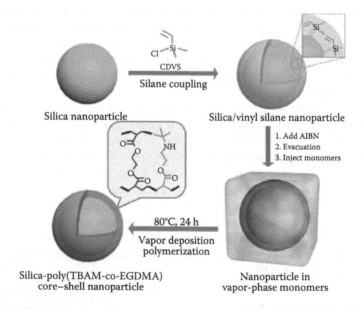

FIGURE 9.1 Schematic diagram of the fabrication of silica-poly(TBAM-co-EGDMA) core–shell nanoparticle. (Song J. et al. [2009] Enhanced antibacterial performance of cationic polymer modified silica nanoparticles. *Chemical Communications* 36, 5418–5420. Reproduced by permission of The Royal Society of Chemistry.)

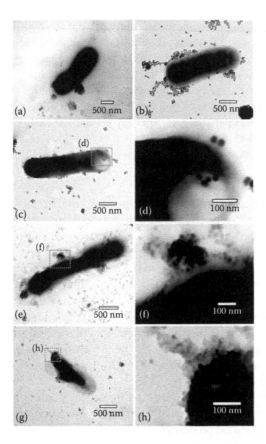

FIGURE 9.2 Transmission electron microscopy images of *E. coli* cells without being treated (a) and treated with the silica/polyrhodanine core–shell nanoparticles with an average size of (b–d) 56 nm, (e and f) 27 nm, and (g and h) 15 nm. (Song J. et al. [2011] Fabrication of silica/polyrhodanine core–shell nanoparticles and their antibacterial properties. *Journal of Materials Chemistry* 21, 19317–19323. Reproduced by permission of The Royal Society of Chemistry.)

9.3.3 HYDROPHOBICITY

Hydrophobicity is a main consideration in the antimicrobial action of polymers. In general, as polymers become more hydrophobic, their incorporation into the lipid membrane is enhanced. Thus, the integrity of the bacterial membrane is more efficiently disrupted. Kuroda and DeGrado [31] studied the antimicrobial and hemolytic activities of amphiphilic polymethacrylate derivatives by alternating the content of hydrophobic groups and molecular weights. However, these authors found that further increases in the mole percentages of butyl methacrylate created hydrophobic polymers that were more likely to experience collapsed polymer chains in water or irreversible aggregation with components of the assay medium, thus preventing antimicrobial action. In another publication, the same group found that antimicrobial activity depended sigmoidally on the mole fraction of the hydrophobic groups [32]. The hemolytic activity of random amphiphilic copolymers increased as the hydrophobic groups increased to level them off at high hydrophobicity values, especially for high-molecular-weight polymers. In addition, a theoretical model was built to analyze the hemolytic activity of polymers. It demonstrated that hemolytic activity can be described as a balance of polymer membrane binding through the partitioning of hydrophobic side chains into lipid layers and the hydrophobic collapsing of polymer chains.

9.3.4 COUNTERION EFFECT

Polymer-associated counterions play a pivotal role in the interaction on the bacterial membrane by altering hydrophobicity. Kanazawa et al. [33] showed that the antimicrobial properties of counterions varied in this order: chloride > tetrafluoride > perchlorate > hexafluorophosphate. However, Chen et al. [10] demonstrated greater antimicrobial activity for bromide than for chloride in polycationic dendrimers. Panarín et al. [34] did not, however, obtain any significant differences in the anions chloride, bromide, and iodide. Dutta et al. [35] carried out variation in the counterions from chloride to organic carboxylates in amino acid–based hydrogelating amphiphiles, and they found out that by changing the counterion, the antimicrobial activity can be modulated. Apart from the increased hydrophobicity of polymers, it is not clear why counterions should have any effect on biocidal activity.

Lienkamp et al. [36] demonstrated that by exchanging the hydrophilic counterions of a ROMP-derived diamine with hydrophobic organic counterions, that polymer had low antimicrobial properties.

9.3.5 EFFECT OF SPACER LENGTH AND ALKYL CHAIN

Recent reports have indicated that synthetic polymers composed of conformationally rigid polymer backbones coupled with regulated facially amphiphilic structures mimic the natural host defense [37]. The antimicrobial activity of these polymers is dependent on spacer length owing to the change occurring in the polymer's conformation and charge density, which vary the interaction with the cytoplasmic membrane [38]. For example, trimethyl-substituted phosphonium salts containing alkyl chains of various lengths with the same hydrophobic structure as common quaternary ammonium salts in order to compare their antibacterial activities were prepared by Kanazawa et al. [39]. For a series of alkyltrimethylphosphonium chlorides used in that study, the cation with the longest alkyl chain (octadecyl) exhibited the greatest activity. However, the results obtained for the phosphonium salts with two long alkyl chains were the opposite of the previous results.

Roy and Das [40] studied five cationic amphiphilic hydrogelators with a quaternary ammonium group of varying alkyl chain length, which exhibited remarkable antimicrobial activity against both Gram+ and Gram− bacteria, as well as biocompatibility with mammalian cells. They found that a minor modification in the alkyl chain of the amphiphile had a dramatic effect on antimicrobial activity. Amphiphiles with an alkyl chain of 12–14 carbons proved to be the most effective against bacteria and were, in most cases, more efficient than widely used traditional antibiotics.

9.4 NANOSTRUCTURED ANTIMICROBIAL POLYMERS

Antimicrobial polymeric nanomaterials are currently being extensively studied for their excellent bactericidal performance, which arises mainly from their increased surface area-to-volume ratio [41]. Nanostructured biomaterials, nanoparticles in particular, have unique physicochemical properties, such as an ultrasmall and controllable size, a large surface-area-to-mass ratio, high reactivity, and a functionalizable structure [42]. Song and Jang [17] published a very interesting review that showed some antimicrobial polymeric structures, as well as synthesis methods and strategies for controlling the shape and size of antimicrobial polymer nanomaterials. Some of the examples offered in that review and other works are provided in this chapter and have been divided into two groups: natural and synthetic antimicrobial polymers.

9.4.1 NATURAL ANTIMICROBIAL POLYMERS

Natural surfaces have been shaped by nature over billions of years of evolution, and it is thought that many of these surfaces might have developed the ability to resist or prevent bacterial colonization [43]. Many of these surfaces perform multiple integrated functions: some examples found in nature are plant leaves, gecko feet, shark skin, insect wings, fish scales, spider silks, and so on [44]. In Sections 9.4.1.1 and 9.4.1.2, the most widely used polymers deriving from nature are shown. We ought to consider that modifications may have been made in order to obtain efficient bactericide polymers. The polymers herein presented have been processed to obtain nanostructures. The main nanostructure-based polymers used for antibacterial purposes are chitosan and its derivatives, antimicrobial peptides.

9.4.1.1 Chitosan Nanoparticles

Chitosan is a polysaccharide derived from chitin, which is a natural product in the exoskeleton of crustaceans, insects, and the cell wall of fungi [45]. This compound is a linear copolymer of (1-4)linked 2-acetamido-2-deoxy-D-glucopyranose and 2-amino-2-deoxy-D-glycopyranose, and it is obtained by the deacetylation of chitin. It is very often used in biomedical applications for its biocompatibility and its low toxicity, as well as its gel-forming capability, high adsorption capacity, and biodegradability [46]. Besides these properties, chitosan has antibacterial, antifungal, and antitumor properties, while its cationic charge is the result of the protonation of its amine groups [45]. The antimicrobial activity of chitosan derivatives containing quaternary ammonium groups, such as N,N,N-trimethyl chitosan, N-propyl-N,N-dimethyl chitosan, and N-furfuryl-N,N-dimethyl chitosan (Figure 9.3), is stronger than chitosan; furthermore, it increases as pH lowers [27].

Recently, this polymer has been made into nanoparticles [47,48]. Qi et al. [47] demonstrated that chitosan nanoparticles have antibacterial activity against *Salmonella choleraesuis*, probably via membrane disruption and leakage of cellular proteins,

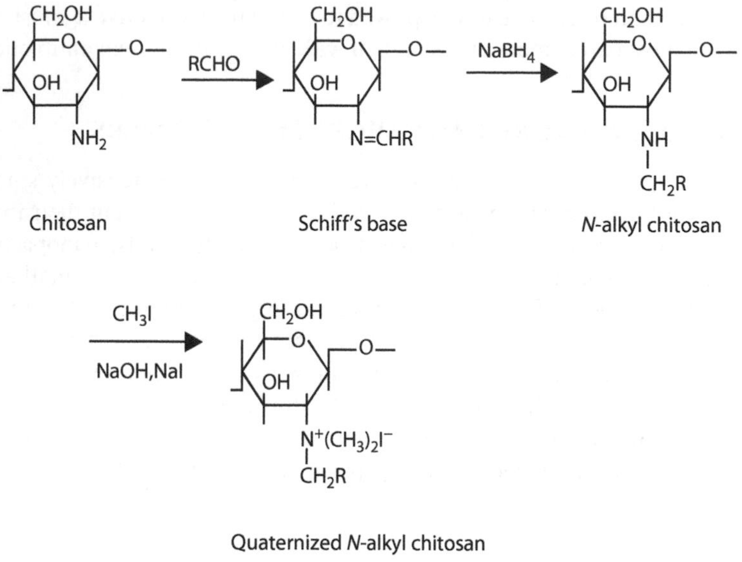

FIGURE 9.3 The scheme of quaternized *N*-alkyl chitosan synthesis. (Reprinted from *Carbohydrate Research*, 22, Jia Z., Shen D., and Xu W., Synthesis and antibacterial activities of quaternary ammonium salt of chitosan, 1–6, Copyright 2001, with permission from Elsevier.)

and that these nanoparticles offer acceptable biocompatibilities for medical applications. Antibacterial cotton treated with chitosan-containing core–shell particles was prepared by surfactant-free emulsion copolymerization in aqueous chitosan. The results show that this material has excellent antibacterial properties with bacterial reduction of more than 99% for *S. aureus* [48]. Other nanostructure-based derivatives are also used for this purpose, such as chitosan tripolyphosphate nanoparticles, as reported in previous studies [49–51].

Chitosan nanoparticles offer several advantages, such as the ability to control the release of active agents and to avoid the use of hazardous organic solvents while fabricating particles since chitosan is soluble in acidic solutions. For this reason, it is extensively used in developing drug delivery systems. Dash et al. [46] built a table that summarizes different types of chitosan-based drug delivery systems. These authors also showed and discussed different chitosan synthesis methods and applications, such as tissue engineering, gene therapy, bioimaging, and green chemistry.

To confer antimicrobial properties to other polymers, they may be mixed with chitosan; polyurethane [52], polyvinylpyrrolidone [53,54], polyethylene oxide [55], and polyethylene terephthalate [56] are examples of such approach where these polymers were blended with chitosan, and the bactericidal activity against *E. coli*, *S. aureus*, and *Klebsiella pneumoniae* was tested with good results. Li et al. [57] showed that the synthesis of quaternized chitosan functionalized with acrylate polyethylene glycol (PEG) side chains produces a nanoporous hydrogel with excellent antimicrobial efficacy against several bacteria. The proposed antimicrobial activity mechanism of the polycationic hydrogel was by the attraction of anionic microbial membrane into the internal nanopores of the hydrogel, which led to microbial membrane disruption and then to microbe death. Chitosan nanoparticles and quaternary ammonium chitosan derivative nanoparticles were also introduced into poly(methyl methacrylate) bone cement with good antimicrobial activity [58].

9.4.1.2 Peptides

Cationic natural antimicrobial peptides are emerging as promising antibiotic agents given their broad-spectrum activities and their ability to combat multidrug-resistant microorganisms [59].

These biomolecules act effectively against highly resistant bacteria such as multidrug-resistant *P. aeruginosa* and MRSA [60]. Some peptides that stand out for their antibacterial activity are cecropin [61], magainin [62], protegrin [63], bactenecin [60], and PR-39 [64]. In addition, peptides with antiviral [65], antiparasitic [65,66], and antifungal characteristics exist [67]; they also exhibit a broad-spectrum antimicrobial activity. The activities of various peptides are presented in Table 9.1.

However, natural peptides are vulnerable to rapid *in vivo* degradation. Some strategies can be employed to solve this problem, such as the synthesis of antimicrobial peptide mimics [68] or the encapsulation of the peptides inside nanoparticles [69]. In this last case, nanostructures prevent the enzymatic and hydrolytic degradation of peptides [70]. Some compounds, such as lipid nanovesicles, phosphatidylcholines, nanofibers, and nanotubes, can be used for this purpose [69].

Self-assembled peptides also offer appealing features as nanostructures for applications in both drug delivery and infection treatment. In some cases, it has been

TABLE 9.1

Activities of Cationic Antimicrobial Peptides and Some Examples of Peptides with Those Activities

Activities of Antimicrobial Peptides	Example Peptides
Broad-spectrum antibacterial	Protegrin, IB-367, MSI-78, indolicidin, CEMA, gramicidin S, polyphemusin
Anti-Gram− bacteria	Polymyxin B
Anti-Gram+ bacteria	HNP1
Synergy with conventional antibiotics	CEMA, magainin II, MSI-78, IB-367
Antifungal	Protegrin, CEMA, indolicidin, gramicidin S, polyphemusin
Synergy with conventional antifungals	Indolicidin
Antiviral (HIV, HSV)	Indolicidin, polyphemusin, protegrin
Anticancer	CEMA, indolicidin
Synergy with conventional anticancer agents	Indolicidin
Antiparasite	Magainin II, indolicidin
Antiendotoxin	CEMA, polyphemusin variants
Wound healing	Magainins, PR39
Chemotactic	HNP-1

Source: *The Lancet Infectious Diseases*, 1(3), Hancock R. E., Cationic peptides: Effectors in innate immunity and novel antimicrobials, 156–164, Copyright 2001, with permission from Elsevier.

demonstrated that nanoparticle formation can enhance antimicrobial activity [71]. These authors published a novel class of core–shell nanoparticles formed by self-assembly amphiphilics with a hydrophobic cholesterol core and strong antimicrobial properties against a range of bacteria, yeasts, and fungi. The synthesized peptide was formed by TAT (which is the minimal amino acid sequence required for membrane translocation) and six arginine residues. Arginine was added to introduce cationic charges in order to improve membrane translocation [72]. The hybrid nanoparticle was improved by adding degradable linkages to render it biocidal and biodegradable [68]. Nanoparticles, which are able to cross the blood–brain barrier in mice, showed a high therapeutic index against *S. aureus* infection. Thus, they are promising antimicrobial agents to treat brain infections and other infectious diseases [71].

Peptide self-immobilization in a bionanocomposite was published by Eby et al. [73] who obtained silica and titania antimicrobial peptide nanoparticles capable of releasing peptides continuously. Antimicrobial activity against *E. coli*, *S. aureus*, *Staphylococcus epidermidis*, and *Candida albicans* was observed. The system provides protection against the proteolytic degradation of the peptide and can be integrated into subcutaneous medical devices for reducing implant-related infections.

Carbon-based nanomaterials, such as carbon nanotubes, graphene, and graphene oxides, have also been reported to be capable of incurring physical and microchemical damage to microbial cells [74]. Hybrid nanostructures can be produced by the conjugation of the antimicrobial peptides with carbon nanotubes to dramatically improve anti-biofilm activity [75]. The multiwalled nanotube (MWNT)–nisin composite showed up to a sevenfold higher antimicrobial property than pristine MWNTs against *E. coli*, *P. aeruginosa*, *S. aureus*, and *B. subtilis*. This composite also has a dramatically improved capability of preventing biofilm formation when deposited as a film and also in suspension. The above-cited authors concluded that this composite can act as an effective economical antimicrobial material. Another example in which carbon nanotubes were used as support are the films on single-walled nanotubes (SWNTs), based on layer-by-layer assembled polyelectrolytes cationic poly(L-lysine) and anionic poly(L-glutamic acid) [76]. In this work, antimicrobial, biodegradable, and biocompatible nanofilm materials were obtained for cell-contacting applications.

9.4.2 NANOSTRUCTURED SYNTHETIC POLYMERS

In the last few years, a variety of surface modification or treatment techniques has emerged for the fabrication of antibacterial compounds, for which purpose polymerization is one of the most important approaches. Nanostructured synthetic polymers can be divided into polymers with own antimicrobial activity and polymers containing antimicrobial organic or inorganic antimicrobial compounds. In the latter case, compounds such as silver, fluoride, or antibiotics can be added to polymers to confer them antimicrobial properties. However, they can often become nonuniform and mechanically weak and can lack long-term stability since leaching time lowers the optimum concentration level and affects antibacterial efficacy [77]. In contrast, antimicrobial polymers with own antimicrobial activity are biocides given their chemical structure and can be long-lasting bactericidal materials. Sections 9.4.2.1 and 9.4.2.2 provide some examples of antimicrobial synthetic polymers, and the most important characteristics of each one are highlighted. This chapter focuses more on polymers with own antimicrobial activity, but it also briefly presents polymers containing low-molecular-weight compounds.

9.4.2.1 Polymers with Own Antimicrobial Activity

Polymers whose antibacterial activity is not attributed to the addition of secondary compounds kill the bacteria directly in contact with their surface. Polyanilines (PANIs), quaternary ammonium compounds, methacrylates, and compounds derived from rhodamine are some examples of the polymers belonging to this category. These compounds can be transformed into nanostructures with improved biocide properties against microorganisms. Surface-modified nanoparticles have received considerable attention as promising biocide agents because of their large surface area. The design of the contact area that interacts with bacteria is a key factor in producing nonleaching antibacterial agents with enhanced bactericidal activity.

Besides, nano-conducting polymers are suitable materials for sensors, and they offer other interesting applications because some possess antimicrobial properties. For example, it is known that PANI is antibacterial in nature. For this reason, PANI can be incorporated into thermoplastics and other materials. However, the use of this polymer in bioapplications entails some problems given its insolubility in organic solvents [78]. These authors reported other alternatives, such as the use of derivatives like poly(naphthylamine) or the copolymerization aniline with other substituted anilines [79,80]. They can be linked to nanoparticles in order to improve their properties, such as antimicrobial activity and better handling. Riaz et al. [28] reported stable PNA nanoparticles and their composites with polyvinyl alcohol (PVA) and polyvinylchloride, which proved effective against Gram+ and Gram– bacteria. In this case, particle size and morphology were found to play a key role in antimicrobial efficiency. The same authors reported that nanostructured PNA with aniline (PNA-co-PANI) and o-toluidine (PNA-co-POT) displayed antimicrobial activity against the bacteria E. coli and S. aureus, and that such activity was much greater than that reported for pristine PANI [81]; they also attributed the bactericide mechanism to their chemical structure and morphology.

Other structures like polycarbonates also have antibacterial properties. A biodegradable and in vivo applicable antimicrobial polymer has been recently synthesized by the metal-free organocatalytic ring-opening polymerization of functional cyclic carbonate in the form of nanoparticles [82]. These authors demonstrated that nanoparticles disrupt microbial walls/membranes selectively and efficiently by inhibiting the growth of Gram+ bacteria, MRSA, and fungi, without inducing significant hemolysis over a wide range of concentrations.

Beyth et al. [83–85] described the synthesis of nanoparticles made from quaternary ammonium cross-linked polyethyleneimine, which was incorporated into dental resin composites during polymerization to result in an antibacterial effect against Streptococcus mutans, the main bacterium causing dental caries. The resin composite maintained its full antibacterial properties over 1 month with no mechanical alterations.

Hybrid antimicrobial materials are compounds that contain two or more combined functional fragments. Antimicrobial macromolecules, which are hybrids, can improve properties such as biocompatibility, antimicrobial activity, and applicability. Some synthetic hybrid antimicrobial polymers based on nanostructures are presented in the following paragraphs.

Melo et al. [86] prepared and characterized hybrid nanoparticles composed of cationic bilayer fragments and polymers carboxymethylcellulose and polydiallyldimethylammonium chloride (PDDA). Bilayer fragments were prepared from the ultrasonic dispersion in water of synthetic and cationic lipid dioctadecyl-dimethylammonium bromide. This composite's antimicrobial activity was checked against *P. aeruginosa* and *S. aureus*. The antimicrobial effect was dependent on the amount of positive charges on particles and was independent of particle size. High potency for PDDA over a range of nanomolar concentrations was also disclosed, with *P. aeruginosa* more sensitive to all the cationic assemblies than *S. aureus*.

Microfibers of self-quaternized block copolymers with strong antibacterial properties were produced by Fu et al. [87]. Polymers poly[((2-dimethylamino)ethyl methacrylate)-co-(glycidyl methacrylate)] and poly(pentachlorophenyl acrylate) were used for the synthesis. Quaternary ammonium salts were generated via *N*-alkylation of tertiary amine groups. The obtained copolymer nanofibers displayed bactericide activity against *E. coli* and *S. aureus* over repeated applications.

Nonleaching material was fabricated by a single-step vapor cross-linking method using vapors of dimethylaminomethylstyrene and ethylene glycol diacrylate. The stable cross-linked copolymer killed bacteria through the disruption of the cell membrane upon surface contact with a reduction in bacterial growth of 99.99%. The strong antibacterial activity of the highly cross-linked coatings indicated that the mobility and length of the antibacterial chain are not critical in determining bactericide activity of the material [88].

To achieve antimicrobial properties, three *N*-halamine additives were introduced into the electrospinning nanofibrous membrane of nylon 6 [89]. The effect of the derivatives, these being chlorinated 5,5-dimetylhydantoin, chlorinated 2,2,5,5-tetramethyl-imidozalidin-4-one, and chlorinated 3-dodecyl-5,5-dimethylhydantoin, was analyzed. The total reduction (below detection limit) of *E. coli* and *S. aureus* was observed in less than 40 min. In this case, chlorine content was also responsible for these strong antibacterial properties. The authors confirmed that no significant leaching of *N*-halamine additives from electrospun nylon 6 was observed.

Inert materials are sometimes used in combination with cationic antimicrobial polymers to form core–shell structures. They offer advantages such as tunable surface functionality, low toxicity, and controllable size. Core–shell nanoparticles combine the properties of a polymer shell with the good colloidal stability of an inorganic core [30]. Silica nanoparticles are often used for this purpose. Cationic polymer–modified silica nanoparticles have enhanced antibacterial performance if compared to bulk polycations [29]. The synthesis of surface-modified silica nanoparticles grafted with acrylate and PEG inhibited the protein adsorption and bacterial adhesion of *S. epidermidis* and *P. aeruginosa* [90]. These coatings were proposed as a new method to mechanically prepare robust films with nonadhesive properties for biomedical applications. The antibacterial activity of nanoparticles based on silica nanoparticles coated with quaternary ammonium cationic surfactant didodecyldimethylammonium bromide was also determined [91]. Particles were highly effective against bacteria, molds, yeast, and the influenza A-H1N1 virus, and they were reused several times. These authors highlighted that nanoparticles can be attached to substrates to form an antimicrobial and antiviral coating. In addition, silica nanoparticles were also modified on the surface by the cationic poly(2-(tert-butylaminoethyl) methacrylate-co-ethylene glycol dimethacrylate) copolymer. The synthesized core–shell nanoparticles showed better antimicrobial activity than free polymers [29]. These silica-polycation core–shell nanoparticles can be used in various applications in the bioadhesive, biofilm, and sterilization fields because they reduce bioadhesion on glass slides. Later, Song et al. [92] synthesized the thin PDMAEMA shells that were formed on the surface of silica nanoparticles via vapor deposition polymerization. The antibacterial performance of these core–shell nanoparticles was effective against both Gram+ and Gram– bacteria. These nanoparticles were active with no further quaternization because of their enlarged surface area. Song and et al. [30] also fabricated polyrhodanime core–shell nanoparticles, which showed excellent biocidal activities against Gram– *E. coli* and Gram+ *S. aureus*. In that paper, nanoparticle size was controlled, and it was found that the smaller the particles, the higher the antimicrobial activity in consequence of the surface-to-volume ratio.

Metallic-based micro- and nanostructured materials, such as copper, zinc, and titanium and their oxides, have also been used to be assembled onto polymers and to construct antibacterial nanoparticles [93,94]. For example, titanium oxide is very popular for producing core–shell nanoparticles. Recently, Kong et al. [95] prepared novel biocidal polymer-functionalized TiO_2 nanoparticles using titania as an initiator. Vinyl monomer mixtures of nontoxic secondary amine-containing biocide-2-(tert-butylamino)ethyl methacrylate and antifouling ethylene glycol dimethacrylate were used for the antimicrobial polymer shell. During UV irradiation, this composite showed improved inhibition of bacterial growth against several bacteria in comparison to pristine TiO_2 nanoparticles.

Carbon nanotubes can be also combined to synthetic antimicrobial polymers. In general terms, SWNTs tend to be more effective than MWNTs. Simmons et al. [96] showed that SWNT combined with the polymer poly(vinylpyrrolidone-iodine) is antimicrobial and a promising material for wound-healing applications. Several other publications using carbon nanotubes can be found in the scientific literature. One very interesting paper was published by Aslan et al. [97] where carbon nanotubes were combined with commonly used biomaterial poly(lactic-coglycolic acid) (PLGA) as a thin film, and they proved very effective against Gram– (*E. coli*) and Gram+ (*S. epidermidis*) bacteria. The authors attributed mechanical disruption and oxidative stress to be the antimicrobial activity mechanism observed.

Magnetic particles are also used in combination with antibacterial polymers. In these cases, the main advantage is the possibility of reuse by collecting nanoparticles with an external magnetic field. Recently, Dong et al. [98] obtained functionalized magnetite nanoparticles with PDMAEMA quaternized with ethyl bromide. On the other hand, the same authors published the synthesis of magnetically separable *N*-halamine nanocomposites through the encapsulation of magnetic silica nanoparticles with an antibacterial *N*-halamine polymer to obtain good antibacterial properties [99].

There are more examples available of antimicrobial nanocomposites containing polymers in an inorganic matrix, for example, based on clays. A nonleaching antimicrobial polyamide nanocomposite based on organoclays and modified with a cationic polymer has been published [100]. The obtained nanocomposites displayed antimicrobial activity and improved mechanical properties, which were dependent on the content of the cationic polymer incorporated into the organoclay. Sodium-montmorillonite clay nanosheets and a poly(diallymethylammonium chloride) composite were investigated as the potential material to construct bone implants given their similar mechanical properties to natural nacre and lamellar bones [101]. This composite, in combination with silver nanoparticles, exhibited antibacterial properties and the almost complete inhibition of *E. coli*.

9.4.2.2 Polymers with Antimicrobial Compounds

Several antimicrobial organic agents, for example, triclosan, chlorhexidine, and rifampicin, have been introduced into polymer nano- and microstructures to confer them antimicrobial activity that they themselves do not have. These compounds can be aggregated in polymer-based nanostructures to confer them the biocide properties. On occasion, the polymer's main function is to produce the controlled delivery of the organic agent.

One of the most widely used antimicrobial agents is triclosan, a potent disinfectant employed in cosmetics and textile applications. This organic compound was incorporated into water-dispersible PVA nanoparticles, thus conferring them antibacterial properties [102]. These authors obtained aqueous nanodispersions with similar properties to solutions, but with better antimicrobial activity.

Another important agent is chlorhexidine. Microparticles of PLGA containing chlorhexidine and its derivates have been shown to possess activity against *Porphyromonas gingivalis* and *Bacteroides forsythus* bacteria [103]. The system described in that paper may prove useful for the localized delivery of chlorhexidine salts and possibly other antimicrobial agents to treat periodontal disease where prolonged controlled delivery is desired.

Rifampicin, an antibiotic for tuberculosis, has also been loaded into PLGA microspheres [104] and nanoparticles [105]. This compound was also loaded into the nanoparticles composed of commercial copolymers such as ethyl acrylate, methyl methacrylate, and a low content of methacrylic acid ester with quaternary ammonium groups [106]. In addition, microparticles containing rifampicin were prepared with poly(3-hydroxybutyrate-co-3-hydroxyvalerate), which led to diminished drug toxicity while maintaining its antimicrobial activity [107].

Besides the addition of organic molecules to polymers, inorganic components can also be added to confer antimicrobial activity to polymers. The most popular inorganic compound for this purpose is probably silver, specifically silver nanoparticles. Silver and its compounds are well known as being antimicrobial against bacteria, viruses, and fungi. Several antimicrobial polymer nanocomposites have been prepared by mixing silver nanoparticles with polymers [2]. By way of example, nanocomposites of polyamide [108] and polypropylene [109] containing silver powder have been produced by melt processing. Silver nanocomposites of poly(acrylamide-co-acrylic acid) hydrogels have also been synthesized [110]. It has been reported that silver frequently act both as a gelation catalyst and as an antimicrobial agent [111].

Copper nanoparticles are also added to polymers to confer them antimicrobial activity. Although copper has been studied less than silver nanoparticles, gaining a better understanding of its properties is well worthwhile. Several authors have used copper nanoparticles in their polymers. Palza et al. [112] synthesized poly(propylene) composites, which were prepared by the melt-mixed approach. This method is very effective as it reduces bacteria to 99.9% in only 4 h. Biocide behavior was completely attributed to the addition of copper nanoparticles. In other cases, encapsulation of copper in polystyrene nanocomposite particles has also been achieved and the Cu/polystyrene nanocomposite particles exhibited antimicrobial activity against a large number of bacteria [113]. These authors concluded that this process is a simple, cheap, and universal way to prepare a variety of other metal polymer nanocomposite material.

Another possibility of using both silver and copper nanoparticles is dual-action polymer/metal nanocomposites. In this case, a combination of the microbial properties of cationic polymers and metal nanoparticles is given synergetically. For example, copper and silver were integrated into polymeric poly(4-vinylpyridine) that had been chemically modified to obtain positively charged particles [114]. The obtained particles displayed dual action against various bacteria, such as *S. aureus*, *P. aeruginosa*, *B. subtilis*, and *E. coli*. These polymeric composite nanoparticles with enhanced bactericide properties can be used in the development of antibacterial surfaces with biocidal activities for a variety of applications.

9.5 MEDICAL APPLICATIONS OF ANTIMICROBIAL POLYMERS

Nosocomial infections have been related to the incidence of thousands of deaths annually in the United Kingdom [115]. For this reason, the use of antimicrobial polymeric nanoparticles in medicine can be very promising. Antimicrobial nanostructures may be used in wound dressings, photodynamic antimicrobial therapy, tissue engineering, artificial organs, dentistry, stem cell scaffoldings, and so on. Medical devices coated with materials with antimicrobial properties have been proposed as a way to diminish microbe adhesion and biofilm formation and to further reduce risk of infection [116].

Major medical implants that can be compromised by infections are of the intravascular, cardiovascular, neurosurgical, orthopedic, ophthalmological, and dental kind [117]. Antimicrobial polymers offer vast applications and opportunities in health care and biomedical implant coatings, including medical devices such as catheters, contact lenses, and stents [118–120].

A large proportion of infections are catheter-related infections. Catheters are medical devices that can be inserted into the body to treat diseases, to perform a surgical procedure, to carry out drug administration, and so forth. They are usually made of flexible polymeric materials, such as silicone and polyurethane [121]. On a catheter surface, a biofilm can be produced, which results in catheter-associated infection [122]. Some papers provide solutions to this problem [123–125], and the addition of polymeric antimicrobial nanoparticles to these devices could be a good alternative.

In addition, significant advances have been made in the use of polymeric nanomaterials in the area of bone and dental implants. Bone cement is employed in orthopedic surgery to join fractured bones or to fix devices in place in dentistry and arthroplasty. Use of metal (silver) nanoparticles provides antimicrobial activity to these materials without impinging on the mechanical and cytotoxic characteristic of the nanocomposite bone cement [6,7]. Moreover, the addition of cationic polymer nanoparticles has also been described; for example, polyethyleneimine nanoparticles incorporated into resin composite cause cell death and trigger biofilm stress *in vivo* [126]. The same authors also added these compounds to bone cement to obtain antimicrobial properties for orthopedic implants.

Drug delivery systems based on antimicrobial nanostructures improve therapeutic efficacy and the safety of drugs since they are delivered at a controlled rate that depends on the requirements of the physiological environment [127]. Drug-loaded nanoparticles can enter host cells through endocytosis. Then, the drug is released to treat microbe-induced intracellular infection. These systems can also be synthesized with controlled composition, shape, size, and morphology. Their surface properties can be manipulated to increase solubility, immunocompatibility, and cellular uptake [128]. The review written by Zhang et al. [42] summarizes some types of polymeric nanoparticles for antimicrobial drug delivery; for example, the antimicrobial activity of amphotericin B–loaded poly(ε-caprolactone) nanospheres coated with a nonionic surfactant showed good therapeutic efficacy against *Leishmania donovani* as compared to the free drug counterparts [129]. Rifampicin-loaded polybutylcyanoacrylate nanoparticles also exhibited enhanced antibacterial activity both *in vitro* and *in vivo* against *S. aureus* and *Mycobacterium avium* [130]; chitosan is also used in this application.

Besides small-molecule drug delivery, antimicrobial polymers can also be utilized to deliver various classes of biomacromolecules, such as peptides, proteins, plasmid DNA, and synthetic oligodeoxynucleotides [128]; for instance, cationic polymers are being actively investigated for gene therapy applications because they are able to form complexes with DNA [131]. Gene therapy is an approach for the treatment or prevention of diseases associated with defective gene expression, which involves the insertion of a therapeutic gene into cells, followed by the expression and production of the required proteins. This approach enables the replacement of damaged genes or the expression inhibition of undesirable genes [131]. In order to achieve this purpose, Wang et al. [132] synthesized new cationic nanoparticles with different amphiphilic cationic copolymers. Another example was published by Saka and Bozkir [133], who carried out a preparation of chitosan and polyethylenimine hybrids modified with PEG nanocomplexes to be used as a gene therapy candidate.

9.6   ENVIRONMENTAL IMPACT AND HUMAN HEALTH

As the range of nanoparticle-based technologies increases, sustainability and environmental impact issues become more important [102]. Some important concerns to be taken into account are the evaluation of long-term chemical risks or benefits, such as environmental persistence, bioaccumulation, and nanoparticle toxicity. In general, inorganic nanoparticles are more environmentally persistent than organic nanomaterials because of their lower degradation. Given their small size, nanoparticles can be widely distributed by air, or even in soil. In soil, large active surfaces give rise to binding to pollutants like heavy metals or organic substances. Depending on the receiving environment, if nanomaterials are not degraded or dissolved, they will tend to aggregate and eventually settle onto the substrate [12].

Many of these polymeric structures also exhibit low toxicity to human cells, a major requirement for biomedical applications [9]. The toxicological properties of nanoparticles are still not well understood. There are several variables (such as chemical composition, size, shape, concentration, rate of degradation, and surface properties) that influence the toxicological profile and the level of selective activity against prokaryotic cells. Growing scientific evidence has reported that free nanoparticles can cross cellular barriers and that exposure to some of these nanoparticles may lead to oxidative damage and inflammatory reactions [134]. For *in vivo* utilization, one of the major drawbacks of polymeric disinfectants, especially nanostructures, is lack of selectivity for bacterial over human cells, which limits their clinical and medicinal utility [31]. The straightforward way of avoiding toxicity when designing novel materials is to use natural cationic polymers (chitosan), or combinations of antimicrobial polymers and appropriate materials, in order to produce good-performing formulations with low toxicity *in vivo* (e.g., biocompatible synthetic polymers such as PMMA with antimicrobial polymers) [9].

REFERENCES

1. Kenawy E. R., Worley S. D., Broughton R. (2007) The chemistry and application of antimicrobial polymer: A state of the art review. *Biomacrolecules* 8, 1359–1384.
2. Muñoz-Bonilla A., Fernandez-García M. (2012) Polymeric materials with antimicrobial activity. *Progress in Polymer Science* 37, 281–339.
3. Spellberg B., Guidos R., Gilbert D., Bradley J., Boucher H. W., Scheld W. M., Bartleet J. G., Edwards J. Jr. (2008) The epidemic of antibiotic-resistant infections: A call to action for the medical community from the Infectious Diseases Society of America. *Clinical Infection Diseases* 46, 155–164.
4. Knetsch M. L. W., Koole L. H. (2011) New strategies in the development of antimicrobial coatings: The example of increasing usage of silver and silver nanoparticles. *Polymers* 3, 340–366.
5. Albers C. E., Hofstetter W., Siebenrock K. A., Landmann R., Klenke F. M. (2013) In vitro cytotoxicity of silver nanoparticles on osteoblasts and osteoclasts at antibacterial concentrations. *Nanotoxicology* 7, 30–36.
6. Prokopovich P., Leech R., Carmalt C. J., Parkin I. P., Perni S. (2013) A novel bone cement impregnated with silver-tiopronin nanoparticles: Its antimicrobial, cytotoxic, and mechanical properties. *International Journal of Nanomedicine* 8, 2227–2237.
7. Prokopovich P., Köbrick M., Brousseau E., Perni S. (2015) Potent antimicrobial activity of bone cement encapsulating silver nanoparticles capped with oleic acid. *Journal of Biomedical Materials Research B.* 103, 273–281. doi:10.1002/jbm.b.33196.
8. Campoccia D., Montarano L., Arciola C. R. (2013) A review of the biomaterials technologies for infection-resistant surfaces. *Biomaterials* 34, 8533–8554.
9. Carmona-Ribeiro A. M., Carrasco L. D. M. (2013) Cationic antimicrobial polymers and their assemblies. *International Journal of Molecular Sciences* 14, 9906–9946.
10. Chen C. Z., Beck-Tan N. C., Dhurjati P., Van Dyk T. K., LaRossa R. A., Cooper S. L. (2000) Quaternary ammonium functionalized poly(propylene imine) dendrimers as effective antimicrobials: Structure-activity studies. *Biomacromolecules* 1, 473–480.

11. Li Q., Mahendra S., Lyon D. Y., Brunet L., Liga M. V., Li D., Alvarez P. J. J. (2008) Antimicrobial nanomaterials for water disinfection and microbial control: Potential application and implications. *Water Research* 42, 4591–4602.
12. Silvestre C., Duraccio D., Cimmino S. (2011) Food packaging based on polymer nanomaterials. *Progress in Polymer Science* 36, 1766–1782.
13. Daly W. H., Guerrini M. M., Culberson D., Macossay J. (1998) *Science and Technology of Polymers and Advanced Materials*. Plenum Press: New York, p. 493.
14. Buchenska J. (1996) Polyamide fibers (PA6) with antibacterial properties. *Journal of Applied Polymer Sciences* 61, 567–576.
15. Paul D. R., Robeson L. M. (2008) Polymer nanotechnology: Nanocomposites. *Polymer* 49, 3187–3204.
16. Applerot G., Perkas N., Amirian G., Girshevitz O., Gedanken A. (2009) Coating of glass with ZnO via ultrasonic irradiation and a study of its antibacterial properties. *Applied Surface Science* 256S, S3–S8.
17. Song J., Jang J. (2013) Antimicrobial polymer nanostructures: Synthetic route, mechanism of action and perspective. *Advances in Colloid and Interface Science* 203, 37–50.
18. Rodrigues L. R., Ligia R. (2011) Inhibition of bacterial adhesion on medical devices. *Bacterial Adhesion: Chemistry, Biology and Physics* 715, 351–367.
19. Dunne W. M. Jr. (2002) Bacterial adhesion: Seen any good biofilms lately? *Clinical Microbiology Reviews* 15, 155–166.
20. Anward H. J., Strap L., Costerton J. W. (1992) Eradication of biofilm cells of *Staphylococcus aureus* with tobramycin and cephalexin. *Canadian Journal Microbiology* 38, 618–625.
21. An Y. H., Dickinson R. B., Doyle R. J. (2000) Mechanisms of bacterial adhesion and pathogenesis of implant and tissue infections. In *Handbook of Bacterial Adhesion: Principles, Methods, and Applications*, An, Yuehuei H., Friedman, Richard J. (Eds.). Humana Press: Totowa, NJ.
22. Williams J. F., Worley S. D. (2000) Infection-resistant nonleachable materials for urologic devices. *Journal of Endourology* 14, 395–400.
23. Denyer S. P. (1995) Mechanisms of action of antibacterial biocides. *International Biodeterioration & Biodegradation* 36, 227–245.
24. Ikeda T., Tazuke S. (1983) Biologically-active polycations-antimicrobial activities of poly(trialkyl(vinylbenzyl)ammonium chloride. *Makromolekulare Chemie-Rapid Communications* 4, 459–461.
25. Ikeda T., Hirayama H., Suzuki K., Yamaguchi H., Tazuke S. (1986) Biologically active polycations, 6. Polymeric pyridinium salts with well-defined main chain structure. *Makromolekulare Chemie* 187, 333–340.
26. Kanazawa A., Ikeda T., Endo T. (1993) Polymeric phosphonium salts as a novel class of cationic biocides. II. Effects of counter anion and molecular weight on antibacterial activity of polymeric phosphonium salts. *Journal of Polymer Science Part A: Polymer Chemistry* 31, 1441–1447.
27. Jia Z., Shen D., Xu W. (2001) Synthesis and antibacterial activities of quaternary ammonium salt of chitosan. *Carbohydrate Research* 22, 1–6.
28. Riaz U., Khan S., Islam M. N., Ahmad S., Ashraf S. M. (2008) Evaluation of antibacterial activity of nanostructured poly(1-naphthylamine) and its composites. *Journal of Biomaterial Sciences Polymer Edition* 47, 643–648.
29. Song J., Kong H., Jang J. (2009) Enhanced antibacterial performance of cationic polymer modified silica nanoparticles. *Chemical Communications* 36, 5418–5420.
30. Song J., Song H., Kong H., Hong J. Y., Jang J. (2011) Fabrication of silica/polyrhodanine core/shell nanoparticles and their antibacterial properties. *Journal of Materials Chemistry* 21, 19317–19323.
31. Kuroda K., DeGrado W. F. (2005) Amphiphilic polymethacrylate derivatives as antimicrobial agents. *Journal of American Chemical Society* 127, 4128–4129.

32. Kuroda K., Caputo G. A., William F. (2009) The role of hydrophobicity in the antimicrobial and hemolytic activities of polymethacrylate derivatives. *Chemistry-A—European Journal* 15, 1123–1133.
33. Kanazawa A., Ikeda T., Endo T. (1993) Polymeric phosphonium salts as a novel class of cationic biocides. 3. Immobilization of phosphonium salts by surface photografting and antibacterial activity of the surface-treated polymer-films. *Journal of Polymer Science Part A: Polymer Chemistry* 31, 1467–1472.
34. Panarín E. F., Solovaskii M. V., Zaikina N. A., Afinogenov G. E. (1985) Biological activity of cationic polyelectrolytes. *Macromolecular Chemistry Supplement* 9, 25–33.
35. Dutta S., Shome A., Kar T., Das P. K. (2011) Counterion-induced modulation in the antimicrobial activity and biocompatibility of amphiphilic hydrogelators: Influence of in-situ-synthesized Ag-nanoparticle on the bactericidal property. *Langmuir* 27, 5000–5008.
36. Lienkamp K., Madkour A. E., Kumar K. N., Nsslein K., Tew G. N. (2009) Antimicrobial polymers prepared by ring-opening metathesis polymerization: Manipulating antimicrobial properties by organic counterion and charge density variation. *Chemical European Journal* 15, 11715–11722.
37. Arnt L., Nüsslein K., Tew G. N. (2004) Nonhemolytic abiogenic polymers as antimicrobial peptide mimics. *Journal of Polymer Sciences, Part A: Polymer Chemistry* 42, 3860–3864.
38. Ikeda T., Tazuke S., Suzuki Y. (1984) Biologically active polycations, 4. Synthesis and antimicrobial activity of poly(trialkylvinylbenzylammonium chloride)s. *Makromolekulare Chemie* 185(5), 869–876.
39. Kanazawa A., Ikeda T., Endo T. (1994) Synthesis and antimicrobial activity of dimethyl and trimethyl substituted phosphonipplicum salts with alkyl chains of various lengths. *Antimicrobial Agents Chemotherapy* 38, 945–952.
40. Roy S., Das P. K. (2007) Antibacterial hydrogels of amino acid-based cationic amphiphiles. *Biotechnology and Bioengineering* 100, 756–764.
41. Engler A. C., Wiradharma N., Ong Z. Y., Coady D. J., Hedrick J. L., Yang Y. Y. (2012) Emerging trends in macromolecular antimicrobials to fight multi-drug-resistant infections. *Nano Today* 7, 201–222.
42. Zhang H., Pornpattanangkul D., Hu C. M. J., Huang C. M. (2010) Development of nanoparticles for antimicrobial drug delivery. *Current Medicinal Chemistry* 17, 585–594.
43. Barthlott W., Neinhuis C. (1997) Purity of the sacred lotus, or escape from contamination in biological surfaces. *Planta* 202, 1–8.
44. Liu K., Jiang L. (2011) Bio-inspired design of multiscale structures for function integration. *Nano Today* 6, 155–175.
45. Rinaudo M. (2006) Chitin and chitosan: Properties and applications. *Progress in Polymer Sciences* 31, 603–632.
46. Dash M., Chiellini F., Ottenbrite R. M., Chiellini E. (2011) Chitosan-A versatile semisynthetic polymer in biomedical applications. *Progress in Polymer Science* 36, 983–1014.
47. Qi L., Xu Z., Jiang X., Hu C., Zou X. (2004) Preparation and antibacterial activity of chitosan nanoparticles. *Carbohydrate Research* 339, 2693–2700.
48. Ye W. J., Xin J. H., Li P., Lee K. L. D., Kwong T. L. (2006) Durable antibacterial finish on cotton fabric by using chitosan-based polymeric core–shell particles. *Journal Applied Polymer Science* 102, 1787–1793.
49. De Campos A. M., Sánchez A., Alonso M. J. (2001) Chitosan nanoparticles: A new vehicle for the improvement of the delivery of drugs to the ocular surface. Application to cyclosporine A. *International Journal of Pharmaceutics* 224, 159–168.
50. Janes K. A., Fresneau M. P., Marazuela A., Fabra A., Alonso M. J. (2001) Chitosan nanoparticles as delivery systems for doxorubicin. *Journal of Controlled Release* 73, 255–267.

51. Xu Y. M., Du Y. M. (2003) Effect of molecular structure of chitosan on protein delivery properties of chitosan nanoparticles. *International Journal of Pharmaceutics* 250, 215–226.
52. Shih C. Y., Huang K. S. (2003) Synthesis of a polyurethane–chitosan blended polymer and a compound process for shrink-proof and antimicrobial woolen fabrics. *Journal of Applied Polymer Science* 88, 2356–2363.
53. Yeh J. T., Chen C. L., Huang K. S., Nien Y. H., Chen J. L., Huang P. Z. (2006) Synthesis, characterization, and application of PVP/chitosan blended polymers. *Journal of Applied Polymer Science* 101, 885–891.
54. Li J., Zivanovic S., Davidson P. M., Kit K. (2010) Characterization and comparison of chitosan/PVP and chitosan/PEO blend films. *Carbohydrate Polymer* 79, 786–791.
55. Zivanovic S., Li J., Davidson P. M., Kit K. (2007) Physical, mechanical, and antibacterial properties of chitosan/PEO blend films. *Biomacromolecules* 8, 1505–1510.
56. Jung K. H., Huh M. W., Meng W., Yuan J., Hyun S. H., Bae J. S., Hudson S. M., Kang I. K. (2007) Preparation and antibacterial activity of PET/chitosan nanofibrous mats using an electrospinning technique. *Journal of Applied Polymer Science* 105, 2816–2823.
57. Li P., Poon Y. F., Li W. F., Shu H. Y., Yeap S. H., Cao Y., Qi X. B., Zhou C. C., Lamrani M., Beuerman R. W., Kang E. T., Mu Y. G., Li C. M., Chang M. W., Leong S. S. J., Chan-Park M. B. (2010) Polycationic antimicrobial and biocompatible hydrogel with microbe membrane suctioning ability. *Nature Materials* 10, 149–156.
58. Shi Z., Neoh K. G., Kang E. T., Wang W. (2006) Antibacterial and mechanical properties of bone cement impregnated with chitosan nanoparticles. *Biomaterials* 27, 2440–2449.
59. Hancock R. E. W., Sahl H. G. (2006) Antimicrobial and host-defence peptides as new anti-infective therapeutic strategies. *Nature Biotechnology* 24, 1551–1557.
60. Hancock R. E. (2001) Cationic peptides: Effectors in innate immunity and novel antimicrobials. *The Lancet Infectious Diseases* 1, 156–164.
61. Gazit E., Miller I. R., Biggin P. C., Sansom M. S. P., Shai Y. (1996) Structure and orientation of the mammalian antibacterial peptide cecropin P1 within phospholipid membranes. *Journal of Molecular Biology* 258, 860–870.
62. Matsuzaki K. (1998) Magainins as paradigm for the mode of action of pore forming polypeptides. *Biochimica et Biophysic Acta* 1376, 391–400.
63. Heller X. T., Waring A. J., Lehrer R. I., Huang H. W. (1998) Multiple states of beta-sheet peptide protegrin in lipid bilayers. *Biochemistry* 37, 17331–17338.
64. Boman H. G., Agerberth B., Boman A. (1993) Mechanisms of action on *Escherichia coli* of cecropin-P1 and PR-39. Antibacterial peptides from pig intestine. *Infection and Immunity* 61, 2978–2984.
65. Jenssen H., Hamill P., Hancock R. E. (2006) Peptide antimicrobial agents. *Clinical Microbiology Reviews* 19, 491–511.
66. Lee D. G., Kim P. I., Park Y., Woo E. R., Choi J. S., Choi C. H., Hahm K. S. (2002) Design of novel peptide analogs with potent fungicidal activity, based on PMAP-23 antimicrobial peptide isolated from porcine myeloid. *Biochemical and Biophysical Research Communications* 293, 231–238.
67. Lee D. G., Kim H. K., Kim S. A., Park Y., Park S. C., Jang S. H., Hahm K. S. (2003) Fungicidal effect of indolicidin and its interaction with phospholipid membranes. *Biochemical and Biophysical Research Communications* 305, 305–310.
68. Chongsiriwatana N. P., Patch J. A., Czyzewski Z. A. M., Dohm M. T. Ivankin A., Gidalevitz D., Zuckermann R. N., Barron A. E. (2008) The role of antimicrobial peptides in preventing multidrug-resistant bacterial infections and biofilm formation. *Proceedings of the National Academy of Sciences* 105, 2794–2799.
69. Brandelli A. (2012) Nanostructures as promising tools for delivery of antimicrobial. *Mini-Reviews in Medicinal Chemistry* 12, 731–741.

70. Ma W., Smith T., Bogin V., Zhang Y., Ozkan C., Ozkan M., Hayden M., Schroter S., Carrier F., Messmer D., Kumar V., Minev B. (2011) Enhanced presentation of MHC class Ia, Ib and class II-restricted peptides encapsulated in biodegradable nanoparticles: A promising strategy for tumor immunotherapy. *Journal of Translational Medicine* 9, 2–10.

71. Liu L. H., Xu K. J., Wang H. Y., Tan P. K. J., Fan W. M., Venkatraman S. S., Li L. J., Yang Y. Y. (2009) Self-assembled cationic peptide nanoparticles as an efficient antimicrobial agent. *Nature Nanotechnology* 4, 457–463.

72. Futaki S., Suzuki T., Ohashi W., Yagami T., Tanaka S., Ueda K., Sugiura Y. (2001) Arginine-rich peptides. An abundant source of membrane-permeable peptides having potential as carriers for intracellular protein delivery. *Journal of Biological Chemistry* 276, 5836–5840.

73. Eby D. M., Farrington K. E., Johnson G. R. (2008) Synthesis of bioinorganic antimicrobial peptide nanoparticles with potential therapeutic properties. *Biomacromolecules* 9, 2487–2494.

74. Hu W. B., Peng C., Luo W., Lv M., Li X., Li D., Huang Q., Fran C. (2010) Graphene-based antibacterial paper. *ACS Nano* 4, 4317–4323.

75. Qi X. B., Poernomo G., Wang K. A., Chen Y. A., Chan-Park M. B., Xu R., Chang M. W. (2011) Covalent immobilization of nisin on multi-walled carbon nanotubes: Superior antimicrobial and anti-biofilm properties. *Nanoscale* 3, 1874–1880.

76. Aslan S., Deneufchatel M., Hashmi S., Li N., Pfefferle L. D., Elimelech M. (2012) Carbon nanotube-based antimicrobial biomaterials formed via layer-by-layer assembly with polypeptides. *Journal of Colloid and Interface Science* 388, 268–273.

77. Hasan J., Crawford R. J., Ivanova E. P. (2013) Antibacterial surfaces: The quest for a new generation of biomaterials. *Trends in Biotechnology* 31, 295–300.

78. Gizdavic-Nikolaidis M. R., Zujovic Z. D., Ray S., Easteal A. J., Bowmaker G. A. (2010) Chemical synthesis and characterization of poly(aniline-*co*-ethyl 3-aminobenzoate) copolymers. *Journal of Polymer Science Polymer Chemistry A* 48, 1339–1347.

79. Borole D. D., Kapadi U. R., Mahulikar P. P., Hundiwale D. G. (2008) Synthesis and characterization of a conducting composite of polyaniline, poly(o-anisidine), and poly(aniline-co-o-anisidine). *Polymer-Plastic Technology and Engineering* 47, 643–648.

80. Gizdavic-Nikolaidis M. R., Bennet J. R., Swift S., Easteal A. J., Ambrose M. (2011) Broad spectrum antimicrobial activity of functionalized polyanilines. *Acta Biomaterialia* 7, 4204–4209.

81. Riaz U., Ashraf S. M. (2012) Evaluation of antibacterial activity of nanostructured copolymers of poly(naphthylamine). *International Journal of Polymeric Materials and Polymeric Biomaterials* 62, 406–410.

82. Nederberg F., Zhang Y., Tan J. P., Xu K., Wang H., Yang C., Gao S., Guo X. D., Fukushima K., Li L., Hedrick J. L., Yang Y. Y. (2011) Biodegradable nanostructures with selective lysis of microbial membranes. *Nature Chemistry* 3, 409–414.

83. Beyth N., Houri-Haddad Y., Baraness-Hadar L., Yudovin-Farber I., Domb A. J., Weiss E. I. (2008) Surface antimicrobial activity and biocompatibility of incorporated poly-ethylenimine nanoparticles. *Biomaterials* 31, 4157–4163.

84. Beyth N., Shvero D. K., Zaltsman N., Houri-Haddad Y., Abramovitz I., Davidi M. P., Weiss E. I. (2013) Rapid kill—Novel endodontic sealer and *Enterococcus faecalis*. *PLoS One* 8, 1–10. doi:10.1371/journal.pone.0078586.

85. Beyth N., Yudovin-Farber I., Bahir R., Domb A. J., Weissa E. (2006) Antibacterial activity of dental composites containing quaternary ammonium polyethylenimine nanoparticles against *Streptococcus mutans*. *Biomaterials* 27, 3995–4002.

86. Melo L. D., Mamizuka E. M., Carmona-Ribeiro A. M. (2010) Antimicrobial particles from cationic lipid and polyelectrolytes. *Langmuir* 26, 12300–12306.

87. Fu G. D., Yao F., Li Z. G., Li X. S. (2008) Solvent-resistant antibacterial microfibers of self-quaternized block copolymers from atom transfer radical polymerization and electrospinning. *Journal of Material Chemistry* 18, 859–867.

88. Ye Y. M., Song Q., Mao Y. (2011) Single-step fabrication of non-leaching antibacterial surfaces using vapor crosslinking. *Journal of Materials Chemistry* 21, 257–262.
89. Tan K., Obendorf S. K. (2007) Fabrication and evaluation of electrospun nanofibrous antimicrobial nylon 6 membranes. *Journal of Membrane Science* 305, 287–298.
90. Holmes P. F., Currie E. P., Thies J. C., van der Mei H. C., Busscher H. J., Norde W. (2009), Surface modified nanoparticles as a new, versatile, and mechanically robust non-adhesive coating: Suppression of protein adsorption and bacterial adhesion. *Journal of Biomedical Material Research* 91, 824–833.
91. Botequim D., Maia J., Lino M. M., Lopes L. M., Simoes P. N., Ilharco L. M., Ferreira L. (2012) Nanoparticles and surfaces presenting antifungal, antibacterial and antiviral properties. *Langmuir* 208, 7646–7656.
92. Song J., Jung Y., Lee I., Jang J. (2013) Fabrication of pDMAEMA-coated silica nanoparticles and their enhanced antibacterial activity. *Journal of Colloid and Interface Science* 407, 205–209.
93. Llorens A., Lloret E., Picouet P. A., Trbojevich R., Fernández A. (2012) Metallic-based micro and nanocomposites in food contact materials and active food packaging. *Trends in Food Science & Technology* 24, 19–29.
94. Seil J. T., Webster T. J. (2012) Antimicrobial applications of nanotechnology: Methods and literature. *International Journal of Nanomedicine* 7, 2767–2781.
95. Kong H., Song J., Jang J. (2010) Photocatalytic antibacterial capabilities of TiO_2-biocidal polymer nanocomposites synthesized by a surface-initiated photopolymerization. *Environmental Science & Technology* 14, 5672–5676.
96. Simmons T. J., Bult J., Hashim D. P., Linhard R. J., Ajayan P. M. (2009) Noncovalent Functionalization as an alternative to oxidative acid treatment of single wall carbon nanotubes with applications for polymer composites. *ACS Nano* 3, 865–870.
97. Aslan S., Loebick C. Z., Kang S., Elimelech M., Pfefferle L. D., Van Tassel P. R. (2010) Antimicrobial biomaterials bases nanotubes dispersed on poly(lactic-co-glycolic acid). *Nanoscale* 2, 1789–1794.
98. Dong H., Huang J., Koepsel R. R., Ye P., Russell A. J., Matyjaszewski K. (2011) Recyclable antibacterial magnetic nanoparticles grafted with quaternized poly(2-dimethylamino)ethyl methacrylate) brushes. *Biomacromolecules* 12, 1305–1311.
99. Dong A., Lan S., Huang J. F., Wang T., Zhao T. Y., Wang W. W., Xiao L. H., Zheng X., Liu F. Q., Gao F. (2011) Preparation of magnetically separable N-halamine nanocomposites for the improved antibacterial application. *Journal of Colloid and Interface Science* 364, 333–340.
100. Nigmatullin R., Gao F. G., Konovalova V. (2009) Permanent, non-leaching antimicrobial polyamide nanocomposites based on organoclays modified with a cationic polymer. *Macromolecular Materials and Engineering* 294, 795–805.
101. Podsiadlo P., Paternel S., Rouillar J. M., Zhang Z., Lee J., Lee J. W., Gulari E., Kotov N. A. (2005) Layer by layer assemble of nacre-like nanostructured composites with antimicrobial properties. *Langmuir* 21, 11915–11921.
102. Zhang H., Wang D., Butler R., Cambell N. L., Long J., Tan B., Duncalf D. J., Foster A. J., Hopkinson A., Taylor D., Angus D., Cooper Al., Rannard S. P. (2008) Formation and enhanced biocidal activity of water-dispersable organic nanoparticles. *Nature Nanotechnology* 3, 506–511.
103. Yue I. C., Proff J., Cortés M. E., Sinisterra R. D., Faris C. B., Hildgen P., Langer R., Shastri V. P. (2004) A novel polymeric chlorhexidine delivery device for the treatment of periodontal disease. *Biomaterials* 25, 3743–3750.
104. Suarez S., O'Hara P., Kazanteseva M., Newcomer C. E., Hopfer R., McMurray D. N., Hickey A. J. (2001) Respirable PLGA microspheres containing rifampicin for the treatment of tuberculosis: Screening in an infectious disease model. *Pharmaceutical Research* 18, 1315–1319.

105. Toti U. S., Guru B. R., Hali M., McPharlin C. M., Wykes S. M., Panyam J., Whittum-Hudson J. A. (2011) Targeted delivered of antibiotics to intracellular chlamydial infections using PLGA nanoparticles. *Biomaterials* 32, 6606–6613.
106. Dillen K., Vandervoort J., Van den Mooter G., Ludwing A. (2006) Evaluation of ciprofloxacin-loaded Eudragit RS100 or RL100/PLGA nanoparticles. *International Journal of Pharmacy* 314, 72–82.
107. Durán N., Alvarenga M. A., Da Silva E. C., Melo P. S., Marcato P. D. (2008) Microencapsulation of antibiotic rifampicin in Poly(3-hydroxybutyrate-co-3-hydroxyvalerate). *Archives of Pharmaceutical Research* 31, 1500–1516.
108. Radheshkumar C., Münstedt H. (2005) Morphology and mechanical properties of antimicrobial polyamide/silver composite. *Material Letters* 59, 1949–1953.
109. Radheshkumar C., Münstedt H. (2006) Antimicrobial polymers from polypropylene/silver composites—Ag+ release measured by anode stripping voltammetry. *Reactive and Functional Polymers* 66, 780–788.
110. Tarnavchyk I., Voronov A., Dohut A., Nosova N., Varvarenko S., Samaryk V., Voronov S. (2009) Reactive hydrogel networks for the fabrication of metal-polymer nanocomposites. *Macromolecular Rapid Communication* 30, 1564.
111. Yates C. C., Whaley D., Babu R., Zhan J. Y., Krishna P., Beckman E., Pasculle A. W., Wells A. (2007) The effect of multifunctional polymer-based gels on wound healing in full thickness bacteria-contaminated mouse skin wound models. *Biomaterials* 28, 3977–3986.
112. Palza H., Gutierrez S., Delgado K., Salazar O., Fuenzalida V., Avila J., Figueroa G., Quijada R. (2010) Toward tailor-made biocide materials based on poly(propylene)/copper nanoparticles. *Macromolecular Rapid Communications* 31, 563–567.
113. Kamrupi I. R., Dolui S. K. (2011) Synthesis of copper-polystyrene nanocomposite particles using water in supercritical carbon dioxide medium and its antimicrobial activity. *Journal of Applied Polymer Science* 120, 1025–1033.
114. Ozay O., Akcali A., Otkun M. T., Silan C., Aktas N., Sahiner N. (2010) P(4-PV) based nanoparticles and composites with dual action as antimicrobial materials. *Colloids Surfaces B Biointerfaces* 79, 460–466.
115. Bhutta A., Gilliam C., Honeycutt M., Schexnayder S., Green J., Moss M., Anand K. J. S. (2007) Reduction of bloodstream infections associated with catheters in pediatric intensive care unit: Stepwise approach. *British Medical Journal* 334, 362–365.
116. Camargo L. F. A., Marra A. R., Buchele G. L., Sogavar A. M. C., Cal R. G. R., de Sousa J. M. A., Silva E., Knobel E. (2009) Double-lumen central venous catheters impregnated with chlorhexidine and silver sulfadiazine to prevent catheter colonisation in the intensive care unit setting: A prospective randomised study. *Journal of Hospital Infection* 72, 227–233.
117. Von Eiff C., Kohnen W., Becker K., Jansen B. (2005) Modern strategies in the prevention of implant-associated infections. *International Journal of Artificial Organs* 28, 1146–1156.
118. Zampa M. F., Araujo I. M. S., Costa V., Costa C. H. N., Santos J. R., Zucolotto V., Eiras C., Leite J. R. S. A. (2009) Leishmanicidal activity and immobilization of dermaseptin 01 antimicrobial peptides in ultrathin films for nanomedicine applications. *Nanomedicine-Nanotechnology Biology and Medicine* 5, 352–358.
119. Li P., Li X., Saravanan R., Li C. M., Leong S. S. J. (2012) Antimicrobial macromolecules: Synthesis methods and future applications. *RSC Advances* 2, 4031–4044.
120. Shukla A., Fleming K. E., Chuang H. F., Chau T. M., Loose C. R., Stephanopoulos G. N., Hammond P. T. (2010) Controlling the release of peptide antimicrobial agents from surfaces. *Biomaterials* 31, 2348–2357.
121. Piccirillo C., Perni S., Gil-Thomas J., Prokopovich P., Wolson M., Pratten J., Parkin I. P. (2009) Antimicrobial activity of methylene blue and toluidine blue O covalently bound to a modified silicone polymer surface. *Journal of Material Chemistry* 19, 6167–6171.

122. Trautner B. W., Darouiche R. O. (2004) Catheter-associated infections—Pathogenesis affects prevention. *Archives of Internal Medicine* 164, 842–850.
123. Noimark S., Dunnill C. W., Kay C. W. M., Perni S., Prokopovich P., Ismail S., Wilson M., Parkin I. P. (2012) Incorporation of methylene blue and nanogold into polyvinyl chloride catheters; A new approach for light-activated disinfection of surfaces. *Journal of Materials Chemistry* 22, 15388–15396.
124. Perni S., Piccirillo C., Pratten J., Prokopovich P., Chrzanowski W., Parkin I. P., Wilson M. (2009) The antimicrobial properties of light-activated polymers containing methylene blue and gold nanoparticles. *Biomaterials* 30, 89–93.
125. Perni S., Prokopovich P. Piccirillo C., Pratten J., Parkin I. P., Wilson M. (2009) Toluidine blue-containing polymers exhibit potent bactericidal activity when irradiated with red laser light. *Journal of Materials Chemistry* 19, 2715–2723.
126. Beyth N., Yudovin-Farber I., Perez-Davidi M., Domb A. J., Weiss E. I. (2010) Polyethyleneimine nanoparticles incorporated into resin composite cause cell death and trigger biofilm stress in vivo. *Proceedings of the National Academic of Sciences of the United States of America* 107, 22038–22043.
127. Kenawy E. R., Bowlin G. L., Mansfield K., Layman J., Simpson D. G., Sanders E. H., Wnek G. J. (2002) Release of tetracycline hydrochloride from electrospun poly(ethylene-co-vinylacetate), poly(lactic acid), and a blend. *Journal of Controlled Release* 81, 57–64.
128. Goldberg M., Langer R., Xinqia J. (2007) Nanostructured materials for applications in drug delivery and tissue engineering. *Journal of Biomaterial Science Polymer Edition* 18, 241–268.
129. Espuelas M. S., Legrand P., Loiseaus P. M., Bories C., Barratt G., Irache J. M. (2002) In vitro antileishmanial activity of amphotericin B loaded in poly(épsilon-caprolactone) nanospheres. *Journal of Drug Targeting* 10, 593–599.
130. Skidan I. N., Gel'perina S. E., Severin S. E., Guliaev A. E. (2003) Enhanced activity of rifampicin loaded with polybutyl cyanoacrylate nanoparticles in relation to intracellularly localized bacteria. *Antibiot Khimioter* 48, 23–26.
131. Eliyahu H., Barenholz Y., Domb A. J. (2005) Polymers for DNA delivery. *Molecules* 10, 34–64.
132. Wang Y. H., Fu Y. C., Chiu H. C., Wang C. Z., Lo S. P., Ho M. L., Liu P. L., Wang C. K. (2013) Cationic nanoparticles with quaternary ammonium-functionalized PLGA-PEG-based copolymers for potent gene transfection. *Journal of Nanoparticle Research* 15, 16, Article no. 2077. doi:10.1007/s11051-013-2077-4.
133. Saka O. M., Bozkir A. (2012) Formulation and in vitro characterization of PEGylated chitosan and polyethylene imine polymers with thrombospondin-I gene bearing pDNA. *Journal of Biomedical Materials Research Part B—Applied Biomaterials* 100B, 984–992.
134. Bownmeester H., Dekkers S., Noordam M. Y., Hagens W. I., Bulder A. S., de Heer C. (2009) Review of health safety aspects of nanotechnologies in food production. *Regulation in Toxicology and Pharmacology* 53, 52–62.

Section III

Nanomaterials in Biosensors

10 Recent Advances in Nanodiagnostic Techniques for Infectious Agents

Muhammad Ali Syed

CONTENTS

ABSTRACT

Infectious diseases have always been a major obstacle to human development and welfare, causing millions of illnesses and deaths in both developing and developed countries with a substantial economic loss. In the modern age of globalization, the massive increase in world population, international travel, and trade has greatly facilitated their spread from one part of the world to other areas. Mankind needs to protect itself against the pathogenic microorganisms they come across in daily life as well as from the horrifying effects of bioterrorism agents. Prevention strategies against infectious agents require reliable, rapid, and accurate detection and identification of causative agents with highest sensitivity, which should be equally available in different parts of the globe, regardless of their economic conditions. Similarly, rapid and early diagnosis of infectious diseases has always remained indispensable for their prompt cure and management, which has stimulated scientists to develop highly sophisticated techniques over centuries and the efforts continue unabated. Conventional microbiological diagnostic techniques such as microscopy, cultural characteristics, biochemical testing, and serology, although reliable, are time consuming, tedious, expensive, less sensitive, and unsuitable for field situations. Nanodiagnostic assays have emerged as a better alternative for early, sensitive, point-of-care, and cost-effective detection of microbial agents. There has been an explosive multidisciplinary research in nanodiagnostics in the last two decades yielding highly fascinating results. This chapter discusses some of the advancements made in the field of nanotechnology-based assays for microbial detection along with providing the basic understanding.

Keywords: Biosensors, Lab-on-a-chip, Microorganisms, Nanoparticles, Quantum dots

10.1 INTRODUCTION

The history of mankind has witnessed massive devastations by infectious diseases (Brachman 2003; Fauci 2001; Syed and Bokhari 2011). The human race has always been found battling with infectious diseases, which is evident from archaeological remains of Egyptian mummies, Hippocrates' writings, and history book chapters on great epidemics in middle-age Europe as well as other areas of the world (Brachman 2003; Wolfe et al. 2007). Communicable diseases have been of particular concern in the era of globalization where international trade and travel has been highly facilitated and practiced. One of the major challenges that contemporary medical science faces today is the spread of infectious diseases from one part of the world to other areas (Hauck et al. 2010). Although mankind has made many remarkable discoveries in the last few decades and has been able to discover cures to numerous diseases such as tuberculosis, malaria, and diarrhea, the great battle against many other diseases continues unabated (Houpikian and Raoult 2002; Pfaller 2001).

Infectious diseases are caused by pathogenic microorganisms (also called infectious agents) that are capable of transmission from one person to another or even from animals and soil; hence, they are the most significant health burden. Developed countries have been successful in reducing the amount of suffering from these diseases; however, they still face the serious challenges of HIV, influenza, food-borne illnesses and hospital-acquired infections, and occasional outbreaks. Most of the suffering and deaths are reported from developing countries of the world because of poor sanitary conditions, substandard health facilities, and malnutrition (Kaittanis et al. 2010).

Early diagnosis of infectious diseases is a prerequisite for prompt treatment and hence protection from progression to advanced stage, which is not only difficult to cure but also communicable to the population. Although massive and dedicated multidisciplinary research in this arena has produced many breakthroughs such as development of highly sophisticated molecular techniques like polymerase chain reaction (PCR), ligase chain reaction, DNA sequencing, DNA hybridization assays, DNA microarrays (Dutse and Yusof 2011; Mairhofer et al. 2009), or commercially available dip stick tests, much more needs to be done for rapid, sensitive, cost-effective, and point-of-care diagnosis of infectious diseases (Syed and Bokhari 2011). Rapid detection of infectious agents from environmental food and water samples is required for both public health and security reasons (Coloma and Harris 2009). Moreover, underdeveloped and resource-poor countries still remain largely deprived of highly sophisticated and valuable molecular techniques in the postgenomics era and demand low-cost devices and systems to be used in remote areas (Syed and Bokhari 2011).

Both classical culture media plate and tube based, as well as modern diagnostic techniques, have served as valuable tools for the diagnosis of infectious diseases. Causative agents of many bacterial diseases may be grown in the microbiology laboratory using culture media and identified by specific cultural characteristics, biochemical testing, serology, and molecular assays. However, each of the diagnostic method has its own advantages and limitations. Test tube–based biochemical and serological testing for the identification of bacterial agents have been in use for almost a century in all parts of the world. However, recent advances of modern molecular techniques have greatly revolutionized infectious disease diagnosis by increasing the sensitivity and reducing the time taken by the laboratory tests (Bissonnette and Bergeron 2012; Muldrew 2009). PCR has successfully occupied its place in many diagnostic laboratories and has emerged as a valuable tool in modern diagnostic laboratories nowadays. Commercially available diagnostic kits manufactured by a number of companies offer rapid and cost-effective diagnosis of many infectious diseases with high sensitivity and specificity (Heo and Hua 2009; Shinde et al. 2012).

Although both conventional and modern molecular diagnostic techniques have been found to be remarkably reliable in the diagnosis of infectious diseases, they are tedious, expensive, and less sensitive in some cases and require skilled personnel, which is unsuitable or unaffordable for many in the field situations (Gehring and Tu 2011; Pfaller 2001; Sanvicens et al. 2009; Syed and Bokhari 2011). In addition, cultivation of slow-growing and fastidious bacteria in the laboratory has always been a challenge where laboratory test results are awaited to start the prompt treatment. Furthermore, a number of bacterial species such as *Treponema pallidum* cannot be grown in the laboratory and hence more sophisticated approaches are required

(Centurion-Lara et al. 1997). Serological assays often fail to produce the desired results because of unavailability of antisera to a wide range of microbial species, poor sensitivity, and higher cost. Moreover, many types of microbial agents may undergo dormant phases in the host and hence become undetectable by the conventionally used diagnostic assays (Speers 2006).

Diagnosis of infectious diseases has been revolutionized by molecular diagnostic techniques by offering rapid diagnostic assays as well as means of detecting antibiotic resistance genes with higher sensitivity and specificity (Mothershed and Whitney 2006; Pfaller 2001; Speers 2006). Real-time PCR (RT-PCR) has been used to determine the drug resistance in both viruses and bacteria, total viral load, and genotyping as well as strain characterization (Pfaller 2001). These modern techniques, although highly sensitive in many cases, are costly and laborious and do not offer an option of point-of-care diagnosis. PCR amplification of microbial gene requires DNA extraction from cells, and it may also produce false-negative and false-positive results (Syed 2014). In addition, many of the aforementioned molecular techniques need trained personnel to operate the sophisticated equipment and hence are unaffordable by most laboratories in underdeveloped and resource-poorer countries. Therefore, microbiologists are in search of ideal alternative strategies for microbial detection and identification bearing highest sensitivity and specificity (Singh et al. 2006; Syed 2014).

Recent research in nanotechnology-based approaches for microbial detection has produced highly fascinating and promising results. Nanomaterials have been highly useful in biological applications, and new disciplines such as nanomedicine and nanobiotechnology have become one of the massively researched areas of science today. High surface-to-volume ratio of these novel materials greatly enhances the sensing of biomolecular interactions by optical, electrical, and electrochemical biosensors. Diagnostic systems having the potential to be automated and miniaturized offering enormous advantage over their counterparts, since they may be used in field situations requiring less complicated protocols (Gabig-Ciminska 2006). Furthermore, popular disposable dip stick assays using gold nanoparticles (Au NPs) seem to be most promising for point-of-care, rapid, sensitive, and cost-effective microbial detection (Syed 2014; Syed and Bokhari 2011).

The newly emerged science of nanotechnology has been merged with another promising field, biosensing, aiming at improving the sensitivity and detection limit of biological events owing to the higher surface area of the sensing surfaces (Liu et al. 2011). Nanostructures such as Au NPs, carbon nanotubes (CNTs), nanowires (NWs), graphene, and others have been used in a number of biosensing applications for the detection of proteins, nucleic acids, and microbial toxins, as well as bacteria and viruses (Doria et al. 2012). Scientists are striving hard to obtain maximum utility of these nanostructures, and multidisciplinary approaches to possible manipulation of materials at submicroscopic and nanoscales for potential applications in life sciences are on their way toward major breakthroughs.

The multidisciplinary field of nanodiagnostics, although in its infancy and still not fully commercialize, will greatly facilitate future microbiologists to develop sensitive and user-friendly devices for microbial detection in their laboratories as well field situations. Scientists from various disciplines have been engaged in designing cutting-edge technologies relying upon novel size-dependent properties of matter of different kinds. The number of research articles published on the latest advancements and breakthroughs in this arena of science is ever increasing. Microbiologists of our time are well aware of the advancements in nanotechnology as well as potential applications in microbiology.

10.2 NANODIAGNOSIS OF INFECTIOUS DISEASES

Although a new discipline, the majority of scientists from various disciplines are familiar with the word *nanotechnology*. It deals with the study of creation, manipulation, and use of materials, systems, and devices having a dimension ranging from 1 to 100 nm (Jianrong et al. 2004; Villaverde 2010). Materials of this size exhibit unique physical and chemical properties because of their higher surface-to-volume ratio, which is different from the larger-sized one (Kaittanis et al. 2010). The spectrum of study of this science is wide, covering both fundamental (such as physics, chemistry, and biology) and applied sciences (such as electronics and materials science) (Kim et al. 2010; Liu 2006). As stated earlier, potential applications of nanotechnology in medicine and biomedical sciences are broad, using the unique features of nanomaterial for the treatment as well as diagnosis of diseases even at the molecular level (Kim et al. 2010). An example of one of many applications of nanotechnology in microbiology is designing nanotechnology-based assay formats for sensitive and early detection of microbial agents or their products (Kim et al. 2010; Kumar et al. 2011a; Liu et al. 2006; Vashist 2013).

Biologists are well aware of nanometer-sized objects, and the electron microscope was in use before nanotechnology became popular. Living systems are composed of a number of nanometer-sized structures such as proteins, DNA, RNA lipids, ligands, receptors, and cell surface molecules. Moreover, viruses present a unique class of nanosized living organisms capable of carrying genetic information and infecting hosts ranging from the largest animals and plants to bacterial cells. Therefore, biologists started their attempts to understand nanometer-sized cellular structures and have been dealing with such small systems for a long time using sophisticated tools like electron microscopes.

The robust sensitivity offered by these nanotechnology-based techniques offers a unique opportunity to understand tiny details of living processes that are difficult to achieve using conventional assay formats. The higher surface-to-volume ratio of the nanomaterials such as Au NPs and CNTs offers a great opportunity to sense biological processes with higher sensitivity. In nanodiagnostic devices, nanomaterials are usually conjugated with a biological species such as antibodies, DNA probes, or aptamers. Nanomaterials conjugated with biomolecules sense and transmit biological information at a minimal period, thereby making them promising material for biosensing applications (Kim et al. 2010). Results of recent studies report the successful use of nanodiagnostic techniques for sensing at a single cell or even at single-molecule-level depth. Furthermore, nanotechnology-based assays fascinate microbiologists by offering the most desired features of rapid, label-free, highly sensitive microbial testing with the option of their onsite utility (Chen et al. 2007; Jain 2003, 2007).

10.3 BIOSENSORS FOR MICROBIAL DETECTION

Since the first use of biosensors in 1960, there has been an explosion in the amount of research carried out in this area of science. Biosensing has emerged as a large scientific field with potential application in diagnostics, environmental monitoring, protein and drug research, among many others (Vo-Dinh and Cullum 2000). The word *biosensor* indicates that the device consists of two parts, that is, a biological and a sensing element. The biological element (e.g., enzyme, antibody, receptor molecule, or DNA probe) recognizes its target, whereas the sensing element transduces the signal into an electronic form so that it can be made interpretable after processing. Biosensors may be classified on the basis of the biomolecules or the transducer. On the basis of type of transducer, they may be classified as electrochemical, optical, ion-sensitive field effect transistors (FETs), thermal detection biosensors, and so forth (Mohanty and Kougdianos 2006). The main types of sensing receptor elements used in biosensors are protein, antibodies, antigen, DNA, enzymes, and other molecules such as lipopolysaccharides, carbohydrates, and glycoproteins (Vo-Dinh and Cullum 2000).

Biosensors are analytical devices used to detect a biological or chemical species or study a biological event. Biosensors may be divided into various types on the basis of the biological element or the type of transducer used. However, biosensors fall into four major categories, namely, electrochemical, optical, acoustic, and calorimetric (Mohanty and Berry 2008). Recent studies report a number of successful attempts to use different types of biosensors for the early detection of microbial agents and their products (Setterington and Alocilja 2012; Syed and Bokhari 2011).

Use of nanomaterials in biosensors introduces many new signal transduction mechanisms in their manufacture that enhance their sensitivity to a greater extent. Because of the submicron size of nanomaterials, they are revolutionizing the field of biosensing, including the one used for the detection and identification of infectious agents (Jianrong et al. 2004).

10.4 MICROFLUIDIC ASSAYS OR LAB-ON-A-CHIP

One of the most fascinating nanodiagnostic techniques for microbiologists is the miniaturized microfluidic systems, also called lab-on-a-chip (LOC). The LOC has gained enormous popularity in the last two decades and has been found to be promising for accurate and point-of-care microbial detection (Chen et al. 2007; Mairhofer et al. 2009). LOC-based assays possess a wide range of applications in rapid, real-time, and simultaneous detection of microbial agents by combining submicroscopic components such as probes, transducers, and chambers of a microfluidic laboratory (Chen et al. 2007; Gabig-Ciminska 2006; Syed 2014). Such systems offer a tremendous advantage of analyzing nano- to microliter-sized volume of the analyte (sample) by automated systems capable of signal enhancement (Dutse and Yusof 2011; Jin et al. 2009). These state-of-the-art devices are suitable for use not only in diagnostic laboratories but also in remote areas of developing countries where diagnostic facilities are scarce or areas such as airports for rapid screening of patients for highly infectious diseases or biowarfare agents (Dutse and Yusof 2011; Mairhofer et al. 2009; Syed 2014).

The highly sophisticated and advanced LOC technology involves a highly multi-disciplinary approach involving a number of scientists from different fields such as microbiology, electronics, chemistry, physics, chemical engineering, and material sciences. The dedicated research resulted in many interesting results and the number of research articles published in this area is ever increasing.

Applications of nanotechnology in the development of LOC have produced amazing results, which are highly promising for the diagnosis of infectious diseases as well as detection of biowarfare agents. A high number of research groups as well as companies are carrying out intense research for developing such miniaturized devices (Liu et al. 2006; Mairhofer et al. 2009). An example of such developments is the work carried out by Liu et al. (2006). They developed an integrated miniaturized portable device capable of simultaneous detection and genotyping of a number of pathogenic bacterial species based on a nucleic acid probe hybridization process. Several other groups have adopted such strategies and produced interesting results by detecting microbial cells up to a single-cell level. In a successful attempt, Ho et al. (2012) developed a microfluidic portable device capable of simultaneous detection of a number of bacterial species causing nosocomial infections and studying their antibiotic resistance patterns in a single assay format. Lee and Yager (2007) developed an LOC DNA microarray for microbial detection from water samples. A number of research groups are engaged in working on using microelectromechanical systems for the simultaneous detection of a number of microbial agents and their metabolic products from clinical as well as food and environmental samples (Dutse and Yusof 2011; Mairhofer et al. 2009).

10.5 NANOMATERIALS IN NANODIAGNOSTICS

As stated previously, nanomaterials are excellent materials for sensing enhancement of advanced and modern devices. Nanoparticles (NPs), CNTs, graphene, and NWs are the best examples of nanomaterials widely used in nanodiagnostic assays for microbial detection and identification (Syed 2014). Some of the most popular nanomaterials along with examples of their successful use are described in Sections 10.5.1 through 10.5.5.

10.5.1 NANOPARTICLES

NPs are one of the major and widely researched applications of nanotechnology in medicine. Apart from their smaller size and higher surface-to-volume ratio, NPs possess many other unique optical magnetic and electronic properties. Furthermore, like other types of nanomaterials, NPs may be easily conjugated with organic molecules, inorganic molecules, and biomolecules of different types. These size- and shape-dependent properties of different types of NPs have been utilized in a number of biosensing strategies for microbial agents. NPs are usually conjugated with a recognition element such as an antibody, nucleic acid probe, enzyme, aptamer, or some other biological species that binds the specific ligand (such as bacteria, virus, toxin, etc.), whereas NPs themselves carry out transduction of the biological event into a measurable signal or act as an optical reporter (Agarwal et al. 2005; Agasti et al.

2010; Liu 2006; Syed 2014; Syed and Bokhari 2011). NPs may be classified on the basis of type of material they are made of: metallic, semiconductor, and polymeric, organic, inorganic, and polymeric NPs. Gold, magnetic, and fluorescent NPs are most commonly used and researched in diagnostic applications and will be described in detail in this chapter with examples of their successful applications (Oh et al. 2011).

10.5.1.1 Gold Nanoparticles

Gold has been an exciting material in nanotechnology because of its excellent optical, electronic, physical, and chemical properties and ease of bioconjugation (Kumar et al. 2011a; Li et al. 2010; Lu et al. 2013; Syed and Bokhari 2011). Au NPs find a wide range of applications among NP-based assays for infectious agents. Au NPs may be easily synthesized in a number of shapes and sizes using a number of protocols and easily functionalized and bioconjugated. The unique size-dependent optical and electronic properties of Au NPs, their inertness in biological fluids, and their stability make them one of the most robust materials used in nanodiagnostics (Bakthawathsalam et al. 2012; Ray et al. 2007; Syed 2014; Syed and Bokhari 2011). Monoclonal antibodies (mAbs), nucleic acid probes, and enzymes are commonly employed bioreceptors, and these molecules may simply be attached to Au NPs after little surface functionalization (Syed and Bokhari 2011). In general, Au NPs have conventionally been used as optical labels, electrochemical markers, surface plasmonic amplifiers, or signal mediators (Halfpenny and Wright 2010; Syed and Bokhari 2011).

Disposable immunochromatographic strips (ICSs) have been extremely popular among microbiologists because of their sensitivity, cost-effectiveness, and rapid results. ICSs have been developed for almost all classes of microorganisms (bacteria, viruses, fungi, algae, and protozoans), microbial toxins, antigens, and antibodies (Syed 2014). The unique feature of ICSs is the appearance of a red line of Au NPs in the case of a positive test soon after applying the sample. This red line appears because of aggregation of colloidal Au NPs that may easily be detected with the naked eye without the aid of any instrumentation. ICSs are the most exciting application of Au NPs in nanodiagnosis for microbial agents that has already reached commercialization (Syed 2014; Syed and Bokhari 2011). Disposable dip stick tests offer portable, cost-effective, reliable, and rapid means of detection of biomolecules and microbial entities from clinical, environmental, and food samples (Syed 2014; Syed and Bokhari 2011; Zarakolu et al. 2002).

ICSs are not new since they have been in use for over a decade and have already reached commercialization. ICSs may easily be developed according to the requirements of the study using specific antibodies or antigens using commercially available membranes and other reagents of analytical grade. The monoclonal IgG antibodies are usually used for the detection of the target antigens because of their specific binding capability (Ho et al. 2004).

A typical ICS consists of a sample pad, conjugate pad, nitrocellulose membrane, and an adsorbent pad (Figure 10.1). Colloidal Au NPs are treated with the mAbs against the microbial antigen to be detected in the sample. The sample pad, made of cellulose, is used to apply the sample, whereas the conjugate pad possesses antibody-conjugated Au NPs (Ab–Au NPs). Once the diluted sample is applied to the sample

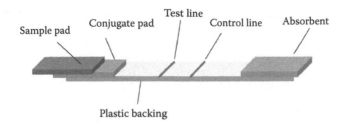

FIGURE 10.1 Diagram of a typical ICS for the detection of microbes or their antigens. The sample is applied to the sample pad made of cellulose, which moves forward to the conjugation pad where antibody-coated colloidal Au NPs are retained. Microbial antigens in the sample react with this complex and form an antigen–Au NP–antibody complex that moves to the test zone made of nitrocellulose where it is captured by a second antibody against the bacterial antigen immobilized in the test zone giving rise to a red line. The control line always appears, because of the presence of anti-IgG antibodies.

pad, it flows to the conjugation pad where it encounters the Ab–Au NP complex resulting in the formation of antibody–antigen–Au NP complex (Ab–Au NP–Agn). This complex moves to the test zone made of nitrocellulose membrane, where it is captured by second antibodies to the same antigen, giving rise to the red color of the test line. The second line in the test zone, called control line, contains anti-IgG antibodies that will capture the Ab–Au NP complex appearing red in both positive and negative test cases (Matsui et al. 2011; Peng et al. 2008; Syed 2014; Zarakolu et al. 2002).

As stated previously, ICSs are easy and economical to prepare in research laboratories. A high number of research publications in the last few years reported the successful use of ICS for bacterial (Blazkova et al. 2011; Huang 2007; Yan et al. 2011), viral (Peng et al. 2008), fungal (Thornton and Clin 2008), parasite antigen (Wang et al. 2011a), and toxin (Ching et al. 2012; Engler et al. 2002) detection with high sensitivity and specificity. Many groups are attempting to improve the sensitivity and the detection limit of these essays. For example, a recent paper by Ching et al. (2012) has reported a detection limit of 5 ng/ml of botulism toxin, one of the most potent toxin and biowarfare agents known to date. Furthermore, many groups have tried to use aptamers as capture molecules instead of antibodies because of their enhanced binding affinity for their ligand (Syed and Pervaiz 2010; Xu et al. 2009).

Tube-based colorimetric assays using Au NPs have also shown interesting results (Figure 10.2). Enormous research data on the use of Au NPs for microbial detection are available. Hybridization probe strategies are among the most popular methods and have the greatest potential for rapid and point-of-care diagnostic applications. DNA may be detected by colorimetric aggregation of Au NPs conjugated with complementary sequence-specific genes of the target organism (Gill et al. 2008; Kalidasan et al. 2013; Kumar et al. 2011a; Ray et al. 2007). In such strategies, microbial DNA sequences are detected using Au NPs conjugated with the complementary sequences. First, microbial double-stranded DNA is denatured so that the complementary sequence may attach to it. Hybridization of DNA conjugated with the target DNA sequence of microbes results in aggregation of the Au

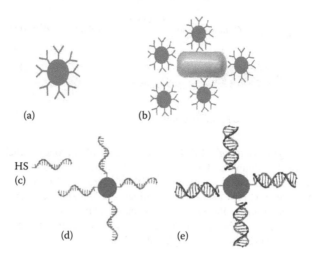

FIGURE 10.2 Au NPs conjugated with different biomolecules: (a) antibodies, (b) antibody-conjugated Au NPs capture bacterial cell, (c) thiolated single-stranded DNA, (d) DNA-conjugated Au NP, (e) DNA-conjugated Au NP hybridizes with the complementary sequence.

NPs visualized with the naked eye (Bakthawathsalam et al. 2012; Gill et al. 2008). Covalent binding of the DNA probe with the Au NPs may be achieved by introducing a thiol group (-SH) to the 3′ or 5′ end of the nucleic acid probe, resulting in stable covalent bond between the Au NP and the probe (Syed and Bokhari 2011). Au NPs aggregated with the target sequence appear red, whereas Au NPs without complementary probes turn purple upon acid-induced aggregation of the Au NPs (Bakthawathsalam et al. 2012).

Au NPs have also been used as fluorescent labels in optical imaging and sensing of cells and biomolecules such as proteins. Extensive research is being carried out on the application of Au NPs for in vivo imaging of cancer cells (Cai et al. 2008). Au NPs may overcome many of the limitations of the classical fluorophores owing to their higher extinction coefficient and broader absorption spectrum in the visible region, which is usually overlapped with the emission wavelength of the Förster or fluorescence resonance energy transfer (FRET) donor (Coto-Garcia et al. 2011; Syed and Bokhari 2011; Yang et al. 2011).

10.5.1.2 Magnetic Nanoparticles

Magnetic nanoparticles (MNPs) attract great attention in biomedicine because of their unique properties. Controllable size ranging from a few nanometers to micrometers, ease of bioconjugation, and their magnetic properties make them ideal material for diagnostics and drug delivery (Chen and Zhang 2012; Pankhurst et al. 2003). MNPs are becoming increasingly popular in nanomedicine because of their higher physical and chemical stability along with magnetic properties and low cost of production (Goeransson et al. 2010; Huang et al. 2010; Koh and Josephson 2009). MNPs have been of importance in microbial detection from clinical samples after conjugation with biomolecules such as antibodies, aptamers, or DNA probes (Ho et al. 2004; Huang et al. 2010). Furthermore, MNPs may also be used for the separation of microbial cells from complex matrices and preparation of bacterial pure cultures for analysis (Padmavathy et al. 2012). Use of superparamagnetic nanoparticles (SPMNPs) is of advantage, because their magnetic properties increase greatly at nanometer size (Cheng et al. 2009; Maalouf et al. 2008; Padmavathy et al. 2012). Surface functionalization of MNPs for bioconjugation is usually achieved using γ-aminopropylethoxysilane (Padmavathy et al. 2012). Furthermore, MNPs may also be coated with silica or a gold shell, whereby the inner magnetic part acts like a core and silica or gold surface forms are the shell. These NPs possess the properties of both magnetic and fluorescent materials (Liu 2006).

An example of the use of MNPs for microbial detection is magnetic relaxation nanosensors (MRNSs), which have been proven to be promising materials for microbial detection with higher sensitivity and specificity. In recent studies, MRNSs employed polymer-coated NPs, which may be conjugated with some biomolecules such as antibodies specific for a microbial agent or its product like a toxin (Kaittanis et al. 2007, 2008, 2012). In a typical assay, binding of bioconjugated MRNSs with their target ligand brings about changes in the sample's magnetic resonance signal, which is directly correlated to the analyte concentration in the sample (Kaittanis et al. 2012). A recent study conducted by Kaittanis et al. (2012) they used MRNSs for the detection of an intracellular parasite, *Mycobacterium avium* ssp. *paratuberculosis* (MAP), from crude samples like blood. They used hybridizing magnetic resonance nanosensors (hMRNSs) for the conserved DNA sequences of MAP. Binding of hMRNSs with the complementary DNA sequence (i.e., IS900) of mycobacterial species resulted in a change in magnetic resonance signal indicating the presence of the microbe. The technique does not require highly purified DNA like in the case of PCR and the test may be performed with minimally processed samples. The presence of this slow-growing intracellular bacterial species may be confirmed in 1 h as compared to culture, which takes an average of 12 weeks (Kaittanis et al. 2012). The same research group also successfully used MRNSs for bacterial antibiotic susceptibility testing in culture media in an attempt to develop a rapid and sensitive assay. They used dextran-coated iron oxide NPs along with a protein with high affinity to carbohydrates (concanavalin A [ConA]) in a competition assay. As expected, the ConA-coated nanosensors responded differently to varying bacterial metabolism of the carbohydrates (Kaittanis et al. 2008).

An example of the promising application of MNPs is their use in water purification systems. MNPs may be used for the removal of microorganisms from water to improve its quality. In such an approach, Huang et al. (2010) used amine-functionalized MNPs for bacterial removal from water samples. The surface of most of the bacterial cells is negatively charged. The amine group on the MNPs confers them positive charge so that they can easily attach the negatively charged bacterial cells. Although it involves nonspecific binding, this strategy possesses great potential for cell enrichment and bacterial removal from water. A study conducted by Lee et al. (2009) used MNPs to detect Bacillus Calmette–Guerin bacteria as a surrogate for *Mycobacterium tuberculosis* (causative agent of tuberculosis) from sputum samples. MNPs bind bacterial cell wall, rendering it superparamagnetic. In the following step, bacteria are concentrated in the microfluidic chamber and the spin time of the whole sample (T2) was measured with nuclear magnetic resonance. They could successfully detect as low as 20 cfu/ml of bacterial cells in 30 minutes.

10.5.1.3 Magnetoresistive Sensors

Magnetoresistive sensors are based on binding of magnetic particles to the sensors' surface as the magnetic field of the MPs brings about changes in the magnetic field of the sensor and therefore changes in electrical current. MPs bind the sensors' surface by either direct or indirect labeling. Direct labeling involves binding through complementary sequences of streptavidin–biotin interaction, whereas indirect labeling is a sandwich ELISA (enzyme-linked immunosorbent assay)–like strategy (Koh and Josephson 2009).

Use of giant magnetoresistance (GMR) sensors has been a powerful strategy in rapid, sensitive, and point-of-care detection of biomolecules. Koets et al. (2009) reported rapid and sensitive detection of *Escherichia coli* DNA using GMR and SPMNPs as detection labels. The double-tagged DNA was used for the study of detection and binding kinetics. Amplification of the target gene was carried using a 5′ biotic forward and 5′ fluorescein reverse primers. DNA was attached to biotin-coated SPMNPs. Amplicon particle complex is captured by the antifluorescein antibodies on the sensor surface and detected by GMP sensors (Koets et al. 2009).

10.5.1.4 Fluorescent Silica Nanoparticles

Silica is composed of a honeycomb-like porous structure having hundreds of pores inside (Chitra and Annadurai 2013). Silica nanoparticles (SNPs) are among the most widely used type of NPs in diagnostic applications. SNPs have emerged as intensively investigated material because of their unique properties such as high surface areas, large pore volumes, tunable pore sizes with a narrow distribution, tunable particle diameters, and ease of synthesis. SNPs have been used by a high number of researchers in their attempts to detect microbial agents with higher sensitivity owing to their robust chemical and optical properties (Wang et al. 2007).

Microbiologists are already familiar with fluorescent microscopes and fluorospectrometry. As soon as fluorescent NPs (FNPs) became available, several applications in the field of diagnostics have been explored (Bau et al. 2011). FNPs, such as silica or organic NPs, may easily be bioconjugated with antibodies, nucleic acid probes, and aptamers and may be used in detecting microbial presence by fluorescence microscope or spectrofluorometer (Wang et al. 2007). Furthermore, dye-doped SNPs present excellent potential for bioanalysis for deep understanding of biological processes and can detect biomolecules in samples with higher sensitivity as compared to other types of FNPs (Bae et al. 2012; Tallury et al. 2010; Wang et al. 2007). Dye-doped FNPs offer advantages over fluorescently labeled antibodies since a single fluorescent SNP (FSNP) may retain thousands of dye molecules in its matrix. Therefore, using these NPs enhances the sensitivity of the assays many hundred-folds. Furthermore, compared to other FNPs, dye-doped or organically modified SNPs offer advantages of photostability and enhanced luminescence. They have been widely used for the imaging of biomolecules such as microbial DNA, antibodies, cell components, and bacterial cells (Pham et al. 2012; Qin et al. 2007).

SNPs offer less aggregation and leakage of the dye as compared to organic NPs. Using appropriate synthesis conditions, thousands of inorganic or organic dye molecules may be incorporated into the matrix of the SNPs (Tallury et al. 2010; Yan et al. 2007). The dye may be either attached to the surface of the NPs or contained inside the particles. However, for imaging purposes, NPs with embedded dye molecules exhibit stronger photostability by being protected from the light (Murcia and Naumann 2005). Furthermore, SNPs may easily be chemically functionalized owing to the versatility of silane chemistry and bioconjugated with antibodies and nucleic acids (Yan et al. 2007). Chemical modification of the NP surface to generate amino or carboxyl groups enables one to covalently attach antibodies to the FNPs (Zhao et al. 2004). Typically, silane surface is coated with alkoxysilane such as carboxy-ethylsilanetriol for the introduction of a carboxyl group and with 3-aminopropyl-triethoxysilane for the amino group (Yan et al. 2007).

The affinity and specificity of the antigen antibody interaction have also been exploited using FSNPs. Different types of cells and proteins have been detected with the help of FSNPs (Yan et al. 2007). Antibody-coated, dye-doped SNPs have shown enhanced sensitivity in immune assays and reduced the detection limit to a single bacterial cell level (Li and Xu 2009; Syed 2014; Zhao et al. 2004). FSNPs may be particularly useful for the detection of fastidious and slow-growing bacteria such as *M. tuberculosis* that require very long incubation periods and special growth requirements.

Like other types of nanomaterials, FNPs have also been successfully used in a number of attempts for microbial detection. In a study conducted by Qin et al. (2007), FSNPs were used for the sensitive detection of *M. tuberculosis* from bacterial mixtures as well as spiked sputum samples. Bacterial cells were first reacted with the mAbs, which were detected by protein A–conjugated RuBpy-doped SNPs. In another study, Tan's group at the University of Florida used FSNPs for multiplexed bacterial monitoring in a single sample (Zhao et al. 2004). Interestingly, the SNPs contained varying concentrations of dye molecules appearing different in color by excitation with the same wavelength. By conjugating each type of these NPs with different antibodies for separate bacterial species, they were able to detect three different bacterial species in the sample, each appearing in a different color (Wang et al. 2007). In a similar study conducted by Ekrami et al. (2011) using mAb against *M. tuberculosis* and protein A–conjugated FNPs, *M. tuberculosis* could easily be detected from sputum samples with 97.1% sensitivity and 91.35% specificity (Syed 2014).

10.5.1.5 Quantum Dots

Semiconductor NPs or quantum dots (QDs) have been one of the most highlighted materials in the last two decades because of their unique size-dependent optoelectronic properties and potential applications in life science research, largely in the field of bioimaging (Bera et al. 2010; Kim et al. 2004; Liandris et al. 2011; Nguyen et al. 2012; Syed 2014). QDs, composed of 100–100,000 atoms (Mazumder et al. 2009), exhibit unique features such as broad absorption spectra, narrower emission bandwidth with size-dependent local maxima (Edgar et al. 2006; Kim and Kim 2012), and enhanced biocompatibility as compared to other nanomaterials (Ma et al. 2010). Furthermore, the interesting feature of the QDs is that different emissions may be excited with the same wavelength, because the emission wavelength is tunable with their size, shape, and composition (Giri et al. 2011). In contrast to QDs, commonly used fluorophores show two drawbacks; first, they have low signal-to-noise ratio, and second, they are not photostable (Edgar et al. 2006).

QDs may also be bioconjugated with DNA probes, antibodies, or other biomolecules. Bioconjugated QDs may offer an excellent opportunity to detect microbial agents because of their unique qualities such as long-term photostability as compared to conventional organic labels (Decho et al. 2008; Edgar et al. 2006). QDs may absorb 10–50 times more photons than the conventional organic dyes at the same excitation photon flux, providing more brightness to the sensing system for microbial detection (Kim and Kim 2012). With minimum interference from autofluorescent particles, enhanced photostability, broader absorption spectra, and ease of bioconjugation, QDs may easily be used for biomolecular analysis as well as for detection of pathogenic agents in complex matrices (Edgar et al. 2006; Liandris et al. 2011; Zhu et al. 2004). QDs with a cadmium selenide (CdSe) core and a zinc sulfide (ZnS) shell have shown excellent fluorescent properties, and they are among the most commonly used and commercially available types of QDs (Valizadeh et al. 2012).

QDs are becoming a popular replacement for dyes in bioanalysis, such as immunoassays and DNA hybridization, having strong potential for microbial detection and identification (Ma et al. 2010; Wang et al. 2012). Furthermore, multicolor QDs may find application in multiplexed assays for simultaneous detection of different microbial species in a given clinical, environmental, or food sample (Hahn et al. 2005). Recent studies on the use of QDs for microbial agents have shown promising agents (Decho et al. 2008; Giri et al. 2011; Liandris et al. 2011; Stringer et al. 2008). To mention a few, Tripp et al. (2008) used mAb-conjugated cadmium telluride (CdTe) QDs for the detection of respiratory syncytial virus, an important cause of lower respiratory tract infection in infants and children as well as elderly and immunocompromised people. In a similar study, Hahn et al. (2005) used CdTe/ZnS core/shell NPs for the detection of an O157:H7 serotype of *E. coli*, a bacterial species of great medical importance to a single-cell level. Attempts have also been made for the simultaneous detection of more than one bacterial species using QDs. For example, Zhao et al. (2009) detected three food-borne pathogenic bacterial species, that is, *Salmonella typhimurium*, *E. coli* O157:H7, and *Shigella flexneri*, using MNPs for cell enrichment and QDs as fluorescent tags.

10.5.2 FRET-BASED BIOSENSORS

FRET has emerged as one of the significant techniques for bioanalysis such as microbial detection and their susceptibility to drugs. FRET is a radiation-less energy transfer from donor fluorophore to acceptor fluorophore (Kim et al. 2008; Mathur et al. 2008; Tsai et al. 2009). FRET biosensors offer quantitative analysis for protein–protein interactions, protein–DNA interactions, conformational studies, and microbial detection with higher sensitivity and specificity (Kattke et al. 2011; Zadran et al. 2012). Molecular beacons (MBs) are an excellent example of FRET biosensors (discussed in Section 10.5.3). Au NPs may also be utilized as fluorescent quencher molecules leading to subpicomolar detection of bioanalytes, which have been proven by both theoretical calculations and experimental work (Halfpenny and Wright 2010; Yang et al. 2011). Furthermore, Au NPs are also considered superquenchers because of their ability to quench a number of fluorophores (Yang et al. 2011) over a long distance (Mayilo et al. 2009).

One of the applications of QDs is their utility as fluorescent donors in FRET-based assays. In a study conducted by Wang et al. (2011b), CdSe/ZnS QDs were used as FRET donors and black hole quenchers were used as FRET acceptors for the detection of the *tst* gene, which encodes toxic shock syndrome toxin in *Staphylococcus aureus* bacteria. They used single-stranded DNA (ssDNA) strands complementary to the *tst* gene conjugated to CdSe/ZnS QDs. A complementary strand tagged with a black hole quencher was used to quench the fluorescence. Detection of the target tst DNA sequences was carried out by adding 10 equivalents of bacterial DNA to the hybrid resulting in the recovery of emission of QDs (Wang et al. 2011b).

10.5.3 MOLECULAR BEACONS

MBs are commonly used for the detection of DNA or RNA sequences. MBs are short, single-stranded nucleotide sequences that fluoresce upon hybridization with the target complementary sequences using FRET phenomenon (Chen et al. 2000; Larios-Sanz et al. 2007; McKillen et al. 2007). The central region of the single-stranded nucleic acid forms the loop of MB, and it is complementary to the target sequence where flanking regions forming stems are complementary to each other (Chen et al. 2000; Tan et al. 2000). A fluorescent moiety is attached to one end of the probe, while nonfluorescent quenchers are attached to the other end (McKillen et al. 2007; Poddar 1999). No fluorescence occurs when the ends of the probes are in proximity, owing to quenching action. The quencher should have its absorption spectrum overlapping with the emission spectrum of the fluorophore. The stem loop structure of the MB opens and hybridizes with the complementary DNA sequences, resulting in the dissociation of the fluorophore from the quencher and hence fluorescence (Figure 10.3) (Chen et al. 2000; Kim et al. 2007a; Poddar 1999; Syed 2014).

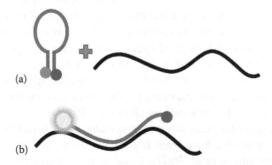

(a)

(b)

FIGURE 10.3 A molecular beacon. Single-stranded DNA sequence having a fluorophore on one side and a quencher on the other end (a). Single-stranded loop region hybridizes with the complementary sequence of the target DNA causing separation of the fluorophore from quencher and hence fluorescence (b).

MBs have also been successfully used for the study of in vivo gene expression in both prokaryotic and eukaryotic cells. Nonetheless, the most common application of MBs is in RT-PCR. RT-PCR utilizes extension of forward and reverse primers as well as MBs complementary to the target sequence to be amplified resulting in the fluorescence. During RT-PCR, a number of amplified DNA segments increase with each round, and therefore, there is an increase in fluorescence, making the technique a quantitative one (Chen et al. 2000; McKillen et al. 2007).

RT-PCR has emerged as a widely used type of PCR in diagnostic and research laboratories for the identification of infectious agents of all types (George et al. 2012; Kim et al. 2007a; Orru et al. 2006; Varma-Basil et al. 2004).

10.5.4 ONE-DIMENSIONAL AND CARBON-DERIVED NANOMATERIALS

One-dimensional (1-D) nanostructures such as CNTs, nanorods, NWs, nanobelts, and nanosprings have become an area of intense research for biosensing applications. These materials have been widely used for nanofabrication owing to their enhanced sensitivity, biocompatibility, and ease of functionalization and preparation. In fact, 1-D structures are the smallest dimension that can be used for efficient electron transport and hence excellent application in nanoscale devices (Kumar et al. 2011b; Wanekaya et al. 2006). Carbon-based nanomaterials, such as 1-D CNTs and two-dimensional (2-D) graphene, have been used in a large number of studies as sensing elements in biosensors for microbial detection owing to their unique properties (Yang et al. 2010). CNTs or graphene-modified electrodes have been proven to be very useful in immobilizing biomolecules for detection of the target microbial species (Qureshi et al. 2009).

10.5.4.1 Carbon Nanotubes

CNTs are considered as the most commonly used building block of nanotechnology (Merkoci 2006). CNTs are the allotropes of carbon having surface-to-volume ratio up to 100,000. CNTs are superior to many nanomaterials because of their unique chemical, thermal, optical, magnetic, surface, and electronic properties as well as unusual strength (Hirlekar et al. 2009; Moon and Kim 2010; Vardharajula et al. 2012). CNTs are widely investigated nanomaterials because of these unique features that may be exploited to develop nanosensors for the study of microbial processes as well as for the detection of biological species with higher sensitivity. Furthermore, CNTs can bind bacterial cells, and their binding affinity may be exploited by using them in bacterial filters (Kim et al. 2007b). CNTs are divided into two main groups, namely, single-walled carbon nanotubes (SWCNTs) and multiple-walled carbon nanotubes on the basis of their structure (Ji et al. 2010).

The highly sensitive bio-nano integrated systems combining CNTs with recognition or catalytic molecules have been remarkable tools for developing biosensors (He and Dai 2006; Zhang et al. 2007). Besides their unique electronic properties, the high surface-to-volume ratio of the CNTs greatly facilitate immobilization of biomolecules such as antibodies, aptamers, oligonucleotides, and proteins without diminishing their structure and bioactivity and, therefore, enhance their sensing capability (He and Dai 2006; Huang et al. 2004; Jain et al. 2012). CNTs are novel material having the capability to promote electron transfer with redox species in electrochemical biosensors (Jain et al. 2012). Furthermore, CNTs may also be functionalized with multiple biomolecules for the simultaneous detection of various microbial species. CNTs may easily be functionalized for many reasons, for example, because of increased solubility, lower toxicity and bioconjugation, and specific binding to the analytes (Vardharajula et al. 2012). Recent studies report their successful use in the development of immunosensors for bacterial detection. Jain et al. (2012) used antibody-conjugated CNTs for electrochemical detection of *Salmonella* bacteria with higher sensitivity and specificity (Jain et al. 2012; Zhang et al. 2007). Moreover, SWCNTs with functionalities such as carboxyl group for covalent binding with proteins have also been developed (Zhang et al. 2007).

1-D SWCNTs (Figure 10.4), also called FETs, may be used to electrically detect biomolecules with extremely high sensitivity. These sensors are useful not only in detecting microbial cells or their products but also in the dynamic detection or release of microbial products in their surroundings (Liu and Guo 2012). As the flow of current is solely on the surface, conductance of SWCNTs is highly sensitive to the electrochemical disturbance imposed by the biomolecular interaction (Huang et al. 2011a). SWCNT-based biosensors have been successfully used for the detection of bacterial cells up to a detection limit of 100 cfu/ml (Huang et al. 2011a; Villamizar et al. 2008). Similarly, SWCNTs have also been used for viral detection; Bhattacharya et al. (2011) used antibody-functionalized CNTs for the detection of avian metapneumovirus, where binding specific antibodies on the CNTs with the viral antigens resulted in a change in conductance.

Bacterial cells possess high binding affinity to carbon nanotube clusters (CNTCs), and this ability has been exploited in bacterial filters (Kim et al. 2007b). CNTCs, with their high binding affinity for bacteria and paramagnetic susceptibility, were explored by Moon and Kim (2010) as universal adsorbents for bacterial cells as well as magnetic separation agents. These two unique features of this class of nanomaterials are particularly useful in bacterial separation and enrichment protocols. In their study, they used CNTCs for binding and capturing bacterial cells of different types, whereas the separation of the bacterial cells was carried out with the help of an external magnet. Such an approach is also helpful in water purification.

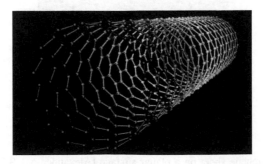

FIGURE 10.4 Single-walled carbon nanotubes (Strock 2006). (Reproduced with permission from Wikipedia; http://upload.wikimedia.org/wikipedia/commons/5/53/Types_of_Carbon _Nanotubes.png.)

10.5.4.2 Graphene

One of the remarkable discoveries in the field of nanotechnology is graphene. Graphene has emerged as one of the most widely investigated nanomaterials since its discovery in 2004. Graphene, a single-atom planar sheet of carbon atoms perfectly arranged in a honeycomb manner (Figure 10.5), possesses a wide range of applications in biosensing because of its extraordinary physical, electrochemical, and optical properties (Mannoor et al. 2012; Syed 2014; Vashist and Venkatesh 2013). This recently discovered 2-D cousin material of the CNTs is believed to be a better alternative to the SWCNTs because of its better electrochemical, electrical, optical, and biocompatibility properties (Mohanty and Berry 2008). Uniform functionalization and immobilization of biomolecules on the graphene surface is achieved through its perfect planar structure. Graphene is an ideal material for biosensing applications because of its electric properties such as high charge mobility and tunable conductance (Huang et al. 2011b).

In the last few years, a number of remarkable efforts have been made to develop graphene-based electrochemical, electrical, and optical biosensors for microbial detection with enhanced sensitivity (Huang et al. 2011b). For example, the graphene-based immunosensor developed by Huang et al. (2011b) for the detection of *E. coli* showed significant conductance increase after exposure to bacterial cells having a detection limit as low as 10 cfu/ml. In another study, Liu et al. (2011) used graphene in the development of electrochemical biosensors for the detection of rotavirus. The graphene film coated on the working electrode possesses excellent electron transfer property. Antibodies to rotavirus were covalently attached to the graphene film and the event of antigen–antibody interaction was monitored with cyclic voltammetry.

In a recent study conducted by Hernandez et al. (2014), graphene oxide was used as a transducer layer whereas aptamers were used as a sensing layer for the construction of potentiometric biosensors for the detection of *S. aureus* up to a detection limit of 1 cfu/ml.

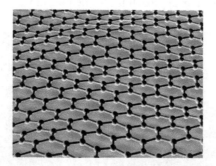

FIGURE 10.5 Graphene sheet on a planar surface (Alexander AIUS 2010). (Reproduced with permission from Wikipedia; http://en.wikipedia.org/wiki/Graphene#mediaviewer/File :Graphen.jpg.)

10.5.5 Nanowires

Like other types of nanomaterials, NW FETs have also been used for the detection of microbial agents and their products in a number of successful studies (Basu et al. 2004; Patolsky et al. 2004). One direct approach to detect the microbial agents is by using semiconductor NW FETs in real time and in a label-free detection manner. For example, NW surface immobilized with antibody brings about change in the conductance upon binding of the target antigen. In a similar study conducted by Patolsky et al. (2004), NWs conjugated with antibodies against influenza A virus were used for conductometric viral detection. Binding and unbinding of the influenza virus with the antibody-modified NWs brought about discrete conductance changes but not with adenoviruses and paramyxoviruses. A similar study was carried out by Zhang et al. (2010) in which a silicon NW-based biosensor was used for the rapid detection of the RT-PCR product of dengue fever virus serotype 2. A peptide nucleic acid probe was attached to the silicon NW, and the complementary nucleic acid sequence of the dengue fever virus amplified using RT-PCR was detected. The results were recorded as change in resistance upon binding of the PCR-amplified fragments of the dengue virus with the probe immobilized on the NWs.

10.6 APTAMERS AS CAPTURE PROBES

mAbs have enjoyed great attention since their introduction because of their extraordinary affinity to their targets. Antibodies have been massively used in biosensing research for the selective binding to their target such as microbial agents or their toxins (Syed and Pervaiz 2010). However, antibodies are very expensive, produced in vivo in animals and may not be produced for every class of molecules such as toxins that may kill the host animals (Lee et al. 2006; Syed and Pervaiz 2010; Tombelli et al. 2005).

Aptamers are ssDNA or RNA sequences synthesized through an in vitro selection and amplification technique, possessing a broader range of applications in therapeutics, biosensing, diagnostics, and research because of their ability to bind their target with higher affinity. Aptamers offer a number of advantages over their antibody counterparts, including their ability to undergo chemical derivatization to prolong their life in bodily fluids and bioavailability in animals. Although aptamers are a recently discovered class of biomolecules, they have become one of the most widely investigated molecules, with a huge number of publications in the last decade. A number of recent studies have used aptamers instead of antibodies as capture probes because of their superior affinity for their target, stability at room temperature, cost-effectiveness, and ease with synthesis and functionalization. Advances in aptamer research have been reviewed elsewhere (Syed and Pervaiz 2010).

10.7 ATOMIC FORCE MICROSCOPY

Atomic force microscopy (AFM) offers advantages over electron microscopy because of its higher resolution, simple protocols of sample preparation, and ease of working in native microbial environments. The most interesting feature of AFM is that it has been used for the study of microbial cell surface structures in great detail under physiological conditions, that is, in a liquid environment (Dufrene 2002).

One of the main problems of using an electron microscope in observing microbial structures is the sample preparation, which not only is a laborious job but also may alter the shape of microbial ultrastructures. Both viral particles and bacterial cells as well as their ultrastructures have been imaged successfully with AFM. Ultracellular structures such as flagella, S layer protein structures, and cell wall, as well as the effects of drugs and enzymes on a bacterial surface may be studied using this type of microscopy. Furthermore, AFM may also potentially be used for the study of cellular growth phases and the effects of drugs on bacterial growth rate in real time under physiological wet conditions, hence making it a promising tool for the study of a single cell (Dufrene 2002; Syed et al. 2009).

In fact, AFM has emerged as more than an imaging technique based on its applications in microbiology. Apart from its applications in imaging cells, their ultrastructures, and single molecules, AFM has also been used for the study of actions of certain drugs on bacterial cells, ligand–receptor interactions, and single-cell studies. An example of the use of AFM in microbiology is the study of *Pseudomonas aeruginosa* and *Pseudomonas putida* biofilms on stainless steel (Dufrene 2002). Touhami et al. (2004) used AFM in combination with thin-section transmission electron microscopy to study the changes occurring in dividing bacteria cell walls, and their results showed a good structural relation using these two techniques (Dufrene 2004). Studies on the physicochemical properties of microbial subcellular structures have usually been difficult because of the very small size of the microorganisms. In recent years, AFM spectroscopy has made it possible to explore many molecular interactions (i.e., hydrophobic or hydrophilic), stiffness of the cell wall, and surface properties such as hydrophobicity. Furthermore, AFM has successfully been used for the study of food quality. AFM measurements provide new insight into the structure–function relationship of food samples (Yang and Wang 2006). In recent years, AFM has been widely used for the study of action of drugs on bacterial cells. Antimicrobial drugs rupturing bacterial cell walls alter cell stiffness and surface roughness, which can be studied using AFM (Chen et al. 2006). Li et al. (2006) have shown the effect of Sushi peptide on Gram-negative bacterial cells using AFM. This is an endotoxin-binding cationic peptide that integrates into the cell by disrupting the cell's outer and inner membranes.

10.8   NANOSENSORS FOR SINGLE-CELL DETECTION

The ultimate goal of nanodiagnostic techniques may possibly be the ultrasensitive detection of biological species to a single-cell or -molecule level. As stated in Section 10.5, different types of nanomaterials have successfully been used for microbial detection at the single-cell level. In situ quantification of pathogenic bacteria or potential bioterrorism agents using sophisticated techniques may ensure safety from possible terrorist attacks. More importantly, the global spread of infectious diseases may be stopped if appropriate and ultrasensitive diagnostic assays are available for prompt and onsite testing. Furthermore, food safety is another serious issue that requires critical testing in the era of enhanced global trade.

The number of publications claiming microbial detection to a single-cell level detection limit has been ever increasing in the last decade. An example of such attempts is the recent publication by Chang et al. (2013) reporting detection of *S. aureus* to a single-cell level using aptamer-conjugated Au NPs and light scattering system. Another recent study conducted by Chung et al. (2013) reported the use of magneto DNA NP system for the rapid simultaneous detection and phenotyping of a number of bacterial strains in a single test with a sensitivity down to a single-cell level. More amazing are papers reporting ultrasensitive detection of nanometer-sized viruses down to a single particle level. One of many such interesting studies is reported by He et al. (2011). They used an ultra-narrow line width whispering gallery microlaser, whose lasting line undergoes frequent splitting upon binding with the nanosized particles such as viruses. They detected influenza virus to a single-virus level detection limit.

10.9 SMARTPHONE MICROSCOPY

One of the most amazing discoveries made in last couple of years is the advent of smartphone microscopes. Highly sophisticated and expensive electron microscopes as well most modern microscopes such as scanning probe microscopes seem to be soon replaced by light, cheap, and handheld microscopes. The capabilities of the world's most powerful microscopes have been brought to compact form, which is one of the biggest breakthroughs of the century (Figure 10.6).

Early or initial attempts were made to combine a piece of magnifying lens with smartphone cameras. However, a recent study conducted by Wei et al. (2013) has reported field portable fluorescent microscopy platform attached to a smartphone capable of imaging 100-nm fluorescent particles as well as fluorescently labeled cytomegaloviruses. This field fluorescent microscopy device may be used for the study of nanometer-sized objects in field settings. Further studies are directed toward an even more simplified form of smartphones capable of imaging viruses and bacterial cells in the environment without requiring complicated protocols. Furthermore, simple molecule imaging is also being speculated using such platforms (Khatua and Orrit 2013).

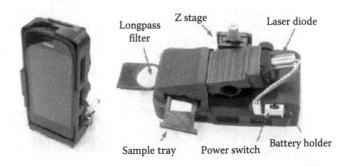

FIGURE 10.6 Smartphone microscope for viruses. (From Q. Wei et al., *ACS Nano*, 7, 9147–9155, 2013. Reproduced with permission.)

10.10 CONCLUSION

Detection and identification of infectious agents have always been a challenging task throughout history. Dedicated efforts continue unabated and enter the era of nanotechnology in the 21st century. Significant advancements in the fields of molecular biology and nanotechnology have made remarkable breakthroughs in the area of microbial diagnosis. Micro- and nanoscale transducers, optical imaging systems, integrated electronic devices, and microbial probes are about to bring about historical breakthroughs in the near future when these technologies enter the phase of massive commercialization at the end-user level. The scientific community seems to have a form of device having features such as miniaturized, automated, portable, cost-effective, and point of care, as well as higher sensitivity and specificity. Furthermore, smart mobile phone–based microscopes integrated with nanotechnology-based assay formats would bring about amazing breakthroughs in life science research. Future microbiologists are expected to be very much familiar with the use of nanotechnology-based techniques and equipment in their laboratories, and it is hoped that the average time taken by each of these diagnostic tests will be reduced significantly. Further, identification of slow-growing and fastidious bacteria is also likely to be made quicker and more sensitive.

ACKNOWLEDGMENT

The author acknowledges the host institution for facilitation in the writing of the manuscript.

CONFLICT OF INTEREST

The author discloses no conflict of interest.

REFERENCES

Agarwal, A., R. A. Tripp, L. J. Anderson and S. Nie. Real-Time Detection of Virus Particles and Viral Protein Expression with Two-Color Nanoparticle Probes, *Journal of Virology*, 79, 8625–8628 (2005).

Agasti, S. S., S. Rana, M. Park, C. K. Kim, C. You and V. M. Rotello. Nanoparticles for Detection and Diagnosis, *Advanced Drug Delivery Reviews*, 62, 316–328 (2010).

Bae, S. W., W. Tan and J. I. Hong. Fluorescent Dye-Doped Silica Nanoparticles: New Tools for Bioapplications, *Chemical Communications*, 48, 2270–2282 (2012).

Bakthawathsalam, P., V. K. Rajendran and J. A. B. Mohammed. A Direct Detection of *Escherichia coli* Genomic DNA Using Gold Nanoprobes, *Journal of Nanobiotechnology*, 10, 1–10 (2012).

Basu, M., S. Seggerson, J. Henshaw, J. Jiang, R. Cordona, C. Lefave, P. J. Boyle, A. Miller, M. Pyqia and S. Basu. Nano-Biosensor Development for Bacterial Detection During Human Kidney Infection: Use of Glycoconjugate-Specific Antibody-Bound Gold Nanowire Arrays (GNWA), *Glycoconjugate Journal*, 21, 487–496 (2004).

Bau, L., P. Tecilla and P. Mancin. Sensing with Fluorescent Nanoparticles, *Nanoscale*, 3, 121–133 (2011).

Bera, D., L. Qian, T. Tseng-Kuan and P. H. Holloway. Quantum Dots and Their Multimodal Applications: A Review, *Materials*, 3, 2260–2345 (2010).

Bhattacharya, M., S. Hong, D. Lee, T. Cui and S. M. Goyal. Carbon Nanotube Based Sensors for the Detection of Viruses, *Sensors and Actuators B*, 155, 67–74 (2011).

Bissonnette, L. and G. Bergeron. Infectious Disease Management through Point-of-Care Personalized Medicine Molecular Diagnostic Technologies, *Journal of Personalized Medicine*, 2, 50–70 (2012).

Blazkova, M., B. Javurkova, L. Fukal and P. Rauch. Immunochromatographic Strip Test for Detection of *Genus cronobacter, Biosensors and Bioelectronics*, 26, 2828–2834 (2011).

Brachman, P. S. Infectious Diseases—Past, Present and Future, *International Journal of Epidemiology*, 32, 684–686 (2003).

Cai, W., T. Gao, H. Hong and J. Sun. Applications of Gold Nanoparticles in Cancer Nanotechnology, *Journal of Nanotechnology Science and Applications*, 1, 17–32 (2008).

Centurion-Lara, A., C. Castro, J. M. Schaffer, W. C. Van Voorhis, C. M. Marra and S. A. Lukehart. Detection of *Treponima pallidum* by a Sensitive Reverse Transcriptase PCR, *Journal of Clinical Microbiology*, 35, 1348–1352 (1997).

Chang, Y. C., C. Y. Yang, R. L. Sun, Y. F. Cheng, W. C. Kao and P. C. Yang. Rapid Single Cell Detection of *Staphylococcus aureus* by Aptamer-Conjugated Gold Nanoparticles, *Scientific Reports*, 3, 1–7 (2013).

Chen, L. and J. Zhang. Bioconjugated Magnetic Nanoparticles for Rapid Capture of Gram Positive Bacteria, *Biosensors and Bioelectronics*, S11, 1–5 (2012).

Chen, W., G. Martinez and A. Mulchandani. Molecular Beacons: A Real Time Polymerase Chain Reaction Assay for Detecting *Salmonella, Analytical Biochemistry*, 280, 166–172 (2000).

Chen, Z., M. G. Mauk, J. Wang, W. R. Abrams, P. L. A. Corstjens, R. S. Niedbala, D. Maladud and H. H. A. Bau. Microfluidic System for Saliva-Based Detection of Infectious Diseases, *Annals New York Academy of Sciences*, 1098, 429–436 (2007).

Chen, Z. Y., X. P. Guo, J. Y. Huang, Y. L. Hong and Q. Zhang. AFM Study of the Effect of Metronidazole on Surface Structures of Sulfate Reducing Bacteria, *Anaerobe*, 12, 106–109 (2006).

Cheng, Y., Y. Liu, J. Huang, K. Li, W. Zhang, Y. Xian and L. Jin. Combining Biofunctional Magnetic Nanoparticles and ATP Bioluminescence for Rapid Detection of *Escherichia coli, Talanta*, 77, 1332–1336 (2009).

Ching, K. H., A. Lin, J. A. McGarvy, L. H. Stanker and R. Hnasko. Rapid and Selective Detection of Botulinum Neurotoxin Serotype-A and -B with a Single Immunochromatographic Test Strip, *Journal of Immunological Methods*, 380, 23–29 (2012).

Chitra, K. and G. Annadurai. Fluorescent Silica Nanoparticles in the Detection and Control of the Growth of Pathogen, *Journal of Nanotechnology*, 2013, 1–7 (2013).

Chung, H. J., C. M. Castro, H. Im, H. Lee and R. Weissleder. A Magneto-DNA Nanoparticle System for Rapid Detection and Phenotyping of Bacteria, *Nature Nanotechnology*, 8, 369–375 (2013).

Coloma, J. and E. Harris. Molecular Genomic Approaches to Infectious Diseases in Resource-Limited Settings, *PLoS Medicine*, 6, 1–6 (2009).

Coto-Garcia, A. M., E. Sotelo-Gonzalez, T. M. Fernandez-Arguelles, R. Pereiro, J. M. Costa-Fernandez and A. Sanz Medel. Nanoparticles as Fluorescent Labels for Optical Imaging and Sensing in Genomics and Proteomics, *Analytical and Bioanalytical Chemistry*, 399, 29–42 (2011).

Decho, A. W., E. M. Beckman, G. T. Chandler and T. Kawaguchi. Application of Photostable Quantum Dots for Indirect Immunofluorescent Detection of Specific Bacterial Serotypes on Small Marine Animals, *Nanotechnology*, 19, 1–4 (2008).

Doria, G., J. Conde, B. Veigas, L. Giestas, C. Almeida, M. Assuncao, J. Rosa and P. V. Bapista. Noble Metal Nanoparticles for Biosensing Applications, *Sensors*, 12, 1657–1687 (2012).

Dufrene, Y. F. Atomic Force Microscopy, a Powerful Tool in Microbiology, *Journal of Bacteriology*, 184 (19), 5205–5213 (2002).

Dufrene, Y. F. Refining Our Perception of Bacterial Surfaces with Atomic Force Microscope (AFM), *Journal of Bacteriology*, 186, 3283–3285 (2004).

Dutse, S. W. and N. A. Yusof. Microfluidics-Based Lab-on-Chip Systems in DNA-Based Biosensing: An Overview, *Sensors*, 11, 5754–5768 (2011).

Edgar, R., M. McKinstry, J. Hwang, A. B. Oppenheim, R. A. Fekete, G. Giulian, C. Merril, K. Nagashima and S. Adhya. High-Sensitivity Bacterial Detection Using Biotin-Tagged Phage and Quantum-Dot Nanocomplexes, *Proceedings of the National Academy of Sciences of the United States of America*, 103, 4841–4845 (2006).

Ekrami, A., A. R. Samarbaf-Zadeh, A. Khosravi, B. Zargar, M. Alavi, M. Amin and A. Kiasat. Validity of Bioconjugated Silica Nanoparticles in Comparison with Direct Smear, Culture, and Polymerase Chain Reaction for Detection of *Mycobacterium tuberculosis* in Sputum Specimens, *International Journal of Nanomedicine*, 6, 2729–2735 (2011).

Engler, K. H., A. Efstratiou, D. Norn, R. S. Kozlov, I. Selga, T. G. Glushkevich, M. Tam, V. G. Melnikov, I. K. Mazurova, V. E. Kim, G. Y. Tseneva, L. P. Titov and R. G. J. George. Immunochromatographic Strip Test for Rapid Detection of Diphtheria Toxin: Description and Multicenter Evaluation in Areas of Low and High Prevalence of Diphtheria, *Journal of Clinical Microbiology*, 40, 80–83 (2002).

Fauci, A. S. Infectious Diseases: Considerations for the 21st Century, *Clinical Infectious Diseases*, 32, 675–685 (2001).

Gabig-Ciminska, M. Developing Nucleic Acid-Based Electrical Detection Systems, *Microbial Cell Factories*, 5, 9 (2006).

Gehring, A. G. and S. I. Tu. High-Throughput Biosensors for Multiplexed Food-Borne Pathogen Detection, *Annual Reviews in Analytical Chemistry*, 4, 151–172 (2011).

George, R., N. Bolus, S. Williams, J. Garner, K. Nugent and M. T. Unlap. A Short Interfering RNA (siRNA) Molecular Beacon for the Detection of Infection, *Journal of Biotechnology and Biomaterials*, 2, 1–6 (2012).

Gill, P., A. Alvandi, H. Abdul-Tehrani and M. Sadeghizadeh. Nanodiagnostic Method for Colorimetric Detection of *Mycobacterium tuberculosis* 16S rRNA, *Diagnostic Microbiology and Infectious Diseases*, 62, 119–124 (2008).

Giri, S., E. A. Sykes, T. L. Jennings and W. C. W. Chan. Rapid Screening of Genetic Biomarkers of Infectious Agents Using Quantum Dot Barcodes, *ACS Nano*, 5, 1580–1587 (2011).

Goeransson, J., T. Z. G. De La Torre, M. Stroemberg, C. Russel, P. Svedlindh, M. Stromme and M. Nilsson. Sensitive Detection of Bacterial DNA by Magnetic Nanoparticles, *Analytical Chemistry*, 82, 9138–9140 (2010).

Hahn, M. A., J. S. Tabb and T. D. Krauss. Detection of Single Bacterial Pathogens with Semiconductor Quantum Dots, *Analytical Chemistry*, 77, 4861–4869 (2005).

Halfpenny, K. C. and D. W. Wright. Nanoparticle Detection of Respiratory Infection, *Nanomedicine and Nanobiotechnology*, 2, 277–290 (2010).

Hauck, T. S., S. Giri, Y. Gao and W. C. W. Chan. Nanotechnology Diagnostics for Infectious Diseases Prevalent in Developing Countries, *Advanced Drug Delivery Reviews*, 64, 438–448 (2010).

He, L., K. S. Ozdemir, J. Zhu, W. Kim and L. Yang. Detecting Single Viruses and Nanoparticles Using Whispering Gallery Microlasers, *Nature Nanotechnology*, 6, 428–432 (2011).

He, P. and L. Dai. Carbon Nanotube Biosensors, *BioMEMS and Biomedical Nanotechnology*, 2006, 171–201 (2006).

Heo, J. and S. Z. Hua. An Overview of Recent Strategies in Pathogen Sensing, *Sensors*, 9, 4483–4502 (2009).

Hernandez, R., C. Valles, A. M. Benito, W. K. Maser, F. X. Rius and J. Riu. Graphene-Based Potentiometric Biosensor for the Immediate Detection of Living Bacteria, *Biosensors and Bioelectronics*, 54, 553–557 (2014).

Hirlekar, R., M. Yamagar, H. Garse, M. Vij and V. Kadam. Carbon Nanotubes and Its Applications: An Overview, *Asian Journal of Pharmaceutical and Clinical Research*, 2, 17–27 (2009).

Ho, J. Y., N. J. Cira, J. A. Crooks, J. Baeza and D. B. Weibel. Rapid Identification of ESKAPE Bacterial Strains Using an Autonomous Microfluidic Device, *PLoS One*, 7 (7), 1–7 (2012).

Ho, K., P. Tsai, Y. Lin and Y. Chen. Using Biofunctionalized Nanoparticles to Probe Pathogenic Bacteria, *Analytical Chemistry*, 76, 7162–7168 (2004).

Houpikian, P. and D. Raoult. Traditional and Molecular Techniques for the Study of Emerging Bacterial Diseases: One Laboratory's Perspective, *Emerging Infectious Diseases*, 8, 122–131 (2002).

Huang, S. H. Gold Nanoparticle-Based Immunochromatographic Assay for the Detection of *Staphylococcus aureus*, *Sensors and Actuators B-Chemistry*, 127, 335–340 (2007).

Huang, T. S., Y. Tzeng, Y. K. Liu, Y. C. Chen, K. R. Walker, R. Guntupalli and C. Liu. Immobilization of Antibodies and Bacterial Binding on Nanodiamond and Carbon Nanotubes for Biosensor Applications, *Diamond Related Materials*, 13, 1098–1102 (2004).

Huang, Y., X. Dong, Y. Liu, L. J. Li and P. Chen. Graphene-Based Biosensors for Detection of Bacteria and Their Metabolic Activities, *Journal of Material Chemistry*, 21, 12358–12362 (2011a).

Huang, Y., H. G. Sudibya and P. Chen. Detecting Metabolic Activities of Bacteria Using a Simple Carbon Nanotube Device for High-Throughput Screening of Anti-Bacterial Drugs, *Biosensors and Bioelectronics*, 26, 4257–4261 (2011b).

Huang, Y. F., Y. F. Wang and X. P. Yan. Amine-Functionalized Magnetic Nanoparticles for Rapid Capture and Removal of Bacterial Pathogens, *Environmental Science and Technology*, 44, 7908–7913 (2010).

Jain, K. K. Application of Nanobiotechnology in Clinical Diagnostics, *Clinical Chemistry*, 53, 2002–2009 (2007).

Jain, K. K. Sensitive Sequence-Specific Molecular Identification System Comprising an Aluminum Micro-Nanofluidic Chip and Associated Real-Time Confocal Detector, *Expert Review of Molecular Diagnostics*, 3, 153–161 (2003).

Jain, S., S. R. Singh, D. Horn, A. V. Davis, M. K. Ram and S. J. Pillai. Development of an Antibody Functionalized Carbon Nanotube Biosensor for Foodborne Bacterial Pathogens, *Biosensors and Bioelectronics*, 2012, S11 (2012).

Ji, S. R., C. Liu, B. Zhang, F. Yang, F. Xu, J. Long, C. Jin, D. L. Fu, Q. X. Ni and X. Yu. Carbon Nanotubes in Cancer Diagnosis and Therapy, *Biochimica et Biophysica Acta*, 1806, 29–35 (2010).

Jianrong, C., M. Yuqing, H. Nongyue, W. Xiaohu and L. Sijiao. Nanotechnology and Biosensors, *Biotechnology Advances*, 22, 505–518 (2004).

Jin, S., B. Yin and B. Ye. Multiplexed Bead-Based Mesofluidic System for Detection of Food-Borne Pathogenic Bacteria, *Applied and Environmental Microbiology*, 75, 6647–6654 (2009).

Kaittanis, C., H. Boukhriss, S. Santra, S. A. Naser and J. M. Perez. Rapid and Sensitive Detection of an Intracellular Pathogen in Human Peripheral Leukocytes with Hybridizing Magnetic Relaxation Nanosensors, *PLoS One*, 7, 1–13 (2012).

Kaittanis, C., S. A. Naser and J. M. Perez. One-Step, Nanoparticle-Mediated Bacterial Detection with Magnetic Relaxation, *Nano Letters*, 7, 380–383 (2007).

Kaittanis, C., S. Nath and J. M. Perez. Rapid Nanoparticle-Mediated Monitoring of Bacterial Metabolic Activity and Assessment of Antimicrobial Susceptibility in Blood with Magnetic Relaxation, *PLoS One*, 3 (9), 1–9 (2008).

Kaittanis, C., S. Santra and J. M. Perez. Emerging Nanotechnology-Based Strategies for the Identification of Microbial Pathogenesis, *Advanced Drug Delivery Reviews*, 62, 408–423 (2010).

268 Biological and Pharmaceutical Applications of Nanomaterials

Kalidasan, K., J. L. Neol and M. Uttamchandani. Direct Visual Detection of *Salmonella* Genomic DNA Using Gold Nanoparticle, *Molecular Biosystems*, 9, 618–621 (2013).

Kattke, M. D., E. J. Gao, K. E. Sapsford, L. D. Stephenson and A. Kumar. FRET-Based Quantum Dot Immunoassay for Rapid and Sensitive Detection of *Aspergillus amstelodami*, *Sensors*, 11, 6396–6410 (2011).

Khatua, S. and M. Orrit. Toward Single-Molecule Microscopy on a Smart Phone, *ACS Nano*, 7, 8340–8343 (2013).

Kim, B. Y. S., J. T. Rutka and W. C. W. Chan. Nanomedicine, *New England Journal of Medicine*, 363, 2434–2443 (2010).

Kim, G. B. and Y. P. Kim. Analysis of Protease Activity Using Quantum Dots and Resonance Energy, *Theranostics*, 2, 127–138 (2012).

Kim, H., M. D. Kane, S. Kim, W. Dominguez, B. M. Applegate and S. Savikhin. A Molecular Beacon DNA Microarray System for Rapid Detection of *E. coli* O157:H7 that Eliminates the Risk of a False Negative Signal, *Biosensors and Bioelectronics*, 22, 1041–1047 (2007a).

Kim, J. H., D. Morikis and M. Ozkan. Adaptation of Inorganic Quantum Dots for Stable Molecular Beacons, *Sensors and Actuators B*, 102, 315–319 (2004).

Kim, J. M., E. V. Shashkov, E. I. Galanzah, N. Kotagiri and P. Zharov. Photothermal Antimicrobial Nanotherapy and Nanodiagnostics with Self-Assembling Carbon Nanotube Clusters, *Lasers in Surgery and Medicine*, 39, 622–634 (2007b).

Kim, Y., D. Sohn and W. Tan. Molecular Beacons in Biomedical Detection and Clinical Diagnosis, *International Journal of Clinical and Experimental Pathology*, 1, 105–116 (2008).

Koets, M., T. V. D. Wijk, J. T. W. M. Van Emeren, A. Van Amerongen and M. W. J. Prins. Rapid DNA Multi-Analyte Immunoassay on a Magneto-Resistance Biosensor, *Biosensors and Bioelectronics*, 24, 1893–1898 (2009).

Koh, I. and L. Josephson. Magnetic Nanoparticle Sensors, *Sensors*, 9, 8130–8145 (2009).

Kumar, A., B. M. Boruach and X. J. Liang. Gold Nanoparticles: Promising Nanomaterials for the Diagnosis of Cancer and HIV/AIDS, *Journal of Nanomaterials*, 2011, 1–17 (2011a).

Kumar, A. M., S. Jung and T. Ji. Protein Biosensors Based on Polymer Nanowires, Carbon Nanotubes and Zinc Oxide Nanorods, *Sensors*, 11, 5087–5111 (2011b).

Larios-Sanz, M., K. D. Kourentzi, D. Warmflash, J. Jones, D. L. Pierson, R. C. Willson and G. E. Fox. 16S rRNA Beacons for Bacterial Monitoring During Human Space Missions, *Aviation Space and Environmental Medicine*, 78, A43–A47 (2007).

Lee, H. H. and P. Yager. Microfluidic Lab-on-a-Chip for Microbial Identification on a DNA Microarray, *Biotechnology and Bioprocess Engineering*, 12, 634–639 (2007).

Lee, H., T. J. Yoon and R. Weissleder. Ultrasensitive Detection of Bacteria Using Core-Shell Nanoparticles and a NMR-Filter System, *Angwandte Chemie International Edition English*, 48, 5657–5660 (2009).

Lee, J. F., G. M. Stovall and A. D. Ellington. Aptamer Therapeutics Advance, *Current Opinion in Chemical Biology*, 10, 282–289 (2006).

Li, A., P. Y. Lee, B. Ho, J. L. Ding and C. T. Lim. Atomic Force Microscopy Study of the Antimicrobial Action of Sushi Peptide on Gram Negative Bacteria, *Biochimica et Biophysica Acta*, 1768, 411–418 (2006).

Li, Y., H. J. Schluesener and S. Xu. Gold Nanoparticle-Based Biosensors, *Gold Bulletin*, 43, 29–41 (2010).

Li, Y. and S. Xu. Highly Sensitive Detection of *Shigella flexneri* Using Fluorescent Silica Nanoparticles, *New Microbiologica*, 32, 377–383 (2009).

Liandris, E., M. Gazouli, M. Andreadou, L. A. Sechi, V. Rosu and J. Ikonomomopoulos. Detection of Pathogenic *Mycobacteria* Based on Functionalized Quantum Dots Coupled with Immunomagnetic Separation, *PLoS One*, 6 (5), 1–6 (2011).

Liu, F., K. S. Choi, T. J. Park, S. Y. Lee and T. S. Seo. Graphene-Based Electrochemical Biosensor for Pathogenic Virus Detection, *Biochip Journal*, 5, 123–128 (2011).

Liu, R. H., S. B. Munro, T. Nguyen, T. Siuda, D. Sucia, M. Bizak, M. Slota, H. S. Fuji, D. Danley and A. McShea. Integrated Microfluidic Custom Array Device for Bacterial Genotyping and Identification, *Journal of Lab Automation*, 11, 360–367 (2006).

Liu, S. and X. Guo. Carbon Nanomaterials Field-Effect-Transistor-Based Biosensors, *NPG Asia Materials*, 4, 1–10 (2012).

Liu, W. T. Nanoparticles and Their Biological and Environmental Applications, *Journal of Bioscience and Bioengineering*, 102, 1–7 (2006).

Lu, X., X. Dong, K. Zhang, X. Han, X. Fang and Y. Zhang. A Gold Nanorods-Based Fluorescent Biosensor for the Detection of Hepatitis B Virus DNA Based on Fluorescence Resonance Energy Transfer, *Analyst*, 138, 642–650 (2013).

Ma, Q., W. Yu and X. Su. Detection of Newcastle Disease Virus with Quantum Dots-Resonance Light Scattering System, *Talanta*, 82, 51–55 (2010).

Maalouf, R., W. M. Hassen, C. Fournier-Wirth, J. Coste and N. Jafrezic-Renault. Comparison of Two Innovative Approaches for Bacterial Detection: Paramagnetic Nanoparticles and Self-Assembled Multilayer Processes, *Microchimica Acta*, 163, 157–161 (2008).

Mairhofer, J., K. Roppert and P. Ertl. Microfluidic Systems for Pathogen Sensing: A Review, *Sensors*, 9, 4804–4823 (2009).

Mannoor, M. S., T. Hu, J. D. Clayton, A. Sengupta, D. L. Kaplan, R. R. Naik, N. Verma, F. G. Omenetto and M. C. McAlpine. Graphene-Based Wireless Bacteria Detection on Tooth Enamel, *Nature Communication*, 3, 1–8 (2012).

Mathur, N., A. Aneja, P. K. Bhatnagar and P. C. Mathur. A New FRET-Based Sensitive DNA Sensor for Medical Diagnostics Using PNA Probe and Water-Soluble Blue Light Emitting Polymer, *Journal of Sensors*, 2008, 1–6 (2008).

Matsui, H., H. Hanaki, M. Inoue, H. Akama, T. Nakae, K. Sunakawa and S. Omura. Development of an Immunochromatographic Strip for Simple Detection of Penicillin-Binding Protein 2, *Clinical Vaccine Immunology*, 18, 248–253 (2011).

Mayilo, S., M. A. Kloster, M. Wunderlich, A. Lutich, T. A. Klar, A. Nichtl, K. Kuerzinger, F. D. Stefani and J. Feldmann. Long-Range Fluorescence Quenching by Gold Nanoparticles in a Sandwich Immunoassay for Cardiac Troponin T, *Nano Letters*, 9, 4558–4563 (2009).

Mazumder, S., R. Dey, M. K. Mitra, S. Mukherjee and G. C. Das. Biofunctionalized Quantum Dots in Biology and Medicine, *Journal of Nanomaterials*, 2009, 1–17 (2009).

McKillen, J., B. Hjertner, A. Millar, F. McNeilly, S. Belak, B. Adair and G. Allan. Molecular Beacon Real-Time PCR Detection of Swine Viruses, *Journal of Virological Methods*, 140, 155–165 (2007).

Merkoci, A. Carbon Nanotubes in Analytical Sciences, *Microchimica Acta*, 152, 157–174 (2006).

Mohanty, N. and V. Berry. Graphene-Based Single-Bacterium Resolution Biodevice and DNA Transistor: Interfacing Graphene Derivatives with Nanoscale and Microscale Biocomponents, *Nano Letters*, 8 (12), 4469–4476 (2008).

Mohanty, S. P. and A. L. Kougdianos. Biosensors: A Tutorial Review, *IEEE XPlore*, 2006, 35–40 (2006).

Moon, H. M. and J. W. M. Kim. Carbon Nanotube Clusters as Universal Bacterial Adsorbents and Magnetic Separation Agents, *Biotechnology Progress*, 26, 179–185 (2010).

Mothershed, E. A. and A. M. Whitney. Nucleic Acid-Based Methods for the Detection of Bacterial Pathogens: Present and Future Considerations for the Clinical Laboratory, *Clinica Chimica Acta*, 363, 206–220 (2006).

Muldrew, K. L. Molecular Diagnostics of Infectious Diseases, *Current Opinions in Pediatrics*, 21, 102–111 (2009).

Murcia, M. J. and C. A. Naumann. Biofunctionalization of Fluorescent Nanoparticles. *Nanotechnologies for the Life Sciences: Biofunctionalization of Nanomaterials* (Kumar, C. S. S. R., ed). Wiley-VCH Verlag GmbH & Co. KGaA, Weinheim (2005).

Nguyen, T. H., T. D. T. Ung, T. H. Vu, T. K. C. Tran, V. Q. Dong, D. K. Dinh and Q. L. Nguyen. Fluorescence Biosensor Based on CdTe Quantum Dots for Specific Detection of H5N1 Avian Influenza Virus, *Advances in Natural Sciences: Nanoscience and Nanotechnology*, 3, 1–5 (2012).

Oh, W., Y. S. Jeong, J. Song and J. Jang. Fluorescent Europium-Modified Polymer Nanoparticles for Rapid and Sensitive Anthrax Sensors, *Biosensors and Bioelectronics*, 29, 172–177 (2011).

Orru, G., M. L. Ferrando, M. Meloni, M. Liciardi, G. Savini and P. D. Santis. Rapid Detection and Quantitation of Bluetongue Virus (BTV) Using a Molecular Beacon Fluorescent Probe Assay, *Journal of Virological Methods*, 137, 34–42 (2006).

Padmavathy, B., A. Patel, R. V. Kumar and B. M. J. Ali. Superparamagnetic Nanoparticles Based Immunomagnetic Separation—Multiplex Polymerase Chain Reaction Assay for Detection of *Salmonella*, *Science of Advanced Materials*, 4, 114–120 (2012).

Pankhurst, Q. A., J. Connolly, S. K. Jones and J. Dobson. Applications of Magnetic Nanoparticles in Biomedicine, *Journal of Physics D: Applied Physics*, 36, R167–R181 (2003).

Patolsky, F., G. Zheng, O. Heyden, M. Lakadamyali and X. Zhuang. Electrical Detection of Single Viruses, *Proceedings of the National Academy of Sciences of the United States of America*, 101, 14017–14022 (2004).

Peng, F., Z. Wang, S. Zhang, R. Wu, S. Hu, Z. Li, X. Wang and D. Bi. Development of an Immunochromatographic Strip for Rapid Detection of H9 Subtype Avian Influenza Viruses, *Clinical Vaccine Immunology*, 15, 569–574 (2008).

Pfaller, M. A. Molecular Approaches to Diagnosing and Mapping Infectious Diseases: Practicality and Costs, *Emerging Infectious Diseases*, 7, 312–318 (2001).

Pham, M. T., T. V. Nguyen, D. T. V. Thi, H. L. N. Thi, K. T. Tong, T. T. Tran, V. H. Chu, J. C. Brochon and H. N. Tran. Synthesis, Photophysical Properties and Application of Dye Doped Water Soluble Silica-Based Nanoparticles to Label Bacteria *E. coli* O157:H7, *Advances in Natural Sciences: Nanoscience and Nanotechnology*, 3, 1–7 (2012).

Poddar, S. K. Detection of Adenovirus Using PCR and Molecular Beacon, *Journal of Virological Methods*, 82, 19–26 (1999).

Qin, D., X. He, K. Wang, X. J. Zhao, W. Tan and J. Chen. Fluorescent Nanoparticle-Based Indirect Immunofluorescence for Detection of *Mycobacterium tuberculosis*, *Journal of Biomedical Biotechnology*, 2007, 1–9 (2007).

Qureshi, A., W. P. Kang, J. L. Davidson and Y. Gurbuz. Review on Carbon-Derived, Solid-State, Micro and Nano Sensors for Electrochemical Sensing Applications, *Diamond Related Materials*, 18, 1401–1420 (2009).

Ray, P. C., G. K. Darbh, A. Ray, J. Walker and W. Hardy. Gold Nanoparticle Based FRET for DNA Detection, *Plasmonics*, 2, 173–183 (2007).

Sanvicens, N., C. Pastells, N. Pascual and M. P. Marco. Nanoparticle-Based Biosensors for Detection of Pathogenic Bacteria, *Trends in Analytical Chemistry*, 28, 1243–1252 (2009).

Setterington, E. B. and E. C. Alocilja. Electrochemical Biosensor for Rapid and Sensitive Detection of Magnetically Extracted Bacterial Pathogens, *Biosensors*, 2, 15–31 (2012).

Shinde, S. B., C. B. Fernandes and V. B. Patravale. Recent Trends in In-Vitro Nanodiagnostics for Detection of Pathogens, *Journal of Controlled Release*, 159, 164–180 (2012).

Singh, A., R. V. Goering, S. Simjee, S. L. Foley and M. J. Zervos. Application of Molecular Techniques to the Study of Hospital Infection, *Clinical Microbiology Reviews*, 19, 512–530 (2006).

Speers, D. J. Clinical Applications of Molecular Biology for Infectious Diseases, *The Clinical Biochemist Reviews*, 27, 39–51 (2006).

Stringer, R. C., S. Schommer, D. Hoehn and S. Grant. A. Development of an Optical Biosensor Using Gold Nanoparticles and Quantum Dots for the Detection of Porcine Reproductive and Respiratory Syndrome Virus, *Sensors and Actuators. B—Chemical*, 134, 427–431 (2008).

Syed, M. A. Advances in Nanodiagnostic Techniques for Microbial Agents, *Biosensors and Bioelectronics*, 51, 391–400 (2014).

Syed, M. A. and S. H. A. Bokhari. Gold Nanoparticle Based Microbial Detection and Identification, *Journal of Biomedical Nanotechnology*, 7, 229–237 (2011).

Syed, M. A. and S. Pervaiz. Advances in Aptamers, *Oligonucleotides*, 20, 215–224 (2010).

Syed M. A., A. S. Bhatti, S. Babar and H. Bukhari. Antibacterial Effects of Silver Nanoparticles on The Bacterial Strains Isolated From Catheterized Urinary Tract Infection Cases. *Journal of Biomedical Nanotechnology*, 5, 209–214 (2009).

Tallury, P., A. Malhotra, L. M. Byrne and S. Santra. Nanobioimaging and Sensing of Infectious Diseases, *Advances Drug Delivery Reviews*, 62, 424–437 (2010).

Tan, W., X. Fang, J. Li and X. Liu. Molecular Beacons: A Novel DNA Probe for Nucleic Acid and Protein Studies, *Chemistry: A European Journal*, 6, 1107–1111 (2000).

Thornton, C. R. and V. Clin. Development of an Immunochromatographic Lateral-Flow Device for Rapid Serodiagnosis of Invasive Aspergillosis, *Vaccine Immunology*, 15, 1095–1105 (2008).

Tombelli, S., M. Minnuni and M. Mascini. Analytical Applications of Aptamers, *Biosensors and Bioelectronics*, 20, 2424–2434 (2005).

Touhami, A., M. H. Jericho and T. J. Beveridge. Atomic Force Microscopy of Cell Growth and Division in *Staphylococcus aureus*, *Journal of Bacteriology*, 186, 3286–3295 (2004).

Tripp, R. A., R. Alvarez, B. Anderson, L. Jones, C. Weeks and W. Chen. Bioconjugated Nanoparticle Detection of Respiratory Syncytial Virus Infection, *International Journal of Nanomedicine*, 2, 117–124 (2008).

Tsai, T. M., Y. H. Cheng, Y. N. Liu, N. C. Liao, W. W. Lu and S. H. Kung. Real-Time Monitoring of Human Enterovirus (HEV)-Infected Cells and Anti-HEV 3C Protease Potency by Fluorescence Resonance Energy Transfer, *Antimicrobial Agents and Chemotherapy*, 53, 748–755 (2009).

Valizadeh, A., H. Mikaeili, M. Samiei, S. M. Farkhani, N. Zarghami, M. Kouhi, A. Akberzadeh and S. Davaran. Quantum Dots: Synthesis, Bioapplications, and Toxicity, *Nanoscale Research Letters*, 7, 1–14 (2012).

Vardharajula, S., S. K. Ali, P. M. Tiwari, E. Eroglu, K. Vig, V. A. Dennis and S. R. Singh. Functionalized Carbon Nanotubes: Biomedical Applications, *International Journal of Nanomedicine*, 7, 5361–5374 (2012).

Varma-Basil, M., H. El-Haj, S. A. E. Marras, M. H. Hazbon, J. M. Mann, N. D. Connell, F. R. Kramer and D. Alland. Molecular Beacons for Multiplex Detection of Four Bacterial Bioterrorism Agents. *Clinical Chemistry*, 50,1060–1062 (2004).

Vashist, S. K. Nanomaterials and Molecular Nanotechnology, *Journal of Nanomaterials and Molecular Nanotechnology*, 2, 1–6 (2013).

Vashist, S. K. and A. G. Venkatesh. Advances in Graphene-Based Sensors and Devices, *Journal of Nanomedicine and Nanotechnology*, 4, 1–2 (2013).

Villamizar, R. A., R. Maroto, F. X. Rius, I. Inza and M. J. Figueras. Fast Detection of *Salmonella infantis* with Carbon Nanotube Field Effect Transistors, *Biosensors and Bioelectronics*, 24, 279–283 (2008).

Villaverde, A. Nanotechnology, Bionanotechnology and Microbial Cell Factories, *Microbial Cell Factories*, 9, 53 (2010).

Vo-Dinh, T. and B. Cullum. Biosensors and Biochips: Advances in Biological and Medical Diagnostics, *Fresenius Journal of Analytical Chemistry*, 366, 540–551 (2000).

Wanekaya, A. K., W. Chen, N. V. Myung and A. Mulchandani. Nanowire-Based Electrochemical Biosensors, *Electroanalysis*, 18, 533–550 (2006).

Wang, D., H. Chen, H. Li, Z. He, X. Ding and L. Deng. Detection of *Staphylococcus aureus* Carrying the Gene for Toxic Shock Syndrome Toxin 1 by Quantum-Dot-Probe Complexes, Journal of Fluorescence, 21, 1525–1530 (2011b).

Wang, L., C. Wu, X. Fan and A. Mustafha. Detection of *Escherichia coli* O157:H7 and *Salmonella* in Ground Beef by a Bead-Free Quantum Dot-Facilitated Isolation Method, *International Journal of Food Microbiology*, 156, 83–87 (2012).

Wang, L., W. Zhao, M. B. O'Donoghue and W. Tan. Fluorescent Nanoparticles for Multiplexed Bacteria Monitoring, *Bioconjugate Chemistry*, 18, 297–301 (2007).

Wang, Y. H., X. R. Li, G. X. Wang, H. Yin, X. P. Cai, B. Q. Fu and D. L. Zhang. Development of an Immunochromatographic Strip for the Rapid Detection of *Toxoplasma gondii* Circulating Antigens, *Parasitology International*, 60, 105–107 (2011a).

Wei, Q., H. Qi, W. Luo, D. Tseng, S. J. Ki, Z. Wan, Z. Goeroes, L. A. Bentoliala, T. T. Wu, R. Sun and A. Ozan. Fluorescent Imaging of Single Nanoparticles and Viruses on a Smart Phone, *ACS Nano*, 7, 9147–9155 (2013).

Wolfe, N. D., C. P. Dunavan and J. Diamon. Origins of Major Infectious Diseases, *Nature*, 447, 279–283 (2007).

Xu, H., X. Mao, Q. Zeng, X. Wang, A. N. Kwade and G. Liu. Aptamer-Functionalized Gold Nanoparticles as Probes in a Dry-Reagent Strip Biosensor for Protein Analysis, *Analytical Chemistry*, 81, 669–675 (2009).

Yan, J., M. C. Estévez, J. E. Smith, E. Wang, X. He, L. Wang and W. Tan. Dye-Doped Nanoparticles for Bioanalysis, *Nano Today*, 2, 44–50 (2007).

Yan, Z. M., J. Zheng, Q. Chen and H. Shen, Development of an Immunochromatographic Strip Test for Rapid Detection of *Vibrio vulnificus*, *NanFang Yi Ke Da Xue Xue Bao*, 31, 894–896 (2011).

Yang, H. and Y. Wang. Application of Atomic Force Microscopy on Rapid Determination of Microorganisms for Food Safety, *Journal of Food Science*, 73, N44–N50 (2006).

Yang, P., S. Yao, W. Wei and J. Cai. An Indirect Immunoassay for Detecting Antigen Based on Fluorescence Resonance Energy Transfer, *American Journal of Analytical Chemistry*, 2, 484–490 (2011).

Yang, W., K. R. Ratinac, S. P. Ringer, P. Thordarson, J. J. Gooding and F. Braet. Carbon Nanomaterials in Biosensors: Should You Use Nanotubes or Graphene? *Angewandte Chemie*, 49, 2114–2138 (2010).

Zadran, S., S. Standley, K. Wong, E. Otiniano, A. Amighi and M. Baudry. Fluorescence Resonance Energy Transfer (FRET)-Based Biosensors: Visualizing Cellular Dynamics and Bioenergetics, *Applied Microbiology and Biotechnology*, 96, 895–902 (2012).

Zarakolu, P., I. Buchanan, M. Tam, K. Smith and W. E. Hook. Preliminary Evaluation of an Immunochromatographic Strip Test for Specific *Treponema pallidum* Antibodies, *Journal of Clinical Microbiology*, 40, 3064–3065 (2002).

Zhang, G. J., L. Zhang, M. J. Huang, Z. H. H. Luo, G. K. I. Tay, E. A. Lim, T. G. Kang and Y. Chen. Silicon Nanowire Biosensor for Highly Sensitive and Rapid Detection of Dengue Virus, *Sensors and Actuators B: Chemical*, 146, 138–144 (2010).

Zhang, Y. B., M. Kanungo, A. J. Ho, P. Freimuth, D. van der Lelie, M. Chen, S. M. Khamis, S. S. Datta, A. T. C. Johnson, J. A. Misewich and S. S., Wong. Functionalized Carbon Nanotubes for Detecting Viral Proteins, *Nano Letters*, 7, 3086–3091 (2007).

Zhao, X., L. R. Hilliard, S. J. Mechery, Y. Wang, R. P. Bagwe, S. Jin and W. Tan. A Rapid Bioassay for Single Bacterial Cell Quantitation Using Bioconjugated Nanoparticles, *Proceedings of the National Academy of Sciences of the United States of America*, 101, 15027–15032 (2004).

Zhao, Y., M. Ye, Q. Chao, N. Jia, Y. Ge and H. Shen. Simultaneous Detection of Multifood-Borne Pathogenic Bacteria Based on Functionalized Quantum Dots Coupled with Immunomagnetic Separation in Food Samples, *Journal of Agricultural Food Chemistry*, 57, 517–524 (2009).

Zhu, L., S. Ang and W. T. Liu. Quantum Dots as a Novel Immunofluorescent Detection System for *Cryptosporidium parvum* and *Giardia lamblia*, *Applied Environmental Microbiology*, 70, 597–598 (2004).

11 Chromogenic Biosensors for Pathogen Detection

Alok P. Das, Bhubaneswari Bal, and Pragyan Smita Mahapatra

CONTENTS

ABSTRACT

Pathogen detection is of prime importance and concern in various sectors such as food, pharmaceutical, health care, and agriculture. Novel biosensing methodologies have been developed for rapid detection of pathogens based on the application of chromogenic substrates with specific enzyme activities. Chromogenic biosensing techniques are fully automated, delivering high selectivity and sensitivity to enhance detection and thus avoiding the need for time-consuming conventional and traditional methods. In addition to rapid detection, the choice of a wide variety of synthetic substrates allows microbial pathogen recognition simultaneously. This chapter deals principally with recent advancements in pathogen detection with particular focus on methods for chromogenic pathogen detection.

Keywords: Biosensors, Nanomaterials, Pathogens, Detection, Commercial application

11.1 INTRODUCTION

Detecting, sensing, and enumerating pathogens are a severe concern, and errors in doing so usually indicate a surplus of dangerous symptoms that, if remaining unnoticed, can result in lethal consequences [1,2]. Sepsis is a life-threatening situation

273

that results in response to a contagion and injures its own cells and organelles. This may result in septic shock, numerous organ failures, and fatality if not detected early. Pyrogen infections along with sepsis have a high mortality rate despite proper remedial and critical care [3]. Recognition of pyrogens is vital for infection control in biological products, biomedical instruments, military operations, environmental monitoring, and food and water security [4]. These are the requirements for a quick and responsive technology for the detection of pathogens in exceptionally minute concentrations [5,6].

Biosensors are condensed diagnostic devices that utilize biomolecules or enzymes to identify precise target analytes in the sample through separate or uninterrupted electrical signal, or spectrometric or luminous indicators [7]. Regardless of their wide range of biomonitoring application, biosensors can be classified into two main groups: (i) high-throughput costly devices and (ii) low-cost, moveable, and simple-to-use devices [8]. Renewed attention brought forth advancement in various approaches for endotoxin recognition, for instance, biomonitoring relying on bioluminescence by use luciferase enzyme [5], fluorescent dyes [9], frequency amplitude responses [10], and pyrogen-specific material such as pyrogen neutralizing proteins [11], pyrogen binding proteins [12], peptides [9], and pyrene derivatives [13]. A complete literature investigation has been carried out over the last 10 years because of the importance of chromogenic biomonitoring-based pyrogen detection (Figure 11.1).

Monitoring of pathogens is vital for infection control in several sectors such as health care products, biomedical equipment, military operations, environmental samples, and food and water safety. A detailed record of pathogenic microorganisms and their corresponding toxin, causal diseases, and causes are mentioned in Table 11.1. With an annual incidence of approximately 18 million worldwide, sepsis is the primary

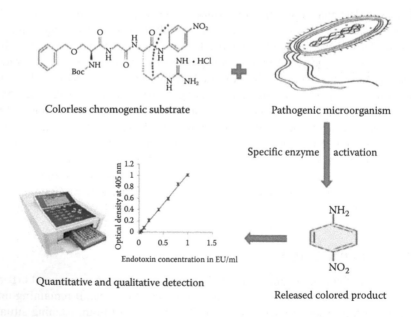

FIGURE 11.1   Mechanism of chromogenic biosensor in pathogen detection.

TABLE 11.1

List of Pathogens with Their Sources, Toxin Produced, Causal Diseases, and Mortality Rate

Pathogenic Organism	Source	Toxin	Disease	Annual Deaths (%)	Reference
Escherichia coli	Contaminated food and water	Endotoxin	Sepsis, cholecystitis, cholangitis	10	[1]
Pasteurella multocida	Animal bite, scratch, or lick	Endotoxin	Osteomyelitis and septic arthritis	20	[14]
Salmonella paratyphi	Contaminated food, poultry	Endotoxin	Salmonellosis	60	[15]
Staphylococcus aureus	Dermal contacts	Endotoxin	Arthritis, pneumonia	5	[14,16]
Listeria monocytogenes	Food contamination	Listeriolysin	Listeriosis	65	[17,18]
Treponema pallidum	Sexual contact	Endotoxin	Syphilis	23	[19]
Coxiella burnetii	Dairy products	Endotoxin	Pneumonia	20	[20]
Yersinia	Dermal contact	Endotoxin	Yersiniosis	5	[21]
Vibrio cholerae	Water contamination	Endotoxin	Diarrhea	70	[22]
Shigella	Contaminated water	Verotoxin	Shigellosis	33	[23,24]
Clostridium perfringens	Contaminated food	Enterotoxin	Food poisoning	24	[25]
Bacillus anthracis	Airborne inhalation	Endotoxin	Anthrax	20	[26]
Brucella suis	Contaminated food	Endotoxin	Flu-like disease, brucellosis	3	[27]
Haemophilus influenzae	Airborne	Endotoxin	Meningitis	10	[28]
Mycobacterium tuberculosis	Contaminated water	Endotoxin	Tuberculosis	0.4	[29]

cause of death in intensive care units, which is a growing concern and a considerable predicament among high-risk patients, with a 30%–40% mortality rate [30]. Mortality rates owing to pyrogenic infection remain elevated and have not changed considerably in the last 10 years (Figure 11.2). According to a previous analysis, global food manufacturing microbiology testing included 738.3 million investigations in 2008, with a market cost of greater than $2 billion. This represents a 17.8% increase in the number of investigations over the last 3 years [31]. The global TIC (Testing, Inspection, and Certification) industry is huge, with revenues of more than $120 billion in 2010.

Biological warfare involves the intentional manipulation of microorganisms and their toxins to bring about infection or death in humans, farm animals, and crops. The appeal of bioterrorism in warfare and in terroristic acts is credited to its small manufacturing costs, easy access, disease-producing capability, easy concealment, and ease in transport [32,33]. Although a huge attempt at developing biosensors is underway, relatively few microorganisms and toxic substances can be detected by available devices [34,35].

Communal and ecological health safety necessitates safe water for consumption, which should be contamination free [36]. Among the microbes distributed in water resources, enteric pathogens are the ones most frequently encountered. As a result, causes of fecal contamination in water for human consumption have to be stringently identified. *Escherichia coli* O157:H7 are usually present at extremely low amounts in ecological waters containing a wide array of microflora [14]. Different techniques are necessary to detect them and these are enormously protracted. Although coliforms are also found in diverse natural environments, drinking water is not a natural environment for them and their existence in drinking water is measured as a probable hazard or symptom of microbiological water quality worsening. Ten to 20 million deaths each year are caused by waterborne pathogens in addition to nonfatal infection [16]. Millions of dollars worth of current documented foods are recalled because of an increase in food poisoning cases, and the need for additional quick, responsive, and

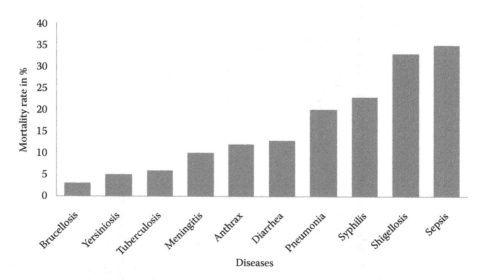

FIGURE 11.2 Graphical representation of diseases and their mortality rate.

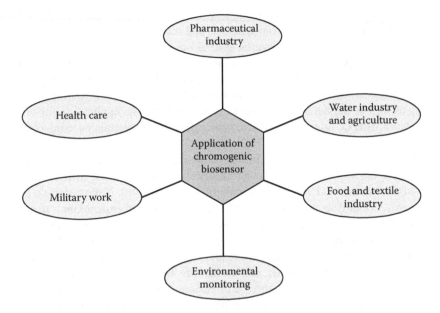

FIGURE 11.3 Diagrammatic representation of application of chromogenic biosensor.

accurate methods of detecting these microbial toxins has increased [17,18]. During 2009–2010, public health departments in the United States reported 1527 food-borne disease outbreaks, resulting in 29,444 cases of illness, 1184 hospitalizations, and 23 deaths. As per Centers for Disease Control and Prevention (CDC) and Food Safety data, norovirus was the cause of most infections, accounting for 42% of outbreaks, followed by *Salmonella*, accounting for 30% of outbreaks. In 2013, the CDC's food poisoning reporting system identified 19,000 related infections, 4200 hospitalizations and 80 deaths among 48 million inhabitants.

Conventional techniques are extremely lengthy, invasive, and burdensome. Efforts are underway to improve the speed and accuracy of biosensors [37]. Development of sensors has always been confronted by new challenges, but this does not deter the prospect of a new sensor-based innovative world. Various sectors demanding rapid pathogen detection and monitoring are presented in Figure 11.3.

11.2 NANOMATERIALS AS BIOSENSORS

The thrust for novel biosensors has improved enormously, signifying a remarkable substitute for the advancement of a competent, rapid, and inexpensive biosensing strategy. In this perspective, nanoparticles (NPs) with unique properties have considerable advantages in the areas of scientific examination, laboratory analysis, ecological monitoring, and food safety [38], with potential opportunities in numerous other fields. Nanotechnology plays a significant role in the development of biosensors with improved sensitivity [39,40]. Nanomaterials exhibit exceptional features because of their quantum size, surface effect, macro-quantum tunnel effect, and electrochemical properties, which make them exceptionally helpful in biosensing applications

[41]. The relevance of NPs in biosensing is strongly associated with their properties that depend on a specific mode from synthesis and subsequent modifications [42], and numerous types of NPs are now available in biosensor-related applications [43–45]. These specific properties of NPs tender a variety of signal transduction modes absent from other materials [46,47]. The choice of NPs is as huge as the range of potential applications in biomonitoring and depends strongly on the use of the biomolecules in sensing as well as the nature of the test to be performed. The applications of several NPs in biosensing cellular organelles and pathogenic microorganisms using biosensing systems are presented in Table 11.2.

The National Nanotechnology Initiative describes nanotechnology as technological progress at the atomic or macromolecular level, with the aim of creating and using structures and devices at a scale of 1–100 nM [48]. Nanomaterials found applications as catalysts, immobilized substrates, or electrochemical labels to extend the biosensing activity with superior sensitivity [49]. Nanomaterials, such as gold nanostructured materials, carbon nanotubes, silicon nanotubes, metal NPs, nanowires, TiO_2 nanowires, and nanoelectrode array, play an important role in biosensing applications such as in food, water, and health care analysis [50]. The sensing ability of the biosensors is enhanced by the use of various nanomaterials such as magnetic NPs, quantum dots, nanochannels, and nanorods [51–54]. From this perspective, the "nanoparticle-based nanobiosensors" are a current and competent group of biosensing systems [55–57]. Recently, vast research has been carried out in alternating

TABLE 11.2
List of Biosensors and Their Nanomaterials for Detection of Pathogenic Bacteria

Biosensor	Nanomaterial Used	Pathogens Detected	Reference
DNA biosensor	Carbon nanotubes, quantum dots	Bacteriophage, *Ganoderma boninense*	[58–61]
Enzymatic biosensors	Gold nanostructured materials	*Listeria monocytogenes*	[62,63]
Field-effect transistor–based biosensors	Carbon nanomaterials, silicon nanowire	Dengue virus infection	[59,64]
Electrochemical biosensor	Gold nanoparticles	*Salmonella, Escherichia coli*	[49,53,65,66]
Acoustic wave biosensors	Au, Pt, CdS, TiO_2, polymers	*E. coli*	[67]
Optical biosensors	Glyconanoparticles, gold nanoparticles	*E. coli, Mycobacterium avium*	[67–69]
Magnetic biosensors	Greigite, iron oxide nanoparticles	*E. coli, M. avium*	[38,67,70]
Graphene-based biosensors	Graphene	*E. coli*	[71]
Glutamate biosensor	Nanoelectrode array	*E. coli*	[72,73]
Impedimetric biosensors	TiO_2 nanowire	*L. monocytogenes, E. coli*	[74,75]

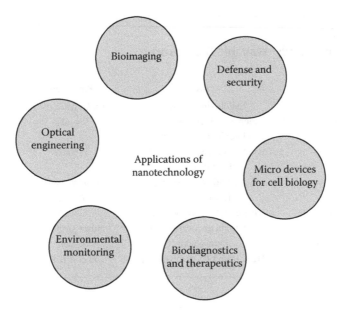

FIGURE 11.4 Application of nanotechnology in various sectors.

electrode surfaces with novel NPs so as to obtain a rapid detection system with superior specificity. This improvement has encouraged research in NP-based biosensors, with applications in areas such as food safety, medical analysis, and environmental monitoring [65,76,77]. The application of nanotechnology in various sectors is explained in Figure 11.4.

11.3 COMMERCIALLY EXISTING CHROMOGENIC SENSORS

Pathogen detection has become a significant requirement because of the large volume of various industrial products being manufactured. Compliance with parameters regarding the levels of pathogen contamination has been made a legal requirement because of the possible adverse biological reactions [78]. Hence, pathogen detection/quantification assumes a notable significance in clinical production, life science, and biomedical research [79]. The commercial availability of a variety of pathogen detection biosensors in the market clearly denotes the inevitability of rapid detection and monitoring of pathogens and their toxins in various sectors [1]. Commercially available chromogenic biosensors are listed in detail in Table 11.3, where every design offers a unique advantage over the previous one. Because of the attention on chromogenic detection, the limulus amebocyte lysate (LAL) assay is considered one of the preferred pathogenic detection systems [80]. A schematic diagram explaining the mechanism of the LAL assay for pathogen detection is provided in Figure 11.5. Alternatives to LAL in the form of kinetic turbidimetric, end point chromogenic, and kinetic chromogenic methods, as well as recombinant factor C attached to fluorescence are available. Among these, the kinetic turbidimetric type presents an inexpensive quantitative method for the detection of pathogen from water and

TABLE 11.3
List of Commercially Available Biosensors

Company	Kit	Pathogen	Detection Limit (EU/ml)
Lonza BioScience	Endotoxin detection	*Escherichia coli*	0.1
Thermo Scientific	Pierce LAL chromogenic endotoxin quantitation kit	*Shigella*	0.1
Gene script	Toxin Sensor Chromogenic LAL endotoxin assay kit	*Yersinia*	0.005
Bioreliance	LAL Endotoxin Testing	*Brucella suis*	0.06
Sigma-Aldrich	E-Toxate Kit	*E. coli*	0.05
Thermo Scientific	Pierce LAL chromogenic endotoxin quantitation kit	*Listeria monocytogenes*	0.1
Associates of Cape Cod	Pyrosate kit	*E. coli*	1.0
InvivoGen	HEK-Blue LPS detection kit	*E. coli* K 12	0.03

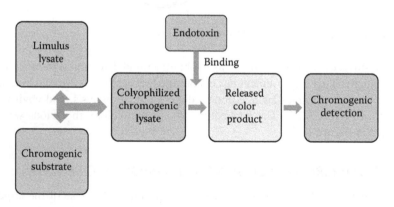

FIGURE 11.5 Schematic diagram explaining the mechanism of LAL assay.

clinical fluids. End point chromogenic LAL provides a smaller amount of product intrusion and more essentially is a quantitative investigation [81]. Kinetic chromogenic LAL has superior sensitivity coupled with little product intrusion (e.g., vaccines and other natural composites). Moving forward, to decrease the dependence on horseshoe crabs lysate, recombinant factor C is attached to fluorescence to reduce false-positive results with enhanced sensitivity [82].

As quick and perceptive recognition of pathogens is a key necessity for scientific works, a colorimetric enzyme–NP conjugate scheme for sensation of microbial contamination has been reported. In this technique, cationic gold NPs featuring quaternary amine head groups are electrostatically bound to the enzyme β-galactosidase (β-Gal), hindering enzyme activity. Pathogenic bacteria attach to the NP and release β-Gal, restoring its activity and providing an enzyme-activated spectrophotometric reading [83]. A new commercial chromogenic method, the βLACTA assay, was

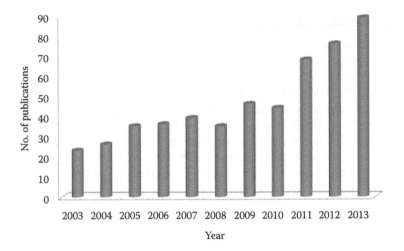

FIGURE 11.6 Graph of a search on the term *chromogenic biosensors* during the period 2003–2013, using the SCI database. This graph clearly depicts a linear increase in manuscripts published on Chromogenic biosensor with the highest number of papers published in the year 2013.

developed to detect nonsusceptibility to ceftazidime in *Pseudomonas aeruginosa.* This swift technique was sensitive (95%) and precise (87%) and offered negative and positive prognostic values of 99% and 100%, respectively [84]. A search on the term *chromogenic biosensors* during the period 2003–2013, using the SCI database, evidently represents a linear increase in manuscripts available on chromogenic biosensors, with the highest number of papers available for the year 2013 (Figure 11.6).

11.4   DETECTION OF PATHOGENS

Pathogen detection is of the utmost importance in many fields demanding rapid sensing and quantifying. Hence, a wide variety of miscellaneous chromogenic methods, using different techniques, has been tested for detecting pathogens or their toxins. Biosensors have been applied for a variety of applications, and chromogenic biosensors have achieved the most significant progress in this area. In this context, chromogenic sensing techniques are based on the change on absorption of UV/visible/ infrared light in response to biochemical reactions.

11.4.1   OPTICAL DETECTION

Optical sensors are largely noted for direct or indirect sensing of microbial strains and their toxins [85]. Access to a large number of substrates and diverse spectrochemical methods has made optical sensors widely available. Optical sensors can detect minute changes in spectophotometric parameters, such as refractive index or turbidity on a transducer surface, and are further differentiated into fluorescence and surface plasmon resonance (SPR) [1].

11.4.2 FLUORESCENCE DETECTION

Fluorescence is an instance in which a fluorophore absorbs light and releases radiance in a visible sequence. Since there is failure of radiative energy, the fluorescent light is always at a longer wavelength than the absorbed light, which is called *Stokes shift* [86,87]. Monitoring of toxins from *Listeria* species using a fluorescent technique has reached a detection limit of 10 ng/ml [88] and can simultaneously detect *E. coli* and *Staphylococcus aureus* with a lower detection limit of 10^2 cells [89]. Additional instantaneous detection has been achieved using CAT-FISH (capture antibody targeted fluorescence in situ hybridization) developed to detect both *E. coli* O157:H7 and *S. aureus* [90]. A chemiluminescence-based pathogen recognition was accounted with a monitoring limit of 0.017–1.6 EU/ml [91], and a luminescence-based sensing technique for endotoxin monitoring has been reported by Hreniak et al. [92] for *Hafnia alvei* PCM 1186 strain. Endotoxin units per milliliter (EU/ml) is a measurement of endotoxin concentration as compared to a precise amount of reference endotoxin; 1 EU/ml is approximately equal to 0.1 ng/ml. A novel pathogen monitoring biosensor using bioluminescence from mutant luciferase enzyme has been reported at a detection limit of 0.0005 EU/ml [5]. A completely innovative colorimetric and fluorometric sensor capable of optical recognition of endotoxin with a detection limit of 270 pM has been reported by Lan et al. [93].

11.4.3 SURFACE PLASMON RESONANCE

SPR is a responsive technique for detecting quantifiable changes in refractive index caused by structural alterations of a thin metal surface [94]. SPR involves the combined oscillation of electrons in a solid or liquid stimulated by incident light. SPR occurs when polarized light hits an electrically conducting exterior at the edge involving two media. This produces electron charge-thickness waves called plasmons, decreasing the intensity of reflected light at a precise angle, called the resonance angle, in proportion to the mass on a sensor surface. SPR-based biosensors are used in detecting *Salmonella* [95], while the use a gold nanorod–based optical DNA biosensor for the detection of pathogens like *Chlamydia trachomatis* has been reported. SPR using bacteriophage as bioreceptors has been successfully used to detect *E. coli* O157:H7 and methicillin-resistant *S. aureus* [96]. Reports on the necessity of endotoxin to CD14 have surfaced, which can later be developed to create a working biosensor [97]. There have also been reports of advanced immediate endotoxin detection using the antibiotic peptide polymyxin B to detect endotoxins with a sensitivity as low as 0.2–0.8 ng/ml [98]. Original techniques with planar interdigital sensors and polymyxin B as bioreceptors are harnessed with a detection limit of 0.05 EU/ml [99]. Recent reports suggest that extremely discriminating microbial biosensors can be designed by inducing a desired microbe metabolic pathway and by adapting them to the substrate of interest, using selected conditions of cell culturing [100].

11.5 CONCLUSION AND OUTLOOK

Conventional pathogen-detecting techniques are responsive but are slow and usually take 24 to 48 h, which makes them unreliable for diagnostic requirements. Hence original methods with novel advances have to be considered to overcome the drawbacks of the existing protocols. Chromogenic sensors escorting with their range of diverse spectrochemical properties, fluorogenic and chromogenic substrates, utilizing specific enzymatic activities are no doubt strong contenders but their elevated price and other intricacy issues fetch them to back foot. Due to its trimness, low cost, reusability, easy disposable, rapid sensing and frequent commercial relevance chromogenic biosensors are of marked accomplishment.

With the potential brought about by the diverse nature of nanomaterials, recent developments in the production and refinement of nanosensors will improve our understanding of these materials and will broaden their usefulness in biosensors. In conclusion, it is clear that nanotechnology will offer numerous advantages for the detection of pathogens, and constant progress of these biosensing technologies will be a particular boon to clinical science. Biosensor technology is not only cost-effective but also lightweight and compact. Certainly, the efficiency and production of compact biosensors as diagnostic devices is a flourishing research area and the potential applications are countless.

REFERENCES

1. A.P. Das, P.S. Kumar, and S. Swain, Recent advances in biosensor based pyrogen detection, *Biosensors and Bioelectronics*, 51, 62–75 (2014).
2. A.P.F. Turner, Biosensors: Sense and sensibility, *Chemical Society Reviews*, 42 (8), 3175–3648 (2013).
3. G. Goscinski, L. Miklos, E. Mats, L. Anders, T. Eva, and S. Jan, Endotoxin neutralization and anti-inflammatory effects of tobramycin and ceftazidime in porcine endotoxin shock, *Critical Care*, 8 (1), R35–R41 (2004).
4. T.Y. Yeo, J.S. Choi, B.K. Lee, B.S. Kim, H.I. Yoon, H.Y. Lee, and Y.W. Cho, Electrochemical endotoxin sensors based on TLR4/MD-2 complexes immobilized on gold electrodes, *Biosensors and Bioelectronics*, 28, 139–145 (2011).
5. K. Noda, H. Goto, Y. Murakami, A.B.F. Ahmed, and A. Kuroda, Endotoxin assay by bioluminescence using mutant firefly luciferase, *Analytical Biochemistry*, 397 (2), 152–155 (2010).
6. W. Su, M. Lin, H. Lee, M. Cho, W. Choe, and Y. Lee, Determination of endotoxin through an aptameter-based impedance biosensor, *Biosensors and Bioelectronics*, 32 (1), 32–36 (2012).
7. A.P.F. Turner, Biosensors: Then and now, *Trends in Biotechnology*, 31, 119–120 (2013).
8. P.V. Mohanan, S. Banerjee, and C.S. Geetha, Detection of pyrogenicity on medical grade polymer materials using rabbit pyrogen, LAL and ELISA method, *Journal of Pharmaceutical and Biomedical Analysis*, 55 (5), 1170–1174 (2011).
9. S. Voss, R. Fischer, G. Jung, K.H. Wiesmüller, and R. Brock, A fluorescence-based synthetic LPS sensor, *Journal of the American Chemical Society*, 129 (3), 554–561 (2007).
10. K.G. Ong, J.M. Leland, K.G.Z. Barrett, M. Zourob, and C.A. Grimes, A rapid highly-sensitive endotoxin detection system, *Biosensors and Bioelectronics*, 21, 2270–2274 (2006).
11. Y. Kaconis, I. Kowalski, J. Howe, A. Brauser, W. Richter, I. Razquin-Olazaran, M. Inigo-Pestana, P. Garidel, M. Rossle, G.M.D. Tejada, T. Gutsmann, and K. Brandenburg, Biophysical mechanisms of endotoxin neutralization by cationic amphiphilic peptides, *Biophysical Journal*, 100 (11), 2652–2661 (2011).

12. J.S. Davis, A.C. Cheng, M. McMillan, A.B. Humphrey, D.P. Stephens, and M.N. Anstey, Sepsis in the tropical Top End of Australia's Northern Territory: Disease burden and impact on Indigenous Australians, *The Medical Journal of Australia*, 194 (10), 519–524 (2011).

13. L. Zeng, J. Wu, Q. Dai, W. Liu, P. Wang, and C.S. Lee, Sensing of bacterial endotoxin in aqueous solution by supramolecular assembly of pyrene derivative, *Organic Letters*, 12 (18), 4014–4017 (2010).

14. J.A. Clark, and A.H. El-Shaarawi, Evaluation of commercial presence-absence test kits for detection of total coliforms, *Escherichia coli*, and other indicator bacteria, *Applied and Environmental Microbiology*, 59, 380–388 (1993).

15. P.L. Cummings, S. Forvillo, and T. Kuo, Salmonellosis-related mortality in the United States, 1990–2006, *Food Borne Pathogenic Disease*, 7 (11), 1393–1399 (2010).

16. Anonymous, Waterborne pathogens kill 10M–20M people/year, *World Water Environmental Engineering*, June 6 (1996).

17. C.W. Donnelly, Listeria monocytogenes: A continuing challenge, *Nutrition Reviews*, 59, 183–194 (2001).

18. W.F. Schlech III, Food borne listeriosis, *Clinical Infectious Disease*, 31, 770–775 (2000).

19. H. Norrgren, S. Andersson, A. Nauclér, F. Dias, I. Johansson, and G. Biberfeld, HIV-1, HIV-2, HTLV-I/II and Treponema pallidum infections: Incidence, prevalence, and HIV-2-associated mortality in an occupational cohort in Guinea-Bissau, *Journal Acquired Immune Deficiency Syndrome Human Retroviral*, 9 (4), 422–428 (1995).

20. K.T. Nielsen, S.S. Nielsen, J.F. Agger, A.B. Christoffersen, and J.S. Agerholm, Association between antibodies to *Coxiella burnetii* in bulk tank milk and perinatal mortality of Danish dairy calves, *Acta Veterinaria Scandinavica*, 53, 64 (2011).

21. Y. Glenn, J.L. Badger, and V.L. Miller, Motility is required to initiate host cell invasion by *Yersinia enterocolitica*, *Infection and Immunity*, 68 (7), 4323–4326 (2000).

22. World Health Organisation Report. Available at http://www.who.int/mediacentre /factsheets/fs330/en/ (2013).

23. P. Bardhan, A.S.G. Faruque, A. Naheed, and D.A. Sack, Decreasing shigellosis-related deaths without *Shigella* spp. specific interventions, *Emerging Infectious Disease*, 16, 11 (2010).

24. M.L. Bennish, and B.J. Wojtyniak, Mortality due to shigellosis: Community and hospital data, *Clinical Infectious Diseases*, 13, 245–251 (1991).

25. J. Bos, L. Smithee, B. McClane, R.F. Distefano, F. Uzal, J.G. Songer, S. Mallonee, and M.J. Crutcher, Fatal necrotizing colitis following a foodborne outbreak of enterotoxigenic *Clostridium perfringens* type A infection, *Clinical Infectious Disease*, 40 (10), e78–e83 (2005).

26. R.C. Spencer, *Bacillus anthracis*, *Journal of Clinical Pathology*, 56 (3), 182–187 (2003).

27. S.S. Harthi, The morbidity and mortality pattern of *Brucella endocarditis*, *International Journal of Cardiology*, 25 (3), 321–324 (1989).

28. O.A. Khair, J.L. Devalia, M.M. Abdelaziz, R.J. Sapsford, H. Tarraf, and R.J. Davies, Effect of Haemophilus influenzae endotoxin on the synthesis of IL-6, IL-8, TNF-alpha and expression of ICAM-1 in cultured human bronchial epithelial cells, *European Respiratory Journal*, 7 (12), 2109–2116 (1994).

29. H. Zhang, F. Huang, W. Chen, X. DU, M.G. Zhou, J. Hu, and L.X. Wang, Estimates of tuberculosis mortality rates in China using the disease surveillance point system 2004–2010, *Biomedical and Environmental Sciences*, 25 (4), 483–488 (2012).

30. J. Blanco, A. Muriel-Bombin, V. Sagredo, F. Taboada, F. Gandia, L. Tamayo, J. Collado, A.D. Garcia-Labattut Carriedo, M. Valledor, M.D. Frutos, M.J. Lopez, A. Caballero, J. Guerra, and B. Alvarez, Incidence, organ dysfunction and mortality in severe sepsis: A Spanish multicentre study, *Critical Care*, 12, 6 (2008).

31. G. Beilei, and M. Jianghong, Advanced technologies for pathogen and toxin detection in foods: Current applications and future directions, *Journal of the Association for Laboratory Automation*, 14, 235 (2009).
32. M.B. Paddle, Biosensors for chemical and biological agents of defense interest, *Biosensors and Bioelectronics*, 11, 1079–1113 (1996).
33. E. Ahanotu, D. Alvelo-Ceron, T. Ravita, and E. Gaunt, Staphylococcal enterotoxin B as a biological weapon: Recognition, management, and surveillance of staphylococcal enterotoxin, *Applied Biosafety*, 11, 120–126 (2006).
34. D.V. Lim, J.M. Simpson, E.A. Kearns, and M.F. Kramer, Current and developing technologies for monitoring agents of bioterrorism and biowarfare, *Clinical Microbiology Reviews*, 18 (4), 583–607 (2005).
35. P. McFadden, Biosensors: Broadband biodetection, Holmes on a chip, *Science*, 297, 2075–2076 (2002).
36. A. Rompre, P. Servais, J. Baudart, M.R.D. Roubin, and P. Laurent, Detection and enumeration of coliforms in drinking water: Current methods and emerging approaches, *Journal of Microbiological Methods*, 49, 31–54 (2002).
37. R.M. Atlas, Biological weapons pose challenge for microbiological community, *ASM News*, 64, 383–388 (1998).
38. A. Merkoc, Nanoparticles-based strategies for DNA, protein and cell sensors, *Biosensors and Bioelectronics*, 26, 1164–1177 (2010).
39. T. Haruyama, Micro- and nanobiotechnology for biosensing cellular responses, *Advance Drug Delivery Review*, 55, 393–401 (2003).
40. K.K. Jain, Nanodiagnostics: Application of nanotechnology in molecular diagnostics, *Expert Review in Molecular Diagnostics*, 3, 153–161 (2003).
41. N.L. Rosi, and C.A. Mirkin, Nanostructures in biodiagnostics, *Chemical Review*, 105, 1547–1562 (2005).
42. S.J. Park, T.A. Taton, and C.A. Mirkin, Array-based electrical detection of DNA with nanoparticle probes, *Science*, 295, 1503–1506 (2002).
43. A. Merkoc, Nanobiomaterials in electroanalysis, *Electroanalysis*, 19, 739–741 (2007).
44. J. Wang, Nanoparticle-based electrochemical DNA detection, *Analytical Chemistry Acta*, 500, 247–257 (2003).
45. A. Merkoc, M. Aldavert, S. Marín, and S. Alegret, New materials for electrochemical sensing V: Nanoparticles for DNA labelling, *Trends in Analytical Chemistry*, 24, 341–349 (2005).
46. A. Ambrosi, M.T. Castaneda, A.J. Killard, M.R. Smyth, S. Alegret, and A. Merkoc, Double-codified gold nanolabels for enhanced immunoanalysis, *Analytical Chemistry*, 79, 5232–5240 (2007).
47. A. Merkoc, M. Aldavert, G. Tarrason, R. Eritja, and S. Alegret, Toward an ICPMS-linked DNA assay based on gold nanoparticles immunoconnected through peptide sequences, *Analytical Chemistry*, 77, 6500–6503 (2005).
48. S.E. McNeil, Nanotechnology for the biologist, *Journal of Leukocyte Biology*, 78, 585–594 (2005).
49. B. Perez-Lopez, and A. Merkoci, Nanomaterials based biosensors for food analysis applications, *Trends in Food Science & Technology*, 22, 625–639 (2011).
50. A. Merkoci, A. Ambrosi, D.L. Escosura, A. Perez, B. Guix, M. Maltez, and S. Marin. Nanomaterials for electroanalysis, *Encyclopedia of Analytical Chemistry*, R.A. Meyers (Ed.). Chichester, doi:10.1002/9780470027318.a9077 (2010).
51. A. Ambrosi, M.T. Castañeda, A. de la Escosura-Muñiz, and A. Merkoci, (Eds.), Gold nanoparticles a powerful label for affinity electrochemical biosensors, Chapter 6, in *Biosensing using Nanomaterials e Bionano*, A. Merkoçi (Ed.). 1st Ed. Wiley-Interscience (2009).

52. Y.H. Lin, S.H. Chen, Y.C. Chuang, Y.C. Lu, T.Y. Shen, and C.A. Chang, Disposable amperometric immunosensing strips fabricated by Au nanoparticles-modified screen-printed carbon electrodes for the detection of foodborne pathogen *Escherichia coli* O157:H7, *Biosensors and Bioelectronics*, 23, 1832–1837 (2008).
53. W. Dungchaia, W. Siangprohb, W. Chaicumpac, P. Tongtawed, and O. Chailapakula, *Salmonella typhi* determination using voltammetric amplification of nanoparticles: A highly sensitive strategy for metalloimmunoassay based on a copper-enhanced gold label, *Talanta*, 77, 727–732 (2008).
54. L.J. Yang, and Y.B. Li, Quantum dots as fluorescent labels for quantitative detection of *Salmonella typhimurium* in chicken carcass wash water, *Journal of Food Protection*, 68 (6), 1241–1245 (2005).
55. N. Sanvicens, C. Pastells, N. Pascual, and M.P. Marco, Nanoparticle-based biosensors for detection of pathogenic bacteria, *Trends in Analytical Chemistry*, 28 (11), 1243–1252 (2009).
56. A. De la Escosura-Muñiz, A. Ambrosi, and A. Merkoc, Electrochemical analysis with nanoparticle-based biosystems, *Trends in Analytical Chemistry*, 27 (7), 568–584 (2008).
57. M.T. Castaneda, A. Merkoc, M. Pumera, and S. Alegret, Electrochemical genosensors for biomedical applications based on gold nanoparticles, *Biosensors and Bioelectronics*, 22, 1961–1969 (2007).
58. S. Cao, J. Chen, X. Jin, W. Wu, and Z. Zhao. Enzyme-based biosensors: Synthesis and applications, in *Biosensor Nanomaterials*, S. Li, J. Singh, H. Li, and I. A. Banerjee (Eds.), Wiley-VCH Verlag GmbH & Co. KGaA, Weinheim, Germany (2011).
59. S. Liu, and G. Xuefeng, Carbon nanomaterials field-effect-transistor-based biosensors, *NPG Asia Materials*, 4, e23 (2012).
60. A. Singh, S. Poshtiban, and S. Evoy, Recent advances in bacteriophage based biosensors for food-borne pathogen detection, *Sensors*, 13, 1763–1786 (2013).
61. S.W. Dutse, N.A. Yusof, H. Ahmad, M.Z. Hussein, Z. Zainal, and R. Hushiarian, DNA-based biosensor for detection of ganoderma boninense, an oil palm pathogen utilizing newly synthesized ruthenium complex [Ru(phen)2(qtpy)]2+ based on a PEDOT-PSS/Ag nanoparticles modified electrode, *International Journal of Electrochemical Science*, 8, 11048–11057 (2013).
62. A. Roberto, S. Luz, R.M. Iost, and F.N. Crespilho, Nanomaterials for biosensors and implantable biodevices, *Nanobioelectrochemistry*, 27–48 (2013).
63. P. Leonard, S. Hearty, J. Brennan, L. Dunnea, J. Quinn, T. Chakraborty, and R.O. Kennedy, Enzyme and microbial technology advances in biosensors for detection of pathogens in food and water, *Enzyme and Microbial Technology*, 32, 3–13 (2003).
64. K. Chena, B.R. Li, and Y.T. Chena, Silicon nanowire field-effect transistor-based biosensors for biomedical diagnosis and cellular recording investigation, *Nano Today*, 6, 131–154 (2011).
65. G.J. Yang, J.L. Huang, W.J. Meng, M. Shen, and X.A. Jiao, A reusable capacitive immunosensor for detection of *Salmonella* spp. based on grafted ethylene diamine and self-assembled gold nanoparticle monolayers, *Analytica Chimica Acta*, 647, 159–166 (2009).
66. X. Zhang, P. Geng, H. Liu, Y. Teng, Y. Liu, and Q. Wang, Development of an electrochemical immunoassay for rapid detection of E. coli using anodic stripping voltammetry based on Cu@Au nanoparticles as antibody labels, *Biosensors and Bioelectronics*, 24, 2155–2159 (2009).
67. M. Yuqing, H. Nongyue, W. Xiaohua, and L. Sijiaoa, Nanotechnology and biosensors Chen Jianrong, *Biotechnology & Advances*, 22, 505–518 (2004).
68. C.E. Boubbou Gruden, and X. Huang, Magnetic glyconanoparticles: A unique tool for rapid pathogen detection, decontamination, and strain differentiation, *Journal of the American, Chemical Society*, 129, 13392–13393 (2007).

69. B.J. Yakes, R.J. Lipert, J.P. Bannantine, and M.D. Porter, Detection of *Mycobacterium avium*, Paratuberculosis by a sonicate immunoassay based on surface-enhanced Raman scattering, *Clinical and Vaccine Immunology*, 15, 227–234 (2008).

70. B.E. Setterington, and C.E. Alocilja, Electrochemical biosensor for rapid and sensitive detection of magnetically extracted bacterial pathogens, *Biosensors*, 2 (1), 15–31 (2012).

71. Y. Huang, X. Dong, Y. Liu, J. Li, and P. Chen, Graphene-based biosensors for detection of bacteria and their metabolic activities, *Journal of Materials Chemistry*, 21, 12358–12362 (2011).

72. L.U. Syed, J. Liu, A.K. Price, Y.F. Li, C.T. Culbertson, and J. Li, Dielectrophoretic capture of *E. coli* cells at micropatterned nanoelectrode arrays, *Electrophoresis*, 32, 2358–2365 (2011).

73. A. Gholizadeh, S. Shahrokhian, A.I. Zad, S.M. Vosoughi, S.D.J. Koohsorkhi, and M. Mehran, Fabrication of sensitive glutamate biosensor based on vertically aligned CNT nanoelectrode array and investigating the effect of CNTs density on the electrode performance, *Analytical Chemistry*, 84 (14), 5932–5938 (2012).

74. R. Wang, W. Dong, C. Ruan, D. Kanayeva, K. Lassiter, R. Tian, and Y. Li, TiO2 nanowire bundle microeectrode based impedance immunosensor for rapid and sensitive detection of Listeria monocytogenes, *Nano Letter*, 9, 4570 (2009).

75. Y. Wang, Z. Ye, and Y. Ying, New trends in impedimetric biosensors for the detection of food borne pathogenic bacteria, *Sensors (Basel)*, 12 (3), 3449–3471 (2012).

76. C. Ozdemir, F. Yeni, D. Odaci, and S. Timur, Electrochemical glucose biosensing by pyranose oxidase immobilized in gold nanoparticle-polyaniline/AgCl/gelatin nanocomposite matrix, *Food Chemistry*, 119, 380–385 (2010).

77. A.C. Vinayaka, S. Basheer, and M.S. Thakur, Bioconjugation of CdTe quantum dot for the detection of 2,4-dichlorophenoxyacetic acid by competitive fluoroimmunoassay based biosensor, *Biosensors and Bioelectronics*, 24, 1615–1620 (2009).

78. R. Pennamareddy, K.J. Prabakar, and J. Pandiyan, *Indian Journal of Science and Technology*, 2 (11), 20–22 (2009).

79. J.L. Ding, and B. Ho, Endotoxin detection from *limulus* amebocyte lysate to recombinant factor C, *Subcellular Biochemistry*, 53, 187–208 (2010).

80. S. Iwanaga, and S. Kawabata, Enzybiotics: Antibiotic enzymes as drugs and therapeutics, *Frontiers in Bioscience*, 3, 973–984 (1998).

81. G.K. Lindsay, P.F. Roslansky, and T.J. Novitsky, Single-step, chromogenic limulus amebocyte lysate assay for endotoxin, *Journal of Clinical Microbiology*, 27, 947–951 (1989).

82. N.S. Tan, M.L. Ng, Y.H. Yau, P.K. Chong, B. Ho, and J.L. Ding, Definition of endotoxin binding sites in horseshoe crab factor C recombinant sushi proteins and neutralization of endotoxin by sushi peptides, *The Federation of American Societies for Experimental Biology Journal*, 14 (12), 1801–1813 (2000).

83. R.O. Miranda, X. Li, L.G. Gonzalez, Z.J. Zhu, B. Yan, U.H.F. Bunz, and V.M. Rotello, Colorimetric bacteria sensing using a supramolecular enzyme–nanoparticle biosensor, *Journal of American Chemical Society*, 133 (25), 9650–9653 (2011).

84. T. Laurent, T.D. Huang, P. Bogaerts, and Y. Glupczynski, Evaluation of the βLACTA test, a novel commercial chromogenic test for rapid detection of ceftazidime-nonsusceptible *Pseudomonas aeruginosa* isolates, *Journal of Clinical Microbiology*, 51 (6), 1951–1954 (2013).

85. S. Okumura, T. Akao, E. Mizuki, M. Ohba, and K. Inouye, Screening of the *Bacillus thuringiensis* Cry1Ac delta-endotoxin on the artificial phospholipid monolayer incorporated with brush border membrane vesicles of *Plutella xylostella* by optical biosensor technology methods, *Journal of Biochemical and Biophysical Methods*, 47 (3), 177–188 (2001).

86. V. Velusamy, K. Arshak, O. Orosynska, K. Oliwa, and C. Adley, An overview of food borne pathogen detection: In the perspective of biosensors, *Biotechnology Advances*, 28, 232–254 (2010).
87. O. Lazcka, F.J.D. Campo, and F.X. Munoz, Pathogen detection: A perspective of traditional methods and biosensors, *Biosensors and Bioelectronics*, 22, 1205–1217 (2007).
88. A. Leung, P.M. Shankar, and R. Mutharasan, A review of fiber-optic biosensors, *Sensors and Actuators B*, 125, 688–703 (2007).
89. X. Xue, J. Pan, H. Xie, J. Wang, and S. Zhang, Quantum dot enabled detection of *Escherichia coli* using a cell-phone, *Talanta*, 77 (5), 1808–1813 (2009).
90. J.M. Stroot, K.M. Leach, P.G. Stroot, and D.V. Lim, Capture antibody targeted fluorescence in situ hybridization (CAT-FISH): Dual labeling allows for increased specificity in complex samples, *Journal of Microbiological Methods*, 88 (2), 275–284 (2012).
91. A.D. Romaschin, D.M. Harris, M.B. Ribeiro, J. Paice, D.M. Foster, P.M. Walker, and J.C. Marshall, A rapid assay of endotoxin in whole blood using autologous neutrophil depend chemiluminescence, *Journal of Immunological Methods*, 212 (2), 169–185 (1998).
92. A. Hreniak, K. Maruszewski, J. Rybka, A. Galmian, and J. Czyewski, A luminescence endotoxin biosensor prepared by the sol–gel method, *Optical Materials*, 26 (2), 141–144 (2004).
93. M. Lan, J. Wu, W. Liu, W. Zhang, J. Ge, H. Zhang, J. Sun, W. Zhao, and P. Wang, Copolythiophene-derived colorimetric and fluorometric sensor for visually supersensitive determination of lipopolysaccharide, *Journal of the American Chemical Society*, 5 (6), 2283–2288 (2012).
94. J.J. Mock, R.T. Hill, Y.J. Tsai, A. Chilkoti, and D.R. Smith, Probing dynamically tunable localized surface plasmon resonances of film-coupled nanoparticles by evanescent wave excitation, *Nano Letter*, 12 (4), 1757–1764 (2012).
95. B. Barlen, S.D. Mazumdar, O. Lezrich, P. Kampfer, and M. Keusgen, Detection of *Salmonella* by surface plasmon resonance, *Sensors*, 7 (8), 1427–1446 (2007).
96. N. Tawil, E. Sacher, R. Mandeville, and M. Meunier, Surface plasmon resonance detection of *E. coli* and methicillin-resistant *S. aureus* using bacteriophages, *Biosensors and Bioelectronics*, 37, 24–29 (2012).
97. M. Burkhardt, A. Lopez Acosta, K. Reiter, V. Lopez, and A. Lees, Purification of soluble CD14 fusion proteins and in use in electrochemiluminescent assay for lipopolysaccharide binding, *Protein Expression and Purification*, 51, 96–101 (2007).
98. S. Ding, B. Chang, C. Wu, C. Chen, and H. Chang, A new method for detection of endotoxin on polymyxin B-immobilized gold electrodes, *Electrochemistry Communications*, 9 (5), 1206–1211 (2007).
99. M.S.A. Rahman, S.C. Mukhopadhyay, P. Yu, J. Goicoechea, I.R. Martis, C.P. Gooneratne, and J. Kosel, Lossy mode resonance optical fiber sensor to detect organic vapors, *Journal of Food Engineering*, 114, 346–360 (2013).
100. M. Urgun-Demirtas, B. Stark, and K. Pagilla, Use of genetically engineered microorganisms (GEMs) for the bioremediation of contaminants, *Critical Reviews in Biotechnology*, 26 (3), 145–164 (2006).

12 Electrochemical Biosensors for Detecting DNA Damage and Genotoxicity

Ali A. Ensafi and Esmaeil Heydari-Bafrooei

CONTENTS

ABSTRACT

Biosensors based on biorecognition events occurring in monolayer or thin-film assemblies on electronic transducers represent an important recent advance in bioelectronics. DNA biosensors constitute an important class of point-of-care diagnostic devices because they are capable of converting the Watson–Crick base pair recognition event signal into an interpretable analytical signal in a shorter time compared with other methods, thereby producing accurate and sensitive results. The emergence of nanotechnology is opening new horizons for the application of nanomaterials in bioelectroanalytical chemistry. The use of nanomaterials in DNA biosensors has taken off rapidly and will surely continue to expand. The unique properties of nanoparticles, nanotubes, and nanowires offer excellent prospects for developing novel nanomaterial-based electrochemical DNA biosensors. Because of their high surface area, nontoxicity, biocompatibility, and charge-sensitive conductance, nanomaterials serve as effective transducers in nanoscale DNA biosensing and bioelectronic devices. This chapter describes new signal amplification and coding strategies for electrochemical DNA damage detection based on the use of nanomaterials.

Keywords: DNA damage, Biosensor, Electrochemical, Genotoxicity, Dendrimers, Carbon nanotubes.

12.1   INTRODUCTION

Electrochemistry is superior in a number of ways to other existing measurement systems. Moreover, electrochemical measurement protocols are suitable for mass fabrication of miniaturized devices. For example, electrochemical biosensors can provide rapid, simple, and low-cost on-field detection. They offer sensitive and selective means of detecting selected DNA sequences, DNA damage, or mutated genes associated with human diseases. DNA-based electrochemical sensors exploit a range of different chemistries, but all take advantage of nanoscale interactions between the target or the damaging agent in solution, the recognition layer, and a solid electrode surface.

It is commonly established that nucleic acid bases undergo reduction and oxidation at the surface of electrodes. Studies of long-chain DNA and RNA molecules have shown that the electrochemical signals of these molecules can be significantly influenced by their ordered higher structures. Electrochemical methods can, therefore, be employed both to detect minor damage to the DNA double helix and to study structural transitions in nucleic acids. Various kinds of nucleic acid interactions can be studied by electrochemical methods. Binding of electroactive substances to DNA can be manifested by changes in their signals. Both electroactive and electroinactive compounds may affect the nucleic acid signals, particularly if their binding results in changes of the DNA structure. It was probably in the 1980s that the first DNA-modified electrode was used, and a few years later, supercoiled DNA, rather than linear DNA, was immobilized on the electrode surface to create a new tool for sensing DNA damage.

Numerous approaches have been developed for electrochemical detection, including direct electrochemistry of DNA, electrochemistry at polymer-modified electrodes, electrochemistry of DNA-specific redox reporters, and electrochemical devices based on DNA-mediated charge transport chemistry. However, electrochemical amplifications with nanoparticles have been identified as one of the best strategies for the enhancement of biosensor sensitivity. Recent studies have demonstrated that nanomaterials not only are capable of enhancing the electrochemical reactivity of important biomolecules but also can promote the electron-transfer reactions of DNA. In addition to enhanced electrochemical reactivity, nanomaterial-modified electrodes have been used to accumulate important biomolecules (e.g., nucleic acids) and to alleviate surface fouling effects. The remarkable sensitivity of nanomaterials to surface adsorbates enables them to be used as highly sensitive nanoscale sensors.

These properties make them extremely attractive for a wide range of applications as electrochemical DNA biosensors. It is the aim of this chapter to describe new signal amplification and DNA immobilization strategies for electrical DNA damage detection based on the use of nanomaterials.

12.2 DNA DAMAGE

DNA is under constant attack from endogenous or exogenous reactive chemical species that produce a wide range of chemical lesions. The relationships between cellular DNA damage caused by endogenous and environmental genotoxic agents, the cellular response, and the development and prevention of human diseases and aging are areas of great current interest in medical, biological, and chemical research [1]. It has been estimated that there are tens of thousands of DNA-damaging events per day suffered by approximately 10^{13} cells within the human body [2] and that DNA damage associated with endogenous species is more extensive (greater than 75%) than that caused by environmental factors [3].

The sources of DNA damage can be divided into three classes. The first class of lesions is attributed to spontaneous causes, which include mechanisms such as deamination of cytosine to uracile, or 5-methyl cytosine leading to thymine or spontaneous depurination or enzyme-mediated base removal that can produce basic sites. Another example is provided by mismatches or insertions/deletions erroneously introduced by polymerases during DNA replication. The second class of lesions is attributed to reactive species endogenously generated by physiological or pathological processes (such as mitochondrial respiration, inflammation, or infectious diseases). These processes can alter DNA's primary structure, for instance, through oxidation of DNA or formation of basic sites. Reactive oxygen species, reactive nitrogen species, or lipid peroxidation products are classic examples of these factors. These reactive intermediates are produced under conditions of oxidative stress, a consequence of normal metabolic activity, and the inflammatory response [3,4]. The third class of lesions is attributed to exogenous physical or chemical agents that are able to generate a large variety of lesions including strand breaks (damaging the phosphodiester backbone of DNA), DNA bulky adducts, or DNA cross-links. For example, ionizing radiation can induce single- and double-strand breaks and exposure to UV light can produce pyrimidine dimers, while a variety of bulky adducts are formed upon DNA interactions with metabolically activated carcinogens such as aromatic amines or polycyclic aromatic hydrocarbons. The principal sources of exogenous alkylating agents are industrial processes, tobacco smoke, and dietary components. It is worth noting that some of these agents are voluntarily administered to cancer patients in order to treat tumors, using strategies such as radiotherapy or alkylating drug-based chemotherapies [4]. The occurrence of lesions in DNA produces structural and dynamic changes in DNA, which impair its function and initiate a complex series of molecular and cellular reactions comprising deleterious events leading to cell death or mutagenesis and defensive mechanisms requiring cell cycle arrest, DNA remodeling, and DNA repair. Different lesions are repaired via different pathways. Damaged bases or base mismatches are excised by the action of N-glycosylases or nucleases (in base excision repair, nucleotide excision repair, or mismatch repair) while highly cytotoxic double-strand breaks are repaired in the course of a mechanism involving DNA recombination. Extensive DNA damage that would be hardly repairable frequently induces programmed cell death (apoptosis). Unrepaired DNA lesions can promote genetic alterations (mutations) that may be linked to an altered phenotype, and, if growth-controlling genes are involved, these mutations can lead to cell transformation and the development of malignant tumors. Proto-oncogenes and tumor suppressor genes may be critical targets for DNA damaging agents.

12.3 CURRENT METHODS OF DNA DAMAGE DETECTION

Detection and analysis of DNA damage are of critical importance in a variety of biological disciplines studying apoptosis, cell cycle and cell division, carcinogenesis, tumor growth, embryogenesis and aging, neurodegenerative and heart diseases, anticancer drug development, and environmental and radiobiological research, among others. Over a period of a few decades, a number of methods have been invented to detect DNA damage in various organisms. To measure DNA damage by most of the currently available chromatographic methods, the isolated DNA is hydrolyzed and the hydrolysate is subsequently prepared for analysis by high-performance liquid chromatography [5–9], gas chromatography [10], or capillary electrophoresis [11] combined with different detection techniques. These methods are highly sensitive, allowing for detection of one damaged base among 10^7 normal ones [7] but may suffer from false positives arising from additional DNA oxidation during sample preparation [5–12]. In some procedures, DNA is exposed to elevated temperatures (e.g., in acidic hydrolysis and in derivatization for gas chromatography–mass spectrometry [GC-MS]) and prooxidant chemicals such as phenol. Therefore, isolation, hydrolysis, and analysis all have the potential to cause further artifactual oxidation of DNA (especially of guanine residues), raising the apparent level of base oxidation products and invalidating the measurement. For example, levels of 8-oxoguanine (8-OHG) (a product of oxidative DNA damage) in acid-hydrolyzed calf thymus DNA by GC-MS techniques are often, but not always, higher than those measured (as 8-OHG) by other methods after enzymic DNA hydrolysis [13,14]. The discrepancy is usually attributed to the artifactual oxidation of guanine during preparation of DNA for GC-MS analysis.

In the other group of techniques, changes in the features of whole DNA molecules (i.e., without complete hydrolysis) upon their damage are monitored. For example, comet assay also called "single cell gel electrophoresis" is a technique for the detection of DNA damage and repair at the level of single cells, which is one of the most advanced techniques introduced to the agricultural sciences in recent years. Isolated DNA from cells are embedded in a thin agarose gel on a microscope slide and unwound in a suitable buffer to be exposed to a weak electric field for attracting broken, negatively charged DNA toward the anode. After electrophoresis, the migrated DNA fragments stained with a fluorescent dye would resemble a shape of a comet observed by fluorescence microscopy. The extent of comet-like shapes would indicate the level of DNA damage in cells. The intensity of comet tail relative to the head would also reflect the extent of DNA damage numerically. Polymerase chain reaction (PCR), halo, terminal deoxyribonucleotidyl transferase–mediated deoxyuridine triphosphate nick end labeling (TUNEL assay), fluorescence in situ hybridization, flow cytometry, Annexin V labeling, immunological assay including immunofluorescent and chemiluminescence thymine dimer detection, immunohistochemical assay, enzyme-linked immunosorbent assay, and radio immunoassay are other methods available for detecting different kinds of DNA damage but with some or other limitations.

12.4   ELECTROCHEMICAL DETECTION OF DNA DAMAGE

Developing accurate assays for DNA damage has attracted increased attention among analytical chemists. The challenge is that any new and fast assay must have sufficient sensitivity to detect one damaged nucleotide in 10^4–10^7 intact nucleotide residues, depending on the type of lesion, in microgram amounts of DNA [15–17].

The development of electrochemical transducer–based devices for determining nucleotide sequences and measuring DNA damage began slowly, but recent progress is encouraging. The main advantages of these devices are their low cost, simple design, small dimensions, and low power requirements. Altered chemical, physicochemical, and structural properties of the damaged DNA are reflected in its redox behavior, which is utilized in numerous DNA damage detection techniques. Electrochemical DNA-based biosensors have been used not only to detect but also to induce and control DNA damage at the electrode surface via electrochemical generation of the damaging (usually radical) species [18]. These devices have been employed to study such chemicals and drugs as niclosamide, adriamycin, benznidazole, thiophene-S-oxide, and nitroderivatives of polycyclic aromatic compounds [19,20].

The electronic transduction of nucleic acid/DNA complexes on electronic transducers such as electrodes or semiconductors could provide a device for DNA damage detection. An electrochemical sensor for detecting DNA damage consists of an electrode with DNA on its surface (Figure 12.1). These devices enable researchers to study the interaction of DNA immobilized on the electrode surface and the analytes in solution, with DNA acting as a promoter between the electrode and the biological molecule under study. Interactions of the surface-confined DNA with a

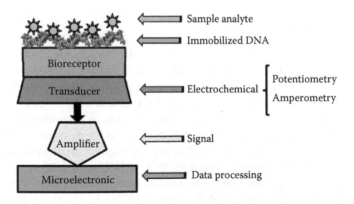

FIGURE 12.1   Schematic diagram showing the main components of a DNA-based electrochemical biosensor.

DNA-damaging agent are converted, via changes in the electrochemical properties of the DNA recognition layer, into measurable electrical signals [21]. The interaction of a number of substances with DNA has been successfully studied using such biosensors, and the interpretation of the results has contributed to the elucidation of the mechanisms by which DNA is damaged by hazardous compounds [22,23].

In using an electrochemical transducer, the analyte must be necessarily electroactive; that is, it should be capable of undergoing heterogeneous electron transfer reactions. The four different bases of DNA (the purines, adenine [A] and guanine [G], and pyrimidines, thymine [T] and cytosine [C]) are all electroactive. At most types of electrodes, deoxyribose and ribose in nucleosides and nucleotides as well as the phosphate groups in the sugar-phosphate backbone are electroinactive unlike the bases that are able to undergo electroreduction or electrooxidation.

A critical issue in the development of a DNA electrochemical biosensor is the sensor material and the degree of surface coverage that influences directly the sensor response. Electrode surface characteristics, therefore, represent an important aspect of the construction of sensitive DNA electrochemical biosensors for rapid detection of DNA interaction and damage. Nucleic acids, and particularly DNA, have been analyzed primarily with liquid mercury and solid carbon electrodes [24–26], including the recently applied boron-doped diamond electrodes [27]. Several studies have also been conducted with other electrodes such as gold, copper, silver, and platinum. More recently, gold, carbon, indium tin oxide (ITO), solid amalgam electrodes, and mercury film electrodes are gaining importance in connection with the development of DNA sensors. Compared to mercury-containing electrodes, the potential windows of most of the solid electrodes are shifted by approximately 1 V to more positive values. The latter electrodes are thus better suited for studying nucleic acid oxidation, while mercury-containing electrodes (both liquid and solid) are better suited for investigating reduction of nucleic acids and their binders. The atomically smooth and highly reproducible surfaces of liquid mercury are particularly suitable for alternating current (ac) impedance measurements, including the impedance spectroscopy, which can provide important information about DNA and RNA interfacial properties (Reference [28] and references therein).

12.4.1 DNA-Modified Electrodes

Earlier DNA biosensor applications typically involved a solution phase (DNA solution) [17,29]. Over the last decade, however, researchers have focused on the ordered structure of DNA onto the sensor surface because of its high sensitivity for detecting the target DNA. For this reason, scientists prefer synthetic and short DNA fragments with known base sequences related to genetic diseases or microorganisms such as viruses and bacteria. Typical DNA probes take 15 to 25 base pairs long that are able to detect their target sequences. Besides the probe, calf thymus and salmon sperm double-stranded or single-stranded DNA (dsDNA and ssDNA, respectively) molecules have also been immobilized onto the recognition element of a biosensor. Looked at from the viewpoint of DNA damage, dsDNA has been used in numerous sensor applications [16] for the detection of DNA damages based on the electrochemical signals of nucleic acids, especially guanine.

DNA immobilization onto the transducer is also a key issue in the construction of biosensing devices. The choice of the immobilization method depends mainly on the biomolecule to be immobilized, the nature of the solid surface, and the transducing mechanism [30]. In addition to the sensitivity of the electrochemical transducer, its ability to provide a stable immobilization environment while retaining its bioactivity must also be considered: a current problem regarding the immobilized biomolecules is the lack of stability and activity in the solid transducer, which is usually overwhelmed by mimicking the in vivo-like environment or the use of spacer arms. Control of the DNA binding surface in terms of surface orientation and coverage is essential for the sensitive monitoring of DNA–DNA and compound–DNA interactions by electrochemistry. The most successful immobilization methods involve adsorption and covalent attachment.

The adsorption method at a controlled potential or without applying a potential, called "wet adsorption" [31,32], is the easiest way to immobilize DNA onto carbon transducers [33,34]. In the adsorption-based immobilization technique, there is no need for special reagents, expensive labeled nucleic acids, or long experimental steps. However, random immobilization of DNA is achieved with this technique and nucleic acids bind weakly onto the surface in parallel layers. Additionally, it is possible to agglomerate DNA onto the surface and the noncovalently bound DNA can be removed from the transducer surface when the electrode is rinsed stringently. Wet adsorption initiates a weak binding that causes easy desorption of the biomolecule from the surface, to leach eventually into the sample solution during measurements. However, dry adsorption also promotes hydrophobic bonds and more stable adsorbed layers on solid surfaces. Furthermore, the adsorption properties of DNA on various supports (e.g., nylon or nitrocellulose) have been known for a long time [35]. The binding forces involving physical adsorption include hydrogen bonds, electrostatic interaction, van der Waals forces, and hydrophobic interactions if water molecules are excluded by dryness [36].

The other method for the immobilization of DNA onto surfaces is covalent attachment. Pividori and Alegret were the first to bind DNA to a pretreated electrode via covalent attachment using carbodiimide molecules [37] followed by binding DNA to the surface from its guanine bases. This method was later improved by adding the N-hydroxysulfosuccinimide reagent in order to activate the carboxyl groups on the carbon electrode. Single-stranded amino-linked DNA or label-free short DNA sequences are thus bound to these groups by their amino tags [38] and deoxyguanosine residues, respectively [37]. On the other hand, covalent agents can also be applied to the untreated carbon surface directly before DNA immobilization onto activated sites of carbodiimide compounds [38].

12.4.2 Detection of DNA Cleavage Using DNA-Based Biosensors

Besides electrophoretic techniques [39–41] and methods based on determination of the ends of polynucleotide chains (such as the TUNEL test [42–44]), cleavage of DNA sugar-phosphate backbone can be detected by electrochemical DNA–based biosensors. These biosensors are based on the strong dependence of accessibility of DNA bases to the transducer surface and DNA conformation and include highly sensitive detection of the strand break formation using mercury electrodes [22,39,45–49] and other techniques suitable for monitoring deeper DNA degradation employing solid (primarily carbon) electrodes [50–54]. These methods are based either on measurements of intrinsic guanine oxidation signal or on application of redox indicators of DNA degradation.

Mercury-based DNA biosensors are able to discriminate between DNA molecules containing and lacking free chain ends when free ends produce specific electrochemical responses under certain conditions. Detection of the strand break at the hanging mercury drop electrode (HMDE) is highly sensitive. By using ac voltammetry, one strand break is detected among more than 2×10^5 nucleotides [51]. In undamaged dsDNA, the nucleobases are secreted in the double helix center, resulting in weak electroactivity of the undamaged DNA and a notable dependence of the intensity of specific DNA signals on the formation of the strand break facilitating communication of the base residues with the mercury surface (reviewed in References [16,22,39,52–55]).

In addition to measurement of intrinsic DNA oxidation response, the redox indicator–based sensor was developed for the detection of DNA strand break using solid electrodes. This technique is based on the selective binding of a metallointercalator $[Co(phen)_3]^{3+}$ to dsDNA at the carbon electrode surface, resulting in enhancement of its voltammetric signals. Deep degradation of DNA during the step of biosensor incubation for a given time (minutes to hours) in the cleavage medium under investigation, after the medium exchange for the follow-up electrochemical measurement, results in a decreased voltammetric response of the metal complex indicator that binds to DNA (such as $[Co(phen)_3]^{3+}$ [56–59]) or into enhancement of the voltammetric response of the negatively charged metal complex like $[Fe(CN)_6]^{3-/4-}$, which is repulsed by the negatively charged DNA layer, depending on the degree of DNA damage [60,61]. Change in the indicator electrochemical response depends on the portion of DNA damaged in the cleavage reaction. Since affinity of the cobalt redox marker to the degraded DNA is much lower than that to the intact dsDNA, the decrease in its voltammetric peak represents the response to the DNA damage. This scheme was applied, for example, in detecting DNA damage by chemical nucleases such as copper, 1,10-phenanthroline complex [50], or in studies of antioxidative properties of yeast polysaccharides [62], flavonoids [51,53], or plant extracts [52].

12.4.3 Detection of Damage to DNA Bases Using DNA-Based Biosensors

The most common and perhaps the most important type of DNA damage is base damage, which occurs at the rate of several thousand base pairs per cell per day in humans [63]. This damage is primarily caused by endogenous metabolic and immune processes rather than environmental toxins, with the exception of UV damage to the skin from sunlight and oxidative damage to lung and blood from smoking [64,65]. Because of the susceptibility of the guanine base to damage by a broad range of genotoxic agents [66–68] and its well-defined electrochemistry at both carbon and mercury electrodes, guanine redox peaks have been frequently utilized as transduction signals in DNA biosensors for the detection of base damage [69–76]. Decrease in the guanine peak current relative to that yielded by intact DNA represents the response to damage to the nucleobase or its release from the polynucleotide chains, which is an event often following modifications within the guanine imidazole ring. Since natural DNA contains many guanine residues, partial decrease in the guanine peaks is usually observed, depending on the extent of DNA damage.

Alkylation of guanine results in a decrease of DNA redox peak guanine measured also by cyclic voltammetry (CV), squarewave voltammetry, or electrochemical impedance spectroscopy (EIS) at the mercury and carbon electrodes. Using this signal, DNA modification by different methylation agents such as dimethyl sulfate (DMS) and mitomycin C (MC) was studied both in solution and at the mercury and carbon surfaces [77,78]. Decrease in the same signal was observed because of DNA modification by thiotepa [76], platinum complexes [79], hydrazine derivatives [70], polychlorinated biphenyls, aflatoxins, anthracenes, acridines, phenol compounds [71,80–82], ultraviolet light [83], arsenic oxide [76], and so on. Besides the low specificity of this type of response, the general problem of relatively low sensitivity is connected with the signal-off approach. These types of DNA sensors are relatively simple, do not require mercury electrodes, and can work with relatively poorly defined, inexpensive, commercially available DNAs.

Better results (regarding sensitivity and obviously specificity as well) can be obtained when a DNA lesion yields products that show characteristic electrochemical activity possessing a new signal. For example, 8-OHG, one of the most abundant products of oxidative DNA damage, is electrochemically oxidized at carbon electrodes at a potential significantly less positive than the parent guanine base [19,20,56]. This approach exhibits much better sensitivity and specificity. Electrooxidation of 8-OHG was recently studied at different solid electrodes, including carbon, gold, platinum, and tin oxide [84]. The oxidation signal of 8-OHG appeared because of the adriamycin-mediated oxidative damage of DNA deposited at the glassy carbon electrode (GCE) [85]. The complexes of osmium (such as $[Os(bipy)_3]^{3+}$) and ruthenium with different redox potentials have been shown as electrocatalysts for 8-OHG and guanine, respectively [86,87].

Chemically modified DNA may acquire specific electrochemical features because of the substances forming bulky adducts with it. A clinically used antitumor agent, MC, covalently binds primarily to G residues, forming interstrand or intrastrand cross-links (Refs. [72,73,88] and references therein). The MC moiety involves reversibly electroreducible quinone moiety. Interactions of acid-activated or reductively activated MC with DNA were investigated by means of CV and EIS [72], including studies of electrochemical MC activation [72,88].

Chemical modification of DNA base residues may be referred to as changes in the DNA double helix structure, including its opening break of the Watson–Crick pairing of the damaged or adjacent bases, formation of base mismatches, and so forth [67,69,74]. These events may influence the behavior of the damaged DNA at electrode surfaces in DNA-based biosensors. For example, the conformational change of DNA arising from its UV-induced damage has been observed to influence the intensity of amperometric signals related to DNA interactions with polypyrrole-modified electrodes [89]. Accessibility of guanine residues for their oxidation at solid electrodes may also be improved because of the disturbance in the dsDNA structure.

Enhancement of the electrocatalytic current of guanine owing to the ruthenium chelate-mediated guanine oxidation or of the electrogenerated chemiluminescence signal [90,91] was reportedly observed as responses to the DNA damage.

DNA base damages can be detected enzymatically using electrochemical DNA–based biosensors. It has been shown that basic sites can be detected by ac voltamme-try at the HMDE after DNA enzymatic digestion by *Escherichia coli exonuclease III* [92,93], an enzyme introducing ssb next to basic lesions, followed by exonu-cleolytic degradation of one strand of DNA. This procedure allowed for the detec-tion of small extents of base changes, not detectable without enzymatic digestion, and was successfully applied to probe base lesions induced by DMS or UV light in living bacterial cells [93]. Multilayer assemblies of cationic redox-active poly-mer films, DNA, and hemoproteins at carbon electrodes have also been designed for testing the genotoxic activity of various chemicals [94]. In these devices, lay-ers of enzymatically active hemoproteins mimic metabolic carcinogen activation processes (e.g., styrene is enzymatically converted to styrene oxide). The activated species diffuse into the DNA layer and attack guanine residues, and the damaged DNA double helix is indicated by using guanine oxidation mediated by the aca-tionic polymeric film.

An electrochemical biosensor using a hairpin DNA with an oxidizable ferrocene label has been introduced for the detection of activities of enzymes such as nucleases (generating single-strand breaks) and DNA ligases (sealing the break) [95]. At a single-strand break in the duplex part of the hairpin structure, the ferrocene-labeled segment was removed under conditions of denaturation with diminution of the cur-rent signal. In the presence of ligase activity, the break was joined, preventing the removal of the ferrocene-labeled segment.

12.4.4 Detection of DNA Association Interactions Using DNA-Based Biosensors

A variety of small molecules are known to interact reversibly with dsDNA through one of the following three modes: (i) electrostatic interactions with the negatively charged nucleic sugar-phosphate structure, (ii) groove binding interactions, or (iii) intercalations between the stacked base pairs of dsDNA [96,97]. A quantitative understanding of the reasons determining the selection of DNA reaction sites is use-ful in designing sequence-specific DNA binding molecules for application in chemo-therapy and in explaining the mechanism involved in the action of neoplastic drugs [98]. It is very important to explain the factors that determine affinity and selectivity in binding molecules to DNA and research on metal ion–nucleic acid complexes advanced when the antitumor activities of platinum (II) compounds were discovered. The action of many carcinogens, cytostatics, environmental pollutants, and so forth involves reversible binding to DNA. DNA association interactions are of interest for chemistry, molecular biology, and medicine, particularly for drug discovery and environmental/medical processes [99,100]. They concern association with both inor-ganic and organic compounds as well as various types of assisted interactions such as metal and metal complex–DNA chemistry [22]. DNA-based biosensors serve as effective screening tools for in vitro tests of this large group of DNA interactions.

Formation of noncovalent DNA complexes with small molecules can be detected via changes in the electrochemical behavior of both the binders and the DNA. Upon binding to large molecules of DNA, apparent diffusion coefficients of the binder decrease, and altered mass transport of these species influences its electrochemical signals [101–105]. This phenomenon has been used to determine association/dissociation constants of the binder–DNA complexes. Peak potentials of the binders may also be changed upon complex formation, depending on the binding mode [106]. Voltammetric studies of complexes and the associates of toxic heavy metals (lead, cadmium [103,107], copper [108,109], mercury [110], nickel [111]) or their complexes ($[Co(NH_3)_6]^{3+}$ [112], dimeric rhodium complexes [113]) with DNA and its components have been studied electrochemically at mercury as well as solid electrodes. Association interactions (and especially intercalations) may induce remarkable changes in the dsDNA conformation, including DNA unwinding and increasing accessibility of the base residues to the environment. These phenomena are often connected with alterations in the intrinsic DNA redox or tensametric signals at carbon or mercury electrodes.

Impedimetric measurements also provide the possibility for detecting electrochemically inactive analytes, which do not bring about noticeable changes in the guanine oxidation current [114,115]. Recently, impedimetry performed in the presence of intercalators has been reported to specify the type of DNA interactions [116].

Electrodes modified with dsDNA have been used as sensors for various reversibly binding substances. Interactions of intercalators or cationic groove binders with the DNA recognition layer result in accumulation of these substances at the DNA-modified electrode, resulting in enhanced binder electrochemical signals. Aromatic amines, important environmental carcinogens, were sensitively detected upon their accumulation within dsDNA anchored at the electrode surfaces [69,81,117].

12.5 NANOMATERIAL-BASED AMPLIFIED ELECTROCHEMICAL DETECTION OF DNA DAMAGE

The high-throughput analysis of DNA damage has enormous diagnostic significance for the early detection of genetic disorders in embryos or newborns or for the continuous detection of mutations that lead to fatal diseases such as cancer. Recent accomplishments in nanotechnology and the discovery of nanoparticles have led to new approaches to the electrochemical detection of DNA damage. Nanomaterials have a number of features such as high surface area, high reactivity, easy dispersibility, and rapid fabrication that make them ideally suited for sensor applications.

12.5.1 DENDRIMERS

The biocompatibility of dendrimers along with their enhanced surface area allows for increased immobilization of DNA on the dendrimer-modified electrode, which can result in a higher sensitivity in the detection of DNA damage [117]. Polyamidoamine (PAMAM) and poly(propylimine) dendrimers possessing amine end groups are highly suitable for use as DNA biosensors. Very few studies on the exploitation of dendrimers in electrochemical DNA biosensors for the detection of DNA damage have been reported in the literature. Recently, a DNA biosensor using a fourth-generation PAMAM dendrimer has been reported [118]. The biosensor was fabricated by immobilizing dsDNA on a thin layer of dendrimer-encapsulated bimetallic nanoparticles (Au-Pd) in a chitosan composite on a GCE (Scheme 1). Using this biosensor as an oxidation target and utilizing a Fenton-type reaction as a method of inducing DNA damage by generating OH radicals, it was possible both to detect DNA damage and to assess the antioxidant capacity of sericin. This was accomplished in two stages. First, a dsDNA/PAMAM-Au-Pd/GCE biosensor was immersed in an acetate buffer to obtain the guanine oxidation peak that was recorded in the acetate buffer as a blank signal (I_{pblank}). Second, another dsDNA/PAMAM-Au-Pd/GCE biosensor was immersed in a reagent solution containing iron/EDTA ions and hydrogen peroxide (Fenton reagent for producing OH radical) in the absence and presence of sericin, respectively. After a short time, the electrode was washed and then immersed in the acetate buffer to obtain the electrochemical response to guanine oxidation. The peak currents in the acetate buffer in the absence (I_{pa}) or presence of an antioxidant (I_{pp}) were recorded. The scavenging percentage of hydroxyl radical (OH) by sericin was calculated using the following equation:

$$\frac{I_{pp} - I_{pa}}{I_{pblank} - I_{pa}} \times 100\%.$$

The prominent feature of the approach is that this linker system is able to enhance the immobilized amount of DNA strands, enlarge the electrochemical signal of DNA indicator, increase the sensitivity for DNA detection, and increase biosensor stability [118].

In another study, the covalent immobilization method was employed to construct a DNA biosensor based on a PAMAM-modified gold electrode using differential pulse voltammetry (DPV) and daunomycin as the electroactive indicator [119]. Chemical modification of the gold electrode was carried out by treatment with mercaptoacetic acid for 2 h at room temperature. The electrode was then immersed in a solution containing appropriate quantities of dendrimer and 1-(3-dimethylaminopropyl)-3-ethylcarbodiimide hydrochloride (EDC). The presence of EDC is very essential for the firm anchorage of the dendrimer to the electrode surface. In the presence of EDC, peptide bond formation takes place between the PAMAM dendrimer molecules and the surface-attached thiol species. Immobilization of DNA was performed by immersing the electrode in the oligonucleotide solution containing EDC in the acetate buffer at pH 5.2 for 10 h. The DPV measurements were conducted from −0.1 to +0.5 V versus SCE in a phosphate buffer solution. The peak current at +0.23 V corresponding to the oxidation of daunomycin was taken as the electrochemical measurement signal. The daunomycin-intercalated DNA duplex electrode gave an increased electrochemical response.

Recently, a DNA biosensor using a first-generation PAMAM dendrimer has been reported [120]. In this study, instead of the gold electrode, a preoxidized GCE was used to form the dendrimer-modified electrode using N-hydroxysuccinimide and EDC as the coupling agents.

The electrochemical impedance technique has been shown to be a useful method for a DNA biosensor using a multinuclear nickel(II) salicylaldimine metallodendrimer platform [121]. Both the preparation of the dendrimer-modified GCE surface and the immobilization of DNA have been effectively accomplished by simple drop-coating procedures. Being electroactive, the metallodendrimer exhibited two redox couples in the phosphate buffer solution. Changes in the impedance signal were taken as indications of DNA damage.

12.5.2 Polymeric Nanoparticles

The most widely investigated polymeric nanomaterials used for biomacromolecule immobilization are conducting polymers including polyaniline (PANI), poly(phenylenevinylene), polypyrrole, polythiophene, polyacetylene, and polyindole [122]. The unique electronic structure of polymeric nanomaterials is responsible for their remarkably high electrical conductivity, ease of processing, low ionization potential, good environmental stability, and high electron affinity. Their conductivity exhibits a strong dependence on solution pH and oxidation state [123]. Conducting polymeric materials retain the exclusive properties of nanomaterials like large surface area and size as well as quantum effects, which add further to their merits for designing and making novel biosensors [123–126]. Regarding biological applications, the thickness and shape of the polymeric film, which is its most important factor in controlling the electrochemical characteristics of transducers, can be readily controlled within the nanometer to micrometer range by modifying the deposition method. These excellent properties of the polymeric nanomaterials provide better signal transduction as well as enhanced sensitivity, selectivity, durability, biocompatibility, direct electrochemical synthesis, and flexibility for the immobilization of biomolecules including DNA [123]. The versatility of these polymers may be determined by the following characteristics: biocompatibility, capability to transduce energy arising from the interaction of the analyte and the analyte-recognizing site into electrical signals that are easily monitored, capability to protect electrodes from interfering materials, and ease of electrochemical deposition on the surface of any type of electrode. Nowadays, polymeric nanomaterials are becoming major tools in nanobiotechnological applications. A thin film of polymeric nanomaterials having both high conductivity and fine structure on the nanoscale is a suitable substrate used for the immobilization of polynucleotides in the electrochemical DNA damage detection.

Ghanbari et al. [127] applied an electrochemically deposited nanostructured polypyrrole film onto a Pt electrode for the immobilization of DNA. Scanning electron microscopy (SEM), CV, and EIS were used to analyze the surface morphology and the analytical characteristics of the electropolymerized polypyrrole film deposited on the Pt electrode. In order to evaluate two types of synthesis methods, they compared the polymer morphologies of films synthesized by the CV (Figure 12.2a) and normal pulse voltammetry (NPV) (Figure 12.2b through h) methods. The SEM images revealed that stocky, rod-like structures were created when the CV method was used and that much finer filamentous structures were created by the NPV one. It was further shown that when DNA was physisorbed onto this PPy nanofiber

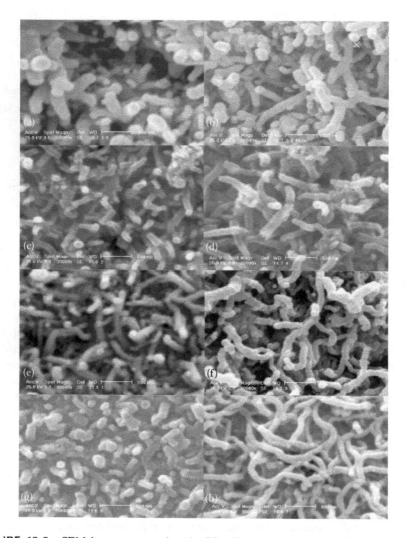

FIGURE 12.2 SEM images comparing the PPy films prepared by (a) CV and (b) NPV (Cpy = 0.1 M, PD = 0.1 s, PI = 6 mV). Synthesis conditions of NPV-prepared PPy films: Cpy (c) 0.02 M; (d) 0.15 M (PD = 0.4 s, PI = 4 mV); PI (e) 2 mV; (f) 10 mV (Cpy = 0.1 M, PD = 0.4 s); PD (g) 0.2 s; (h) 0.4 s (Cpy = 0.1 M, PI = 4 mV). PI, pulse increment; PD, pulse duration; Cpy, concentration of pyrrole. (License No. 3375440889869)

film–coated Pt electrode, the resulting electrochemical biosensor was able to detect DNA–spermidine interactions using the oxidation of guanine in the DNA. The NPV method enabled Ppy nanofiber films of higher electroactivity to be prepared owing to the higher specific surface area (Figure 12.2b through h). Ramanavicius et al. [128] reported the potential pulse technique as the most suitable method for the preparation of nanostructured Ppy with entrapped biomolecules. The potentiostatic and potentiodynamic method of electropolymerization was also used to prepare Ppy nanofibers [129]. Electrodes prepared by the potentiostatic procedure showed higher

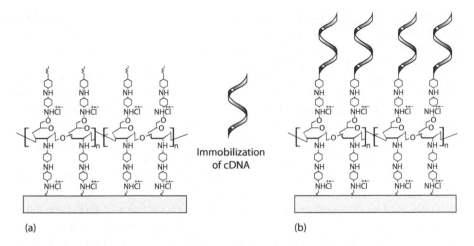

(a)   (b)

FIGURE 12.3 Schematic presentation of the (a) fabrication of CHIT-co-PANI/ITO electrode; (b) immobilization of DNA over CHIT-co-PANI/ITO electrode. (License No. 3384730775054)

responses to the oxidation of dsDNA than the electrodes prepared by potentio-dynamic methods.

DNA was also covalently attached onto PANI nanotubes synthesized on the graphite electrode [130]. The collective effect of PANI nanotubes and the enhanced conductivity led to the extremely high sensitivity of the biosensor in detecting DNA damage. A DNA biosensor has also been reportedly prepared using the copolymer of PANI and chitosan (Figure 12.3) [131]. The biosensor showed enhanced electron transfer properties, which was attributed to the combination of PANI's excellent conductivity and the cationic character of chitosan. PANI nanowires have also been synthesized electrochemically on the surface of GCE [132] and phosphate-ended DNAs covalently attached onto the amino groups of PANI nanowires.

12.5.3 Metal and Metal Oxide Nanoparticles

Electrochemical detection of DNA damage using DNA biosensors can be tailored to become extremely sensitive devices with a high multiplexing capability. When combined with the unique electrical properties of metal nanoparticles, they make electrical detection systems that provide excellent prospects for designing DNA damage detection devices. Nanoparticles have been extensively used for the immobilization of biomolecules [133]. In addition to their biocompatibility, they can produce a unique microenvironment that gives rise to improved freedom of orientation for affinity binding with advantages over planar substrates, increased surface area for higher probe loading capacities, and enhanced diffusion of amplification agents. Modification of electrode surfaces with nanoparticles can be carried out by simple electrostatic adsorption or by covalent attachments such as chemical cross-linking, electron beam or UV light irradiation, and electrodeposition [134–136]. Electrostatic adsorption is straightforward and the particle size can be strictly controlled in the preceding chemical synthesis of the nanoparticle. These surfaces, however, are unstable and subject to particle desorption. Nanoparticles covalently cross-linking to a surface can be quite versatile because of the large range of functional groups available for cross-linking. However, the prerequisite to the process is surface modification in order to avoid hindering electrochemical signals to the electrode. Nanoparticle synthesis from electron beam and UV light irradiation does not suffer from the insulating effects of covalent cross-linking; however, these methods can be expensive and time consuming. Electrochemical deposition of nanoparticles, on the other hand, is a simple and facile method to create nanoparticle-modified surfaces while the final nanoparticle size and surface density can be controlled by varying the deposition time, potential, and metal ion concentration in solution.

Metal oxide nanoparticles are often applied to immobilize biomolecules, while semiconductor nanoparticles are often used as labels or tracers. Among the nanomaterials used as components in biosensors, gold nanoparticles (AuNPs) are much explored for developing DNA-based biosensors because of their capability to increase electronic signals when a biological component is maintained in contact with the nanostructured surface. AuNPs, with a diameter of 1–100 nm, have a high surface-to-volume ratio and a high surface energy to allow the stable immobilization of a large amount of biomolecules retaining their bioactivity. Moreover, AuNPs permit fast and direct electron transfer between a wide range of electroactive species and electrode materials [137–141]. In addition to AuNPs that offer new paths for DNA biosensor development, other metal nanoparticles extensively explored include silver, platinum, palladium, copper, cobalt, zirconia, and titanium [142,143].

Generally, in order to bind to AuNPs, the oligonucleotides need modification with special functional groups that can interact strongly with AuNPs. Thiol groups are the most widely used for DNA and gold linkages. A few years ago, our team developed an amperometric DNA-based sensor for the detection of chronic lymphocytic leukemia [144]. We immobilized thiol-modified probe oligonucleotides at the 5'-phosphate end on the AuNP-modified electrode surface. It was found that the high surface-to-volume ratio of AuNPs greatly enhanced the hybridization of the target DNA. Some other functional groups have also been investigated. Cai et al. immobilized [145] an oligonucleotide with a mercaptohexyl group at the 5'-phosphate end onto AuNPs 16 nm in diameter, which was self-assembled on a cystamine-modified gold electrode. The saturated immobilization quantity of DNA on the modified electrode was approximately 10 times greater than that on a bare gold electrode. DNA damage induced by perfluorooctane sulfonate (PFOS) was further developed on a nanoporous bionic interface [146]. The interface was formed by assembling DNA on AuNPs that were embedded in a nanoporous overoxidized polypyrrole film. DNA damage owing to PFOS was proved using electrochemistry and x-ray photoelectron spectroscopy and was investigated by detecting the DPV response of methylene blue (MB), which was used as the electroactive indicator in the system.

It has been shown that the interaction of anticancer drugs with DNA and RNA bases in the presence of nanotitanium dioxide is enhanced [147]. The results indicate that the presence of TiO_2 nanoparticles obviously increased the binding affinity of dacarbazine to DNA and specific DNA bases, resulting in significantly enhanced detection sensitivity. Liu et al. developed sol-gel-derived TiO_2/ITO electrode based on photooxidized adsorbed dsDNA. In their study, MB was used to electrochemically monitor structural changes in dsDNA. They used this bioelectrode for the evaluation of the antioxidant properties of glutathione and gallic acid [148].

Zirconia is a technologically important material that has recently attracted considerable interest in electrochemical biosensor development since its surface has both oxidizing and reducing properties, as well as acidic and basic properties. Liu et al. developed a sol-gel-derived ZrO_2 DNA-modified GCE to investigate the effect of lanthanide concentration on its electron transfer behavior [149]. Chitosan is a biopolymer that has been widely used as an effective dispersant of ZrO_2 nanoparticles and carbon nanotubes (CNTs) because of its adhesive nature. The resulting biocompatible nanocomposite of multiwalled CNTs (MWCNTs)/nano-ZrO_2/chitosan has been utilized for the covalent immobilization of DNA for DNA hybridization detection [150]. The advantage of zirconia (ZrO_2) and gold nanoparticle (NG) film-modified GCE in the immobilization of DNA has been demonstrated by Zhang et al. for the construction of DNA biosensors [151]. The NG/GCE was obtained by dipping the pretreated GCE in nanogold colloid and then electrodepositing at 1.5 V for 700 s. Zirconia was immobilized to the NG/GCE by further cyclic voltammetric scanning in an aqueous electrolyte of $ZrOCl_2$ and KCl between −1.1 and +0.7 V at a scan rate of 20 mV/s for 10 consecutive cycles. The immobilization of ssDNA on the electrode surface was carried out as follows: the ZrO_2/NG/GCE was immersed in 2.0 mL Tris–HCl buffer (pH 7.0) solution containing ssDNA and then electrodeposited at 0.8 V for 400 s. After that, the electrode was rinsed three times with Tris–HCl buffer. Thus, the probe-captured electrode (ssDNA/ZrO_2/NG/GCE) was ready for use. The schematic representation of the immobilization of DNA on the ZrO_2/NG/GCE is shown in Figure 12.4.

A new approach based on Cu_2O hollow microspheres consisting of Cu_2O nanoparticles was developed by Zhu et al. for the fabrication of an electrochemical DNA biosensor of hepatitis B virus. They found that the hollow Cu_2O nanoparticles greatly enhanced the immobilization of the DNA probe on the electrode surface and improved the sensitivity of DNA biosensors [152]. The carbon ionic liquid electrode modified with Fe_2O_3 microspheres and self-doped PANI nanofibers (a copolymer of aniline and m-aminobenzene sulfonic acid) was used for the immobilization of the probe DNA [153]. The strong adsorption ability of Fe_2O_3 microspheres and the excellent conductivity of the self-doped PANI nanofibers enhanced the sensitivity of the DNA biosensor.

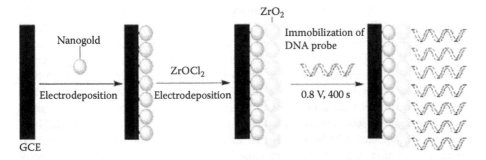

FIGURE 12.4 Schematic representation of the immobilization of DNA on ZrO_2/NG/GCE. (License No. 3384730465268)

12.5.4 CARBON NANOTUBES

Modification of CNTs with nucleic acids constitutes a very promising area for the development of devices for DNA damage detection, gene therapy, drug discovery and delivery, and so forth. The application of CNTs in electrochemical DNA biosensors is quite promising for many reasons: CNTs constitute novel platforms for DNA immobilization with important electrochemical transducing properties and high specific surface area which not only can increase the quantity of DNA attached but also can concentrate a great number of electroactive nanoparticles to amplify DNA damage detection [154,155]. The more basic techniques used for DNA immobilization on CNTs are physisorbed multisite attachment and covalent anchoring (single point linkage). In the latter case, typical schemes are provided by the conjugation of DNA terminal functional groups with functional groups in the CNT surface via the carbodiimide chemistry, streptavidin/biotin interactions, and so forth. In general, DNA is physisorbed on CNTs by wrapping the tube, with the bases (a polar region of the molecule) in close contact with the hydrophobic walls of CNTs whereas the phosphate backbone faces the solution [156,157].

CNT functionalization is a prerequisite to the application of such CNT nanostructures. Functionalization allows the immobilization of biomolecules on CNTs to occur. This encourages the use of nanotubes as potentially new types of biosensor materials. One of the most common schemes for covalent functionalization is the use of carbodiimide chemistry, which consists of generating carboxylic groups at the edges of the CNT (electrode) followed by coupling with NH_2-containing species (biomolecules) through the formation of a covalent amide bond [158]. This procedure has been extensively used for the attachment of amine-terminated DNA aptamers. Noncovalent functionalization relies on physical adsorption that is based on weak interactions (e.g., hydrogen bonding, π–π stacking, electrostatic forces, van der Waals forces, and hydrophobic interactions). It is particularly attractive because it offers the possibility for attaching chemical handles, which preserves the sp^2 nanotube structure and, consequently, avoids effects on the electronic network.

CNTs can help strengthen the DNA signal response to be distinguished from the background noise owing to surface area effects. In some cases, a decrease in oxidation overpotential has also been reported [158–160]. Pacios Pujadó compared DNA oxidation on novel upright CNT microelectrodes and GCEs modified by randomly dispersed CNTs [161]. The electrochemical responses of Poly-G physically adsorbed on CNT microelectrodes, on CNT-modified glassy carbon, and on glassy carbon were traced by DPV. The results showed that the presence of CNTs remarkably increased the guanine oxidation current because of the increased adsorption of Poly-G provided by the higher surface area of the CNTs. Well-defined DPV profiles are also observed in the case of CNT microelectrodes. This indicates that direct electrochemistry of DNA guanine at a CNT-modified electrode provided significantly enhanced voltammetric signals as compared to that at the unmodified electrode [161]. Wang et al. detected 100 fmol of breast cancer BRCA1 gene using the enhanced guanine oxidation signal at a CNT-modified GCE [162]. Pedano et al. have recently fabricated a CNT paste electrode using MWNT for the adsorption and electrochemical oxidation of nucleic acids [163]. Yim et al. [164] designed DNAzyme–MWCNT conjugates with the help of streptavidin modification onto CNT conjugates using carbodiimide chemistry for the proper and selective binding of biotinylated DNAzyme to streptavidin-coated surfaces.

Recently, we exploited the capability of poly(diallyldimethylammonium chloride) (PDDA) and chitosan to disperse MWCNTs for the immobilization of DNA to MWCNT-modified graphite electrodes [79,165–170]. PDDA is a water-soluble and quaternary ammonium, cationic polyelectrolyte that usually acts as a positively charged colloid when dissolved in aqueous solutions. In this study, doubly distilled water with a pH less than 7.0 was used to dissolve the PDDA. Positively charged PDDA and chitosan were easily coated on the negatively charged surface of the MWCNTs by electrostatic interaction. PDDA molecules combine considerably well with DNA to form DNA films because it is a strong, linear cationic polyelectrolyte. The MWCNTs not only display unique electron transfer properties that induce the conductivity of PDDA and improve electron transfer characteristics, they also increase the amount of PDDA deposited on the electrode. Electrochemical oxidation of codeine and morphine bonded on dsDNA/MWCNTs–PDDA/pencil graphite electrode (PGE) was used to obtain an analytical signal. Both molecules were electrochemically oxidized owing to the presence of phenolic and amino groups in their structures when DPV was used at a PGE [165]. When DNA was added to the solution, the electrochemical signal of codeine and morphine decreased and shifted to more negative and positive potentials, respectively. The interaction modes were identified as electrostatic for codeine and intercalation for morphine with two anodic peaks of codeine merging into them when DNA concentration increased. At high DNA concentrations, a sharp anodic wave was observed for codeine with a clear distinction between codeine and morphine oxidation peaks.

In another work, {MWCNTs/PDDA/DNA}$_2$ layer-by-layer films were prepared to detect DNA damage induced by radicals generated from sulfite autoxidation using CV and EIS [167]. The change in the peak potential separation (ΔEp) and the charge transfer resistance (Rp) after incubation of the DNA biosensor in the damaging solution for a certain time were used as indicators of DNA damage. It was found that sulfite in the presence of Co(II), Cu(II), Cr(VI), Fe(III), and Mn(II) caused damage to DNA while neither sulfite alone nor metal ions alone did have the same effect. The results suggest that sulfite is rapidly autoxidized in the presence of Co(II), Cu(II), Cr(VI), Fe(III), and Mn(II), producing radicals that cause the DNA damage. These radicals can be ranked in a descending order of their ability to induce DNA damage with sulfite as follows: Fe(III) > Co(II) > Cu(II) > Cr(VI) > Mn(II). DNA damage induced by sulfite plus Co(II), Cr(VI), or Fe(III) was inhibited by primary alcohols, but no such effect was observed when superoxide dismutase and tert-butyl alcohol were used.

Recently, our team developed a DNA detection method using electrochemical DNA biosensor with {MWCNTs/PDDA/dsDNA}$_2$ film on the graphite electrode and MB as an indicator (Figure 12.5) [165]. To detect the DNA damage, the modified electrode was immersed into MB solution to load MB into the dsDNA present on the surface of the electrode. The DPV of the loaded MB on the electrode showed a sharp peak at −0.230 V versus Ag/AgCl. In a blank solution, the MB loaded into the films was gradually released from the electrode surface, but the complete reloading of MB into the films was realized by immersing the electrode into the MB solution

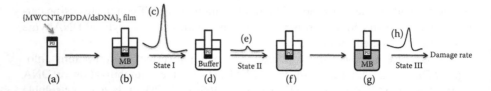

FIGURE 12.5 Schematic diagram of the procedure of loading/releasing/reloading of MB in/out of the {MWCNTs/PDDA/dsDNA}$_2$ layer-by-layer films and the corresponding DPV detection: (a) assembling of {MWCNTs/PDDA/dsDNA}$_2$ film; (b) loading of MB; (c) DPV scan in the buffer solution; (d) releasing of MB in the blank buffer; (e) DPV scan in the buffer; (f) incubation in the damaging solution; (g) reloading of MB; and (h) DPV scan in the buffer solution. (License No. 3375440409981)

again, indicating the good reversibility of MB incorporation. However, after incubation of the DNA-modified electrode in the solution of a known genotoxic agent (glutathione, chromium(VI) plus hydrogen peroxide), the damaged MWCNTs/PDDA/dsDNA films did not return to their original form and fully loaded state by reloading MB, thereby showing smaller DPV peak currents.

In yet another work, an electrochemical protocol was described for the direct monitoring of genotoxicity of catecholics. In this work, catechol was encapsulated on MWCNTs (CA@MWCNT) through continuous CV on the surface of PGE [169]. Subsequently, a DNA-functionalized biosensor (DNA/CA@MWCNT/PGE) was prepared and characterized for the detection and investigation of DNA damage induced by radicals generated from catecholics. Such procedures lead to strong adsorption (immobilization) of CA as the damaging agent on carbon surfaces. We used EIS to investigate the oxidative DNA damage induced by CA in the presence of metal ions. Furthermore, we inspected the role of glutathione and plumbagin in preventing DNA damage.

12.6 CONCLUSION

The use of nanomaterials in electrical DNA damage detection has taken off rapidly and will surely continue to expand. Because of their high surface area, nontoxicity, biocompatibility, and charge-sensitive conductance, nanomaterials serve as effective transducers in nanoscale DNA biosensing and bioelectronic devices. Such nanomaterial-based DNA assays and devices are expected to have a major impact on clinical diagnostics, environmental monitoring, and food safety. They exhibit a number of key features including high sensitivity, exquisite selectivity, fast response time, and rapid recovery (reversibility) as well as the potential for integration of arrays on a massive scale, which put them far above other sensor technologies available today. The high sensitivity of these nanoparticle-based electrical systems heralds the prospects of detecting DNA damage without the need for PCR amplification. It is expected that future innovative research will lead to new particle-based electrical detection strategies that, when coupled with other major technological advances, will result in effective, easy-to-use, handheld portable devices for DNA diagnostics.

ACKNOWLEDGMENTS

The authors wish to thank the Research Council of Isfahan University of Technology, the Center of Excellence in Sensor and Green Chemistry, and the Iranian Nanotechnology Initiative Council for their support.

REFERENCES

1. C. Li, C.B. Thompson, DNA Damage, Deamidation and Death, *Science*, 2002, 1346–1347.
2. S. Jackson, and J. Bartek, The DNA-Damage Response in Human Biology and Disease, *Nature*, 461, 1071–1078 (2009).
3. T. Lindahl, and D.E. Barnes, Repair of Endogenous DNA Damage, *Cold Spring Harb. Symp. Quant. Biol.*, 65, 127–133 (2000).
4. R. De Bont, and N. van Larebeke, Endogenous DNA Damage in Humans: A Review of Quantitative Data, *Mutagenesis*, 19, 169–185 (2004).
5. P.C. Dedon, and S.R. Tannenbaum, Reactive Nitrogen Species in the Chemical Biology of Inflammation, *Arch. Biochem. Biophys.*, 423, 12–22 (2004).
6. T.G. England, A. Jenner, O.I. Aruoma, and B. Halliwell, Determination of Oxidative DNA Base Damage by Gas Chromatography-Mass Spectrometry. Effect of Derivatization Conditions on Artifactual Formation of Certain Base Oxidation Products, *Free Radic. Res.*, 29, 321–330 (1998).
7. G. Guetens, G. De Boeck, M. Highley, A.T. Van Oosterom, and E.A. De Bruijn, Oxidative DNA Damage: Biological Significance and Methods of Analysis, *Crit. Rev. Clin. Lab. Sci.*, 39, 331–457 (2002).
8. H.J. Helbock, K.B. Beckman, M.K. Shigenaga, P.B. Walter, A.A. Woodall, H.C. Yeo, and B.N. Ames, DNA Oxidation Matters: The HPLC-Electrochemical Detection Assay of 8-Oxo-Deoxyguanosine and 8-Oxo-Guanine, *Proc. Natl. Acad. Sci. U.S.A.*, 95, 288–293 (1998).
9. H. Kasai, A New Automated Method to Analyze Urinary 8-Hydroxydeoxyguanosine by a High-Performance Liquid Chromatography-Electrochemical Detector System, *J. Radiat. Res.*, 44, 185–189 (2003).
10. A. Weimann, D. Belling, and H.E. Poulsen, Quantification of 8-oxo-guanine and Guanine as the Nucleobase, Nucleoside and Deoxynucleoside Forms in Human Urine by High-Performance Liquid Chromatography-Electrospray Tandem Mass Spectrometer, *Nucleic Acids Res.*, 30, e7 (2002).
11. A. Jenner, T. England, O. Aruoma, and B. Halliwell, Measurement of Oxidative DNA Damage by Gas Chromatography-Mass Spectrometry: Ethanethiol Prevents Artifactual Generation of Oxidized DNA Bases, *Biochem. J.*, 331, 365–369 (1998).
12. S. Inagaki, Y. Esaka, M. Sako, and M. Goto, Analysis of DNA Adducts Bases by Capillary Electrophoresis with Amperometric Detection, *Electrophoresis*, 22, 3408–3412 (2001).
13. J. Cadet, C. D'ham, T. Douki, J.P. Pouget, J.L. Ravanat, and S. Sauvaigo, Facts and Artifacts in the Measurement of Oxidative Base Damage to DNA, *Free Radic. Res.*, 29, 541–550 (1998).
14. J. Lunec, ESCODD: European Standards Committee on Oxidative DNA Damage, *Free Radic. Res.*, 29, 601–608 (1998).
15. A. Collins, ESCODD (European Standards Committee on Oxidative DNA Damage) Comparison of Different Methods of Measuring 8-oxoguanine as a Marker of Oxidative DNA Damage, *Free Radic. Res.*, 32, 333–341 (2000).

16. E. Palecek, Modern polarographic (Voltammetric) techniques in biochemistry and molecular biology, In *Topics in Bioelectrochemistry Bioenergetics*, Vol. 5, G. Milazzo, ed., John Wiley, Chichester, UK, 1983, pp. 65–155.
17. J.M. Sequaris, Analytical voltammetry of biological molecules, In *Wilson Wilson's Comprehensive Analytical Chemistry*, Vol. 27, Analytical Voltammetry, G. Svehla, ed., Elsevier, Amsterdam, 1992, pp. 143–150.
18. E. Palecek, From Polarography of DNA to Microanalysis with Nucleic Acid-Modified Electrodes, *Electroanalysis*, 8, 7–14 (1996).
19. M. Fojta, Detecting DNA damage with electrodes, In *Electrochemistry of Nucleic Acids Proteins: Towards Electrochemical Sensors for Genomics Proteomics*, E. Palecek, F. Scheller, J. Wang, eds., Elsevier, Amsterdam, 2005, pp. 386–431.
20. F.C. Abreu, M.O.F. Goulart, and A.M.O. Brett, Detection of the Damage Caused to DNA by Niclosamide Using an Electrochemical DNA-Biosensor, *Biosens. Bioelectron.*, 17, 913–919 (2002).
21. A.M.O. Brett, V.C. Diculescu, A.M. Chiorcea-Paquim, and S.H.P. Serrano, DNA-electrochemical biosensors for investigating DNA damage, In *Electrochemical Sensors Analysis*, S. Alegret, A. Merkoci, eds., Elsevier, Amsterdam, 2007, pp. 413–438.
22. C.M.A. Brett, and A.M.C.F. Oliveira Brett, *Electrochemistry. Principles, Methods Applications*, Oxford University Press, UK, 1993.
23. M. Fojta, Electrochemical Sensors for DNA Interactions and Damage, *Electroanalysis*, 14, 1449–1463 (2002).
24. M. Fojta, L. Havran, R. Kizek, and S. Billová, Voltammetric Microanalysis of DNA Adducts with Osmium tetroxide,2,2′-bipyridine Using a Pyrolytic Graphite Electrode, *Talanta*, 56, 867–874 (2002).
25. G. Marrazza, I. Chianella, and M. Mascini, Disposable DNA Electrochemical Biosensors for Environmental Monitoring, *Anal. Chim. Acta*, 387, 297–307 (1999).
26. G. Marrazza, I. Chianella, and M. Mascini, Disposable DNA Electrochemical Sensor for Hybridization Detection, *Biosens. Bioelectron.*, 14, 43–51 (1999).
27. J. Wang, J.R. Fernandes, and L.T. Kubota, Polishable and Renewable DNA Hybridization Biosensors, *Anal. Chem.*, 70, 3699–3702 (1998).
28. C. Prado, G.U. Flechsig, P. Grundler, J.S. Foord, F. Marken, and R.G. Compton, Electrochemical Analysis of Nucleic Acids at Boron-Doped Diamond Electrode, *Analyst*, 127, 329–332 (2002).
29. E. Palecek, and B.D. Frary, A Highly Sensitive Pulse-Polarographic Estimation of Denatured Deoxyribonucleic Acid in Native Deoxyribonucleic Acid Samples, *Arch. Biochem. Biophys.*, 115, 431–436 (1966).
30. E. Palecek, and M. Fojta, *Bioelectronics: From Theory to Applications*, Wiley, Germany, 2005.
31. J.F. Cassidy, A.P. Doherty, and J.G. Vos, Amperometric methods of detection, In *Principles of Chemical Biological Sensors*, D. Diamond, ed., John Wiley & Sons, Toronto, 1998.
32. A. Erdem, M.I. Pividori, M. del Valle, and S. Alegret, Rigid Carbon Composites: A New Transducing Material for Label-Free Electrochemical Genosensing, *J. Electroanal. Chem.*, 567, 29–37 (2004).
33. D. Ozkan, A. Erdem, P. Kara, K. Kerman, B. Meric, J. Hassmann, and M. Ozsoz, Allele-Specific Genotype Detection of Factor V Leiden Mutation from Polymerase Chain Reaction Amplicons Based on Label-Free Electrochemical Genosensor, *Anal. Chem.*, 74, 5931–5936 (2002).
34. A. Erdem, K. Kerman, B. Meric, U.S. Akarca, and M. Ozsoz, DNA Electrochemical Biosensor for the Detection of Short DNA Sequences Related to the Hepatitis B Virus, *Electroanalysis*, 11, 586–588 (1999).

35. J. Wang, X.H. Cai, G. Rivas, H. Shiraishi, P.A.M. Farias, and N. Dontha, DNA Electrochemical Biosensor for the Detection of Short DNA Sequences Related to the Human Immunodeficiency Virus, *Anal. Chem.*, 68, 2629–2634 (1996).
36. E. Southern, K. Mir, and M. Shchepinov, Molecular Interactions on Microarrays, *Nat. Genet. Supp.*, 21, 5–9 (1999).
37. M.I. Pividori, and S. Alegret, Electrochemical Genosensing Based on Rigid Carbon Composites. A Review, *Anal. Lett.*, 38, 2541–2565 (2005).
38. K.M. Millan, and S.R. Mikkelsen, Sequence-Selective Biosensor for DNA Based on Electroactive Hybridization Indicators, *Anal. Chem.*, 65, 2317–2323 (1993).
39. M.S. Yang, M.E. McGovern, and M. Thompson, Genosensor Technology and the Detention of Interfacial Nucleic Acid Chemistry, *Anal. Chim. Acta*, 346, 259–275 (1997).
40. M. Fojta, and E. Palecek, Upercoiled DNA-Modified Mercury Electrode: A Highly Sensitive Tool for the Detection of DNA Damage, *Anal. Chim. Acta*, 342, 1–12 (1997).
41. P. Boublikova, M. Vojtiskova, and E. Palecek, Determination of Submicrogram Quantities of Circular Duplex DNA in Plasmid Samples by Adsorptive Stripping Voltammetry, *Anal. Lett.*, 20, 275–291 (1987).
42. J.P. Pouget, T. Douki, M.J. Richard, and J. Cadet, DNA Damage Induced in Cells by Gamma and UV Radiation as Measured by HPLC/GC-Ms and HPLC-EC and Comet Assay, *Chem. Res. Toxicol.*, 13, 541–549 (2000).
43. P. Olive, R. Dur, J. Raleigh, C. Luo, and C. Aquino-Parsons, Comparison between the Comet Assay and Pimonidazole Binding for Measuring Tumour Hypoxia, *Br. J. Cancer*, 83, 1525–1531 (2000).
44. A. Migheli, Electron Microscopic Detection of DNA Damage Labeled by TUNEL, *Methods Mol. Biol.*, 203, 31–39 (2002).
45. D. Loo, TUNEL Assay. An Overview of Techniques, *Methods Mol. Biol.*, 203, 21–30 (2002).
46. M. Fojta, l. Havran, and E. Palecek, Chronopotentiometric Detection of DNA Strand Breaks with Mercury Electrodes Modified with Supercoiled DNA, *Electroanalysis*, 9, 1033–1034 (1997).
47. M. Fojta, T. Kubicarova, and E. Palecek, Cleavage of Supercoiled DNA by Deoxyribonuclease I in Solution and at the Electrode Surface, *Electroanalysis*, 11, 1005–1012 (1999).
48. M. Fojta, V. Stankova, E. Palecek, J. Mitas, and P. Koscielniak, A Supercoiled DNA-Modified Mercury Electrode-based Biosensor for the Detection of DNA Strand Cleaving Agents, *Talanta*, 46, 155–161 (1998).
49. M. Fojta, T. Kubicarova, and E. Palecek, Electrode Potential-Modulated Cleavage of Surface-Confined DNA by Hydroxyl Radicals Detected by an Electrochemical, *Biosens. Bioelectron.*, 15, 107–115 (2000).
50. M. Fojta, L. Havran, T. Kubicarova, and E. Palecek, Electrode Potential-Controlled DNA Damage in the Presence of Copper Ions and Their Complexes, *Bioelectrochemistry*, 55, 25–27 (2002).
51. M. Bukova, J. Labuda, J. Sandula, L. Krizkova, I. Stepanek, and Z. Durackova, Detection of Damage to DNA and Antioxidative Activity of Yeast Polysaccharides at the DNA-Modified Screen-Printed Electrode, *Talanta*, 56, 939–947 (2002).
52. O. Korbut, M. Buckova, J. Labuda, and P. Grundler, Voltammetric Detection of Antioxidative Properties of Flavonoids Using Electrically Heated DNA Modified Carbon Paste Electrode, *Sensors*, 3, 1–10 (2003).
53. J. Labuda, M. Buckova, L. Heilerova, A. Caniova-Ziakova, E. Brandsteterova, J. Mattusch, and R. Wennrich, Detection of Antioxidative Activity of Plant Extracts at the DNA-Modified Screen-Printed Electrode, *Sensors*, 2, 1–10 (2002).
54. J. Labuda, M. Buckova, L. Heilerova, S. Silhar, and I. Stepanek, Evaluation of the Redox Properties and Anti/Pro-Oxidant Effects of Selected Flavonoids by Means of a DNA-Based Electrochemical Biosensor, *Anal. Bioanal. Chem.*, 376, 168–173 (2003).

55. E. Palecek, Polarographic techniques in nucleic acid research, In *Progress in Nucleic Acid Research Molecular Biology*, Vol. 18, W.E. Cohn, ed., Academic Press, New York, 1976, pp. 151–213.
56. E. Palecek, M. Fojta, F. Jelen, and V. Vetterl, In *The Encyclopedia of Electrochemistry*, Vol. 9, Bioelectrochemistry, A.J. Bard, M. Stratsmann, eds., Wiley-VCH, Weinheim, 2002, pp. 365–429.
57. J. Labuda, M. Fojta, F. Jelen, and E. Palecek, Towards electrochemical sensors for genomics and proteomics, In *Encyclopedia of Sensors*, C.A. Grimes, E.C. Dickey, M.V. Pishko, eds., American Scientific Publishers, Stevenson Ranch, CA, 2006, pp. 201–228.
58. J. Labuda, K. Bubnicova, L. Kovalova, M. Vanickova, J. Mattusch, and R. Wennrich, Voltammetric Detection of Damage to DNA by Arsenic Compounds at a DNA Biosensor, *Sensors*, 5, 411–423 (2005).
59. R. Ovadekova, S. Jantova, S. Letasiova, and J. Labuda, Nanostructured Electrochemical DNA Biosensors for Detection of the Effect of Berberine on DNA from Cancer Cells, *Anal. Bioanal. Chem.*, 386, 2055–2062 (2006).
60. J. Galova, G. Ziyatdinova, and J. Labuda, Disposable Electrochemical Biosensor with Multiwalled Carbon Nanotubes—Chitosan Composite Layer for the Detection of Deep DNA Damage, *Anal. Sci.*, 24, 711–716 (2008).
61. J. Galova, R. Ovadekova, A. Ferancova, and J. Labuda, Disposable DNA Biosensor with the Carbon Nanotubes–Polyethyleneimine Interface at a Screen-Printed Carbon Electrode for Tests of DNA Layer Damage by quinazolines, *Anal. Bioanal. Chem.*, 394, 855–861 (2009).
62. J. Labuda, R. Ovadekova, and J. Galova, DNA-Based Biosensor for the Detection of Strong Damage to DNA by the Quinazoline Derivative as a Potential Anticancer Agent, *Microchim. Acta*, 164, 371–377 (2009).
63. M. Bukova, J. Labuda, J. Sandula, L. Krizkova, I. Stepanek, and Z. Durackova, Detection of Damage to DNA and Antioxidative Activity of Yeast Polysaccharides at the DNA-Modified Screen-Printed Electrode, *Talanta*, 56, 939–947 (2002).
64. T. Lindahl, Instability and Decay of the Primary Structure of DNA, *Nature*, 362, 709–715 (1993).
65. S.K. Das, Harmful Health Effects of Cigarette Smoking, *Mol. Cell Biochem.*, 253, 159–165 (2003).
66. B.N. Ames, L.S. Gold, and W.C. Willett, The Causes and Prevention of Cancer, *Proc. Natl. Acad. Sci. U.S.A.*, 92, 5258–5265 (1995).
67. M.G. Blackburn, and M.J. Gait, *Nucleic Acids in Chemistry Biology*, IRL Press, New York, 1990.
68. O.D. Scharer, Chemistry and Biology of DNA Repair, *Angew. Chem., Int. Ed.*, 42, 2946–2974 (2003).
69. E.C. Friedberg, DNA Damage and Repair, *Nature*, 421, 436–440 (2003).
70. M. Mascini, I. Palchetti, and G. Marrazza, DNA Electrochemical Biosensors, *Fresenius J. Anal. Chem.*, 369, 15–22 (2001).
71. J. Wang, M. Chicharro, G. Rivas, X.H. Cai, N. Dontha, P.A.M. Farias, and H. Shiraishi, DNA Biosensor for the Detection of Hydrazines, *Anal. Chem.*, 68, 2251–2254 (1996).
72. F. Lucarelli, A. Kicela, I. Palchetti, G. Marrazza, and M. Mascini, Electrochemical DNA Biosensor for Analysis of Wastewater Samples, *Bioelectrochemistry*, 58, 113–118 (2002).
73. C. Teijeiro, P. Perez, D. Marin, and E. Palecek, Cyclic Voltammetry of Mitomycin C and DNA, *Bioelectrochem. Bioenerg.*, 38, 77–83 (1995).
74. P. Perez, C. Teijeiro, and D. Marin, Interactions of Surface-Confined DNA with Electroreduced Mitomycin C Comparison with Acid-Activated Mitomycin C, *Chem. Biol. Interact.*, 117, 65–81 (1999).

75. D. Marin, P. Perez, C. Teijeiro, and E. Palecek, Interactions of Surface-Confined DNA with Acid-Activated Mitomycin C, *Biophys. Chem.*, 75, 87–95 (1998).
76. D. Marin, R. Valera, E. de la Red, and C. Teijeiro, Electrochemical Study of Antineoplastic Drug Thiotepa Hydrolysis to Thiol Form and Thiotepa—DNA Interactions, *Bioelectrochem. Bioenerg.*, 44, 51–56 (1997).
77. J. Wang, G. Rivas, M. Ozsos, D.H. Grant, X.H. Cai, and C. Parrado, Microfabricated Electrochemical Sensor for the Detection of Radiation-Induced DNA Damage, *Anal. Chem.*, 69, 1457–1460 (1997).
78. F. Jelen, M. Tomschik, and E. Palecek, Adsorptive Stripping Square-Wave Voltammetry of DNA, *J. Electroanal. Chem.*, 423, 141–148 (1997).
79. A.A. Ensafi, M. Amini, and B. Rezaei, Impedimetric DNA-Biosensor for the Study of Anti-Cancer Action of Mitomycin C: Comparison between Acid and Electroreductive Activation, *Biosens. Bioelectron.*, 59, 282–288 (2014).
80. V. Brabec, DNA Sensor for the Determination of Antitumor Platinum Compounds, *Electrochim. Acta*, 45, 2929–2932 (2000).
81. F. Lucarelli, I. Palchetti, G. Marrazza, and M. Mascini, Electrochemical DNA Biosensor as a Screening Tool for the Detection of Toxicants in Water and Wastewater Samples, *Talanta*, 56, 949–957 (2002).
82. G. Chiti, G. Marrazza, and M. Mascini, Electrochemical DNA Biosensor for Environmental Monitoring, *Anal. Chim. Acta*, 427, 155–164 (2001).
83. M. Mascini, Affinity Electrochemical Biosensors for Pollution Control, *Pure Appl. Chem.*, 73, 23–30 (2001).
84. M. Ozsoz, A. Erdem, P. Kara, K. Kerman, and D. Ozkan, Electrochemical Biosensor for the Detection of Interaction Between Arsenic Trioxide and DNA Based on Guanine Signal, *Electroanalysis*, 15, 613–619 (2003).
85. J. Langmaier, Z. Samec, and E. Samcova, Electrochemical Oxidation of 8-Oxo-2′-Deoxyguanosine on Glassy Carbon, Gold, Platinum and Tin(IV) Oxide Electrodes, *Electroanalysis*, 15, 1555–1560 (2003).
86. A.M.O.B. Rett, M. Vivan, I.R. Fernandes, and J.A.P. Piedade, Electrochemical Detection of In Situ Adriamycin Oxidative Damage to DNA, *Talanta*, 56, 959–970 (2002).
87. E. Palecek, and F. Jelen, Electrochemistry of nucleic acids, In *Electrochemistry of Nucleic Acids Proteins: Towards Electrochemical Sensors for Genomics Proteomics*, E. Palecek, F. Scheller, J. Wang, eds., Elsevier, Amsterdam, 2005, pp. 74–174.
88. D.H. Johnston, K.C. Glasgow, and H.H. Thorp, Electrochemical Measurement of the Solvent Accessibility of Nucleobases Using Electron Transfer between DNA and Metal Complexes, *J. Am. Chem. Soc.*, 117, 8933–8938 (1995).
89. E.C. Friedberg, Biological Responses to DNA Damage: A Perspective in the New Millennium, *Cold Spring Harb. Symp. Quant. Biol.*, 65, 593–602 (2000).
90. J. Wang, M. Jiang, and A.N. Kawde, Flow Detection of UV Radiation-Induced DNA Damage at a Polypyrrole-Modified Electrode, *Electroanalysis*, 13, 537–540 (2001).
91. L. Dennany, R.J. Forster, and J.F. Rusling, Simultaneous Direct Electrochemiluminescence and Catalytic Voltammetry Detection of DNA in Ultrathin Films, *J. Am. Chem. Soc.*, 125, 5213–5218 (2003).
92. J. Mbindyo, L. Zhou, Z. Zhang, J.D. Stuart, and J.F. Rusling, Detection of Chemically Induced DNA Damage by Derivative Square Wave Voltammetry, *Anal. Chem.*, 72, 2059–2065 (2000).
93. E. Palecek, Local Supercoil-Stabilized DNA Structures, *Crit. Rev. Biochem. Mol. Biol.*, 26, 151–226 (1991).
94. K. Cahova-Kucharikova, M. Fojta, T. Mozga, and E. Palecek, Use of DNA Repair Enzymes in Electrochemical Detection of Damage to DNA Bases In Vitro and in Cells, *Anal. Chem.*, 77, 2920–2927 (2005).

95. J.F. Rusling, Sensors for genotoxicity and oxidized DNA, In *Electrochemistry of Nucleic Acids Proteins: Towards Electrochemical Sensors for Genomics Proteomics*, E. Palecek, F. Scheller, J. Wang, eds., Elsevier, Amsterdam, 2005, pp. 433–449.

96. G. Zauner, Y. Wang, M. Lavesa-Curto, A. MacDonald, A.G. Mayes, R.P. Bowater, and J.N. Butt, Tethered DNA Hairpins Facilitate Electrochemical Detection of DNA Ligation, *Analyst*, 130, 345–349 (2005).

97. E. Palecek, and M. Fojta, Detecting DNA Hybridization Damage, *Anal. Chem.*, 73, 74A–83A (2001).

98. A. Erdem, Nanomaterial-Based Electrochemical DNA Sensing Strategies, *Talanta*, 74, 318–325 (2007).

99. I.K. Larsen, Intercalating agents, In *A Textbook of Drug Design Development*, P. Krosgaard-Larsen, H. Bundgaard, eds., Harwood Academic Publishers, Germany, 1991, p. 192.

100. A. Erdem, and M. Ozsoz, Electrochemical DNA Biosensors Based on DNA-Drug Interactions, *Electroanalysis*, 14, 965–974 (2002).

101. N. Hadjiliadis, and E. Sletten, *Metal Complex–DNA Interactions*, Blackwell Publishing Ltd., Chichester, UK, 2009.

102. M.T. Carter, M. Rodriguez, and A.J. Bard, Voltammetric Studies of the Interaction of Metal Chelates with DNA. 2. Tris-chelated Complexes of Cobalt(Iii) and Iron(II) with 1,10-Phenanthroline and 2,2′-bipyridine, *J. Am. Chem. Soc.*, 111, 8901–8911 (1989).

103. M. Rodriguez, and A.J. Bard, Electrochemical Studies of the Interaction of Metal Chelates with DNA. 4. Voltammetric and Electrogenerated Chemiluminescent Studies of the Interaction of tris(2,2′-bipyridine)osmium(II) with DNA, *Anal. Chem.*, 62, 2658–2662 (1990).

104. W. Sufen, P. Tuzhi, and C.F. Yang, Electrochemical Studies for the Interaction of DNA with an Irreversible Redox Compound—Hoechst 33258, *Electroanalysis*, 14, 1648–1653 (2002).

105. S. Wang, T.Z. Peng, and C.F. Yang, Investigation of the Interaction of DNA and Actinomycin D by Cyclic Voltammetry, *J. Electroanal. Chem.*, 544, 87–92 (2003).

106. S. Wang, T. Peng, and C.F. Yang, Investigation on the Interaction of DNA and Electroactive Ligands Using a Rapid Electrochemical Method, *J. Biochem. Biophys. Methods*, 55, 191–204 (2003).

107. J.M. Sequaris, and M. Esteban, Cyclic Voltammetry of Metal/Polyelectrolyte Complexes: Complexes of Cadmium and Lead with Deoxyribonucleic Acid, *Electroanalysis*, 2, 35–41 (1990).

108. J.M. Sequaris, and J. Swiatek, Interaction of DNA with Pb^{2+}: Voltammetric and Spectroscopic Studies, *Bioelectrochem. Bioenerg.*, 26, 15–28 (1991).

109. F. Jelen, B. Yosypchuk, A. Kourilova, L. Novotny, and E. Palecek, Label-Free Determination of Picogram Quantities of DNA by Stripping Voltammetry with Solid Copper Amalgam or Mercury Electrodes in the Presence of Copper, *Anal. Chem.*, 74, 4788–4793 (2002).

110. P.A.M. Farias, A.D. Wagener, and A.A. Castro, Ultratrace Determination of Adenine in the Presence of Copper by Adsorptive Stripping Voltammetry, *Talanta*, 55, 281–290 (2001).

111. R.F. Johnston, D.M. Lewis, and J.Q. Chambers, Accumulation of Hg(II) by Adsorbed Polyuridylic Acid: Differentiation of Coordinated Hg(II) and Covalently Mercurated Species, *J. Electroanal. Chem.*, 466, 2–7 (1999).

112. J.L.M. Alvarez, J.A.G. Calzon, and J.M.L. Fonseca, Electrocatalytic Effects of Deoxyribonucleic Acids, Adenine and Guanine on the Reduction of Ni(II) at a Mercury Electrode, *J. Electroanal. Chem.*, 457, 53–59 (1998).

113. M. Fojta, R. Doffkova, and E. Palecek, Determination of Traces of RNA in Submicrogram Amounts of Single- or Double-Stranded DNAs by Means of Nucleic Acid-Modified Electrodes, *Electroanalysis*, 8, 420–426 (1996).
114. E.D. Gil, S.H.P. Serrano, E.I. Ferreira, and L.T. Kubota, Electrochemical Evaluation of Rhodium Dimer-DNA Interactions, *J. Pharm. Biomed. Anal.*, 29, 579–584 (2002).
115. E. Katz, and I. Willner, In *Technology Performance*, V. Mirsky, ed., Springler-Verlag, Berlin, 2004, pp. 67–106.
116. J.Y. Park, and S.M. Park, DNA Hybridization Sensors Based on Electrochemical Impedance Spectroscopy as a Detection Tool, *Sensors*, 9, 9513–9532 (2009).
117. M. Gebala, L. Stoica, S. Neugebauer, and W. Schuhmann, Label-Free Detection of DNA Hybridization in Presence of Intercalators Using Electrochemical Impedance Spectroscopy, *Electroanalysis*, 21, 325–331 (2009).
118. A.M. Caminade, C. Padie, R. Laurent, A. Maravel, and J.M. Majoral, Uses of Dendrimers for DNA Microarrays, *Sensors*, 6, 901–914 (2006).
119. P. Qian, S. Ai, H. Yin, and J. Li, Evaluation of DNA Damage and Antioxidant Capacity of Sericin by a DNA Electrochemical Biosensor Based on Dendrimer-Encapsulated Au-Pd/Chitosan Composite, *Microchim. Acta*, 168, 347–354 (2010).
120. N. Zhu, Y. Gu, Z. Chang, P. He, and Y. Fang, PAMAM Dendrimers-Based DNA Biosensors for Electrochemical Detection of DNA Hybridization, *Electroanalysis*, 18, 2107–2114 (2006).
121. W.J. Shi, S.Y. Ai, J.H. Li, and L.S. Zhu, Electrochemical Biosensor Based on Dendrimer Immobilized Deoxyribonucleic Acid, *Chinese J. Anal. Chem.*, 36, 335–338 (2008).
122. O. Arotiba, A. Ignaszak, R. Malgas, A.A. Amir, P.C.L. Baker, S.F. Mapolie, and E.I. Iwuoha, An Electrochemical DNA Biosensor Developed on Novel Multinuclear Nickel(II) Salicylaldimine Metallodendrimer Platform, *Electrochim. Acta*, 53, 1689–1696 (2007).
123. B.D. Malhotra, A. Chaubey, and S.P. Singh, Prospects of Conducting Polymers in Biosensors, *Anal. Chim. Acta*, 578, 59–74 (2006).
124. H. Peng, L. Zhang, C. Soeller, and J.T. Sejdic, Conducting Polymers for Electrochemical DNA Sensing, *Biomaterials*, 30, 2132–2148 (2009).
125. A. Malinauskas, J. Malinauskiene, and A. Ramanavicius, Conducting Polymer-Based Nanostructurized Materials: Electrochemical Aspects, *Nanotechnology*, 16, R51–R62 (2005).
126. L. Xia, Z. Wei, and M. Wan, Conducting Polymer Nanostructures and their Application in Biosensors, *J Colloid Interface Sci*, 341, 1–11 (2009).
127. K. Ghanbari, S.Z. Bathaieb, and M.F. Mousavi, Electrochemically Fabricated Polypyrrole Nanofiber-Modified Electrode as a New Electrochemical DNA Biosensor, *Biosens. Bioelectron.*, 23, 1825–1831 (2008).
128. A. Ramanavicius, A. Ramanaviciene, and A. Malinauskas, Electrochemical Sensors Based on Conducting Polymer-Polypyrrole, *Electrochim. Acta*, 51, 6025–6037 (2006).
129. A. Ozcan, Y. Sahin, M. Ozsoz, and S. Turan, Electrochemical Oxidation of ds-DNA on Polypyrrole Nanofiber Modified Pencil Graphite Electrode, *Electroanalysis*, 19, 2208–2216 (2007).
130. H. Chang, Y. Yuan, N. Shi, and Y. Guan, Electrochemical DNA Biosensor Based on Conducting Polyaniline Nanotube Array, *Anal. Chem.*, 79, 5111–5115 (2007).
131. A. Tiwari, and S. Gong, Electrochemical Detection of a Breast Cancer Susceptible Gene Using cDNA Immobilized Chitosan-co-Polyaniline Electrode, *Talanta*, 77, 1217–1222 (2009).
132. N. Zhu, Z. Chang, P. He, and Y. Fang, Electrochemically Fabricated Polyaniline Nanowire-Modified Electrode for Voltammetric Detection of DNA Hybridization, *Electrochim. Acta*, 51, 3758–3762 (2006).

133. S.J. Guo, and S.J. Dong, Biomolecule-Nanoparticle Hybrids for Electrochemical Biosensors, *TrAC-Trends Anal. Chem.*, 28, 96–109 (2009).
134. E. Katz, and I. Willner, Integrated, Nanoparticle–Biomolecule Hybrid Systems: Synthesis, Properties, and Applications, *Angew. Chem. Int. Ed.*, 43, 6042–6108 (2004).
135. G. Schmid, and L.F. Chi, Metal Clusters and Colloids, *Adv. Mat.*, 10, 515–526 (1998).
136. S.G. Kwon, and T. Hyeon, Colloidal Chemical Synthesis and Formation Kinetics of Uniformly Sized Nanocrystals of Metals, Oxides, and Chalcogenides, *Acc. Chem. Res.*, 41, 1696–1709 (2008).
137. S. Hrapovic, Y. Liu, K.B. Male, and J.H.T. Luong, Electrochemical Biosensing Platforms Using Platinum Nanoparticles and Carbon Nanotubes, *Anal. Chem.*, 76, 1083–1088 (2004).
138. C.Y. Liu, and J.M. Hu, Hydrogen Peroxide Biosensor Based on the Direct Electrochemistry of Myoglobin Immobilized on Silver Nanoparticles Doped Carbon Nanotubes Film, *Biosens. Bioelectron.*, 24, 2149–2154 (2009).
139. Z. Li, X. Wang, G. Wen, S. Shuang, C. Dong, M.C. Paau, and M.M. Choi, Application of Hydrophobic Palladium Nanoparticles for the Development of Electrochemical Glucose Biosensor, *Biosens. Bioelectron.*, 26, 4619–4623 (2011).
140. A.P. Baioni, M. Vidotti, P.A. Fiorito, and S.I.C. de Torresia, Copper Hexacyanoferrate Nanoparticles Modified Electrodes: A Versatile Tool for Biosensors, *J. Electroanal. Chem.*, 622, 219–224 (2008).
141. A. Salimi, R. Hallaj, and S. Soltanian, Fabrication of a Sensitive Cholesterol Biosensor Based on Cobalt-oxide Nanostructures Electrodeposited onto Glassy Carbon Electrode, *Electroanalysis*, 21, 2693–2700 (2009).
142. I. Robert, A. Reynolds, C.A. Mirkin, and R.L. Letsinger, Homogeneous, Nanoparticle-Based Quantitative Colorimetric Detection of Oligonucleotides, *J. Am. Chem. Soc.*, 122, 3795–3796 (2000).
143. R. Jin, G. Wu, Z. Li, C.A. Mirkin, and G.C. Schatz, What Controls the Melting Properties of DNA-Linked Gold Nanoparticle Assemblies?, *J. Am. Chem. Soc.*, 125, 1643–1654 (2003).
144. A.A. Ensafi, M. Taei, H.R. Rahmani, and T. Khayamian, Sensitive DNA Impedance Biosensor for Detection of Cancer, Chronic Lymphocytic Leukemia, Based on Gold Nanoparticles/Gold Modified Electrode, *Electrochim. Acta*, 56, 8176–8183 (2011).
145. Cai, C. Xu, P. He, and Y. Fang, Colloid Au-Enhanced DNA Immobilization for the Electrochemical Detection of Sequence-Specific DNA, *J. Electroanal. Chem.*, 510, 78–85 (2001).
146. L. Lu, L. Xu, T. Kang, and S. Cheng, DNA Damage Due to Perfluorooctane Sulfonate Based on Nano-Gold Embedded in Nano-Porous Poly-Pyrrole Film, *Appl. Surf. Sci.*, 284, 258–262 (2013).
147. S. Liu, and A. Chen, Coadsorption of Horseradish Peroxidase with Thionine on TiO_2 Nanotubes for Biosensing, *Langmiur*, 21, 8409–8413 (2005).
148. J. Liu, C. Roussel, G. Lagger, P. Tacchini, and H.H. Girault, Antioxidant Sensors Based on DNA-Modified Electrodes, *Anal. Chem.*, 77, 7687–7694 (2005).
149. S.Q. Liu, J.J. Xu, and H.Y. Chen, ZrO_2 Gel-Derived DNA-Modified Electrode and the Effect of Lanthanide on its Electron Transfer Behavior, *Bioelectrochemistry*, 57, 149–154 (2002).
150. Y. Yang, Z. Wang, M. Yang, J. Li, F. Zheng, G. Shen, and R. Yu, Electrical Detection of Deoxyribonucleic Acid Hybridization Based on Carbon-Nanotubes/Nano Zirconium Dioxide/Chitosan-Modified Electrodes, *Anal. Chim. Acta*, 584, 268–274 (2007).
151. W. Zhang, T. Yang, C. Jiang, and K. Jiao, DNA Hybridization and Phosphinothricin Acetyltransferase Gene Sequence Detection Based on Zirconia/Nanogold Film Modified Electrode, *Appl. Surf. Sci.*, 254, 4750–4756 (2008).

152. A.A. Ansari, R. Singh, G. Sumana, and B.D. Malhotra, Sol–Gel Derived Nano-Structured Zinc Oxide Film for Sexually Transmitted Disease Sensor, *Analyst*, 13, 997–1002 (2009).

153. W. Zhang, T. Yang, X. Li, D. Wang, and K. Jiao, Conductive Architecture of Fe_2O_3 Microspheres/Self-Doped Polyaniline Nanofibers on Carbon Ionic Liquid Electrode for Impedance Sensing of DNA Hybridization, *Biosens. Bioelectron.*, 25, 428–434 (2009).

154. J. Wang, Carbon-Nanotube Based Electrochemical Biosensors: A Review, *Electroanalysis*, 17, 7–14 (2005).

155. S.N. Kim, J.F. Rusling, and F. Papadimitrakopoulos, Carbon Nanotubes for Electronic And Electrochemical Detection of Biomolecules, *Adv. Mater.*, 19, 3214–3228 (2007).

156. D. Tasis, N. Tagmatarchis, A. Bianco, and M. Prato, Chemistry of Carbon Nanotubes, *Chem. Rev.*, 106, 1105–1136 (2006).

157. M.L. Carot, R.M. Torresi, C.D. Garcia, M.J. Esplandiu, and C.E. Giacomelli, Electrostatic and Hydrophobic Interactions Involved in CNT Biofunctionalization with Short ss-DNA, *J. Phys. Chem. C*, 114, 4459–4465 (2010).

158. J. Kong, H.T. Soh, A.M. Cassell, C.F. Quate, and H. Dai, Synthesis of Individual Single-Walled Carbon Nanotubes on Patterned Silicon Wafers, *Nature*, 395, 878–881 (1998).

159. P. He, Y. Xu, and Y. Fang, Applications of Carbon Nanotubes in Electrochemical DNA Biosensors, *Microchim. Acta*, 152, 175–186 (2006).

160. J. Wang, M. Li, Z. Shi, N. Li, and Z. Gu, Electrochemistry of DNA at Single-Wall Carbon Nanotubes, *Electroanalysis*, 16, 140–144 (2004).

161. M. Pacios Pujadó, Carbon Nanotubes as Platforms for Biosensors with Electrochemical Electronic Transduction, Springer Theses, Springer-Verlag Berlin Heidelberg, 2012. doi:10. 1007/978-3-642-31421-6_5.

162. J. Wang, A.N. Kawde, and M. Musameh, Carbon-Nanotube-Modified Glassy Carbon Electrodes for Amplified Label-Free Electrochemical Detection of DNA Hybridization, *Analyst*, 128, 912–916 (2003).

163. M.L. Pedano, and G.A. Rivas, Adsorption and Electrooxidation of Nucleic Acids at Carbon Nanotubes Paste Electrodes, *Electrochem. Commun.*, 6, 10–16 (2004).

164. T.J. Yim, J. Liu, Y. Lu, R.S. Kane, and J.S. Dordick, Highly Active and Stable DNAzyme-Carbon Nanotube Hybrids, *J. Am. Chem. Soc.*, 127, 12200–12201 (2005).

165. A.A. Ensafi, M. Amini, and B. Rezaei, Detection of DNA Damage Induced by Chromium/Glutathione/H_2O_2 System at MWCNTs–Poly(diallyldimethylammonium Chloride) Modified Pencil Graphite Electrode Using Methylene Blue as an Electroactive Probe, *Sens. Actuators B*, 177, 862–870 (2013).

166. A.A. Ensafi, E. Heydari-Bafrooei, and B. Rezaei, Different Interaction of Codeine and Morphine with DNA: A Concept for Simultaneous Determination, *Biosens. Bioelectron.*, 41, 627–633 (2013).

167. A.A. Ensafi, E. Heydari-Bafrooei, and M. Amini, DNA-Functionalized Biosensor for Riboflavin Based Electrochemical Interaction on Pretreated Pencil Graphite Electrode, *Biosens. Bioelectron.*, 31, 376–381 (2012).

168. A.A. Ensafi, E. Heydari-Bafrooei, and B. Rezaei, DNA-Based Biosensor for Comparative Study of Catalytic Effect of Transition Metals on Autoxidation of Sulfite, *Anal. Chem.*, 85, 991–999 (2013).

169. A.A. Ensafi, M. Amini, and B. Rezaei, Assessment of Genotoxicity of Catecholics Using Impedimetric DNA-Biosensor, *Biosens. Bioelectron.*, 53, 43–50 (2014).

170. A.A. Ensafi, M. Amini, and B. Rezaei, Biosensor Based on ds-DNA Decorated Chitosan Modified Multiwall Carbon Nanotubes for Voltammetric Biodetection of Herbicide Amitrole, *Colloids Surf. B.*, 109, 45–51 (2013).

13 *In Vivo* Molecular Imaging with Quantum Dots
Toward Multimodality and Theranostics

Sarah P. Yang, Shreya Goel, and Weibo Cai

CONTENTS

ABSTRACT

Nanotechnology can profoundly affect cancer diagnosis and patient management in the future. Quantum dots (QDs), with their myriad advantages over conventional organic fluorescent dyes on the one hand, and potential toxicity and instability in biological environment on the other, present a very intriguing field of research. In this chapter, we aim to summarize the progress in the use of molecularly targeted QD-based nanoprobes for *in vivo* imaging applications. We discuss the current state-of-the-art synthesis, surface modification, bioconjugation methodologies, and the recent advances in QD technology. We then highlight specific examples of actively targeted QDs including multifunctional and theranostic nanosystems, concluding the chapter with a brief overview of the challenges and future directions for this promising class of nanoprobes in molecular imaging.

Keywords: Quantum dots (QDs), Nanotechnology, Cancer, Molecular imaging, Near-infrared fluorescence, Tumor targeting, Multimodality imaging, Theranostics

13.1 INTRODUCTION

Because of their small size, nanomaterials can provide significant advantages for molecular imaging and therapeutic applications. As they are typically orders of magnitude smaller than human cells, nanoparticles (NPs) can interact with biomolecules both on the surface and inside the cells in unprecedented manners. When conjugated with targeting moieties, NPs can be employed to interrogate specific molecular and cellular events in living systems. As such, nanotechnology has the ability to revolutionize disease diagnosis and treatment.

Molecular imaging is defined as "the non-invasive visualization, characterization and measurement of biological processes at the cellular and molecular level in humans and other living systems" (Mankoff 2007). Molecular imaging technologies have improved drastically over the last two decades and now include tools such as magnetic resonance imaging (MRI), computed tomography (CT), positron emission tomography (PET), single-photon emission CT, fluorescence/bioluminescence, and ultrasound. In recent years, a variety of NPs, including magnetic NPs (Amstad et al. 2009; Chaughule et al. 2012; Yu et al. 2008), quantum dots (QDs) (Cai and Hong 2012; Cai et al. 2006; Dubertret et al. 2002; Gao et al. 2004, 2010a,b; Sun et al. 2012), carbon nanotubes (Robinson et al. 2012; Shi et al. 2007; Tao et al. 2012), gold NPs (Kim et al. 2007; Lee et al. 2008; Yigit and Medarova 2012), and graphene-based nanomaterials (Gollavelli and Ling 2012; Hong et al. 2012a,b), have been studied for molecular imaging applications.

In this chapter, we will summarize the recent progress in the use of molecularly targeted QD-based nanoprobes for *in vivo* imaging applications. We will first briefly discuss the properties of the ideal imaging probe and the synthesis and surface modification approaches for *in vivo* applications of QDs. We will then give a brief overview of passive and active targeting followed by a detailed discussion on the use of targeted QDs for *in vivo* targeted imaging. We will also describe examples of QD-based nanoprobes for multifunctional applications. We will conclude the chapter by discussing the challenges and future directions for applications of QDs in the biomedical arena.

13.2 SYNTHESIS AND SURFACE MODIFICATION OF QDs FOR IMAGING APPLICATIONS

13.2.1 THE IDEAL IMAGING PROBE

The ideal probe for *in vivo* optical imaging has sustained fluorescence, long circulation lifetime, high biocompatibility, low toxicity, and minimal nonspecific uptake (Zhu et al. 2013a). Because of their attractive optical and electronic properties, QDs have attracted significant attention for optical imaging applications (Resch-Genger et al. 2008). Typically, QDs are semiconductor nanocrystals composed of II–IV (e.g., CdSe, CdTe) or III–V (e.g., InP, InAs) groups of elements. Often, the core material is coated with a semiconductor shell (e.g., CdS, ZnSe, ZnS) to improve the photoluminescence properties and reduce the leaching of the heavy metal core (Dif et al. 2008; Talapin et al. 2004).

Many of the unique properties of QDs arise as a result of quantum confinement. When the dimensions of an NP are less than that of the Bohr radius or the approximate diameter of the exciton (~5.3 nm), electron confinement occurs. As a result, nanomaterials of this size have a number of unique properties (Efros 1982). For instance, the band gap energy increases, allowing the NP to absorb light at higher wavelengths (i.e., higher energy); as the diameter of CdSe QDs decreases from 20 to 2 nm, the band gap energy increases from 1.7 to 2.4 eV (730 to 520 nm) (Alivisatos 1996). Thus, by controlling particle size, QDs with wide absorption range and narrow, symmetric emission spectra can easily be developed (Delehanty et al. 2009; Michalet et al. 2005; Murphy et al. 2006). Additionally, the high quantum yields (QY >90%), long fluorescence lifetime (>10 ns), and large effective Stokes shift (>200 nm) of QDs make them suitable for both single-molecule tracking and multiplexed imaging (Resch-Genger et al. 2008). Because of their resistance to photobleaching and chemical degradation, QDs have also been widely used for long-term imaging studies (Cai et al. 2007b).

A variety of factors (e.g., size, charge, concentration, and stability) can influence the toxicity of a nanomaterial. For QDs, toxicity can result from core degradation, free radical generation, and interaction with subcellular components and proteins (Geszke-Moritz and Moritz 2013). To address the potential for toxicity and improve biocompatibility, QDs have been functionalized with or encapsulated within biocompatible molecules (e.g., polymers, liposomes, and inorganic silica) (Jayagopal et al. 2007; Loginova et al. 2012; Nicolas et al. 2011) and Cd-free QDs (e.g., $CuInS_2$, InP, InAs, Si QDs, C-dots) have been developed (Cao et al. 2007; Cassette et al. 2010; Deng et al. 2012; Erogbogbo et al. 2011; Gao et al. 2010b, 2012; Li et al. 2009; Sun et al. 2006; Zhou et al. 2007a).

13.2.2 SYNTHESIS

While a variety of methods have been developed for the synthesis of QDs, the majority of the methods can be classified into two categories: organometallic synthesis and aqueous synthesis. In the organometallic method, the QDs are synthesized in an organic solvent such as trioctylphosphine oxide (TOPO), with a high boiling point and high coordinating capacity for the metal and chalcogen components of the QD (Peng and Peng 2001; Qu et al. 2001; Smith et al. 2006; Talapin et al. 2001). The advantages of this approach are that the QDs possess nearly perfect crystal structures, have high fluorescence QY, and narrow size distributions. However, this approach is costly and labor intensive. Furthermore, it poses problems for biological applications as the QDs must be transferred from the organic solvent to an aqueous matrix before use. Strategies such as ligand exchange and coating with a water-soluble shell have been developed for this purpose, but they often cause a significant loss in fluorescence signal.

The synthesis of QD via the aqueous route generally involves three main steps (Lesnyak et al. 2013). First, metal/thiol complexes are formed by dissolving a metal salt in water and then adding the thiol of interest. Second, a chalcogen is injected into the metal/thiol solution forming the MeX precursor. Finally, heating or microwave irradiation is employed to facilitate nucleation and QD growth. While QDs synthesized via this route generally have lower quantum yield and broader size distribution, the method is typically simpler, more reproducible, and more biocompatible than the organometallic approach (Kalasad et al. 2009; Law et al. 2009; Rogach et al. 1996; Zhu et al. 2013b; Zou et al. 2008).

13.2.3 Surface Modification

For *in vivo* applications of nanomaterials, surface modification can be used to increase suspension stability and to reduce toxicity in biocompatible matrices. Surface modification can also protect the materials from degradation and, in the case of QDs, fluorescence quenching. For QDs with hydrophobic surfaces (i.e., those prepared via the organometallic route), the surface must be rendered hydrophilic before use in *in vivo* applications. Approaches to render QDs hydrophilic include surface ligand exchange, phospholipid encapsulation, and surface silanization (Wang et al. 2012a). In these processes, the surface of the QDs is coated with molecules that contain both hydrophilic and hydrophobic regions. The hydrophobic regions bind to the QD surface while the hydrophilic regions provide aqueous stability.

For surface ligand exchange, the hydrophobic surfactant molecules are replaced with bifunctional molecules (Li et al. 2009; Park et al. 2011). These molecules typically contain thiols as the surface anchoring hydrophobic groups and carboxyl or hydroxyl moieties as the hydrophilic end groups. Examples include cysteine (Choi et al. 2007; Liu et al. 2007; Lowe et al. 2012; Tian et al. 2012), polyethylene glycol (PEG) (Al-Jamal et al. 2009; Choi et al. 2009; Schipper et al. 2009), and glutathione (Tiwari et al. 2009). Another approach is to encapsulate the QDs within phospholipid micelles (Al-Jamal and Kostarelos 2011; Dubertret et al. 2002; Li et al. 2012; Travert-Branger et al. 2008, 2011). In this process, the phospholipids and amphiphilic di- and triblock polymers are dispersed in solution so that they can self-assemble around the QDs. This method is advantageous because it does not alter the QD surface, allowing the optical properties to be retained. The third strategy employs surface silanization, wherein QDs are coated with an inorganic silica shell, a class of highly biocompatible material (Bruchez et al. 1998; Szabo and Vollath 1999). In this technique, the surface ligands are exchanged with thiol-derived silanes. The silanes are typically cross-linked to increase stability, even over a broad pH range, and reduce toxicity (Zhu et al. 2013b).

In addition, ligands such as PEG, a commercially available polymer, can be coated on the QD surface (Lee et al. 2010; Pellegrino et al. 2004). In general, PEGylation increases NP biocompatibility by reducing the interactions between the particle and serum proteins (Karakoti et al. 2011). PEG is believed to increase the shielding of surface charge, particle hydrophilicity, and the repulsion forces between PEG molecules as well as decrease the interfacial free tension of NPs. Moreover, the high surface density of PEG is thought to prevent surface binding by serum proteins. Together, these effects can reduce interactions with serum proteins.

Several groups have examined how PEGylation affects the biocompatibility of QDs (Al-Jamal et al. 2009; Ballou et al. 2004; Schipper et al. 2009). For instance, Ballou et al. (2004) functionalized ZnS/CdSe core/shell QDs with an amphiphilic polymer (polyacrylic acid; amp) or the same coating conjugated with methoxy-terminated PEG of various molecular weights (mPEG-750 QDs, mPEG-5000 QDs). They found that the QDs with the largest PEG coating had the longest circulation time. In fact, the circulating lifetime of the mPEG-5000 QDs was >50 min while that of the amp and mPEG-750 QDs was <12 min (Ballou et al. 2004).

In another study, Schipper et al. examined how surface modification with PEG-2000 influenced the biodistribution of commercially available CdSe/ZnS QDs, which are coated with a proprietary polymer (QDpoly) to make them water soluble (Schipper et al. 2009). Both PEG-conjugated (QDpolyPEG) and unconjugated QDpoly showed different biodistribution patterns. For instance, uptake into the liver and spleen was slower for the conjugated QDs (QDpolyPEG, 6 min; QDpoly, 1 min). Thus, surface modification with PEG was found to increase the circulation half-life of QDs as well as reduce their uptake into organs of the RES, making QDs more suitable for *in vivo* imaging applications.

Other studies have used PEG in combination with other polymers for surface modification of QDs. For instance, polymer-coated semiconductor QDs have been reported for ultrasensitive and multiplexed imaging of molecular targets *in vivo* (Gao et al. 2004). Hydrophobic CdSe/ZnS core/shell QDs were synthesized through the organometallic method using TOPO as the coordinating ligand and then coated with PEG and an ABC triblock copolymer containing hydrophobic (polybutylacrylate and polyethylacrylate) and hydrophilic (polymethacrylic) regions. Reduced aggregation and fluorescence loss of QDs were observed during both storage in physiological buffer and *in vivo* imaging applications.

In addition to PEG, other biocompatible coatings have been employed for surface modification of QDs (Cao et al. 2012; Kim et al. 2011; Wen et al. 2012). For example, CdTe/CdSe core/shell QDs encapsulated within poly(lactic-co-glycolic acid) nanospheres were found to be distinguishable from the background autofluorescence in as little as 1 h postinjection (p.i.). Furthermore, QDs were detected *in vivo* for up to 48 h p.i. (Kim et al. 2011). In another study, hydrophobic PbS QDs were coated with an amphiphilic polymer forming *N*-succinyl-*N'*-octyl nanomicelles. These QD-containing nanomicelles caused low toxicity and accumulated more specifically within tumor tissues (Cao et al. 2012).

13.2.4 STRATEGIES FOR BIOCONJUGATION

Once hydrophilic, a number of strategies can be employed for conjugation of QDs with biomolecules (e.g., EDC/NHS coupling, thiol–maleimide reaction, streptavidin–biotin binding, metal–histidine interactions, etc.). One of the most common methods for bioconjugating QDs is through coupling reagents such as ethyl(dimethylaminopropyl) carbodiimide (EDC) and N-hydroxysuccinimide (NHS) (Hua et al. 2006). In this approach, an amide bond is formed between a carboxyl and an amino group. One drawback of this approach is that nonspecific cross-linking can occur because there are several carboxyl and amino groups on a single biomolecule. This can reduce the activity of the biomolecule because there are fewer groups available for biological processes.

Another strategy for conjugation of QDs with biomolecules is the thiol–maleimide reaction. This reaction is more specific than EDC/NHS coupling since it involves only the thiol groups on the surface of the biomolecule. This reaction employs a heterobifunctional cross-linking agent, sulfo-succinimidyl-4-(N-maleimidomethyl) cyclohexane-1-carboxylate, which contains an NHS ester on one end and a maleimide group on the other (Hermanson 2008). The ester reacts with amino groups on the surface of the QDs while the maleimide can be conjugated with thiolated biomolecules.

The streptavidin–biotin interaction is another strategy commonly used for the bioconjugation of QDs (Allen et al. 2010; Chen et al. 2012a; Maldiney et al. 2012). Streptavidin is a nonglycosylated protein produced by the bacterium *Streptomyces avidinii* while biotin is a water-soluble vitamin (vitamin B_7) and is essential for cell growth, fatty acid production, and the metabolism of fats and amino acids. This strategy relies on the high affinity of streptavidin for biotin; binding can occur directly between streptavidin-functionalized QDs and biotinylated proteins/peptides or streptavidin can be used as a bridge between biotinylated QDs and biomolecules.

Another strategy for surface modification is metal–histidine binding (Bae et al. 2009; Park et al. 2010). In this approach, nickel nitrilotriacetic acid (Ni–NTA), commonly used for isolation and purification of proteins, is conjugated to the QD surface through a Ni^{2+} complexation reaction. The Ni–NTA complex can then bind to histidine-tagged proteins. This method increases the aqueous stability of QDs because the NTA ligand contains tricarboxylates.

13.3 *IN VIVO* ACTIVE TARGETING WITH QDs

13.3.1 PASSIVE VERSUS ACTIVE TARGETING

NPs can be designed to target tumors *in vivo* through either passive or active targeting (Figure 13.1). Passive targeting relies on the convection and diffusion of materials through the body (Danhier et al. 2010). Tumor blood vessels often have excessive angiogenesis and hypervasculature, a lack of pericytes, defective vascular architecture, inconsistent blood flow, and a lack of lymphatic vessels; together, these abnormalities lead to enhanced vascular permeability and reduced drainage from the tumor. As such, nanomaterials can extravasate from the blood vessels into the interstitial space within the tumor and remain there. This phenomenon, known as the enhanced permeability and retention (EPR) effect, has been the gold standard

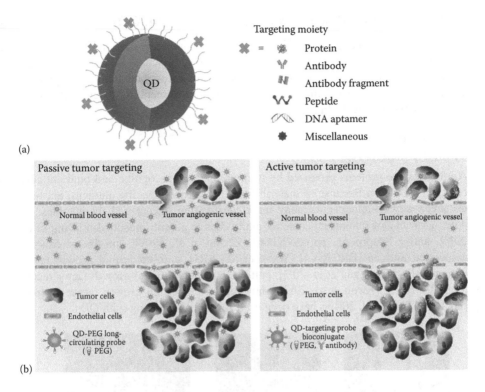

(a)

(b)

FIGURE 13.1 Schematic illustrating (a) the targeting moieties employed for *in vivo* targeted imaging applications with QDs and (b) passive (via leaky tumor vasculature) and active targeting (via high-affinity binding between QD–antibody conjugates and tumor antigens). (Adapted from X.H. Gao et al., *Nature Biotechnology*, 22, 969–976, 2004.)

for tumor-targeted drug design. As such, it is the guiding principle for the design of many NP-based imaging agents and therapeutics (Maeda et al. 2009).

However, there are limitations to EPR-based targeting schematics for NP-based therapies. In general, particles need to be between 10 and 100 nm in diameter to avoid renal clearance but maintain their ability to extravasate. Particles should be uncharged or anionic to avoid renal clearance. Because the degree of tumor angiogenesis and vasculature varies with tumor type and location, the extent of passive targeting will vary between different tissues and tumor types (Danhier et al. 2010).

Because of these drawbacks, active targeting with nanomaterials has been investigated for molecular imaging and therapeutic applications. Active targeting can be achieved by attaching targeting ligands to the surface of the NP, which then bind to receptors at the target site (Pirollo and Chang 2008). Receptors are typically overexpressed on either the tumor cells or the tumor vasculature, but not on normal cells. Thus, NPs are directed to specific locations within the body. While binding to the tumor cell can lead to cellular uptake by the NPs, binding to the tumor endothelium does not require extravasation of the NP and many of the endothelial markers of interest are present on a variety of tumor types.

13.3.2 Targeting Moieties for *In Vivo* Imaging with QDs

To minimize nonspecific uptake during *in vivo* active tumor-targeting applications, QDs have been conjugated with a variety of targeting moieties. Most of the moieties fall into two main categories: proteins (including antibodies and antibody fragments) and peptides. Other less common moieties include aptamers, folic acid (FA)/folate, and polymers (Figure 13.1a).

13.3.2.1 Proteins

13.3.2.1.1 Antibodies

Antibodies are proteins produced by immune cells to recognize and bind antigens on foreign objects. Because of their ability to recognize specific antigens, antibodies are a key component in many targeted imaging agents and therapeutics. To date, a variety of human monoclonal antibodies (e.g., anti-mesothelin [Ding et al. 2011], anti-α-fetoprotein, anti-AVE1642 [Zhang et al. 2009], anti–breast cancer–associated antigen [BRCAA-1] [Wang et al. 2011], anti–epidermal growth factor receptor [EGFR] [Yang et al. 2011], anti–vascular endothelial growth factor receptor [VEGFR-2] [Kwon et al. 2013], anti–human epidermal growth factor receptor [HER-2] [Tada et al. 2007]) have been used for active targeting with QDs.

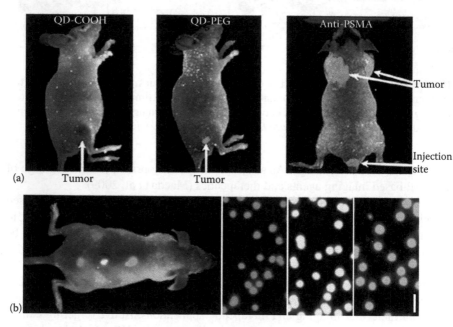

FIGURE 13.2 (a) Spectrally resolved *in vivo* fluorescence images of C4-2 human prostate tumor–bearing mice using QD probes with three different surface modifications: carboxylic acid groups, PEG groups, and PEG–PSMA Ab conjugates. (b) Multicolor capability of QD imaging. Images of multicolor QD–encoded microbeads emitting green, yellow, and red light (right) and *in vivo* imaging of subcutaneously injected microbeads on a host mouse (left). The scale bar represents 1 μm. (Adapted from X.H. Gao et al., *Nature Biotechnology*, 22, 969–976, 2004.)

One of the first *in vivo* imaging studies with antibody-conjugated QDs was published in 2004 (Figure 13.2). Gao et al. conjugated CdSe/ZnS core/shell QDs with the antibody against prostate-specific membrane antigen (PSMA), a membrane glycoprotein that is strongly expressed in tumor neovasculature (Gao et al. 2004). Enhanced accumulation was achieved within 2 h p.i. when anti-PSMA-conjugated QDs were intravenously delivered and retained in C4-2 tumor xenografts. On the other hand, only weak tumor signal was detected with QDs modified with carboxylic acid and PEG groups, even after 6 and 24 h p.i., respectively (Figure 13.2a). Using both subcutaneous injection of QD-tagged cancer cells and systemic injection of multifunctional QD probes, sensitive and multicolor fluorescence imaging of cancer cells was also made possible under *in vivo* conditions (Figure 13.2b).

Another antibody of interest for molecular imaging and therapeutic applications is directed against EGFR. EGFR is a cell surface receptor for the epidermal growth factor (EGF) protein family and is often overexpressed in various types of cancer including oral squamous cell carcinoma (OSCC) and head and neck squamous cell carcinoma and has been widely used as a targeting moiety (Kalyankrishna and Grandis 2006; Rogers et al. 2005). For example, near-infrared (NIR) CdTe/ZnS core/shell QDs conjugated with anti-EGFR antibody have shown promising prospects in *in vivo* imaging of OSCC and development of personalized surgical therapies (Yang et al. 2011). Fluorescence signals were clearly observed from BcaCD885 tumor xenografts, and maximal signal-to-noise ratio was observed from 15 min to 6 h p.i. On the other hand, fluorescence signal did not surpass background with unconjugated QDs or after blocking with EGF before QD administration.

13.3.2.1.2 Antibody Fragments

While considered the gold standard for many targeted imaging and therapeutic agents, antibodies may not be the ideal targeting moiety for *in vivo* imaging with QDs. Only a handful of antibodies can be conjugated to the surface of each particle given their relatively large size, thereby hampering the sensitivity of the probe. Also, antibodies may hinder the penetration of QDs into solid tumors. Given these issues, antibody fragments have been examined as alternative targeting moieties. Several studies have utilized single-chain antibody fragments (ScFv), which consist of antibody heavy- and light-chain variable domains connected by a flexible peptide linker, for *in vivo* imaging with QDs. While these fragments are much smaller than intact antibodies (25 kDa vs. 150 kDa), they still possess the high binding affinity and antigen specificity of intact antibodies (Zhou et al. 2007b).

For instance, when block copolymer-coated CdSe/ZnS core/shell QDs were conjugated with ScFv-EGFR, a large number of ScFv-EGFR QDs were found to selectively home into orthotopic PaCa-2 pancreatic tumors (Yang et al. 2009). In contrast, very few QDs were detected in tumors from mice that received unconjugated QDs. Furthermore, compared to unconjugated QDs, markedly lower levels of ScFv-EGFR QDs were detected in the lungs and kidneys. Similarly, in another study, commercially available, PEGylated CdSe/ZnS core/shell QDs were functionalized with anti-c-Met ScFv; c-Met is a receptor tyrosine kinase that is associated with cancer cell proliferation, migration, invasion, and tumor angiogenesis (Lu et al. 2011). Significantly higher signal intensity and tumor-to-normal tissue ratios were obtained in H1993 tumor xenografts anti-c-Met-scFv-coupled

QDs than with unconjugated QDs at both 6 and 24 h p.i. Similar results were obtained with scFv-GRP78-conjugated CdSe/ZnS core/shell QDs (Xu et al. 2012). GRP78 is a member of the heat shock protein family and is crucial for cancer cell proliferation and angiogenesis. QD-GRP78 scFv bioconjugates not only aided in multicolor fluorescence imaging but also showed breast cancer growth inhibition in MDA-MB-231 xenografts.

13.3.2.1.3 Other Proteins

Antibodies and antibody fragments are not the only type of protein used as targeting ligands. For example, natural cell surface ligands, such as EGF, have strong affinity for specific targets, making them ideal targeting moieties. EGF is found in many tissues and functions by binding to the EGFR on the cell surface. EGF is involved in DNA synthesis, cell growth, proliferation, and differentiation, and its overexpression is associated with a variety of cancers (Cai et al. 2008a). When conjugated with EGF, CdSe/ZnS QDs were found to accumulate within HCT116 tumor xenografts in 1 to 6 h p.i. (Diagaradjane et al. 2008). On the other hand, unconjugated QDs did not accumulate within the tumor, indicating that EGFR-specific binding and not increased vascular permeability of tumors, was responsible for the enhanced uptake.

13.3.2.2 Peptides

Peptides, or short chains of linked amino acids, have been used in a large number of *in vivo* targeted imaging studies for several reasons. Their small size allows a number of peptides to be attached to a single molecule. Furthermore, they are easy to synthesize, have low immunogenicity, and are tolerant to a variety of reaction conditions. The first study to evaluate *in vivo* tumor targeting with peptide-conjugated QDs did so more than a decade ago (Akerman et al. 2002). ZnS-capped CdSe QDs were conjugated with three different peptides: GFE, which binds to endothelial cells in lung blood vessels; F3, which binds to blood vessels and tumor cells; and LyP-1, which binds to lymphatic vessels and tumor cells. F3- and LyP-conjugated QDs accumulated in MDA-MB-435 tumor xenografts with F3–QDs colocalizing with lectin, a blood vessel marker, and LyP-1–QDs colocalizing with the lymphatic vessel marker, podoplanin. Similarly, GFE–QDs accumulated in the lungs, confirming the ability of peptide-coated QDs to home to their targets *in vivo*. None of the QDs were detected in the brain, heart, kidney, and skin. This was the first study to demonstrate that peptides could be used for *in vivo* tumor imaging and that QDs could be targeted to distinct biological structures.

Since this pioneering study, the majority of peptide-based QD studies have utilized the peptide, arginine–glycine–aspartate (RGD). RGD is a cellular recognition and attachment moiety for a variety of extracellular matrix proteins including integrins (Wang et al. 2012a). Applications of RGD range from disease diagnosis to drug development and tissue engineering because of its small size, low immunogenicity, and simple, inexpensive synthesis. For tumor targeting, RGD peptides are often used to target integrin $\alpha_v\beta_3$, which is overexpressed in the endothelial cells of tumor neovasculature in many cancer types (e.g., bone, brain, skin, lung, and breast) (Cai and Chen 2008; Cai et al. 2008b). To date, a number of studies have established the tumor-targeting ability of QDs when conjugated with RGD (Cai et al. 2006; Gao et al. 2010b; Huang et al. 2013; Li et al. 2012; Mukthavaram et al. 2011; Smith et al. 2010; Yong 2010; Yong et al. 2009, 2010). In general, studies employing QDs consisting of II–IV groups of elements saw significantly higher levels of tumor accumulation when conjugated with the RGD peptide (i.e., active targeting) than with unconjugated QDs (i.e., passive targeting). Nonspecific QD uptake was also observed in the liver and spleen owing to accumulation in the reticuloendothelial system but was generally reduced with RGD conjugation. Accumulation generally occurred rapidly and reached a maximum within a couple of hours. Within 24–48 h, background levels were reduced through renal and hepatic clearance; hence, targeted QD imaging was improved.

To reduce the potential for toxicity, recent studies have examined the use of RGD-conjugated Cd-free QDs for *in vivo* imaging (Erogbogbo et al. 2011; Gao et al. 2012). RGD-conjugated, biocompatible silicon (Si) semiconductor-based QDs demonstrated increasing luminescence intensity in Panc-1 tumor xenografts with time while nonconjugated SiQDs showed no tumor uptake (Figure 13.3). In fact, the total

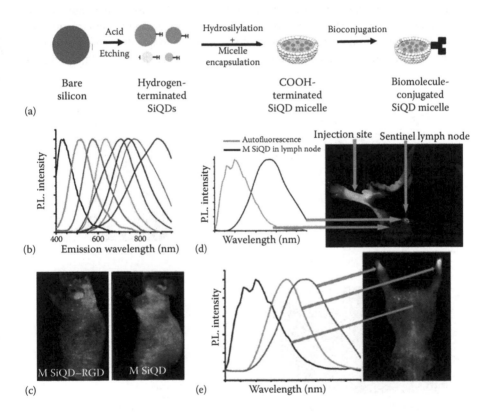

FIGURE 13.3 (a) Schematic illustrating the synthesis and surface functionalization of silicon QDs (SiQDs). (b) Normalized emission spectra from SiQDs (2–8 nm) excited by a single source (365 nm). Red shifts from 450 to 900 nm were observed with increasing particle size. (c) *In vivo* luminescence imaging of Panc-1 tumor–bearing mice injected with SiQD–RGD or SiQD (40 h p.i.). (d) Sentinel lymph node imaging after localization of SiQDs in an axillary position. Autofluorescence is indicated in green and the unmixed SiQD signal is in red. (e) *In vivo* multiplex NIR imaging capability of SiQDs subcutaneously injected in the lower limbs of a mouse. Autofluorescence is indicated in green and the unmixed SiQD signal is in red and yellow. (Adapted from F. Erogbogbo et al., *ACS Nano*, 5, 413–423, 2011.)

luminescence intensity for the conjugated SiQDs was 186 times higher than that for the unconjugated SiQDs. The conjugated SiQDs had lower liver and spleen uptake than unconjugated particles. Furthermore, these NPs could also be used for sentinel lymph node mapping and multicolor NIR imaging in live mice, thereby maintaining the key advantages of QD-based imaging methods. In another study, dendron-coated InP QDs with RGD dimers were found to drastically enhance the contrast of SKOV-3 tumor xenografts than the nonconjugated QDs at 24 h p.i. (Gao et al. 2012).

13.3.2.3 Other Targeting Moieties

13.3.2.3.1 Aptamers

Aptamers are short oligonucleotide acid or peptide sequences that bind to specific targets. Aptamers are rapidly cleared from the body, have low immunogenicity, and can be easily synthesized via chemical methods *in vitro*. Because of these advantages, this new class of targeting moiety is of interest in molecular imaging and therapeutics (Hong et al. 2011). To date, only a couple of studies have conjugated aptamers to QDs for *in vivo* imaging applications (Savla et al. 2011; Zhang et al. 2013). In one report,

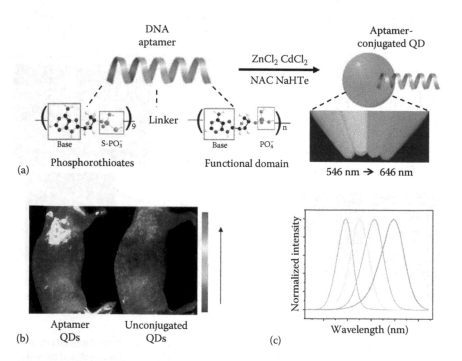

FIGURE 13.4 (a) Schematic illustrating the one-pot synthesis of DNA aptamer-conjugated QDs, depicting the structure of phosphorothioates and the functional domain (b). Fluorescence images of A459 tumor–bearing mice injected with aptamer-conjugated QDs and unconjugated QDs. (c) Normalized emission spectra (above) and representative photograph (below) of aptamer-conjugated QDs with controllable maximum emission wavelengths ranging from 546 to 646 nm, under UV irradiation. (Adapted from C. Zhang et al., *Analytical Chemistry*, 85, 5843–5849, 2013.)

aptamer-functionalized Zn^{2+}-doped CdTe QDs were synthesized via a facile one-pot hydrothermal route and applied for active tumor-targeted imaging *in vitro* and *in vivo* (Figure 13.4). The aptamers were specific to MUC1, or mucin 1, a glycoprotein that lines epithelial cells in the lungs, stomach, intestines, and eyes. Moreover, the over-expression of MUC1 has been associated with a variety of carcinomas (e.g., colon, breast, ovarian, lung, and pancreatic cancers). The QDs showed high quantum yield, good photostability, and highly specific tumor targeting in A549 xenografts in mice.

13.3.2.3.2   Folate/Folic Acid

Folate is the naturally occurring form of the water-soluble vitamin B_9. FA is a syn-thetically produced form of the same vitamin. Folate/FA is crucial for DNA syn-thesis, repair, and methylation and for RNA synthesis. As the alpha form of the folate receptor (FR-α) is overexpressed on many epithelial cancers, folate/FA have been used as targeting moieties for a variety of molecular imaging and targeting applications (Kularatne and Low 2010). In fact, folate/FA ligands have been used in a handful of *in vivo* imaging studies with QDs (Chen et al. 2012b; Deng et al. 2012; Liu et al. 2012; Wang et al. 2012b; Xue et al. 2012; Yang et al. 2011). In one study, CdTe/ZnS core/shell QDs encapsulated within amphiphilic triblock copoly-mer micelles and conjugated with FA were used to target Panc-1 tumor xenografts in mice. The optical and colloidal stability of the QDs were preserved, and the formula-tion specifically targeted the tumor site. Very low fluorescence was detected in the tumors of mice administered with the unconjugated QD micelles. Additionally, *ex vivo* analysis showed high fluorescence within the tumor but not with other tissues upon FA-QD micelle administration.

13.3.2.3.3   Polymers

Certain polymers can also act as targeting moieties for *in vivo* applications. For instance, hyaluronic acid (HA) has been used for *in vivo* imaging with graphene QDs (GQDs) (Abdullah Al et al. 2013; Bhang et al. 2009; Ossipov 2010). HA is a glycos-aminoglycan that is found throughout the connective, epithelial, and neural tissues. It is important for cell proliferation and migration and is involved in the progression of certain cancers. Abdullah et al. observed significant accumulation of HA-conjugated GQDs within A549 tumor xenografts whereas tumor accumulation was much lower with unconjugated GQDs (Abdullah Al et al. 2013). Furthermore, uptake in the liver and kidney was much lower with HA–GQDs than with unconjugated GQDs.

13.4   MULTIFUNCTIONAL QDs FOR MOLECULAR IMAGING AND THERAPEUTICS

13.4.1   MULTIMODALITY QDs

While a number of studies have established the excellent abilities of QDs as fluo-rescent probes for *in vivo* active tumor targeting, single imaging modality often is not enough to obtain all the necessary information. For instance, fluorescence imaging lacks the ability for quantification and deep tissue penetration. On the other hand, MRI has excellent soft tissue contrast and resolution but lacks sensitivity while

PET has excellent sensitivity, quantitation, and tissue penetration but relatively low resolution. For these reasons, multimodality probes that combine multiple imaging techniques into a single probe have been developed (Cai and Chen 2008). In addition, multimodal agents allow cross-modality verification, which can provide more accurate data than possible with a single modality alone. In fact, many QD-based nanoprobes have been designed and evaluated for these applications.

In MRI, protons are excited with a strong magnetic field and the relaxation signals of the proton spins are detected and converted to images. Superparamagnetic iron oxide NPs (SPIONs) are emerging as probes for *in vivo* MRI because they can cause local field inhomogeneities resulting in shortened relaxation times. Recently, a number of dual-modality probes consisting of SPIONs and QDs have been developed for optical imaging and MRI. Fluorescent magnetic NPs (FMNPs) in which CdTe QDs and Fe_3O_4 NPs were encapsulated within a 3-aminopropyltriethoxysilane shell have been reported (Wang et al. 2011). This shell was then conjugated with anti-BRCAA1 antibody. Using noninvasive fluorescence imaging and MRI, the MGC-803 tumor xenografts were easily delineated from the surrounding tissue. *Ex vivo* analysis at 12 h p.i. revealed significant accumulation of the FMNPs within the tumor while little accumulation was observed in other organs (e.g., liver, lung, spleen, and heart). They confirmed accumulation of the FMNPs within the tumor with MRI. In fact, significant change in T2 signal intensity was observed in some regions of tumors at 12 h p.i.

In another study, a multilayered multimodal, core/shell nanoprobe (MQQ probe) was designed in which Fe_3O_4 MNPs (MRI) and CdSe/ZnS and CdSeTe/ CdS core/shell QDs (visible and NIR fluorescent [NIRF] imaging) were encapsulated within multiple silica layers and then conjugated with anti-HER2 antibody for breast cancer–specific targeting (Ma et al. 2012). Intense fluorescence signals were observed within the KPL-4 tumor xenografts at 48 h p.i. Using MRI, they confirmed the presence of FMNPs within the tumor. In fact, T2-weighted MRI indicated that the anti-HER2-conjugated MQQ probes were primarily located in the peripheral regions around the tumor blood vessels. This synthetic strategy presents an easy way to prepare a variety of the multimodality probes with different NPs and functional molecules.

In PET imaging, gamma rays emitted by the positron emitting radiolabeled probe are detected and converted to a 3D image (Gambhir 2002). Because this technique is highly sensitive and provides excellent tissue penetration, it is widely used in cancer diagnosis, staging, and evaluation of therapeutic efficacy (Alauddin 2012; Eary et al. 2011; Grassi et al. 2012; Vach et al. 2011). While ^{18}F ($t_{1/2}$ = 110 min) is the most commonly used radioisotope in clinical applications, isotopes with longer half-lives (e.g., ^{64}Cu [$t_{1/2}$ = 12.7 h], ^{86}Y [$t_{1/2}$ = 14.7 h], ^{89}Zr [$t_{1/2}$ = 78.1 h]) are often used for *in vivo* animal studies.

The initial targeted dual-modality QD probes for *in vivo* optical and PET imaging involved labeling of CdTe QDs with cRGD peptide and $VEGF_{165}$ moieties to target tumor angiogenesis (Cai et al. 2007a; Chen et al. 2008). A macrocyclic chelating agent, DOTA (1,4,7,10-tetraazacyclododecane-*N,N',N",N'''*-tetraacetic acid), was introduced onto amine-functionalized QDs, which in turn complexed with ^{64}Cu radioisotope for PET imaging. A dual PET/NIRF probe can overcome the qualitative or semiquantitative nature of optical imaging and can allow for a more accurate assessment of the pharmacokinetics and tumor-targeting efficacy of QDs. DOTA–QD–VEGF conjugates showed enhanced tumor vasculature targeting (Chen et al. 2008). VEGFR-specific uptake of targeted QDs was observed in U87MG glioma xenografts, confirmed by excellent correlation between *ex vivo* PET and NIRF organ imaging (Figure 13.5b and c). Furthermore, histological examination revealed that DOTA–QD–VEGF primarily targeted the tumor vasculature through specific VEGF–VEGFR binding and that little extravasation occurred. This bifunctional approach renders higher degree of accuracy for the quantitative targeted NIRF imaging in deep tissue. Vasculature-specific targeting of QDs with little extravasation was again observed.

More recently, CdSe/ZnS QDs encapsulated in amphiphile polysorbate 60 were developed, which also contained the chelator NOTA (1,4,7-triazacyclononane-*N,N',N''*-triacetic acid) (Lee et al. 2012). The QDs were subsequently radiolabeled with ^{68}Ga ($t_{1/2}$ = 68 min) and conjugated with cRGD. Using noninvasive fluorescence imaging, they observed higher accumulation of RGD–QDs than unconjugated QDs in U87MG tumor xenografts, which was confirmed with PET imaging.

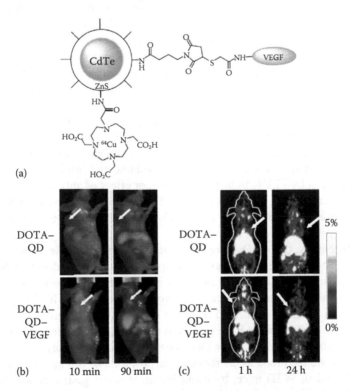

FIGURE 13.5 (a) Schematic illustrating the structure of DOTA–QD–VEGF conjugates, radiolabeled with ^{64}Cu, which allows for PET imaging. (b) Time-dependent *in vivo* NIRF imaging of U87MG tumor–bearing mice injected with DOTA–QD–VEGF and DOTA–QD. (c) Whole-body coronal PET images of U87MG tumor–bearing mice injected with ^{64}Cu–DOTA–QD and ^{64}Cu–DOTA–QD–VEGF. White arrows indicate tumor. (Adapted from K. Chen et al., *Eur J Nucl Med Mol Imaging*, 35, 2235–2244, 2008.)

Tumor-to-muscle ratio of RGD–QDs in U87MG tumor xenografts was 3.5:1, indicating specific targeting of the nanoconjugates. To further examine the targeting specificity of these materials, they compared the uptake of RGD–QDs in mice bearing U87MG and A431 tumor xenografts expressing high and low levels of integrin αvβ3, respectively. With optical and PET imaging, they observed higher QD accumulation in U87MG tumors than in A431 tumors (U87MG tumor-to-A431 tumor ratio ~5.5:1).

13.4.2 THERANOSTICS

Theranostics is an emerging field that combines disease diagnosis with therapy and drug delivery. Given their small size, large surface area, and ability to undergo surface modification, nanomaterials are an ideal platform for theranostic applications. To date, a handful of studies have examined QDs for theranostic applications (Lu et al. 2011; Nurunnabi et al. 2010; Ruan et al. 2012; Xu et al. 2012).

A number of these studies have employed anti-HER2 for *in vivo* targeting and treatment with QDs (Nurunnabi et al. 2010; Ruan et al. 2012). Anti-HER2 is a monoclonal antibody that interferes with the HER2, human EGFR 2. Also known as Herclon, Herceptin, and trastuzumab, anti-HER2 is used to target and treat breast cancer. In breast cancer, the HER2 pathway is often overstimulated, causing rapid tumor cell proliferation (Nurunnabi et al. 2010). As a cancer therapeutic, anti-HER2 functions by binding to the HER2 receptor, causing cell cycle arrest and, thus, reducing proliferation and suppressing angiogenesis.

In one such study, CdTe/CdSe core/shell QDs encapsulated within polymer micelles and conjugated with anti-HER2 antibody (130–150 nm) were tested against MDA-MB 231 breast tumors (Figure 13.6) (Nurunnabi et al. 2010). Anti-HER2 QD micelles were found to drastically reduce the volume and inhibit the growth of the tumor xenografts by 77.3%. In fact, the antitumor effect of anti-HER2 QD micelles was higher than that of anti-HER2 alone. This antitumor activity coincided with rapid and sustained accumulation of the QDs within the tumor, allowing for simultaneous imaging.

In another study, CdTe QDs were conjugated with ribonuclease A (RNase A) and anti-HER2 (Ruan et al. 2012). RNase A is an enzyme that degrades the RNA within cancer cells, inhibiting mRNA translation and protein synthesis, which leads to apoptosis. Using noninvasive optical imaging, subcutaneous MGC-803 gastric cancer xenografts could be delineated from the surrounding background tissue within 3 h p.i. *Ex vivo* analysis at 24 h p.i. indicated that the QDs primarily accumulated in the tumor tissues with much fewer QDs located in spleen, kidney, heart, lung, and liver. To evaluate the probe for therapeutic purposes, an *in situ* gastric cancer model was established in SCID mice, by using bioluminescent gastric cancer tissues. In anti-HER2 QD–treated animals, bioluminescence signals remained constant while signals in the control group increased over time, indicating that anti-HER2 QDs reduced tumor growth. Furthermore, mice treated with anti-HER2 QDs had longer survival time (>11 weeks) than control-treated mice (8 weeks).

Antibody fragments have also been used as targeting and therapy agents in theranostic applications. For instance, the antibody fragment ScFv GrP79-H19 was conjugated

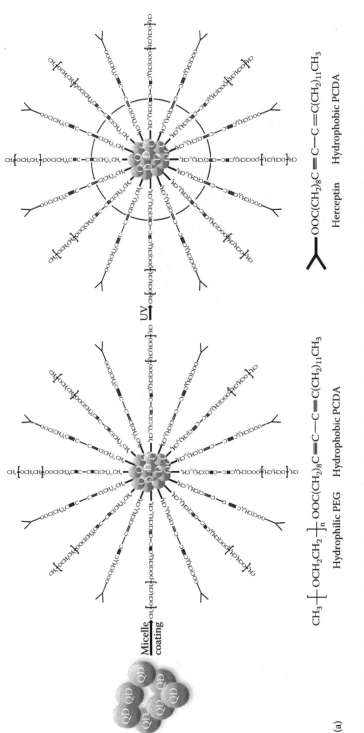

(a)

$$CH_3 \!-\!\!\left[\!OCH_2CH_2\!\right]_n\!\!-\!\!OOC(CH_2)_8C \equiv C\!-\!C \equiv C(CH_2)_{11}CH_3$$

Hydrophilic PEG   Hydrophobic PCDA

$$OOC(CH_2)_8C \equiv C\!-\!C \equiv C(CH_2)_{11}CH_3$$

Herceptin   Hydrophobic PCDA

FIGURE 13.6 (a) Schematic depicting the surface functionalization and bioconjugation of anti-HER2 to NIR QD-loaded micelles. *(Continued)*

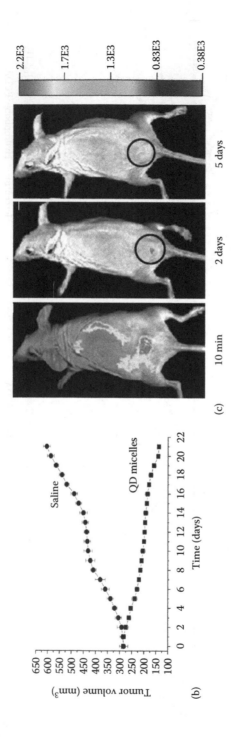

FIGURE 13.6 (CONTINUED) (b) Tumor volume on 0, 7, 14, and 21 days posttreatment with anti-HER2 QD micelles and saline. (c) Time-dependent *in vivo* fluorescence imaging of MDA-MB-231 tumor–bearing mice (indicated by black circle) injected with anti-HER2 QD micelles. (Adapted from M. Nurunnabi et al., *Biomaterials,* 31, 5436–5444, 2010.)

to CdSe QDs (Xu et al. 2012). GRP78 is a stress response chaperone, located within the endoplastic reticulum shown to be involved in cancer cell proliferation and angiogenesis and is overexpressed in a variety of cancers including breast and prostate (Arap et al. 2004). The bioconjugates were effectively internalized by the cancer cells and upregulated phophosphate-AKT-ser473. The growth of MDA-MB-231 tumor xenografts in mice treated with ScFv-GRP78 QDs was significantly inhibited (~74%) when compared to those treated with unconjugated QDs. Furthermore, QDs were found within the tumor cells of mice still showing measurable tumor mass but not in other organs (e.g., kidney, heart, liver, spleen, and lung) using multicolor fluorescence imaging.

13.5 CONCLUSION AND FUTURE PERSPECTIVES

Nanotechnology provides new tools to significantly enhance our understanding and management of every phase of disease diagnosis and therapy. Especially, in the field of molecular imaging, nanomaterials have touched upon every single modality. QDs remain one of the most widely studied probes for both *in vitro* and *in vivo* imaging. Numerous breakthroughs in synthesis and surface modification strategies have given impetus to advances in *in vivo* targeted imaging and simultaneous therapeutic applications in small animals. Because of their inherent advantages over conventional fluorescent dyes, such as tunable and narrow emission spectrum, greater fluorescence intensity, and photostability, QDs promise significant contributions in both basic sciences and clinical applications. Moreover, QDs emitting multiple wavelengths in the NIR region have extended the horizon of possible clinical applications with multiplex imaging.

Despite the intensive research efforts and the remarkable progress made over the two decades, QDs have only achieved a fraction of their initially projected potential until now. *In vivo* toxicity and instability of QDs, inefficient delivery, and lack of *in vivo* quantification are few of the major roadblocks in the translation of QDs to clinical settings. Reduced optical penetration depth limits their applications to tissues close to the surface, further hindering their direct translation to *in vivo* imaging. Moreover, conflicting results regarding their *in vivo* pharmacokinetics and biodistribution have compounded the problem. Several surface modification strategies, described above, have been adopted to reduce the potential toxicity and increase the overall blood circulation time of QDs. Biopolymer coatings have been found to protect QDs from *in vivo* degradation. However, such coatings lead to an increase in size and affect the ADME (absorption, distribution, metabolism, and excretion) properties of the QD conjugates. Thus, development of robust surface chemistries and their careful optimization are equally critical.

In vivo targeted imaging can be instrumental in overcoming inefficient delivery and off-target toxicities associated with QDs. As such, the choice of targeting ligand is very important. An ideal ligand for QD-based nanoprobes should keep the overall size small, should be stable and easy to synthesize, and can be attached to the platform in large numbers (multivalency effect). Moreover, owing to poor extravasation of QDs, vasculature (instead of cell-based) targeting could be more effective and must be explored thoroughly in the future. All these criteria can be easily fulfilled by small peptides, antibody fragments, molecules, and aptamers, which can be easily designed and optimized for such purposes. Multitarget imaging, by incorporating different ligands on the QD surface, is another novel area that can further improve their clinical translatability.

In addition, as with other nanomaterials, QDs can provide a multifunctional nanoplatform for multimodality imaging and theranostics. Dual-modality agents such as fluorescence/MRI or fluorescence/PET should be particularly interesting for future imaging applications. In fact, combining more than two techniques like in a fluorescence/MRI/PET trimodal probe can effectively provide excellent sensitivity and quantitative ability (stemming from PET), anatomical information (from MRI), and *ex vivo* validation capabilities (from optical) at the same time. Combining both multimodality imaging and therapeutic components into a theranostic agent can allow specific delivery of the therapeutic agent in desired dose to the target site and its accurate noninvasive measurement. However, challenges remain and multidisciplinary efforts will be needed to develop and optimize QD-based nanoplatforms to fully realize their potential in defining the future paradigms in cancer prevention, diagnosis, therapy, and patient management.

ACKNOWLEDGMENTS

This work is supported, in part, by the University of Wisconsin, Madison, the National Institutes of Health (NIBIB/NCI 1R01CA169365 and P30CA014520), the Department of Defense (W81XWH-11-1-0644), and the American Cancer Society (125246-RSG-13-099-01-CCE).

REFERENCES

Abdullah Al N., J.-E. Lee, I. In, H. Lee, K.D. Lee, J.H. Jeong, S.Y. Park, Target Delivery and Cell Imaging Using Hyaluronic Acid-Functionalized Graphene Quantum Dots, *Molecular Pharmaceutics*, 10, 3736–3744 (2013).

Akerman M.E., W.C.W. Chan, P. Laakkonen, S.N. Bhatia, E. Ruoslahti, Nanocrystal Targeting In Vivo, *Proceedings of the National Academy of Sciences of the United States of America*, 99, 12617–12621 (2002).

Alauddin M.M., Positron Emission Tomography (Pet) Imaging with (18)F-Based Radiotracers, *American Journal of Nuclear Medicine and Molecular Imaging*, 2, 55–76 (2012).

Alivisatos A.P., Semiconductor Clusters, Nanocrystals, and Quantum Dots, *Science*, 271, 933–937 (1996).

Allen P.M., W. Liu, V.P. Chauhan, J. Lee, A.Y. Ting, D. Fukumura, R.K. Jain, M.G. Bawendi, Inas(Zncds) Quantum Dots Optimized for Biological Imaging in the Near-Infrared, *Journal of the American Chemical Society*, 132, 470–471 (2010).

Al-Jamal W.T., K.T. Al-Jamal, B. Tian, A. Cakebread, J.M. Halket, K. Kostarelos, Tumor Targeting of Functionalized Quantum Dot-Liposome Hybrids by Intravenous Administration, *Molecular Pharmaceutics*, 6, 520–530 (2009).

Al-Jamal W.T., K. Kostarelos, Liposomes: From a Clinically Established Drug Delivery System to a Nanoparticle Platform for Theranostic Nanomedicine, *Accounts of Chemical Research*, 44, 1094–1104 (2011).

Amstad E., S. Zurcher, A. Mashaghi, J.Y. Wong, M. Textor, E. Reimhult, Surface Functionalization of Single Superparamagnetic Iron Oxide Nanoparticles for Targeted Magnetic Resonance Imaging, *Small*, 5, 1334–1342 (2009).

Arap M.A., J. Lahdenranta, P.J. Mintz, A. Hajitou, A.S. Sarkis, W. Arap, R. Pasqualini, Cell Surface Expression of the Stress Response Chaperone GRP78 Enables Tumor Targeting by Circulating Ligands, *Cancer Cell*, 6, 275–284 (2004).

Bae P.K., K.N. Kim, S.J. Lee, H.J. Chang, C.K. Lee, J.K. Park, The Modification of Quantum Dot Probes Used for the Targeted Imaging of His-Tagged Fusion Proteins, *Biomaterials*, 30, 836–842 (2009).

Ballou B., B.C. Lagerholm, L.A. Ernst, M.P. Bruchez, A.S. Waggoner, Noninvasive Imaging of Quantum Dots in Mice, *Bioconjugate Chemistry*, 15, 79–86 (2004).

Bhang S.H., N. Won, T.-J. Lee, H. Jin, J. Nam, J. Park, H. Chung, H.-S. Park, Y.-E. Sung, S.K. Hahn, B.-S. Kim, S. Kim, Hyaluronic Acid-Quantum Dot Conjugates for In Vivo Lymphatic Vessel Imaging, *ACS Nano*, 3, 1389–1398 (2009).

Bruchez M., M. Moronne, P. Gin, S. Weiss, A.P. Alivisatos, Semiconductor Nanocrystals as Fluorescent Biological Labels, *Science*, 281, 2013–2016 (1998).

Cai W., K. Chen, Z.-B. Li, S.S. Gambhir, X. Chen, Dual-Function Probe for Pet and Near-Infrared Fluorescence Imaging of Tumor Vasculature, *Journal of Nuclear Medicine*, 48, 1862–1870 (2007a).

Cai W., X. Chen, Multimodality Molecular Imaging of Tumor Angiogenesis, *Journal of Nuclear Medicine*, 49, 113S–128S (2008).

Cai W., H. Hong, In a "Nutshell": Intrinsically Radio-Labeled Quantum Dots, *American Journal of Nuclear Medicine and Molecular Imaging*, 2, 136–140 (2012).

Cai W., A.R. Hsu, Z.B. Li, X. Chen, Are Quantum Dots Ready for In Vivo Imaging in Human Subjects?, *Nanoscale Research Letters*, 2, 265–281 (2007b).

Cai W., G. Niu, X. Chen, Imaging of Integrins as Biomarkers for Tumor Angiogenesis, *Current Pharmaceutical Design*, 14, 2943–2973 (2008b).

Cai W., G. Niu, X. Chen, Multimodality Imaging of the Her-Kinase Axis in Cancer, *European Journal of Nuclear Medicine and Molecular Imaging*, 35, 186–208 (2008a).

Cai W.B., D.W. Shin, K. Chen, O. Gheysens, Q.Z. Cao, S.X. Wang, S.S. Gambhir, X.Y. Chen, Peptide-Labeled Near-Infrared Quantum Dots for Imaging Tumor Vasculature in Living Subjects, *Nano Letters*, 6, 669–676 (2006).

Cao J., H. Zhu, D. Deng, B. Xue, L. Tang, D. Mahounga, Z. Qian, Y. Gu, In Vivo NIR Imaging with PbS Quantum Dots Entrapped in Biodegradable Micelles, *Journal of Biomedical Materials Research Part A*, 100A, 958–968 (2012).

Cao L., X. Wang, M.J. Meziani, F. Lu, H. Wang, P.G. Luo, Y. Lin, B.A. Harruff, L.M. Veca, D. Murray, S.-Y. Xie, Y.-P. Sun, Carbon Dots for Multiphoton Bioimaging, *Journal of the American Chemical Society*, 129, 11318–11319 (2007).

Cassette E., T. Pons, C. Bouet, M. Helle, L. Bezdetnaya, F. Marchal, B. Dubertret, Synthesis and Characterization of Near-Infrared Cu-in-Se/Zns Core/Shell Quantum Dots for In Vivo Imaging, *Chemistry of Materials*, 22, 6117–6124 (2010).

Chaughule R.S., S. Purushotham, R.V. Ramanujan, Magnetic Nanoparticles as Contrast Agents for Magnetic Resonance Imaging, *Proceedings of the National Academy of Sciences India Section a-Physical Sciences*, 82, 257–268 (2012).

Chen K., Z.-B. Li, H. Wang, W. Cai, X. Chen, Dual-Modality Optical and Positron Emission Tomography Imaging of Vascular Endothelial Growth Factor Receptor on Tumor Vasculature Using Quantum Dots, *European Journal of Nuclear Medicine and Molecular Imaging*, 35, 2235–2244 (2008).

Chen L., X. Zhang, G. Zhou, X. Xiang, X. Ji, Z. Zheng, H. He, H. Wang, Simultaneous Determination of Human Enterovirus 71 and Coxsackievirus B3 by Dual-Color Quantum Dots and Homogeneous Immunoassay, *Analytical Chemistry*, 84, 3200–3207 (2012a).

Chen L.-N., J. Wang, W.-T. Li, H.-Y. Han, Aqueous One-Pot Synthesis of Bright and Ultrasmall CdTe/CdS Near-Infrared-Emitting Quantum Dots and Their Application for Tumor Targeting In Vivo, *Chemical Communications*, 48, 4971–4973 (2012b).

Choi H.S., B.I. Ipe, P. Misra, J.H. Lee, M.G. Bawendi, J.V. Frangioni, Tissue- and Organ-Selective Biodistribution of NIR Fluorescent Quantum Dots, *Nano Letters*, 9, 2354–2359 (2009).

Choi H.S., W. Liu, P. Misra, E. Tanaka, J.P. Zimmer, B.I. Ipe, M.G. Bawendi, J.V. Frangioni, Renal Clearance of Quantum Dots, *Nature Biotechnology*, 25, 1165–1170 (2007).

Danhier F., B. Ucakar, N. Magotteaux, M.E. Brewster, V. Preat, Active and Passive Tumor Targeting of a Novel Poorly Soluble Cyclin Dependent Kinase Inhibitor, Jnj-7706621, *International Journal of Pharmaceutics*, 392, 20–28 (2010).

Delehanty J.B., H. Mattoussi, I.L. Medintz, Delivering Quantum Dots into Cells: Strategies, Progress and Remaining Issues, *Analytical and Bioanalytical Chemistry*, 393, 1091–1105 (2009).

Deng D., Y. Chen, J. Cao, J. Tian, Z. Qian, S. Achilefu, Y. Gu, High-Quality Cuins2/Zns Quantum Dots for In Vitro and In Vivo Bioimaging, *Chemistry of Materials*, 24, 3029–3037 (2012).

Diagaradjane P., J.M. Orenstein-Cardona, N.E. Colon-Casasnovas, A. Deorukhkar, S. Shentu, N. Kuno, D.L. Schwartz, J.G. Gelovani, S. Krishnan, Imaging Epidermal Growth Factor Receptor Expression In Vivo: Pharmacokinetic and Biodistribution Characterization of a Bioconjugated Quantum Dot Nanoprobe, *Clinical Cancer Research*, 14, 731–741 (2008).

Dif A., E. Henry, F. Artzner, M. Baudy-Floc'h, M. Schmutz, M. Dahan, V. Marchi-Artzner, Interaction between Water-Soluble Peptidic CdSe/ZnS Nanocrystals and Membranes: Formation of Hybrid Vesicles and Condensed Lamellar Phases, *Journal of the American Chemical Society*, 130, 8289–8296 (2008).

Ding H., K.-T. Yong, W.-C. Law, I. Roy, R. Hu, F. Wu, W. Zhao, K. Huang, F. Erogbogbo, E.J. Bergey, P.N. Prasad, Non-Invasive Tumor Detection in Small Animals Using Novel Functional Pluronic Nanomicelles Conjugated with Anti-Mesothelin Antibody, *Nanoscale*, 3, 1813–1822 (2011).

Dubertret B., P. Skourides, D.J. Norris, V. Noireaux, A.H. Brivanlou, A. Libchaber, In Vivo Imaging of Quantum Dots Encapsulated in Phospholipid Micelles, *Science*, 298, 1759–1762 (2002).

Eary J.F., D.S. Hawkins, E.T. Rodler, E.U. Conrad, 3rd, (18)F-Fdg Pet in Sarcoma Treatment Response Imaging, *American Journal of Nuclear Medicine and Molecular Imaging*, 1, 47–53 (2011).

Efros A.L., Interband Absorption of Light in a Semiconductor Sphere, *Soviet Physics Semiconductors-USSR*, 16, 772–775 (1982).

Erogbogbo F., K.-T. Yong, I. Roy, R. Hu, W.-C. Law, W. Zhao, H. Ding, F. Wu, R. Kumar, M.T. Swihart, P.N. Prasad, In Vivo Targeted Cancer Imaging, Sentinel Lymph Node Mapping and Multi-Channel Imaging with Biocompatible Silicon Nanocrystals, *ACS Nano*, 5, 413–423 (2011).

Gambhir S.S., Molecular Imaging of Cancer with Positron Emission Tomography, *Nature Reviews Cancer*, 2, 683–693 (2002).

Gao J., K. Chen, R. Luong, D.M. Bouley, H. Mao, T. Qiao, S.S. Gambhir, Z. Cheng, A Novel Clinically Translatable Fluorescent Nanoparticle for Targeted Molecular Imaging of Tumors in Living Subjects, *Nano Letters*, 12, 281–286 (2012).

Gao J., K. Chen, R. Xie, J. Xie, S. Lee, Z. Cheng, X. Peng, X. Chen, Ultrasmall Near-Infrared Non-Cadmium Quantum Dots for In Vivo Tumor Imaging, *Small*, 6, 256–261 (2010a).

Gao J., K. Chen, R. Xie, J. Xie, Y. Yan, Z. Cheng, X. Peng, X. Chen, In Vivo Tumor-Targeted Fluorescence Imaging Using Near-Infrared Non-Cadmium Quantum Dots, *Bioconjugate Chemistry*, 21, 604–609 (2010b).

Gao X.H., Y.Y. Cui, R.M. Levenson, L.W.K. Chung, S.M. Nie, In Vivo Cancer Targeting and Imaging with Semiconductor Quantum Dots, *Nature Biotechnology*, 22, 969–976 (2004).

Geszke-Moritz M., M. Moritz, Quantum Dots as Versatile Probes in Medical Sciences: Synthesis, Modification and Properties, *Materials Science & Engineering C-Materials for Biological Applications*, 33, 1008–1021 (2013).

Gollavelli G., Y.-C. Ling, Multi-Functional Graphene as an In Vitro and In Vivo Imaging Probe, *Biomaterials*, 33, 2532–2545 (2012).

Grassi I., C. Nanni, V. Allegri, J.J. Morigi, G.C. Montini, P. Castellucci, S. Fanti, The Clinical Use of Pet with (11)C-Acetate, *American Journal of Nuclear Medicine and Molecular Imaging*, 2, 33–47 (2012).

Hermanson G.T., Quantum Dot Nanocrystals, in: G.T. Hermanson (Ed.) *Bioconjugate Techniques*, Academic Press, New York, 2008, pp. 455–463.

Hong H., S. Goel, Y. Zhang, W. Cai, Molecular Imaging with Nucleic Acid Aptamers, *Current Medicinal Chemistry*, 18, 4195–4205 (2011).

Hong H., K. Yang, Y. Zhang, J.W. Engle, L. Feng, Y. Yang, T.R. Nayak, S. Goel, J. Bean, C.P. Theuer, T.E. Barnhart, Z. Liu, W. Cai, In Vivo Targeting and Imaging of Tumor Vasculature with Radiolabeled, Antibody-Conjugated Nanographene, *ACS Nano*, 6, 2361–2370 (2012a).

Hong H., Y. Zhang, J.W. Engle, T.R. Nayak, C.P. Theuer, R.J. Nickles, T.E. Barnhart, W. Cai, In Vivo Targeting and Positron Emission Tomography Imaging of Tumor Vasculature with Ga-66-Labeled Nano-Graphene, *Biomaterials*, 33, 4147–4156 (2012b).

Hua X.-F., T.-C. Liu, Y.-C. Cao, B. Liu, H.-Q. Wang, J.-H. Wang, Z.-L. Huang, Y.-D. Zhao, Characterization of the Coupling of Quantum Dots and Immunoglobulin Antibodies, *Analytical and Bioanalytical Chemistry*, 386, 1665–1671 (2006).

Huang H., Y.-L. Bai, K. Yang, H. Tang, Y.-W. Wang, Optical Imaging of Head and Neck Squamous Cell Carcinoma In Vivo Using Arginine-Glycine-Aspartic Acid Peptide Conjugated Near-Infrared Quantum Dots, *Oncotargets and Therapy*, 6, 1779–1787 (2013).

Jayagopal A., P.K. Russ, F.R. Haselton, Surface Engineering of Quantum Dots for In Vivo Vascular Imaging, *Bioconjugate Chemistry*, 18, 1424–1433 (2007).

Kalasad M.N., A.K. Rabinal, B.G. Mulimani, Ambient Synthesis and Characterization of High-Quality CdSe Quantum Dots by an Aqueous Route, *Langmuir*, 25, 12729–12735 (2009).

Kalyankrishna S., J.R. Grandis, Epidermal Growth Factor Receptor Biology in Head and Neck Cancer, *Journal of Clinical Oncology*, 24, 2666–2672 (2006).

Karakoti A.S., S. Das, S. Thevuthasan, S. Seal, Pegylated Inorganic Nanoparticles, *Angewandte Chemie-International Edition*, 50, 1980–1994 (2011).

Kim D., S. Park, J.H. Lee, Y.Y. Jeong, S. Jon, Antibiofouling Polymer-Coated Gold Nanoparticles as a Contrast Agent for In Vivo X-Ray Computed Tomography Imaging, *Journal of the American Chemical Society*, 129, 7661–7665 (2007).

Kim J.S., K.J. Cho, T.H. Tran, M. Nurunnabi, T.H. Moon, S.M. Hong, Y.-K. Lee, In Vivo Nir Imaging with CdTe/CdSe Quantum Dots Entrapped in PLGA Nanospheres, *Journal of Colloid and Interface Science*, 353, 363–371 (2011).

Kularatne S.A., P.S. Low, Targeting of Nanoparticles: Folate Receptor, *Methods in Molecular Biology*, 624, 249–265 (2010).

Kwon H., J. Lee, R. Song, S.I. Hwang, J. Lee, Y.-H. Kim, H.J. Lee, In Vitro and In Vivo Imaging of Prostate Cancer Angiogenesis Using Anti-Vascular Endothelial Growth Factor Receptor 2 Antibody-Conjugated Quantum Dot, *Korean Journal of Radiology*, 14, 30–37 (2013).

Law W.-C., K.-T. Yong, I. Roy, H. Ding, R. Hu, W. Zhao, P.N. Prasad, Aqueous-Phase Synthesis of Highly Luminescent CdTe/ZnTe Core/Shell Quantum Dots Optimized for Targeted Bioimaging, *Small*, 5, 1302–1310 (2009).

Lee J., Y. Choi, K. Kim, S. Hong, H.-Y. Park, T. Lee, G.J. Cheon, R. Song, Characterization and Cancer Cell Specific Binding Properties of Anti-EGFR Antibody Conjugated Quantum Dots, *Bioconjugate Chemistry*, 21, 940–946 (2010).

Lee S., E.-J. Cha, K. Park, S.-Y. Lee, J.-K. Hong, I.-C. Sun, S.Y. Kim, K. Choi, I.C. Kwon, K. Kim, C.-H. Ahn, A Near-Infrared-Fluorescence-Quenched Gold-Nanoparticle Imaging Probe for In Vivo Drug Screening and Protease Activity Determination, *Angewandte Chemie-International Edition*, 47, 2804–2807 (2008).

Lee Y.K., J.M. Jeong, L. Hoigebazar, B.Y. Yang, Y.-S. Lee, B.C. Lee, H. Youn, D.S. Lee, J.-K. Chung, M.C. Lee, Nanoparticles Modified by Encapsulation of Ligands with a Long Alkyl Chain to Affect Multispecific and Multimodal Imaging, *Journal of Nuclear Medicine*, 53, 1462–1470 (2012).

Lesnyak V., N. Gaponik, A. Eychmueller, Colloidal Semiconductor Nanocrystals: The Aqueous Approach, *Chemical Society Reviews*, 42, 2905–2929 (2013).

Li L., T.J. Daou, I. Texier, C. Tran Thi Kim, L. Nguyen Quang, P. Reiss, Highly Luminescent Cuins2/Zns Core/Shell Nanocrystals: Cadmium-Free Quantum Dots for In Vivo Imaging, *Chemistry of Materials*, 21, 2422–2429 (2009).

Li Y., Z. Li, X. Wang, F. Liu, Y. Cheng, B. Zhang, D. Shi, In Vivo Cancer Targeting and Imaging-Guided Surgery with Near Infrared-Emitting Quantum Dot Bioconjugates, *Theranostics* 2, 769–776 (2012).

Liu L., K.-T. Yong, I. Roy, W.-C. Law, L. Ye, J. Liu, J. Liu, R. Kumar, X. Zhang, P.N. Prasad, Bioconjugated Pluronic Triblock-Copolymer Micelle-Encapsulated Quantum Dots for Targeted Imaging of Cancer: In Vitro and In Vivo Studies, *Theranostics*, 2, 705–713 (2012).

Liu Y.-S., Y. Sun, P.T. Vernier, C.-H. Liang, S.Y.C. Chong, M.A. Gundersen, Ph-Sensitive Photoluminescence of CdSe/ZnSe/ZnS Quantum Dots in Human Ovarian Cancer Cells, *Journal of Physical Chemistry C*, 111, 2872–2878 (2007).

Loginova Y.F., S.V. Dezhurov, V.V. Zherdeva, N.I. Kazachkina, M.S. Wakstein, A.P. Savitsky, Biodistribution and Stability of CdSe Core Quantum Dots in Mouse Digestive Tract Following Per Os Administration: Advantages of Double Polymer/Silica Coated Nanocrystals, *Biochemical and Biophysical Research Communications*, 419, 54–59 (2012).

Lowe S.B., J.A.G. Dick, B.E. Cohen, M.M. Stevens, Multiplex Sensing of Protease and Kinase Enzyme Activity Via Orthogonal Coupling of Quantum Dot Peptide Conjugates, *ACS Nano*, 6, 851–857 (2012).

Lu R.-M., Y.-L. Chang, M.-S. Chen, H.-C. Wu, Single Chain Anti-C-Met Antibody Conjugated Nanoparticles for In Vivo Tumor-Targeted Imaging and Drug Delivery, *Biomaterials*, 32, 3265–3274 (2011).

Ma Q., Y. Nakane, Y. Mori, M. Hasegawa, Y. Yoshioka, T.M. Watanabe, K. Gonda, N. Ohuchi, T. Jin, Multilayered, Core/Shell Nanoprobes Based on Magnetic Ferric Oxide Particles and Quantum Dots for Multimodality Imaging of Breast Cancer Tumors, *Biomaterials*, 33, 8486–8494 (2012).

Maeda H., G.Y. Bharate, J. Daruwalla, Polymeric Drugs for Efficient Tumor-Targeted Drug Delivery Based on EPR-Effect, *European Journal of Pharmaceutics and Biopharmaceutics*, 71, 409–419 (2009).

Maldiney T., M.U. Kaikkonen, J. Seguin, Q. le Masne de Chermont, M. Bessodes, K.J. Airenne, S. Yla-Herttuala, D. Scherman, C. Richard, In Vitro Targeting of Avidin-Expressing Glioma Cells with Biotinylated Persistent Luminescence Nanoparticles, *Bioconjugate Chemistry*, 23, 472–478 (2012).

Mankoff D.A., A Definition of Molecular Imaging, *Journal of Nuclear Medicine*, 48, 18N–21N (2007).

Michalet X., F.F. Pinaud, L.A. Bentolila, J.M. Tsay, S. Doose, J.J. Li, G. Sundaresan, A.M. Wu, S.S. Gambhir, S. Weiss, Quantum Dots for Live Cells, In Vivo Imaging, and Diagnostics, *Science*, 307, 538–544 (2005).

Mukthavaram R., W. Wrasidlo, D. Hall, S. Kesari, M. Makale, Assembly and Targeting of Liposomal Nanoparticles Encapsulating Quantum Dots, *Bioconjugate Chemistry*, 22, 1638–1644 (2011).

Murphy J.E., M.C. Beard, A.G. Norman, S.P. Ahrenkiel, J.C. Johnson, P.R. Yu, O.I. Micic, R.J. Ellingson, A.J. Nozik, PbTe Colloidal Nanocrystals: Synthesis, Characterization, and Multiple Exciton Generation, *Journal of the American Chemical Society*, 128, 3241–3247 (2006).

Nicolas J., D. Brambilla, O. Carion, T. Pons, I. Maksimovic, E. Larquet, B. Le Droumaguet, K. Andrieux, B. Dubertret, P. Couvreur, Quantum Dot-Loaded Pegylated Poly(Alkyl Cyanoacrylate) Nanoparticles for In Vitro and In Vivo Imaging, *Soft Matter*, 7, 6187–6193 (2011).

Nurunnabi M., K.J. Cho, J.S. Choi, K.M. Huh, Y.-H. Lee, Targeted Near-Ir Qds-Loaded Micelles for Cancer Therapy and Imaging, *Biomaterials*, 31, 5436–5444 (2010).

Ossipov D.A., Nanostructured Hyaluronic Acid-Based Materials for Active Delivery to Cancer, *Expert Opinion on Drug Delivery*, 7, 681–703 (2010).

Park J., J. Nam, N. Won, H. Jin, S. Jung, S. Jung, S.-H. Cho, S. Kim, Compact and Stable Quantum Dots with Positive, Negative, or Zwitterionic Surface: Specific Cell Interactions and Non-Specific Adsorptions by the Surface Charges, *Advanced Functional Materials*, 21, 1558–1566 (2011).

Park H.-Y., K. Kim, S. Hong, H. Kim, Y. Choi, J. Ryu, D. Kwon, R. Grailhe, R. Song, Compact and Versatile Nickel-Nitrilotriacetate-Modified Quantum Dots for Protein Imaging and Forster Resonance Energy Transfer Based Assay, *Langmuir*, 26, 7327–7333 (2010).

Pellegrino T., L. Manna, S. Kudera, T. Liedl, D. Koktysh, A.L. Rogach, S. Keller, J. Radler, G. Natile, W.J. Parak, Hydrophobic Nanocrystals Coated with an Amphiphilic Polymer Shell: A General Route to Water Soluble Nanocrystals, *Nano Letters*, 4, 703–707 (2004).

Peng Z.A., X.G. Peng, Formation of High-Quality CdTe, CdSe, and CdS Nanocrystals Using CdO as Precursor, *Journal of the American Chemical Society*, 123, 183–184 (2001).

Pirollo K.F., E.H. Chang, Does a Targeting Ligand Influence Nanoparticle Tumor Localization or Uptake?, *Trends Biotechnol*, 26, 552–558 (2008).

Qu, L.H., Z.A. Peng, X.G. Peng, Alternative Routes toward High Quality CdSe Nanocrystals, *Nano Letters*, 1, 333–337 (2001).

Resch-Genger U., M. Grabolle, S. Cavaliere-Jaricot, R. Nitschke, T. Nann, Quantum Dots Versus Organic Dyes as Fluorescent Labels, *Nature Methods*, 5, 763–775 (2008).

Robinson J.T., G. Hong, Y. Liang, B. Zhang, O.K. Yaghi, H. Dai, In Vivo Fluorescence Imaging in the Second Near-Infrared Window with Long Circulating Carbon Nanotubes Capable of Ultrahigh Tumor Uptake, *Journal of the American Chemical Society*, 134, 10664–10669 (2012).

Rogach A.L., L. Katsikas, A. Kornowski, D.S. Su, A. Eychmuller, H. Weller, Synthesis and Characterization of Thiol-Stabilized CdTe Nanocrystals, *Berichte Der Bunsen-Gesellschaft-Physical Chemistry Chemical Physics*, 100, 1772–1778 (1996).

Rogers S.J., K.J. Harrington, P. Rhys-Evans, P.O. Charoenrat, S.A. Eccles, Biological Significance of C-Erbb Family Oncogenes in Head and Neck Cancer, *Cancer and Metastasis Reviews*, 24, 47–69 (2005).

Ruan J., H. Song, Q. Qian, C. Li, K. Wang, C. Bao, D. Cui, Her2 Monoclonal Antibody Conjugated RNase-A-Associated CdTe Quantum Dots for Targeted Imaging and Therapy of Gastric Cancer, *Biomaterials*, 33, 7093–7102 (2012).

Savla R., O. Taratula, O. Garbuzenko, T. Minko, Tumor Targeted Quantum Dot-Mucin 1 Aptamer-Doxorubicin Conjugate for Imaging and Treatment of Cancer, *Journal of Controlled Release*, 153, 16–22 (2011).

Schipper M.L., G. Iyer, A.L. Koh, Z. Cheng, Y. Ebenstein, A. Aharoni, S. Keren, L.A. Bentolila, J.Q. Li, J.H. Rao, X.Y. Chen, U. Banin, A.M. Wu, R. Sinclair, S. Weiss, S.S. Gambhir, Particle Size, Surface Coating, and Pegylation Influence the Biodistribution of Quantum Dots in Living Mice, *Small*, 5, 126–134 (2009).

Shi D., Y. Guo, Z. Dong, J. Lian, W. Wang, G. Liu, L. Wang, R.C. Ewing, Quantum-Dot-Activated Luminescent Carbon Nanotubes Via a Nano Scale Surface Functionalization for In Vivo Imaging, *Advanced Materials*, 19, 4033–4037 (2007).

Smith A.M., G. Ruan, M.N. Rhyner, S.M. Nie, Engineering Luminescent Quantum Dots for in vivo Molecular and Cellular Imaging, *Annals of Biomedical Engineering*, 34, 3–14 (2006).

Smith B.R., Z. Cheng, A. De, J. Rosenberg, S.S. Gambhir, Dynamic Visualization of RGD-Quantum Dot Binding to Tumor Neovasculature and Extravasation in Multiple Living Mouse Models Using Intravital Microscopy, *Small*, 6, 2222–2229 (2010).

Sun M., D. Hoffman, G. Sundaresan, L. Yang, N. Lamichhane, J. Zweit, Synthesis and Characterization of Intrinsically Radiolabeled Quantum Dots for Bimodal Detection, *American Journal of Nuclear Medicine and Molecular Imaging*, 2, 122–135 (2012).

Sun Y.P., B. Zhou, Y. Lin, W. Wang, K.A.S. Fernando, P. Pathak, M.J. Meziani, B.A. Harruff, X. Wang, H.F. Wang, P.J.G. Luo, H. Yang, M.E. Kose, B.L. Chen, L.M. Veca, S.Y. Xie, Quantum-Sized Carbon Dots for Bright and Colorful Photoluminescence, *Journal of the American Chemical Society*, 128, 7756–7757 (2006).

Szabo D.V., D. Vollath, Nanocomposites from Coated Nanoparticles, *Advanced Materials*, 11, 1313–1316 (1999).

Tada H., H. Higuchi, T.M. Wanatabe, N. Ohuchi, In Vivo Real-Time Tracking of Single Quantum Dots Conjugated with Monoclonal Anti-Her2 Antibody in Tumors of Mice, *Cancer Research*, 67, 1138–1144 (2007).

Talapin D.V., S. Haubold, A.L. Rogach, A. Kornowski, M. Haase, H. Weller, A Novel Organometallic Synthesis of Highly Luminescent CdTe Nanocrystals, *Journal of Physical Chemistry B*, 105, 2260–2263 (2001).

Talapin D.V., I. Mekis, S. Gotzinger, A. Kornowski, O. Benson, H. Weller, CdSe/CdS/ZnS and CdSe/ZnSe/ZnS Core-Shell-Shell Nanocrystals, *Journal of Physical Chemistry B*, 108, 18826–18831 (2004).

Tao H., K. Yang, Z. Ma, J. Wan, Y. Zhang, Z. Kang, Z. Liu, In Vivo NIR Fluorescence Imaging, Biodistribution, and Toxicology of Photoluminescent Carbon Dots Produced from Carbon Nanotubes and Graphite, *Small*, 8, 281–290 (2012).

Tian B., W.T. Al-Jamal, J. Van den Bossche, K. Kostarelos, Design and Engineering of Multifunctional Quantum Dot-Based Nanoparticles for Simultaneous Therapeutic-Diagnostic Applications, *Multifunctional Nanoparticles for Drug Delivery Applications: Imaging, Targeting, and Delivery*, 345–365 (2012).

Tiwari D.K., S.-I. Tanaka, Y. Inouye, K. Yoshizawa, T.M. Watanabe, T. Jin, Synthesis and Characterization of Anti-Her2 Antibody Conjugated CdSe/CdZnS Quantum Dots for Fluorescence Imaging of Breast Cancer Cells, *Sensors*, 9, 9332–9354 (2009).

Travert-Branger N., F. Dubois, O. Carion, G. Carrot, B. Mahler, B. Dubertret, E. Doris, C. Mioskowski, Oligomeric PEG-Phospholipids for Solubilization and Stabilization of Fluorescent Nanocrystals in Water, *Langmuir*, 24, 3016–3019 (2008).

Travert-Branger N., F. Dubois, J.-P. Renault, S. Pin, B. Mahler, E. Gravel, B. Dubertret, E. Doris, in situ Electron-Beam Polymerization Stabilized Quantum Dot Micelles, *Langmuir*, 27, 4358–4361 (2011).

Vach W., P.F. Hoilund-Carlsen, B.M. Fischer, O. Gerke, W. Weber, How to Study Optimal Timing of PET/CT for Monitoring of Cancer Treatment, *American Journal of Nuclear Medicine and Molecular Imaging*, 1, 54–62 (2011).

Wang J., S. Han, D. Ke, R. Wang, Semiconductor Quantum Dots Surface Modification for Potential Cancer Diagnostic and Therapeutic Applications, *Journal of Nanomaterials*, (2012a).

Wang K., J. Ruan, Q. Qian, H. Song, C. Bao, X. Zhang, Y. Kong, C. Zhang, G. Hu, J. Ni, D. Cui, BRCAA1 Monoclonal Antibody Conjugated Fluorescent Magnetic Nanoparticles for In Vivo Targeted Magnetofluorescent Imaging of Gastric Cancer, *Journal of Nanobiotechnology*, 9, 23 (2011).

Wang W., D. Cheng, F. Gong, X. Miao, X. Shuai, Design of Multifunctional Micelle for Tumor-Targeted Intracellular Drug Release and Fluorescent Imaging, *Advanced Materials*, 24, 115–120 (2012b).

Wen C.-J., L.-W. Zhang, S.A. Al-Suwayeh, T.-C. Yen, J.-Y. Fang, Theranostic Liposomes Loaded with Quantum Dots and Apomorphine for Brain Targeting and Bioimaging, *International Journal of Nanomedicine*, 7, 1599–1611 (2012).

Xu W., L. Liu, N.J. Brown, S. Christian, D. Hornby, Quantum Dot-Conjugated Anti-GRP78 Scfv Inhibits Cancer Growth in Mice, *Molecules*, 17, 796–808 (2012).

Xue B., D.-W. Deng, J. Cao, F. Liu, X. Li, W. Akers, S. Achilefu, Y.-Q. Gu, Synthesis of NAC Capped near Infrared-Emitting CdTeS Alloyed Quantum Dots and Application for In Vivo Early Tumor Imaging, *Dalton Transactions*, 41, 4935–4947 (2012).

Yang K., F.-J. Zhang, H. Tang, C. Zhao, Y.-A. Cao, X.-Q. Lv, D. Chen, Y.-D. Li, In-Vivo Imaging of Oral Squamous Cell Carcinoma by EGFR Monoclonal Antibody Conjugated near-Infrared Quantum Dots in Mice, *International Journal of Nanomedicine*, 6, 1739–1745 (2011).

Yang L., H. Mao, Y.A. Wang, Z. Cao, X. Peng, X. Wang, H. Duan, C. Ni, Q. Yuan, G. Adams, M.Q. Smith, W.C. Wood, X. Gao, S. Nie, Single Chain Epidermal Growth Factor Receptor Antibody Conjugated Nanoparticles for In Vivo Tumor Targeting and Imaging, *Small*, 5, 235–243 (2009).

Yigit M.V., Z. Medarova, In Vivo and Ex Vivo Applications of Gold Nanoparticles for Biomedical Sers Imagingi, *American Journal of Nuclear Medicine and Molecular Imaging*, 2, 232–241 (2012).

Yong K.-T., Biophotonics and Biotechnology in Pancreatic Cancer: Cyclic RGD-Peptide-Conjugated Type II Quantum Dots for In Vivo Imaging, *Pancreatology*, 10, 553–564 (2010).

Yong K.-T., R. Hu, I. Roy, H. Ding, L.A. Vathy, E.J. Bergey, M. Mizuma, A. Maitra, P.N. Prasad, Tumor Targeting and Imaging in Live Animals with Functionalized Semiconductor Quantum Rods, *ACS Applied Materials & Interfaces*, 1, 710–719 (2009).

Yong K.-T., I. Roy, W.-C. Law, R. Hu, Synthesis of cRGD-Peptide Conjugated Near-Infrared CdTe/ZnSe Core-Shell Quantum Dots for In Vivo Cancer Targeting and Imaging, *Chemical Communications*, 46, 7136–7138 (2010).

Yu M.K., Y.Y. Jeong, J. Park, S. Park, J.W. Kim, J.J. Min, K. Kim, S. Jon, Drug-Loaded Superparamagnetic Iron Oxide Nanoparticles for Combined Cancer Imaging and Therapy in Vivo, *Angewandte Chemie-International Edition*, 47, 5362–5365 (2008).

Zhang C., X. Ji, Y. Zhang, G. Zhou, X. Ke, H. Wang, P. Tinnefeld, Z. He, One-Pot Synthesized Aptamer-Functionalized CdTe:Zn^{2+} Quantum Dots for Tumor-Targeted Fluorescence Imaging In Vitro and In Vivo, *Analytical Chemistry*, 85, 5843–5849 (2013).

Zhang H., X. Zeng, Q. Li, M. Gaillard-Kelly, C.R. Wagner, D. Yee, Fluorescent Tumour Imaging of Type I IGF Receptor In Vivo: Comparison of Antibody-Conjugated Quantum Dots and Small-Molecule Fluorophore, *British Journal of Cancer*, 101, 71–79 (2009).

Zhou J., C. Booker, R. Li, X. Zhou, T.-K. Sham, X. Sun, Z. Ding, An Electrochemical Avenue to Blue Luminescent Nanocrystals from Multiwalled Carbon Nanotubes (MWCNTs), *Journal of the American Chemical Society*, 129, 744–745 (2007a).

Zhou Y., C.D. Daryl, H. Zou, M.E. Hayes, G.P. Adams, D.B. Kirpotin, J.D. Marks, Impact of Single-Chain Fv Antibody Fragment Affinity on Nanoparticle Targeting of Epidermal Growth Factor Receptor-Expressing Tumor Cells, *Journal of Molecular Biology*, 371, 934–947 (2007b).

Zhu Y., H. Hong, Z.P. Xu, Z. Li, W. Cai, Quantum Dot-Based Nanoprobes for in vivo Targeted Imaging, *Current Molecular Medicine*, 13, 1549–1567 (2013b).

Zhu Y., Z. Li, M. Chen, H.M. Cooper, G.Q. Lu, Z.P. Xu, One-Pot Preparation of Highly Fluorescent Cadmium Telluride/Cadmium Sulfide Quantum Dots under Neutral-Ph Condition for Biological Applications, *Journal of Colloid and Interface Science*, 390, 3–10 (2013a).

Zou L., Z. Gu, N. Zhang, Y. Zhang, Z. Fang, W. Zhu, X. Zhong, Ultrafast Synthesis of Highly Luminescent Green- to Near Infrared-Emitting CdTe Nanocrystals in Aqueous Phase, *Journal of Materials Chemistry*, 18, 2807–2815 (2008).

14 Surface Modifications by Polymers for Biosensing Applications

Laura Sola, Chiara Finetti, Paola Gagni,
Marcella Chiari, and Marina Cretich

CONTENTS

ABSTRACT

The advancement of microfabrication techniques has led to the development of miniaturized and fully integrated solid-phase analytical devices that allow one to perform studies of complex cellular processes, high-throughput screening, and parallel diagnostic detection. They imply a scaling down of the entire analytical process while maintaining high sensitivity. Considering their tiny dimensions, the surface properties of the microdevices must be carefully tailored to maximize probe immobilization and target binding efficiency and to reduce background noise. Polymeric coatings for modifying/functionalizing substrates are one of the most effective ways for tailoring surface characteristics and conferring the properties described above. Here, we present a nonexhaustive review of the state-of-art surface derivatization methods for biosensing applications by polymeric coatings focusing on applications of such coatings in microarray technology, microfluidics, DNA sequence characterization, and nanoparticles.

Keywords: Polymer, Coating, Surface Chemistry, Biosensing, Microarrays, Microfluidics, Nanoparticles

14.1 INTRODUCTION

In the fields of medical, environmental, and chemical sciences, there is an increasing need for the selective identification of specific molecules in complex mixtures of related substances. The development of techniques based on molecular recognition events that allow measurements of the concentration of certain compounds in complex mixtures is of great interest. Furthermore, in recent years, biosensing of changes in conformation of proteins and DNA sequences upon external stimuli or interactions with other molecules as gained increasing interest to shed light on biological mechanisms such as protein synthesis and gene regulation.

Recent progresses in microfabrication techniques have led to the development of miniaturized and fully integrated solid-phase analytical devices that allow one to perform entire experiments, studies of complex cellular processes, high-throughput screening, and parallel diagnostic detection. They imply a scaling down of the entire analytical process (time, sample and reagent volumes, costs) while maintaining very high sensitivity. Considering their tiny dimensions, the aforementioned surfaces must be perfectly designed and controlled in order to maximize probe immobilization and target binding efficiency, to reduce background noise, and to prevent nonspecific molecular interaction.

When the modification of a suitable substrate must be performed to promote covalent attachment of DNA sequences of proteins at specific locations, the control of surface chemical–physical characteristics is of remarkable importance in order to maximize probe density immobilization and to maintain their native and functional conformation. Besides, in order to obtain accurate analysis and optimization of the *signal-to-noise* ratio, the surface chemistry should minimize hydrophobic interactions, which are the main source of biomolecule-specific binding.

Therefore, there are several surface requirements that must be taken into account in biosensing applications:

* The surface must contain functional groups for the easy immobilization of molecules of interest.
* The binding between the biomolecule and the solid surface must be strong enough to retain the molecule on the surface during the entire biosensing experiment.
* The surface must be inherently inert and resist nonspecific adsorption.
* The coupling chemistry should allow the control of biomolecule orientation.
* The local chemical environment must allow the immobilized molecules to retain the native conformation and its functionality.

The use of polymeric materials for modifying/functionalizing substrates is one of the most effective ways for tailoring surface characteristics and conferring the properties described above.

What follows is a nonexhaustive review of the state-of-art surface derivatization methods for biosensing applications with special emphasis on polymeric coatings.

After an introduction to the different types of polymer-based functionalizations, the chapter will focus on applications of such coatings in microarray technology, microfluidics, DNA sequence characterization, and nanoparticles.

14.1.1 SURFACE COATING: STATE OF THE ART

Thin coatings applied to the surface of materials can improve the properties of objects dramatically as they allow control of the interaction of a material with its environment. This has been known to man more or less empirically for several thousand years. Lacquer generated from tree sap was used as a protective coating for wooden objects. Varnishes, enamels, and coatings from pitch and balsam were used by Egyptians to render waterproof ships. Lacquer and varnish coatings were applied to homes and ships for decoration and as protective measures against adverse environmental conditions. In modern times, the coatings industry is a multibillion dollar business and, especially if the value of the protected objects is considered, a very important contribution to the world economy. Today, however, the application range of coatings extends much beyond the simple decoration and protection aspects, and functional coatings have become an enabling technology in a wide variety of different high-tech areas. Fields in which such high-tech coatings are applied range from computer chips (Thompson et al. 1994) and hard disk manufacturing (Rühe et al. 1996) to the use of special coatings in biomedical and aviation applications (Tirrell et al. 2002).

When considering such applications, thin organic coatings are applied to control the interactions between the material and its environment. Examples of interface properties that can be controlled by deposition of a thin organic film onto a surface include friction adhesion, adsorption of molecules from the surrounding environment, or wetting with water or other liquids (Grest 1997; Klein et al. 1994). In medical applications, coatings allow control of the interaction of biological cells and biomolecules with artificial materials in order to enhance the biocompatibility of an implant or to avoid the nonspecific adsorption of proteins onto the active surfaces of an analytical device (Ratner et al. 1996). In addition, the application of functional coatings allows the coverage of a surface with groups that interact with other molecules in their environment through specific molecular recognition processes.

Depending on the type of interaction between the molecules that are constituents of the coating and the substrate that is to be modified, two classes of strategies for the deposition of thin organic coatings can be distinguished. In one of these, the molecules interact with the substrate by physical forces (Fleer et al. 1993; Jones and Richards 1999), while the other class consists of molecules that are attached to the surfaces through chemical bonds. In the latter case, a monomolecular layer or a surface-attached network is strongly ("irreversibly") attached to the surface.

A number of technologically relevant coating techniques rely on physical interactions between the deposited molecules and the substrate, including (a) painting/droplet evaporation, (b) spray coating, (c) spin coating, and (d) dip coating.

In contrast to such processes, more sophisticated coating techniques have been developed, including the Langmuir–Blodgett technique (Mathauer et al. 1992), the adsorption of monomolecular layers of homo- and block copolymers (Halperin et al. 1992) from solution, and the layer-by-layer (LBL) (Decher 2002) technique in which multilayer stacks of oppositely charged polyelectrolytes are deposited onto a (charged) substrate.

The films obtained by physical interactions owing to low stability can be subjected to destruction by (1) desorption during solvent exposure, (2) displacement by molecules that have stronger interaction with the surface, (3) dewetting (for films above the glass transition temperature, Tg), and (4) delamination (for films below Tg).

An alternative to improve stability of coatings even in very adverse conditions is to use coatings covalently attached to the surface. The price that must be paid for an enhanced stability of the system is a more complicated coating procedure and the requirement to choose the coating conditions more carefully, so that the surface reaction proceeds in high yield and with limited side reactions. A frequently employed strategy for the preparation of well-controlled surface layers makes use of small molecules with a reactive head group that is amenable to form a covalent bond with a corresponding chemical moiety on the surface, which is to be modified. Such layers are commonly called self-assembled monolayers (SAMs) (Ulman 1991). Examples are silanes anchored on silanol groups of glass surfaces, phosphates or phosphonate on metal(oxide)s, and thiols or disulfides on noble metal surfaces (gold surfaces). By this approach, stable coatings can be obtained, which may have a strong degree of positional and orientational order. If such molecules expose a specific chemical moiety or a biochemically active group, it is possible to obtain a more or less strict two-dimensional (2D) arrangement of these functionalities (Xia and Whitesides 1998). Examples are molecules that contain "ligands" as recognition sites in bioaffinity assays. In this way, surfaces can be generated (e.g., on top of the transducer of a biosensor) that very specifically bind proteins from solution (Kambhampati et al. 2001; Knoll et al. 2000). The intrinsic limitations of this strictly 2D arrangement of the functional groups are evident: the maximal surface density of the functional moieties is limited by the surface area cross section causing a limited accessibility of functionalities. One obvious solution to the above problem is the extension into the third dimension, that is, the use of polymers carrying the functional groups along the chain, thus generating higher cross-sectional densities of these groups and simultaneously guaranteeing good accessibility.

14.1.2 Polymeric Modification of Surfaces

Most approaches aimed at attaching polymers to a surface use a system where the polymer carries an "anchor" group either as an end group or along the side chain. This anchor group can react with appropriate sites on the substrate surface, thus yielding surface-attached monolayers of polymer molecules (termed *grafting to*) (Figure 14.1) (Tsubokawa et al. 1989a). Another straightforward technique is to carry out a polymerization reaction in the presence of a substrate onto which monomers had been attached (Hashimoto et al. 1982). During the polymerization reaction, the surface-anchored monomers are incorporated into growing polymer chains (Figure 14.1).

Although *grafting to* reactions are easy to perform, it should be noted that several complications arise from their use for the functionalization of a surface. The anchor groups present in the polymer chain and the sites exposed onto the surface must not compete or react with the polymer functional groups. Another complication inherent to *grafting to* processes is the intrinsic limitation of the coating thickness. When the surface coverage increases, the polymer concentration at the interface quickly becomes larger than the concentration of the polymer in solution. Additional chains, which are to be attached to the surface, must diffuse against this concentration gradient. Moreover, in order to accommodate further chains, they must change from coil conformation in solution to a stretched ("brush-like") conformation at the surface. Hence, the higher is the graft density of the chains at the surface, the stronger the entropy penalty is rapidly precluding the attachment of further chains.

The term *polymer brush* refers to a system in which the polymer chains are attached by one end to a surface. Despite the fact that the *grafting to* method provides polymers attached in such a fashion, because of the problems discussed above, it is not able to produce dense films with chains stretched away from the surface. When polymer molecules are tethered to a surface, three basic cases must be distinguished

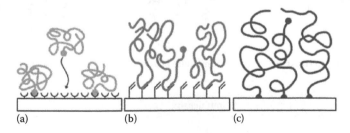

(a)   (b)   (c)

FIGURE 14.1 Schematic illustration of different processes used for the attachment of polymers to surfaces: (a) "grafting to"; (b) grafting via incorporation of surface-bound monomeric units; (c) "grafting from/surface-initiated polymerization."

depending on the graft density of the attached chains (Fleer et al. 1993; Jones and Richards 1999) (Figure 14.2):

a. If the distance between two anchoring sites is larger than the size of the surface-attached polymers, the segments of the individual chains do not feel each other and behave more or less like a single chain in solution assuming a "mushroom" conformation (dilute brush).

Completely different cases are obtained if the chains are attached to the surface at such short distances between the anchor points that the polymer molecules overlap. With increasing graft density, graft chains will be obliged to stretch away from the surface, forming the so-called polymer brush.

b. Polymer brushes may be categorized into two groups different in graft density. One is the "semidilute" brush (Figure 14.2), in which polymer chains overlap with each other but the free energy of interaction between the chains is not so high.

c. The other category is the "concentrated brush" or the high-density brush (Figure 14.2), for which the higher-order interactions should be taken into account. In this regime, the segments of the chains try to avoid each other as much as possible and minimize segment–segment interactions by stretching away from the surface.

From the stretching of the polymer chains perpendicular to the surface, several new physical phenomena arise. Examples are ultralow friction surfaces (Klein et al. 1993) in which materials coated with surface-attached polymer chains do not become wetted by free polymer, even if the surface-attached and the free chains are chemically identical. Another characteristic of concentrated polymer brushes is noted to be the size-exclusion effect (Yoshikawa et al. 2006), in which the graft chains are highly extended and highly oriented so that large molecules, sufficiently

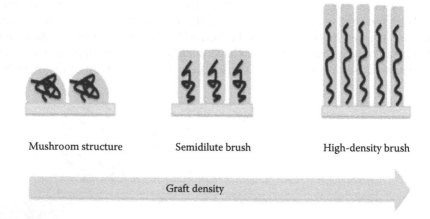

Mushroom structure   Semidilute brush   High-density brush

Graft density

FIGURE 14.2 Development of grafted surfaces from a mushroom structure to a high-density polymer brush: with increasing graft density, graft chains will be obliged to stretch away from the surface, forming the so-called polymer brush.

large compared with the distance between the nearest neighbor graft points, are physically excluded from the entire brush layer. In addition, in the case of functional brush polymers, high densities of functional groups can be obtained at the surface of the substrate through moving from the strictly 2D arrangement of these groups present in typical surfaces to a more three-dimensional (3D) situation. An example that illustrates such behavior is the attachment of DNA probe molecules to surface-attached polymer chains, which can significantly enhance the sensitivity of a DNA chip (Pirri et al. 2006).

The abovementioned *grafting to* method, giving limited graft densities, allows obtaining polymer chains in a "mushroom" conformation and, in the best case, semi-dilute brushes.

An effective method to prepare high-density brushes is the *grafting from* method, that is, the graft polymerization starting with initiating sites fixed on the surface. In this technique, the addition of monomer to growing chain ends or to primary radicals is not strongly hindered by the already grafted chains in a good solvent condition. Therefore, this technique is more promising to produce a polymer film with a larger thickness and a higher graft density than the *grafting to* technique (Prucker and Rühe 1998a,b; Tsubokawa et al. 1989b). The polymerization process obtained by the *grafting from* approach is also defined as surface-initiated polymerization, a very attractive method for the generation of well-defined polymeric architectures with high density of brushes customized with desirable properties.

14.1.3 APPLICATION AS NOVEL BIOINTERFACE

Attractive application of polymer brushes is directed toward a biointerface to tune the interaction of solid surfaces with biologically important materials such as proteins and cells. For example, it is important to prevent surface adsorption of proteins through nonspecific interactions, because the adsorbed protein often triggers a biofouling, for example, the deposition of biological cells, bacteria, and so on.

In an effort to understand the process of protein adsorption, the interaction between proteins and brush surfaces has been modeled (Figure 14.3a): similarly to the interaction with particles, the interaction with proteins is simplified into three generic modes. One is the primary adsorption, in which a protein (or modeled particle) diffuses into the brush and adsorbs on the surface. The secondary adsorption is the adsorption of a protein at the outermost (free) surface of swollen brushes. The last one is the tertiary adsorption, which is caused by the interaction of proteins with the polymer segments within the brush.

For relatively small proteins, primary adsorption induced by a short-range attraction at the surface is important and will be repressed by an increase in graft density. For larger proteins, which hardly diffuse into the brush and cannot approach the substrate surface by a steric or osmotic repulsion between the brush and protein, the secondary adsorption is predominated by van der Waals attraction with the outermost (free) surface of the brush. This mode can be suppressed by increasing the brush thickness. Well-defined high-density polymer brushes achievable by surface-initiated living radical polymerization (see below) would produce surfaces with (i) a size-exclusion limit (Figure 14.3b) set for a very low molecular weight (Yoshikawa

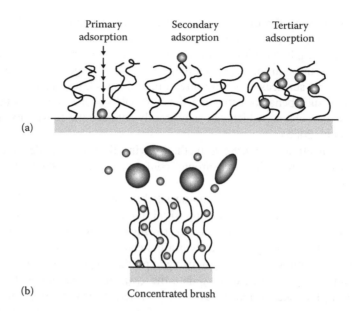

(a)

(b)   Concentrated brush

FIGURE 14.3 (a) Surface adsorption modes of proteins through nonspecific interactions; (b) size-exclusion effect of concentrated brush. (Reprinted with permission from C. Yoshikawa et al., Protein repellency of well-defined, concentrated poly(2-hydroxyethyl methacrylate) brushes by the size-exclusion effect, *Macromolecules*, 39, 2284–2290. Copyright 2006 American Chemical Society.)

et al. 2006), (ii) a strong repulsion force against compression, (iii) effectively tunable properties of the outermost (free) surface by introducing functional moieties or short block segments at the end of graft chains, (iv) grafting of functional polymers including hydrophilic polymers and polyelectrolytes, and (v) precise design of a variety of chain architectures such as hyperbranched and cross-linked graft chains.

For many applications of polymer brushes, it is not simply protection against mechanical or chemical damage that is important. Rather, where the polymer layer acts as a barrier against contact with the environment, a more specific chemical response to the surrounding medium is desirable. Examples of this situation include layers into which DNA, protein molecules, or complexing agents are chemically incorporated (Rühe and Knoll 2002). To this end, polymers with desired functional groups can be formed directly from the corresponding monomers (Pirri et al. 2006). An alternative would be first to generate a brush from a simple and inexpensive precursor monomer containing a reactive group, and this can then be transformed into the final moiety (Rühe and Knoll 2002).

It is quite evident that, in principle, the direct approach is much simpler as the desired brush can be prepared in a one-step reaction. A requirement is that the functional group is compatible with the polymerization process used for brush formation.

The use of "living" polymerization reaction, that is, reaction where the number of active or dormant and thus potentially active species remains more or less constant on the time scale of the polymerization reaction, allows the generation of brushes that carry at the end pointing away from the surface a functional group or brushes that consist of a copolymer. Another interesting system is generated by block copolymer in which a first inert polymeric segment is anchored onto the surfaces and a second functional polymeric segment is exposed at the environment: this system provides a suitable substrate for the arrangement of the biological macromolecules (oligonucleotides, proteins, peptides) in order to be recognized by microarray technology.

14.2 COATINGS FOR MICROARRAY SUPPORTS

One of the most powerful analytical tools for biomolecular recognition is the so-called microarray technology, which implies an orderly arrangement of probes with known identity used to determine complementary targets in solutions. In the microarray technology, it is of the utmost importance to immobilize biomolecules onto the surface. Polymeric coatings, usually referred to as 3D chemistries, provide a homogeneous surface derivatization with a high concentration of reactive groups and an increased capacity of binding molecules of interest. Furthermore, in the field of biosensing, they act as linkers distributing the bound probe molecules also in the axial position, thus causing a faster reaction with the target involved in biomolecular recognition. Additionally, 3D scaffold properties can be tailored for specific applications.

Microarray analyses were developed at first for DNA investigation. Building a DNA microarray involves the immobilization of thousands of oligonucleotides directly on a chip either by photolithographic methods (Lipshutz et al. 1999) or by spotting (Lashkari et al. 1997) in order to analyze mRNA transcript levels expressed under various conditions. However, it is known that the mRNA expression level and the corresponding protein abundances (or activities) do not always correlate because of changes in translation rates and protein lifetimes (Anderson and Seilhamer 1997; Gygi et al. 1999). Furthermore, the analysis of mRNA transcripts does not take into account posttranslational modifications, such as proteolysis, phosphorylation, glycosylation, or acetylation, although many signaling pathways mediate such structural alterations. Therefore, the motivation to overcome such difficulties has led to the development of promising technology that allows large-scale analysis of proteins in a parallel and miniaturized fashion.

Over the past decade, the combination of 2D gel electrophoresis/mass spectrometry (MS) has been the major tool in comprehensive proteomic studies; in this process, the proteome is resolved and each spot is analyzed by MS or MS/MS. The resolution of this method is good enough to separate evenly protein isoforms that are modified by posttranslational processes (e.g., phosphorylation [Kaufmann et al. 2001], glycosylation [Taniguchi et al. 2001], and deamination [Sarioglu et al. 2000]). There are, however, several limitations, such as (1) automation of the processes involved, (2) the detection of scarce proteins, (3) low reproducibility, (4) time-consuming protocols, and (5) difficulties in separation of hydrophobic membrane proteins and basic or high-molecular-mass proteins (Molloy et al. 2002; Patton 1999; Santoni et al. 2000). Another combination for proteome study is the liquid chromatography/MS method, in which it is possible to combine ion-exchange, reversed-phase, and affinity-based separations to improve the resolution of each protein species. Although these two technologies theoretically offer a complete coverage of the proteome, they still lack the properties of parallelization and miniaturization that are required for high-throughput screening of proteins. In order to comply with these characteristics, an alternative technology, the so-called protein microarray/chip, has emerged (Fung 2004; Kambhampati 2003). The protein microarray comprises a large number of capture agents that selectively bind to the proteins of interest on solid surfaces. As in the case of nucleic acid microarrays, both multiplexation and miniaturization are achieved relative to traditional methods, thus dramatically increasing the amount of data that can be obtained per volume of biological sample. For example, when 100 µl of sample is applied to a flat surface with 10,000 spatially and biochemically distinct features (e.g., each one being derivatized with a different antibody), then it would be possible to obtain up to 10,000 data points in just one experiment. By comparison, a conventional 96-well ELISA-type assay would only produce a single data point from the same amount of sample.

A general scheme of a typical array experiment is shown in Figure 14.4: a large set of capture ligands (DNA, protein, or peptide probes) is arranged on a solid func- tionalized support using a robot (spotter) able to spot few nanoliters of a probe solu- tion. After washing and blocking surface unreacted sites, the array is probed with a sample containing (among a variety of unrelated molecules) the counterparts (target) of the molecular recognition event under study. If an interaction occurs, a signal is revealed on the surface by a variety of detection techniques. One of the most impor- tant is the scanning of fluorescent-labeled target molecules that allows the detection of a large number of binding events in parallel.

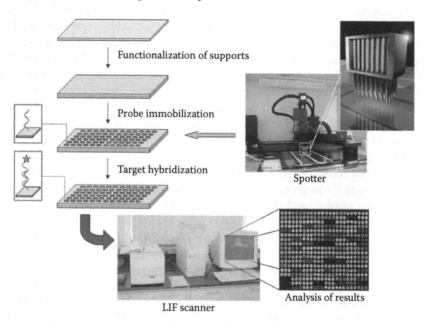

FIGURE 14.4 General scheme of a typical microarray experiment. A set of capture ligands is arrayed on a functionalized support using a robot able to spot a few nanoliters of each probe solution. After blocking surface unreacted sites, the array is probed with a sample contain- ing the counterparts (target) of the molecular recognition event under study. If an interaction occurs, a signal is revealed by fluorescence scanning.

14.2.1 DNA Microarrays

In the early 1990s, the demand for new tools to cope with the enormous quantity of genomic information arose (Thube et al. 2009). Such a necessity led to the development of microarray technology as it was revealed to be, since its very first application, a powerful technique for analyzing thousands of genes of several biological systems.

Briefly, microscopic drops of DNA oligonucleotides, each containing picomoles of specific DNA (e.g., short section of a gene, DNA segments), are deposited onto a surface to hybridize cDNA or cRNA samples. The actual construction of microarrays involves the immobilization or in situ synthesis of DNA probes onto the specific test sites of the solid support or substrate material. High-density DNA contains hundreds of thousands of oligonucleotides immobilized onto a surface. The system, developed at Affymetrix, uses photolitographic techniques to carry out parallel synthesis of several oligos directly onto the solid support, enabling large-scale production. Microelectronic arrays have been developed by Nanogen; they are able to produce reconfigurable electric fields allowing transport of charged DNA/RNA, and then, upon reversing the electric field, an electronic stringency effect occurs, improving hybridization. Several other methods to obtain microarrays are reported in literature, such as synthesis in situ, ink-jet printing, and spotting.

Probes have to be carefully designed considering some aspects, such as probe length, melting temperature and avoiding repetitive motifs, regions that are likely to incur in secondary structure (in the case of mRNA), or cross-hybridization to sequences other than the target ones (Stoughton 2005).

DNA microarrays have attracted scientists' interest because of their potential in clinical diagnostics, genotyping, determination of disease-relevant genes, detection of single nucleotide polymorphisms (SNPs), and posttranslational modifications. For example, De Saizieu et al. measured the relative transcript levels of 100 *Streptococcus pneumoniae* genes during the development of natural competence and during stationary phase (De Saizieu et al. 1998).

DNA microarray is now widely used in virology: 25 common genotypes of human papillomavirus have been identified (Li et al. 2008). The ability to characterize and subclassify tumors has improved thanks to this technology that allows tumor gene expression profile, analysis of multiple gene interaction in cancer, detection of DNA methylation, alterations, allelic association, cancer predisposition genes, oncogenes, and tumor suppressor genes. Microarray analysis of microbial pathogens has potential use in food safety, for example, Cretich et al. (2009a) developed a genomic microarray for the detection of pathogens in milk. Another useful application of DNA microarray is the identification of resistant genes in infectious agents that cause drug or antibiotic resistance, thus helping in developing new drugs.

14.2.2 Protein Arrays

Protein-detecting microarrays have gained interest in the last few years; they mainly allow performance of two different types of analyses, depending on their purposes for protein detection. One is to determine the abundances of proteins of interest in complex protein mixtures with highly specific capture agents for each target protein, for example, by antigen–antibody interactions. The other is to find out the functions of proteins of interest, including protein–protein interactions, receptor–ligand interactions, enzymatic activities, and so on. Hence, protein arrays generally fall into the following categories (Cretich et al. 2014):

1. Function arrays
2. Detection arrays (or analytical arrays)

In protein function arrays (which are generally aimed at discovering protein function in fundamental research), a large set of purified proteins or peptides or even an entire proteome is spotted and immobilized. The array is then used for parallel screening of a range of biochemical interactions. Protein function arrays (Blackburn and Hart 2005) can be used to study the effect of substrates or inhibitors on enzyme activities (Zhu et al. 2003), protein–drug or hormone effector interactions (Kim et al. 2005), or epitope mapping studies (Chiari et al. 2005). In an another kind of protein arrays, usually referred to as reverse-phase microarrays (Zhu and Snyder 2003), tissues, cell lysates, or serum samples are spotted on the surface and probed with one antibody per analyte for a multiplex readout. The reverse-phase microarray falls, generally, in the category of function microarray.

In protein detection microarrays, an array of affinity reagents (antigens or antibodies), rather than the native proteins themselves, is immobilized on a support and used to determine protein abundances in a complex matrix such as serum. Analytical arrays can be used to assay antibodies (for diagnosis of allergy or autoimmunity diseases) or to monitor protein expression on a large scale.

The microarray assay format is ideally suited to the panel of tests that are emerging from the proteomic and genomic initiatives because this method of highly parallel testing is more rapid than serial assays. At the forefront of emerging tests that are suited to a protein microarray format are tests for autoimmune diseases, detection of cytokines, and assessing of allergic responses. A commercially available protein microarray for allergy diagnosis, ImmunoCAP ISAC by Phadia (www.phadia.com), is, for instance, one of the first examples of a protein microarray that really entered into routine clinical analysis.

14.2.3 MICROARRAY SUPPORTS

The aim of microarrays is the study of molecular interactions occurring between two partners: one contained in a liquid sample and one immobilized on a solid support. The chemistry used for the immobilization of probe molecules on the substrate plays a significant role in the success of any experiment. This is particularly true with protein arrays. Unlike DNA, proteins tend to bind to surfaces in a nonspecific manner and, in doing so, sometimes lose their biological activity (Chiari et al. 2005). The surfaces typically used for immobilization of DNA are rarely suitable for proteins because of the biophysical differences between the two classes of bioanalytes.

Therefore, the attributes for a substrate used to immobilize proteins are different from those for a DNA microarray. The key requirements of the surface hosting a protein microarray assay are as follows:

1. Provision of an optimal binding capacity of capture ligands (probes).
2. Retention of biological activity of capture ligands (proteins tend to unfold when immobilized onto a support, in order to allow internal hydrophobic side chains to form hydrophobic bonds with the solid surface).
3. Accessibility of the ligand by the interaction partner (protein–surface interactions reduce the accessibility of the target, possibly leading to false-negative results). This issue is particularly important for peptide micro-arrays because of the small molecular mass of capture ligands.
4. Low degree of aspecific interaction (the achievement of a low degree of aspecific binding is extremely difficult when the sample is a complex mix-ture of thousands of molecules such as serum).

This is of outstanding importance because the abundance of some proteins in plasma is very low (sometimes lower than 1 pg/ml) and their detection is very prob-lematic. Therefore, one of the paramount challenges of manufacturing a viable pro-tein chip is the correct choice of a solid surface and the development of a surface chemistry that is compatible with a diverse set of proteins while maintaining their integrity, native conformation, and biological function.

14.2.3.1   Characteristics of the Supports

The final performance of a microarray biochip strongly depends on parameters related to the immobilization process itself. These include the following:

- The chemical and physical properties of the surface, as they influence both specific and nonspecific binding of target and nontarget biomolecules
- The distance between the immobilized probes and the chip surface
- The orientation of the immobilized proteins, which might impair binding, especially to large analytes such as proteins
- The density of the probes on the surface, which determines the chip's sen-sitivity and limit of detection

The selection of the solid surface employed for generating the protein chip depends on the intended application. For example, gold surfaces are often used for the development of biosensors with electrochemical and surface plasmon resonance (SPR) readout (Lee et al. 2005) because of their outstanding electrical conductivity and convenient functionalization by means of thiol chemisorption. In contrast, glass and silicon are typically preferred for optical sensors because of their transparency (in the case of glass) and low intrinsic fluorescence. In general, these surfaces are characterized by their chemical homogeneity and stability, their controllable surface properties (such as polarity and wettability), their reactivity toward a wide range of chemical functionalities, and the reproducibility of surface modification.

14.2.3.2   Planar Chip Surfaces

Glass slides are the favored surfaces for microarrays for a number of reasons such as availability, cost, flatness, rigidity, transparency, and amenability of the surface to chemical modification (Holloway et al. 2002). Methodologies for functionalizing glass slides with chemical groups have been reported for the development of small-molecule and DNA microarrays (MacBeth et al. 1999; Pirrung 2002). The main method for functionalization of glass slides uses reactive silanol groups (Si-OH) on the glass surface that can be generated by pretreatment of the surface with, for example, piranha solution (H_2O_2/H_2SO_4) or NaOH solution or oxygen plasma. Organofunctional silanes of the general structure $(RO)_3Si(CH_2)_nX$ or trichlorosilanes are then used to introduce new functional groups on the surface (Sagiv 1980). A large variety of silane reagents are commercially available, bearing amine, thiol, carboxy, epoxide, and other functional groups for subsequent modification steps. Various protocols for silanization can be found in the literature, employing deposition of silanes from organic solutions, from aqueous solutions, from gas phase, or by chemical vapor deposition (Benters et al. 2001). Dendrimers are compounds with branched chemical structures that carry a range of chemically reactive groups at their periphery; they have been applied for surface derivatization to create a larger functional surface area. The dendritic structure can either be synthesized in situ by derivatization of the surface with multifunctional linkers (Beier and Hoheisel 1999) or be generated by direct surface modification with a presynthesized branched structure, such as polyamidoamine (Ajikumar et al. 2007), phosphine (Le Berre et al. 2003), or poly(propylene imine) dendrimers (Pathak et al. 2004).

14.2.3.3 Chips with 3D Matrices

Instead of spotting probes onto a 2D solid surface, molecules can diffuse into a porous matrix formed by polymer membranes or hydrogels. These matrices show a high capacity for protein immobilization and can provide a more homogeneous "natural" aqueous environment than flat surfaces, thus preventing denaturation of proteins. However, they suffer from problems related to mass transport effects and sometimes high background signals. Traditional membrane materials that have been used are nitrocellulose and nylon, the latter providing greater physical strength and binding capacity. Protein attachment to nylon is also generally more stable than to nitrocellulose: nylon allows for positive or negative electrostatic interactions or photocross-linking, while nitrocellulose is believed to bind proteins by means of hydrophobic interactions (Del Campo and Bruce 2005). Further improvement of mechanical stability is offered by anodically oxidized porous alumina. This material offers readily available surface chemistries, in particular silanization methods, which can lead to higher densities of biomolecular probes, and thus to higher sensitivity in array applications (Lemeer et al. 2007).

Polymeric hydrogels represent hydrophilic matrices into which proteins can diffuse, leading to 100-fold higher capacity of immobilization than it is found for planar surfaces (Timofeev et al. 1996). Covalent attachment of the gels to solid surfaces allows for generation of stable microarray chips. For example, agarose and acrylamide can be photopolymerized onto a surface functionalized with acrylic groups (Guschin et al. 1997). Subsequently, the polymer can be activated with hydrazine or ethylenediamine to generate amine groups on the surface (Piletsky et al. 2003). Other examples of polymeric gel surfaces that can be used for the immobilization of proteins involve polysaccharides, such as chitosan or dextran (Piehler et al. 1996). Chitosan is an amine-modified, natural, nontoxic polysaccharide, and it is biodegradable. Because of its pH-responsive properties, it can simultaneously be immobilized onto glass supports and bind proteins through electrostatic interactions. Dextran is a complex branched polysaccharide consisting of glucose molecules joined into chains of varying lengths. Dextran hydroxy groups can be oxidized to aldehyde functionalities that can then be covalently immobilized onto amine-functionalized supports, and unreacted aldehyde groups can be further used for protein immobilization. Supramolecular hydrogels composed of glycosylated amino acids have recently been introduced as surface materials for protein arrays (Kiyonaka et al. 2004). Biodegradable polyesters, such as poly(L-lactic acid) and its various copolymers with lactic acid and glycolic acid, have also been studied as surfaces for biological applications (Yoon et al. 2002).

14.2.3.4 Design Principles for Minimizing Nonspecific Adsorption

In contrast to DNA microarray applications, nonspecific binding represents a major obstacle in the development of protein microarray assays. The quality of a microarray assay is determined not only by the desired binding events between biomolecules but also, to a large extent, by the suppression of undesired, nonspecific binding of analytes and other components within the biological sample. As nucleic acids are uniformly negatively charged, spontaneous adsorption to a given surface is much easier for proteins, which can adsorb through electrostatic, van der Waals, and Lewis acid–base forces as well as through hydrophobic interactions and conformational changes (Hlady and Buijs 1996). Such nonspecific binding can give rise to background signals and thus to low signal-to-noise ratios. Effective reduction of nonspecific adsorption has been achieved by careful selection of the surface material, for instance, by using naturally occurring surfaces such as elastin (Nath et al. 2004), sarcosine (Ostuni et al. 2001), agarose (Ponten and Stolt 1980), cellulose (Carter 1965), and polysaccharides (Luk et al. 2000; Ostuni et al. 2001), or by using synthetic polymeric surfaces such as fluorocarbon polymers and molecules (Ko et al. 2005; Vargo et al. 1995), polyethylene glycol (PEG) (Groll et al. 2004; Michel et al. 2005), poly(vinyl alcohol) (Batra et al. 2005; Sugawara and Matsuda 1995), or polyelectrolytes (Mendelsohn et al. 2003; Michel et al. 2005; Yam et al. 2006). One particularly versatile approach to suppressing nonspecific adsorption is based on surfaces that present oligo(ethylene glycol) derivatives (Dilly et al. 2006; Hoffmann et al. 2006; Mrksich et al. 1995). A thorough study by Whitesides and Prime showed that crystalline helical and amorphous forms of SAMs of oligo(ethyleneglycol)-functionalized alkanethiolates on gold are resistant to protein adsorption (Prime and Whitesides 1993). It is hypothesized that binding of interfacial water by the ethylene glycol layer is important for the ability of the SAM to resist protein adsorption (Chen et al. 2005). However, the susceptibility of ethylene glycol chains to autoxidation limits their long-term application. Surface phospholipids also minimize nonspecific binding. Their strong hydration capacity, achieved by electrostatic interaction, is postulated to be responsible for this effect (Chen et al. 2005). The zwitterionic properties of monolayers of, for example, oligophosphorylcholine SAMs result in suppression of kinetically irreversible nonspecific adsorption of proteins, but unfortunately, phosphorylcholine monolayers are not very stable. In an attempt to further rationalize the design of surfaces resistant to protein adsorption, Whitesides et al. formulated a hypothesis relating the preferential exclusion of a "solute" to its ability to render surfaces resistant to the adsorption of proteins. When elements of known osmolytes (organic compounds affecting osmosis) or kosmotropes (organic compounds contributing to the stability and structure of water–water interactions) were incorporated into alkanethiolates such as betaine, taurine, or hexamethylphosphoramide, SAMs of these compounds displayed improved protein repellence (Kane et al. 2003). Although these elaborate approaches have proven to be effective for minimizing nonspecific adsorption, it must be clearly stated that the old-fashioned blocking of reactive surface sites by the addition of blocking agents such as the bovine serum albumin protein, skim milk powder, or other reagents and the presence of surfactants such as Tween-20 and sodium dodecyl sulfate (SDS) are usually indispensable to the suppression of nonspecific protein adsorption (Crowther 1995).

14.2.3.5 Polymer Coatings

The reactivity of a chip surface is determined by the functional groups it displays. The density of the reactive groups is one important factor controlling the amount of protein that can be immobilized on a specific surface area and thus consequently influences the limit of detection attainable with the particular chip. For example, the direct attachment of a protein to a surface without a spacer can cause steric constraint of the protein's reactivity or interaction capability compared to the protein in solution. Moreover, multiple direct contacts with the surface can induce denaturation or partial denaturation and thus a decrease in activity. By introducing a spacer between the protein and the reactive group on the surface, these effects can be minimized.

In general, proteins offer many functional groups, mainly in the amino acid side chains, that are suitable for immobilization purposes. Such functional groups can be used to covalently couple proteins to surfaces by a range of different reactions.

In the case of DNA, sequences can be synthetically modified at one end to expose a functional group that easily reacts with the derivatized surface.

In an attempt to obtain a suitable polymer coating with high capacity for probe immobilization offering a homogeneous "natural" aqueous environment, a hydrophilic copolymer made of N,N-dimethylacrylamide, N-(acryloyloxy)succinimide, and 3-(trimethoxysilyl)propyl methacrylate (copoly(DMA–NAS–MAPS)), first reported for the preparation of low-density DNA microarrays, was developed (Pirri et al. 2004). The synthesis of the polymer, as reported in Sola et al. (2012), is schematized in Figure 14.5. The innovative aspect in this approach relies in the fact that the polymer self-adsorbs onto the glass surface very quickly, simply by immersing glass slides in a diluted aqueous solution of the polymer and without time-consuming glass pretreatments. Therefore, the coating procedure provides a fast and inexpensive method for producing hydrophilic functional surfaces bearing active esters, able to react with amino groups of modified DNA, proteins, and peptides. The copoly(DMA–NAS–MAPS) coating was used on glass in the assessment of rheumatoid factor in human serum samples (Cretich et al. 2004), on poly(dimethylsiloxane) (PDMS) (Cretich et al. 2008), nitrocellulose (Cretich et al. 2009a), and silicon for high-sensitivity protein assays (Cretich et al. 2009b; Gagni et al. 2013). The results have demonstrated that the immobilized probes maintain an active conformation and are easily accessible; moreover, after the assay, the slides exhibited a very low

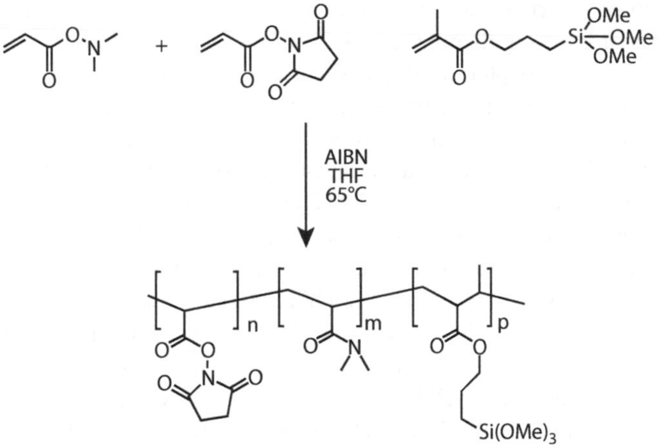

FIGURE 14.5 Synthesis of poly(DMA–co-NAS–co-MAPS) as described in Sola et al. (2012).

background. The polymeric surface was also tested as a peptide microarray support in an epitope mapping study (Chiari et al. 2005). This study suggested that although the copoly(DMA–NAS–MAPS) slides bind the capture molecule in a random conformation, the aqueous microenvironment created by the polymeric coating provided a good accessibility of the ligand.

14.3 SMART COATING FOR DNA SWITCHING CONTROL

A smart coating is a system able to respond to a stimulus, based on predefined functionalities, providing a smart feedback. In other words, it is an active coating, sensitive to an external stimulus, that changes its physical or chemical properties, preferably in a reversible way, and able to work as a sensor or actuator.

Stimuli-responsive coating is of enormous interest in several fields, such as the development of micro- and nanofluidic devices, self-cleaning surfaces, tissue engineering, and sensor devices.

The response of a polymer, as a consequence of the modification of pH, temperature, electric field, ultraviolet (UV) wavelength, or solvent, typically includes a variation of its chain dimension, secondary structure, solubility, intramolecular association, and hydrophobicity/hydrophilicity. In most cases, the physical/chemical phenomenon that provokes the response is the formation or destruction of secondary forces (such as hydrogen bonds or hydrophobic and electrostatic interactions) or simple chemical reactions (e.g., acid–base reactions). In other cases, the response is more dramatic and includes bond brakeage of polymer backbone or cross-linking groups (Roy et al. 2010).

These smart surfaces gain tremendous relevance when applied to biosensors because the ability to modulate a biomolecule activity on a surface enables the development of sensitive, disposable, microfluidic devices for real-time bioanalytical analysis and bioseparations (Mendes 2008).

The design of smart surfaces is based on the use of materials forming SAMs or polymer films or by using them as a foundation to attach stimuli-responsive materials. In particular, this chapter highlights the use of polymer coatings that can change their properties by chemical, electrical, thermal, and optical impulse.

One of the most known and widely used switchable polymer is poly(*N*-isopropylacrylamide) (pNIPAM), a thermo-responsive polymer that has a low critical solution temperature (LCST) of 32°C when in aqueous solutions: below this temperature, pNIPAM is soluble in an extended and swelled conformation. When the temperature increases above the LCST, the polymer collapses, excluding the aqueous solvent from its polymer chain. This behavior is attributed to the presence of hydrogen bonds between the amide groups and water molecules that are broken at high temperature (Mendes 2008) and is schematized in Figure 14.6.

Thanks to its behavior, pNIPAM has been widely exploited as coating for cell culture dishes (Kushida et al. 1999). Cells in fact establish strong hydrophobic interactions with the collapsed pNIPAM; therefore, a decrease in the culture temperature, below the LCST, results in their detachment from the dish. This feature can be exploited to remove cells from a culture instead of using mechanical dissociation or enzymatic digestion. pNIPAM was also found to be useful to regulate the adhesion of other biomolecules such as bacterial protein, peptide, and steroids (Mendes 2008). As a consequence of such a regulatory behavior, it has been exploited to develop a microfluidic device with the ability to absorb proteins from a solution and to release them on demand by changing the temperature of the pNIPAM-coated silicon chip. Gold wires have been used as heaters that could be heated separately so that restricted areas of the chip could be regulated (Mendes et al. 2007).

A precise control of biomolecule activity onto a surface can be achieved also by stimulating a polymer coating by UV light. For example, the azobenzene molecule undergoes a cis–trans isomerization when illuminated with a wavelength of 300–400 nm so that the stable trans form isomerizes, reversibly, to the cis state. This transition is accompanied by a shape modification as the trans isomer is more linear with respect to the cis one. Hayashi et al. (2007) have incorporated azobenzene moieties into a peptide immobilized on a carboxymethyl dextran–coated gold chip:

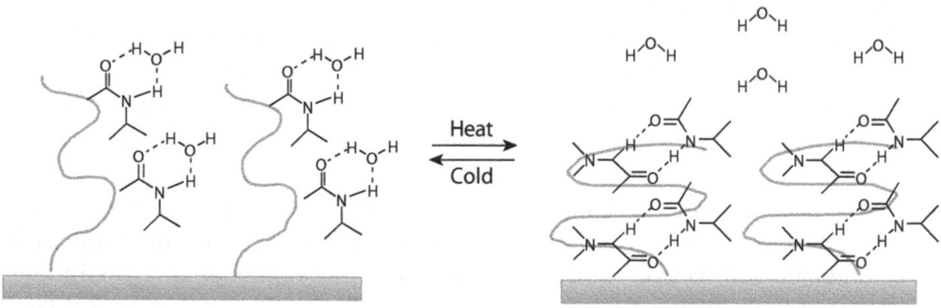

FIGURE 14.6 Diagram illustrating the temperature-induced switching of a pNIPAM-modified surface. pNIPAM chains are shown forming intermolecular hydrogen bonds with water molecules at temperatures below the LCST (left) and forming intramolecular hydrogen bonds between C=O and N–H.

the binding of the peptide to its RNA aptamer was finely regulated thanks to the conformational changes of azobenzene.

Polymer brush coatings can change their conformation because of the combination of entropic repulsion between polymer chains: this behavior has offered the possibility to generate responsive films on both planar surfaces and nanoparticles. In the case of homopolymer brushes, the responsive behavior originates from the properties of the polymer chains and their grafted density, while when considering block copolymer brushes, the stimuli-responsive behavior is due to the phase segregation of the single blocks, specifically when the solvent affinities of the two blocks are different. This process is schematized in Figure 14.7. Phase segregation of mixed polymer brushes (when two or more different polymers are grafted to the same surface) causes the switching of the spatial distribution of the polymer chains, which differently expose their functional groups, thus switching between the properties of the two single constituent of the coating (Cohen et al. 2010). For example, a mixed polymer brush coating made of poly(styrene) and poly(2-vinylpyridine) varies its surface composition and, as a consequence, its wettability when treated with different solvents (Draper et al. 2004).

These combinations of different behaviors broaden the switch range of properties. For example, the balance among electrostatic, steric, and hydrophobic forces can be achieved exposing to external stimuli a triblock coating made of poly(styrene-block-2-vinylpyridine-block-ethylene oxide) (Cohen et al. 2010).

Stimuli-responsive polymer coatings facilitate the transduction mechanism in biosensors. For example, Tokareva et al. (2004) showed the tuning of plasmon resonance coupling between gold nanoparticles and gold substrates mediated by a brush layer of poly(2-vinylpyridine), becoming a highly sensitive pH-responsive sensor.

Hydrogels have become very attractive because of their swelling properties: switching between open and closed pores offers the opportunity to regulate the transportation or accommodation of chemicals, biomolecules, and nanoparticles. For example, poly(2-vinylpyridine) gel films show pH-dependent porosity. At the same time, it is sensitive to cholesterol molecules and this response is used to regulate the permeability of electrochemically active ions across a gel grafted on the surface of an electrode (Cohen et al. 2010). Microlenses with tunable focal lengths, made of pNIPAM and poly(acrylic acid), are able to autofocus under external pressure: the regulation of the focal length is controlled by the shrunken or swollen material refractive index variation, caused by protonation/deprotonation of the acidic groups, temperature modification, and cross-linking/decross-linking events. These tunable microlenses can be introduced into microfluidic devices.

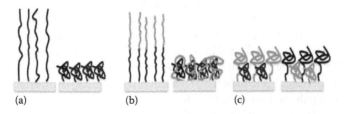

(a)   (b)   (c)

FIGURE 14.7 Illustration of various architectures and responsive behavior of polymers: (a) single-component homopolymer brushes; (b) block copolymer brushes; (c) mixed brushes.

One of the major applications of smart surfaces in biosensors concerns DNA-based analytical platforms and the investigation of protein–DNA interactions. Protein–DNA interactions play a crucial role in many biological processes, including gene expression. Even though they are not very well understood, these conformation changes play a critical role in transcription.

In Section 14.3.1, we highlight the recent achievements made in the development of smart surfaces for DNA studies.

14.3.1　DNA Switch Biosensors

DNA-based analytical platforms have found their way into the scientific world, providing remarkable improvements in bioanalytics, healthcare, biosensing, and diagnostics. Despite the versatility they demonstrated in biomolecular recognition, DNA-tethered surface potential has not been entirely exploited yet. Nature offered the cue to go beyond: biomolecules undergo conformational changes as a consequence of molecular binding and recognition, which is an easily exploited feature. Only a little more than a decade ago, it was observed that DNA responds to externally applied electrical potentials (Kelley et al. 1998), and since then, the development of systems that can manipulate DNA behavior under a certain stimulus has gained a lot of interest, giving birth to the so-called DNA switching nanomachines. These platforms have great potentialities in several fields, such as biomolecular sensing or intelligent drug delivery. The basic mechanisms by which many DNA nanomachines induce motion are through conformational changes in DNA that result from environmental changes in pH (Liu et al. 2006; Meng et al. 2009; Yang et al. 2010) and ionic strength (He et al. 2005) or through the binding of signaling molecules (Yurke et al. 2000). Such nanomachines were, for example, previously used to induce bending of cantilevers (Shu et al. 2005): DNA conformational changes to a quadruplex shape (i-motif) were monitored as a bending of the microcantilevers. Xia et al. (2008), taking cue from membrane acid-sensing ion channels, reported their use as gates for synthetic nanopores. Conical solid nanopores are synthesized to contain, in their inner part, i-motif DNA structures, sensible to pH variations, and as a consequence, nanopores can be easily opened and closed by changing buffer (Figure 14.8). DNA nanoswitch array finds use in the detection of local pH or metal ion concentration. Liu et al. (2006) have developed a sensor on which i-motif, fluorescently labeled DNA is tethered to a gold surface, and as a consequence of pH variations, DNA loses its quadruplex shape and unfolds vertically, allowing detection of fluorescence, which is quenched while in the i-motif configuration as depicted in Figure 14.9.

To date, several platforms utilize orientation changes of surface-immobilized DNA induced by the modulation of an electric potential to control the surface charge of the sensor (Kaiser and Rant 2010; Yang et al. 2010). The characteristic behavior of the DNA switching, such as the switching amplitude (the difference between upright and horizontal orientations) or switching dynamics, is influenced by buffer pH, ionic strength, and temperature (Kaiser and Rant 2010; Rant et al. 2004). In fact, charged objects in solutions containing salts are completely screened by these free ions that create a layer, whose length (Debye length) is inversely proportional to ionic strength. In the case of very high ionic strength, electric interactions are almost

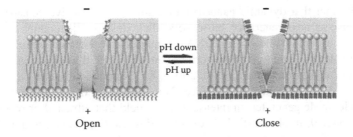

FIGURE 14.8   Scheme of the nanopores containing i-motif DNA structures that can be easily opened or closed by varying the pH buffer. (Reprinted with permission from F. Xia et al., Gating of single synthetic nanopores by proton-driven DNA molecular motors, *J. Am. Chem. Soc.*, 130, 8345–8350. Copyright 2008 American Chemical Society.)

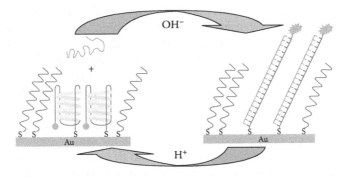

FIGURE 14.9   Schematic presentation of the reversible actuation of the immobilized motor DNA array on a microcontact printing patterned surface. At low pH, the motor DNA adopts its closed i-motif structure, which brings the fluorophore close to the gold surface and quenches its fluorescence. At high pH, the i-motif unfolds and hybridizes with its complementary strand in solution to form a rigid duplex, which lifts up the fluorophore away from the gold surface and becomes highly fluorescent. (Reprinted with permission from D. Liu et al., A reversible pH-driven DNA nanoswitch array, *J. Am. Chem. Soc.*, 128, 2067–2071. Copyright 2006 American Chemical Society.)

completely suppressed and double-stranded DNA assumes a standing position while single-stranded DNA tends to coil and to assume a compressed state; conversely, at low ionic strength, the charges along the DNA sequence are not shielded anymore and electrostatic repulsions occur, causing single-stranded DNA to stiff and extend vertically upon the surface, representing the only way to manipulate single-stranded oligonucleotides (Kaiser and Rant 2010). Additionally, the switching amplitude is influenced by conformation changes of the immobilized DNA, making it possible to detect DNA hybridization or denaturation (Rant et al. 2007) or to utilize the platform for high-throughput characterization of the DNA sequence dependence on conformation changes that are induced by DNA binding proteins such as transcription factors (Spuhler et al. 2010). DNA conformational investigations mostly require induced orientation of the surface-immobilized DNA in a standing position to observe any of its possible variation (Spuhler et al. 2010). DNA switching motors represent the most attractive system to obtain a controlled orientation of oligonucleotides. However, despite the fact that dynamic nanostructures are very attractive considering their potential use as next-generation biosensors, their design still remains a challenge. Up to know, except for a few cases, DNA orientation and switching mainly implicate alternating electric field to a gold electrode, on which the thiol-functionalized DNA probes were end-grafted. Rant et al. (2007), for example, developed a platform to study DNA orientation on a gold surface. The application of an electric potential to the gold electrode generates an intense electric field that attracted or repelled fluorescently labeled, thiol-modified oligonucleotides, causing its orientation. It is well known that gold causes quenching of fluorescence; thus, by measuring fluorescence intensity, it was possible to determine occurring conformational changes (Figure 14.10). Similarly, Meng et al. introduced a platform that exploited the presence of cysteine on the gold surface to orient DNA. Because of the cysteine isoelectric point, which changes the pH value of the buffers, interactions between DNA and the surface vary, causing DNA extension or collapse (Meng et al. 2009). To our knowledge, independently from the mechanism of DNA switching, all the supports used are mainly gold electrodes. This is because attaching thiol-modified oligonucleotides is a very easy and fast process. Only few cases report the use of different materials, such as poly(ethylene terephthalate) (PET) (Xia et al. 2008), using carboxy-amine coupling chemistry. Unfortunately, these systems totally lack surface chemistry control, which may have some limitations: for example, control of probe density is not simple and effortless. Usually, a spacer, such as mercaptoethanol, is required, but in other cases, some other expedients can be used, for example, electrical desorption applying high negative potentials (Kaiser and Rant 2010). An example of polymeric coating able to orient correctly DNA strands is reported by Spuhler et al. who designed a covalently bound smart coating composed of neutral and ionizable monomers, so that the surface charge density can be perfectly controlled by changing buffer pH. As a consequence of net charge variation, DNA was precisely regulated and its orientation was quantified with subnanometer precision (Spuhler et al. 2012). Additionally, the precise measured height changes can provide further information about protein–DNA complexes: if the orientation of surface-bound double-stranded DNA probes is known, then the height change gives the position of protein binding on the DNA sequence. Conversely, if the orientation and the binding positions are known, then the fluorophore height changes allow measurement of the conformation changes induced by protein binding (Figure 14.11).

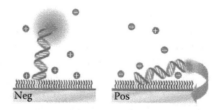

FIGURE 14.10 Scheme of DNA switching caused by the application of an electric potential. When a negative potential is applied to the gold electrode, the negative charges repel the negatively charged DNA. Conversely, a positively charged electrode attracts DNA.

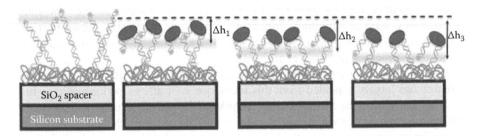

FIGURE 14.11 Measurement platform for the high-throughput measurement of protein–DNA interactions. The mean height of fluorophore tags on immobilized dsDNA probes is precisely measured. Protein binding induces conformation changes in the immobilized DNA, which permits protein binding without labeling the protein. The known orientation of dsDNA probes permits measurement of the protein binding location and of the induced conformation changes.

14.4 LAB-ON-A-CHIP MICROFLUIDIC DEVICES

The rapid and accurate determination of chemical or biological parameters represents one of the major issues in several research and production fields, such as environmental analysis, diagnostic chemical synthesis, and biotechnology. Very often, the sample or compound of interest constitutes only a minor part of the complex mixture taken into account; hence, it has to be perfectly distinguished from the background. Moreover, sometimes, samples are not available in high concentration; thus, very sensitive analytical techniques are required to study them. In the late 1980s, the so-called total chemical analysis system (TAS) was proposed to overcome this issue: this strategy carries out precisely and automatically a sequence of processes such as sampling, sample transportation, separation, and detection.

In the last 20 years, improvements and progress in microfabrication techniques have widely attracted the scientific world. The application of these principles to TAS has led to a fully integrated analytical system on a micrometer scale. The concept was first introduced by Manz et al. in 1990 (Manz et al. 1990) who named it miniaturized total chemical analysis system (µTAS). Considering their potential and role, a second definition of these analytical systems is Lab on a Chip (LoC): they are, in fact, hybrid microanalytical devices that collect various processes on a single platform. They basically integrate fluidic and electronic constituents, containing, on the same chip, microchannels, microvalves, sensing components, microelectrodes, thermal elements, optical apparatus, and micromixers, thus allowing performance of a series of processes or, in some cases, an entire experiment on the same, miniaturized platform. As a consequence, scientists have evaluated the possibility of applying this technology in diagnostics, food quality assessment, cell analysis, genetic mapping, protein analysis, and bioassay. They have gained a lot of importance in drug discovery, for example, in clinical trial studies, drug syntheses, and pharmaceutical formulations and in evaluating the synergic effect of coadministered medicines.

The main advantages of LoC are compactness, portability, process automation, low power consumption, minimal use of samples and reagents, and reduced risk of contamination. Besides their small dimensions, LoC systems support a variety of processes, such as sampling, dispensing, mixing, concentrating, amplification, separation, and detection. Moreover, they allow parallel sample processing and high-throughput screening (Kovarik et al. 2013).

LoC devices have found several fields of application. In general, biomedical research has largely benefited from this technique as it allows performance of full classical analysis but on a smaller scale. Thanks to the use of electrical and mechanical micropumps, separation of biomolecules, cells, and nanoparticles can be managed by exploiting transportation methods based on sample charge and size. LoC devices display high efficiency in mixing reagent and samples in a very precise manner owing to reduced liquid volumes. Both active mixing (such as electrokinetic or magnetically driven mixers) and passive mixing can be used. In particular, passive mixing can be achieved in twisted microchannels where fluid turbulence is created. Temperature gradients can be easily created in these platforms, inside the microchannels: this enables, for example, repeatable temperature cycles and thus DNA amplification by means of PCR reactions (Kovarik et al. 2013). Genomic research requires a specialized analytical technique, the so-called microarray technology, which can be fully integrated into these systems. Furthermore, capillary electrophoresis can also be easily performed in microchannels: because of the tiny dimensions, surface-to-volume ratio increases significantly and electrophoretic forces become more significant, enabling fast and efficient separations. The ultimate goal of LoC devices is their evolution into point-of-care tests (POCTs). A POCT is defined as any medical test close to the patient: in the doctor's office, by the hospital bed, or at home. The most common ones are glucose tests, rapid streptococcal tests, and pregnancy tests.

14.4.1 DEVICE DESIGN, MANUFACTURING, AND MATERIALS

Design of a LoC involves, as a first step, a series of numerical simulation to foresee the components' behavior and performance. It is fundamental to investigate the functionality of a muticomponent microfluidic platform implemented with complicated sample analysis.

LoC should be modular and should combine elementary fluidic components like micropumps, microvalves, reservoirs, and microchannels to allow a straightforward process. Its design should allow uncomplicated assembly and easy maintenance. Manufacturing procedures are very similar to microelectronic chip fabrication. Photolithography remains the main technique to pattern microfluidic and electric features. It implies the use of a photomask and UV light, and it enables the production of small features maintaining high-quality aspects (Kovarik et al. 2013).

Soft lithography is an alternative based on direct printing or molding of different materials. In this case, elastomers (such as PDMS) are used instead of rigid photomasks.

In the early years of μTAS, the dominant materials applicable for microfluidic device fabrication were inorganic materials, such as silicon, glass, and quartz. All of these materials are widely used in the microelectronics industry and standard microfabrication techniques have already been well developed. Nowadays, among these materials, silicon is seldom used for microfluidic devices because it is not transparent to visible and UV light for optical detection. In comparison, glass has been the major inorganic material used in microfluidic device fabrication because it has good optical, mechanical, electrical insulating, and thermal properties. In addition, glass surfaces are easy to modify because surface chemistries have been well established. Even though quartz, a pure form of silicon dioxide, has superior physical properties over other inorganic materials for microfabrication, it is not widely used in microfluidic device fabrication because of its high cost and difficult fabrication requirements.

Unfortunately, these materials are very expensive and require cumbersome fabrication techniques. As a consequence, new materials have been recently introduced for the fabrication of microfluidic devices. Cyclic olefin copolymer, PET, polycarbonate, PDMS, and polytetrafluoroethylene are currently used to fabricate disposable microfluidic devices via plastic machining technologies such as injection molding, casting, and embossing.

The control of the surface properties of these systems is fundamental to obtain optimal analytical performance: the hydrophobicity of the materials reduces their wettability and complicates the introduction of aqueous solutions into narrow channels and, at the same time, makes the material unsuitable for use with biological samples. It is known that proteins irreversibly interact with surfaces by means of electrostatic and hydrophobic interactions, leading to poor analytical performance. As a consequence, it is very important to modify the surface of these polymeric materials to decrease their hydrophobicity and obtain better biocompatibility.

Several modification methods have been reported in literature, but the most commonly used are divided into three categories: gas-phase methods, wet chemical processes, and a combination of the two. The gas-phase methods include plasma oxidation, UV irradiation, and chemical vapor deposition. The first two processes induce a chemical modification of the surfaces by introducing new functional groups, while the third hides the undesirable characteristic of the materials by the deposition of vapors onto the surfaces. Oxygen plasma, for example, reacts with methyl groups on the surface, generating silanol groups similar to silicon oxide (Makamba et al. 2003). On the contrary, UV irradiation, starting from air oxygen, generates ozone, which interacts with the surface resulting in the formation of hydroxy groups (Efimenko et al. 2002). Even though these processes are very easy to perform, their main drawback is the fast aging of the treated material. For example, plasma degrades a thin layer of the material, producing low-molecular-weight polymer chains that are dissolved when in contact with liquids. Another issue is the instability of the process: PDMS recovers its hydrophobicity after a short time because of the migration of uncured monomers from the bulk to the surface (Berdichevsky et al. 2004). The chemical vapor deposition process implies the chemical reaction of gas reagents in an environment activated by heat, light, and plasma followed by the formation of a stable product on the surface as powder or films (Choy 2003).

Wet chemical modification processes include the use of suspensions or solutions, which cause the adsorption of the solute through electrostatic interactions or chemical reaction with the functional groups of the surface. Films obtained by physical interactions of molecules with the substrate are usually unstable, because of the desorption caused by the exposure to organic solvents or the replacement of other molecules that can form a more stable interaction with the surface. Surface modification through the LBL technique or the deposition of polyanions and polycations is an emerging simple and efficient method for controlling the coating thickness on the nanoscale. The LBL coating consists in the adsorption of polyelectrolyte layers (macromolecules bearing charged moieties along their chain) of opposite charge, leading to a highly reproducible nanostructured multilayer (Kolasinska et al. 2009). The process shows a series of advantages as it consists in the spontaneous adsorption of solutions onto the surface, but the obtained film is not very stable and the interactions between biomolecules and polyelectrolytes are very likely to happen. Furthermore, the material that has to be coated needs to be charged as well. This issue has been solved by treating PDMS with polycations such as poly(diallyldimethylammonium chloride) or chitosan: they interact with PDMS through hydrophobic interactions leading to a first charged layer, which is able to adsorb others (Wang et al. 2006).

Another approach implies the dynamic modification of surfaces using surfactants, a very fast and simple process that involves the use of amphiphilic molecules added to the analysis running buffer. The hydrophobic chain of the surfactant adsorbs onto the hydrophobic surface, while the polar chain remains in contact with the solution. Several surfactants have been taken into consideration, such as SDS, dodecanol polyoxyethylene (Brij35), sodium deoxycholate, phosphatidic acid, and polyethylene oxide (Dou et al. 2004; Garcia et al. 2005). The success of the treatment depends on the surfactant concentration and the adsorption characteristics because the chain can adopt different orientations on the surface. In order to increase antifouling properties, the surfactant concentration must be slightly inferior to the critical micellar concentration, because in this way, a dense single layer deposits onto the surface, thus preventing the interactions of biomolecules. If the concentration is too high, a double layer of molecules adsorbs onto the surfaces but the polar chains are not efficiently exposed, or in other cases, micelles and aggregates are formed and adsorbed onto the surfaces, reducing the efficacy of the treatment.

Unfortunately, the functionality and stability of coatings obtained using these approaches depend on many factors that are difficult to control, such as both the polyelectrolyte ionic strength and concentration, type of solvent, temperature, pH, and so on (Ariga et al. 2007).

Another approach to improve the surface properties of microfluidic devices is silanization, a process based on the condensation of silanol groups via the oxidation of functional alkoxy- or chlorosilanes (Figure 14.12). The silanization process is

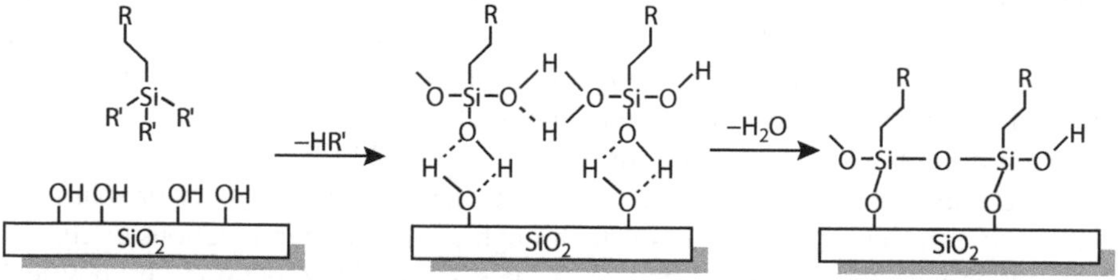

FIGURE 14.12 Scheme of the silanization process. Aliphatic chains bind to hydroxy groups on the surface by means of hydrogen bonds. Removal of water stabilizes the binding by the formation of covalent bonds. A number of polymers bearing reactive functionalities have been grafted onto silanized PDMS.

divided into three phases: aliphatic chains are attracted onto the surface through the alkoxysilane groups, which act as a polar moiety of an amphiphilic molecule. The presence of water hydrolyzes those groups, which can bind to the hydroxy groups of the surface by the formation of hydrogen bonds. Finally, removal of water using reduced pressure and high temperature stabilizes the binding by the formation of covalent bonds (Silberzan et al. 1991).

A number of polymers bearing reactive functionalities have been grafted onto silanized PDMS. For instance, O-[(N-succinimidyl)succinyl]-O-mPEG, poly(dimethyl-acrylamide co-glycidyl methacrylate) (poly(DMA-GMA)), poly(vinylpyrrolidone)-g-glycidyl methacrylate (PVP-g-GMA), and poly(vinyl alcohol)-g-glycidyl methacrylate (PVA-g-GMA) have been covalently grafted onto APTES-modified PDMS surfaces (Zhou et al. 2010). These polymers are attached to the surface owing to the reactivity of surface functionalities to the chemically reactive polymer groups. Both these and other processes combining UV or plasma treatments with graft polymerization rely on the reproducibility of silanization, which is known to be difficult to control even on glass, which is the most reactive material for organosilanes (Vansant et al. 1995). Zilio et al. (2014) have introduced a simple process that combines gas phase and wet chemical modification.

Several plastic materials have been treated with plasma and then immersed into a diluted solution of a dimethylacrylamide-based polymer solution. The coating procedure is easy, fast, and robust and provides hydrophilic functional films covalently bound to the surface. In this work, it was found that polymers bearing silane groups are effective at forming thin films on different thermoplastics as well as on PDMS. The presence of silane groups pending from the polymer backbone is critical for stabilizing the coating on a number of plastics. The coatings reported in this work are very stable to harsh conditions such as organic solvents and high temperature, and in general, the hydrophobicity of the thermoplastic materials used diminished water contact angles from approximately 100° to 80° or 40°.

14.4.2 BIOSENSING IN MICROFLUIDICS STRUCTURES

Combination of biosensors and microfluidics chips enhances analytical capability, widening the scope of possible applications. The role of microfluidics in biomedical analysis was recently reviewed (Gervais et al. 2011; Sackmann et al. 2014).

Microfluidic methods are being developed to perform a variety of diagnostic tests with built-in analysis capabilities. When a microarray is embedded in a microfluidic structure, polymers are efficient means to immobilize the capturing probes and suppress nonspecific adhesion of proteins. For example, a sensitive flow-through micro-array immunoassay device was developed (Liu et al. 2011) in which a poly[glycidyl methacrylate-co-poly(ethylene glycol) methacrylate] (P(GMA-co-PEGMA)) brush is coated on a glass slide through a surface-initiated atom transfer radical polymerization to immobilize capture proteins. The integrated device was realized by laminating the protein-arrayed slide onto a double-sided adhesive tape–attached poly(methyl methacrylate) microfluidic structure. The parallel microarray-based device was designed to perform immunoassays for simultaneous analysis of samples demonstrating reduced total assay time over the static microarray immunoassay. The rapid and sensitive detection can be mainly ascribed to the P(GMA-co-PEGMA)-brushed substrate, of which both the hydrophilicity from its PEG component and the binding capability from its GMA moiety result in higher protein loading capacity, lower nonspecific adsorption, and higher antibody–antigen binding efficiency.

In general, each component of a TAS microdevice requires a specific functionalization depending on its role in the assay, with each modification contributing to the success of the analysis. Hydrophilicity/hydrophobicity is needed to direct fluids in the microchannels; biosensing areas usually require stable immobilization of the probes; microreactors necessitate coatings to prevent nonspecific adhesion of the enzymes and other reaction components; cell-based analytical devices need antifouling properties in some of their areas. An example of the flexibility in tailoring surface properties provided by polymer chemistry is illustrated by the work by Samuel et al. (2010). In this work, a versatile pathway for the generation of polymer-based microfluidic devices with tailor-made surface chemistry was described. A photochemical process was used to covalently bind polymers onto surfaces of hot embossed microchannels. The microfluidics chips have the format of a compact disk (CD) made of polymethylmethacrylate and polyethylene-co-norbornene. Thin films of polymers containing photoactive benzophenone units were deposited onto the surface of the devices and irradiated with UV light leading to the surface attachment of ultrathin polymer networks. In contrast to their unmodified CDs, the microfluidic channels coated with hydrophilic, photoattached layers can be filled in a straightforward manner with water by capillary forces. Channels coated by thin films of poly(ethyloxazoline) demonstrated resistance to nonspecific protein adhesion. Generation of hydrophobic patches inside the modified microfluidic channels using benzophenone-containing fluoropolymers allowed the generation of passive microfluidic valves to direct fluid motion in the CDs.

14.5 POLYMER-COATED NANOPARTICLES FOR BIOSENSING

Nowadays, nanoparticles have great importance in basic and applied research in different kinds of fields such as optics and electronics. In the last 20 years, the synthesis and the characterization of nanoparticles have experienced a rapid progress (Burda et al. 2005; Park et al. 2007; Tenne 2003). Colloidal inorganic nanocrystals are promising materials because of their unique size-dependent properties and have found broad application in analytical chemistry (Alivisatos et al. 1998; Efros and Rosen 2000; Moriarty 2001). Thanks to their chemical and physical properties, they can be used to construct novel and improved sensing devices, including electrochemical sensors and biosensors that offer great promise in terms of high performance (high sensitivity and selectivity), high speed, miniaturization, and low cost.

Many kinds of nanoparticles, such as metal, oxide, and semiconductor nanocrystals, have been used for different kinds of biosensors where nanoparticles play different roles. One of the most important functions provided by nanoparticles in biosensor construction includes the immobilization of biomolecules, retaining their bioactivity and increasing their stability. In fact, because of their large specific surface area and high surface free energy, nanoparticles can adsorb biomolecules strongly or, as well described earlier, they can be functionalized, exploiting the functional groups embedded in the polymer shell. Crumbliss et al. (1992) exploited colloidal gold as a biocompatible enzyme immobilization matrix suitable for the fabrication of enzyme electrodes. Electrochemical immunosensors based on the immobilization of antigen or antibody on nanoparticles are extensively studied; for example, an amperometric immunosensor for the sensitive detection of hepatitis B surface antigen was designed exploiting gold nanoparticles for the bioconjugation (Zhuo et al. 2005). Besides gold nanoparticles, other types of nanoparticles such as silver and silica (Cai et al. 2001) have also been used for the immobilization of antibodies and antigens. DNA molecules can be immobilized on nanoparticles for the construction of electrochemical DNA sensors. For this purpose, it is necessary to modify the DNA strands with special functional groups that can interact strongly with nanoparticles (Cai et al. 2001). Important functions that nanoparticles can provide into electrochemical sensors and biosensors are based on their excellent catalytic properties and conductivity. In particular, metal nanoparticles such as gold and platinum nanoparticles exhibit good catalytic properties and have been used in electrochemical analysis (Raj et al. 2003; You et al. 2003) or on biosensors for enhanced electron transfer properties (Liu et al. 2003).

Gold nanoparticles are the most frequently used among all the metal nanoparticle labels available (Dequaire et al. 2000), and they represent an excellent nanoplatform to develop methods for biosensing. They can be employed for a wide range of applications, ranging from chemical to biological samples, as demonstrated by many research groups (Burda et al. 2005; Daniel and Astruc 2004; Homola 2008; Njoki et al. 2007). A distinctive feature of gold nanoparticles is the SPR absorption, which is due to the strong vibrant color of their colloidal solution. This particular property provides enhancement of SPR biosensor response (Matsui et al. 2005). In addition to their unique SPR effect, surface-enhanced Raman scattering detection represents an important application, where gold nanoparticles are used as probes for single molecules (Kneipp et al. 1997; Krug et al. 1999; Morasso et al. 1998; Nie and Emery 1997; Rodriguez et al. 2010).

Luminescent semiconductors or nanocrystals or quantum dots (QDs) are a recently developed class of nanomaterial whose unique photophysical properties help create a new generation of robust fluorescent biosensors. In fact, they are suitable for bioassays thanks to the possibility of being excited at almost any wavelength below the band edge. This peculiarity, combined with high photobleaching resistance and multiplexing capabilities, makes them attractive to biologists for use in fluorescence assays, in place of the common organic fluorophores that have numerous drawbacks (Resch-Genger et al. 2008). The widespread use of QDs in a myriad of biosensing applications including immunoassays, nucleic acid detection, resonance energy-transfer studies, clinical/diagnostic assays, and cellular labeling was recently summarized (Sapsford et al. 2006). QDs on immunoassay detection have been widely studied; for instance, they are used in immunoassays for the rapid detection of protein toxins in clinical, environmental, and food/water security-based applications. Their size-tunable photoluminescence coupled with the broad absorption spectra has allowed multiplexed immunoassays (Goldman et al. 2004) for the simultaneous detection of four toxins: cholera toxin, ricin, Shiga-like toxin, and staphylococcal enterotoxin B. In this assay, the unique photophysical properties of

QDs play a fundamental role because specific antibodies for each of the toxins are coupled to a different-color QD representing a real, new, and advantageous approach for optical biosensing.

QDs were recently used to amplify detection signal in interferometric biosensors based on dual-polarization interferometry for immunoglobulin E in serum (Platt et al. 2014). Moreover, QDs have become advantageous reporters in microarray technology (Nichkova et al. 2007; Sapsford et al. 2011). The performance of CdSe/ZnS QDs in comparison with the fluorescent dye Alexa 647 as fluorescent tags in a sandwich immunoassay microarray was explored to detect ApoE, a potential biomarker of Alzheimer's disease (Morales-Narvaez et al. 2012). The authors obtained up to a sevenfold enhancement in the limit of detection when compared with a conventional ELISA assay and up to a fivefold enhancement when compared with Alexa 647 as reporter in microarray format.

The use of QDs provides benefits in DNA microarray as well. These include gene expression monitoring, mutation detection, and SNP typing. In particular, they allow the simultaneous comparison of different genomes or genetic markers facilitating pathogen identification and cancer diagnosis/evaluation. Gerion et al. in 2002 demonstrated specific hybridization of four different QD–DNA conjugates on surfaces containing complementary DNA strands (Gerion et al. 2002) and later the same group studied the use of QD–DNA conjugates for the simultaneous detection of hepatitis B and C genotypes and SNP detection (Gerion et al. 2003).

The use of QDs in microarray technology improved biosensing performance and accelerated incorporation of this technology into real-world bioanalytical scenarios for applications in diagnostics, safety, security, and environmental monitoring.

14.5.1 NANOPARTICLE COATING

The usefulness of nanoparticles in biomedical applications depends on the ability to manipulate their surface chemistry while maintaining their properties identical to the features that they have in the organic solvents where they are mostly synthesized. Therefore, the development of methods that can provide small, biocompatible, monodisperse, and chemically reactive nanoparticles stable in water is a key factor for their use in biomedical applications. As a matter of fact, nanocrystals can be synthesized either in aqueous solution starting from various materials such as Au (Schmid and Lehnert 1989), CdTe and CdSe (Rogach et al. 2004), and Fe_3O_4 (Berger et al. 1999) or in organic solvents starting from Au (Fink et al. 1998), CdTe and CdSe (Peng and Peng 2001), and Fe_3O_{4S} (Sun and Zeng 2002). However, various synthetic approaches in organic solvent at high temperature are widely used to provide control over size and shape (Manna et al. 2000) and in order to obtain highly crystalline and monodisperse nanocrystals. This involves their surface being coated with different hydrophobic surfactant molecules (e.g., trioctylphosphine oxide [–TOPO–] or hexadecylamine [–HDA–]) that provide their hydrophobicity and protect them from further growth and from the external environment.

Several methods exist for converting hydrophobic nanocrystals into hydrophilic particles, which is a prerequisite for biological applications as mentioned earlier (Potapova et al. 2003). Currently, there are three common strategies to transfer nanoparticles from organic solvents into aqueous solutions (Anderson et al. 2008): molecular exchange, use of amphiphilic molecules, and polymer coating.

The technique of molecular exchange is probably the simplest method to change the solubility of a nanoparticle (Chan and Nie 1998; Freeman et al. 1995; Mattoussi et al. 2000). In this method, an external molecule (e.g., mercaptoacetic acid) is added to a solution of nanoparticles in a specific solvent (e.g., chloroform), allowing the competition for binding sites onto the nanoparticles' surface with the original surface ligand (e.g., TOPO or HDA). When the surface ligand is displaced by the external molecule, the polarity and surface chemistry of the nanoparticles are altered, making the nanoparticles hydrophilic and displaying on the surface carboxylic acid groups useful for conjugation. However, this method requires adsorption of surface ligands that could desorb from the surface leading to nanoparticles' aggregation.

In an alternative strategy, an amphiphilic molecule (e.g., phospholipids) can be exploited. The interaction of its hydrophobic portion with the nanoparticles' surface causes the exhibition of hydrophilic functionalities on the nanoparticles' surface (Dubertret et al. 2002; Pellegrino et al. 2004; Wu et al. 2003; Yu et al. 2007). Microspheres (e.g., silica nanoparticles), liposomes, or hydrogels can be exploited in order to incorporate nanoparticles for the modification of their polarity and functionality (Darbandi et al. 2005; Gao and Nie 2003; Han et al. 2001), but these encapsulated structures could be large in comparison to the original size of the nanoparticle.

The inclusion of hydrophobic nanoparticles in an amphiphilic polymeric shell (Dubertret et al. 2002; Pellegrino et al. 2004) is advantageous compared to other approaches, as the nanoparticles are simply wrapped in a polymeric shell thanks to the interactions between the alkyl chains of the surfactant coating and the hydrophobic regions of the polymer. The advantage of this method over the ligand exchange protocols is that it can be used regardless of the type of surfactant and of the specific inorganic material that forms the nanocrystal core. Therefore, this procedure is easily extendable to many different types of hydrophobic nanoparticles. Moreover, the phase transfer from organic solvents into aqueous solution using amphiphilic polymers confers long-term colloidal stability to nanoparticles, helping them retain their major physical properties (such as, for instance, the fluorescence of CdSe/ZnS QDs and the magnetic moment of Fe_2O_3 and $CoPt_3$ nanoparticles). Basically, when an amphiphilic polymer is employed, the solubilization mechanism consists of an interdigitation of the polymer hydrophobic segments with the surfactants on the nanoparticles' surface, leaving the polar polymer backbone exposed to the environment with the hydrophilic groups protruding from the surface. Pellegrino et al. (2004) described a general strategy that allows the phase transfer of the hydrophobically capped nanocrystals from organic to aqueous solution by wrapping an amphiphilic polymer around the particles (Figure 14.13). In particular, hydrophobic nanocrystals of various materials such as $CoPt_3$ (Shevchenko et al. 2002), Au (Fink et al. 1998), CdSe/ZnS (Dabbousi et al. 1997), and Fe_2O_3 (Hyeon et al. 2001) have been water solubilized through this strategy. This simple and general protocol exploits the nonspecific hydrophobic interactions between the alkyl chains of poly(maleic anhydride alt-1-tetradecene) and the nanocrystal surfactant molecules. The attachment of the polymer onto the particle surface is highly stable because of the numerous contact points mediated by hydrophobic interaction; moreover, the stability can be further improved by cross-linking

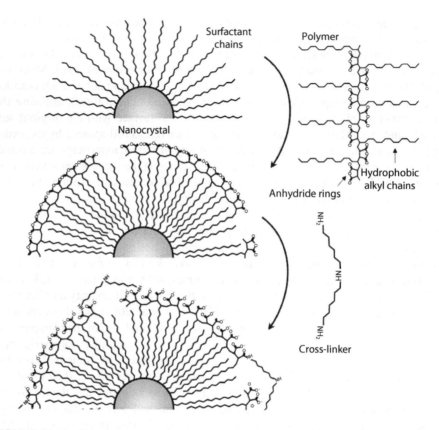

FIGURE 14.13 Scheme of the polymer coating procedure: the hydrophobic alkyl chains of the polymer intercalate with the surfactant coating. The anhydride rings are located on the surface of the polymer-coated nanocrystal and they are opened by the amino end groups of the cross-linker molecule linking the individual polymer chains. The surface of the polymer shell becomes negatively charged, stabilizing the particles in water by electrostatic repulsion. (Reprinted with permission from T. Pellegrino et al., Hydrophobic nanocrystals coated with an amphiphilic polymer shell: A general route to water soluble nanocrystals, *Nano Lett.*, 4, 703–707. Copyright 2004 American Chemical Society.)

of the polymer shell (Jiang et al. 2006; Kang and Taton 2005; Pellegrino et al. 2004). In this case, addition of bis(6 aminohexyl)amine results in the cross-linking of the polymer chains around each nanoparticle (Figure 14.12). The surface of the polymer shell becomes negatively charged, upon hydrolyzation of the unreacted anhydride groups stabilizing the particles in water by electrostatic repulsion.

Yu et al. (2007) demonstrated the use of poly(maleic anhydride-alt-1-octadecene) to water-solubilized magnetic, semiconductor, and metallic nanoparticles. Disappointingly, this particular amphiphilic polymer is no longer commercially available.

Other groups have also demonstrated the synthesis of an amphiphilic polymer and studied wrapping and solubilization of nanoparticles in aqueous solvents (Luccardini et al. 2006; Wang et al. 2007; Wu et al. 2003). Other types of amphiphilic polymers currently under investigation include block copolymers (e.g., polystyrene-*b*-poly(acrylic acid) [Schabas et al. 2008] and poly(methyl methacrylate)–poly(ethyleneoxide) [Smith et al. 2006]) and amphiphilic hyperbranched polyethylenimine (Nann 2005). These authors not only describe methods for the phase transfer of colloidal nano-crystals QDs, they also underline the advantages of the use of amphiphilic polymers as they provide coatings with considerably higher integrity and stability, reducing the QDs' sensitivity to oxygen and light (Nida et al. 2008). In fact, for semiconductor nanoparticles, the extent of passivation is particularly important, significantly affect-ing the photoluminescent properties, especially quantum yield. This fluorescence dependence on surface features is crucial to retain optical properties for biological imaging applications. The amphiphilic particle coatings not only enable the phase transfer of the nanoparticles from organic solvents to aqueous solution but also serve as a versatile platform for chemical modification and bioconjugation (Wu et al. 2003; Yu et al. 2007).

Polymers bearing carboxylic acid and amine functional groups facilitate attach-ment of biomolecules, allowing the use of polymer-coated nanoparticles in a variety of applications including protein detection and cell labeling. Although the presence of surfactant molecules on nanoparticles' surface is necessary, they may also ren-der nanoparticles hydrophobic or prevent the nanoparticles from undergoing further chemical functionalization. Furthermore, the surfactant layer may be unstable to subsequent processing and conjugation chemistry. Lin et al. (2008) describe a proce-dure allowing a direct embedding of functional groups (such as PEG, organic fluoro-phore, sugar, and biotin) in the polymer shell without the need of post-bioconjugation chemistry. This strategy is based on coupling functional molecules in organic solvent to the polymer before the actual embedding of the particles in the polymer. Following this protocol, molecules that are not soluble in aqueous solution can be grafted on the particle surface as the coupling is performed in organic solvents. In this way, no addi-tional reagents are needed for the coupling. In traditional approaches, cross-linkers such as EDC (1-ethyl-3-(3-dimethylamino propyl)carbodiimide) have to be used to add functionality to the particle surface involving a postmodification of polymer-coated nanoparticles in aqueous solution (Sperling et al. 2006).

The importance of a robust approach to obtain colloidally stable, water-soluble, small, biocompatible, and monodisperse nanoparticles with flexible surface chem-istry is also described by Finetti et al. (2014). In this work, a robust approach, schematized in Figure 14.14, for phase transfer into water and functionalization of

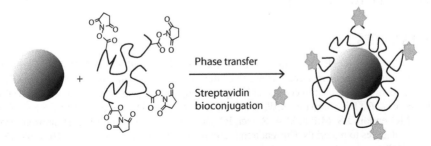

Phase transfer

Streptavidin bioconjugation

FIGURE 14.14 Schematic representation of one-pot phase transfer of the CdSe–ZnS QDs by derivatization with copoly(DMA–NAS–MAPS) and bioconjugation with streptavidin.

QDs for use as fluorescent tags and multifunctional nanoscaffolds for bioimaging, sensing, and therapeutics was developed. Also, in this work, a functional amphiphilic copolymer, copoly(DMA–NAS–MAPS), is employed (Pirri et al. 2004). The method is very straightforward, as functional bioligands, such as proteins, can be directly immobilized onto the nanocrystal surface, exploiting the active ester groups of the coating polymer by means of a peptide bond formed during QD solubilization. Unlike most of the published methods, the proposed functionalization approach does not require coupling agents and multistep reactions since a phase-transfer and surface derivatization of colloidal nanocrystals by a one-pot procedure is provided. The polymer-coated QDs obtained with this method demonstrated that hydrophobic nanoparticles embedded in a shell of amphiphilic polymers with incorporated functional groups show the same colloidal properties of the previously published nanoparticles with no functional groups in their shells.

14.6 CONCLUSION

The successful application of polymer coatings is a versatile method to fine-tune the characteristics of surfaces for molecular recognition. In recent years, a variety of innovative methods have been introduced to modify biosensors, LoC devices, and nanoparticles. Some methods require sophisticated control of reaction such as in the creation of brush polymeric surfaces whereas other coatings are simple and straightforward. New routes will be introduced in the near future for the production of new surfaces and hybrid materials with a pivotal role in a wide range of areas such as interfacial reactions, biomedical devices/implants, and biosensors. Stimuli-responsive polymers and antifouling coatings are expected to assume a preeminent position in future scenarios.

ACKNOWLEDGMENTS

This work was partially financed by MIUR (Italian Ministry of University and Research) through NEMATIC (Project no. RBFR12OO1G), by EU through FP7 NADINE (NAnosystems for early DIagnosis of NEurodegenerative Diseases) Project Contract no. 246513, by Regione Lombardia (Project LOCSENS ID no. 30071637), and by the POR-FESR Regione Lombardia & Cariplo Foundation (Project MINER ID 42708181, ID 2013-1738).

REFERENCES

Ajikumar P.K., J.K. Ng, Y.C. Tang, J.Y. Lee, G. Stephanopoulos and H.P. Too, Carboxyl-terminated dendrimer-coated bioactive interface for protein microarray: High-sensitivity detection of antigen in complex biological samples, *Langmuir*, 23, 5670–5677 (2007).

Alivisatos A.P., P.F. Barbara, A.W. Castleman, J. Chang, D.A. Dixon, M.L. Klein, G.L. McLendon, J.S. Miller, M.A. Ratner, P.J. Rossky, S.I. Stupp and M.E. Thompson, From molecules to materials: Current trends and future directions, *Adv. Mater.*, 10, 1297–1336 (1998).

Anderson L. and J. Seilhamer, A comparison of selected mRNA and protein abundances in human liver, *Electrophoresis*, 18, 533–537 (1997).

Anderson R.E. and W.C.W. Chan, Systematic investigation of preparing biocompatible, single, and small ZnS-capped CdSe quantum dots with amphiphilic polymers, *ACS Nano*, 2, 1341–1352 (2008).

Ariga K., J.P. Hill and Q. Ji, Structure and rheology of reverse micelles in dipentaerythrityl tri-(12-hydroxystearate)/oil systems, *Phys. Chem. Chem. Phys.*, 9, 2319–2340 (2007).

Batra D., S. Vogt, P.D. Laible and M.A. Firestone, Self-assembled mesoporous polymeric networks for patterned protein arrays, *Langmuir*, 21, 10301–10306 (2005).

Beier M. and J.D. Hoheisel, Versatile derivatisation of solid support media for covalent bonding on DNA-microchips, *Nucleic Acids Res.*, 27, 1970–1977 (1999).

Benters R., C.M. Niemeyer and D. Wöhrle, Dendrimer-activated-solid supports for nucleic acid and protein microarrays, *Chembiochem*, 2, 686–694 (2001).

Berdichevsky Y., J. Khandurina and A. Guttman, UV/zone modification of poly(dimethylsiloxane) microfluidic channels, *Sens. Actuators B Chem.*, 97, 402–408 (2004).

Berger P., N.B. Adelman, K.J. Beckman, D.J. Campbell, A.B. Ellis and G.C. Lisensky, Preparation and properties of an aqueous ferrofluid, *J. Chem. Educ.*, 76, 943–948 (1999).

Blackburn J.M. and D.J. Hart, Fabrication of protein function microarrays for systems-oriented proteomic analysis, *Methods Mol. Biol.*, 310, 197–216 (2005).

Burda C., X. Chen, R. Narayanan and M.A. El-Sayed, Chemistry and properties of nanocrystals of different shapes, *Chem. Rev.*, 105, 1025–1102 (2005).

Cai H., C. Xu, P. He and Y. Fang, Colloid Au-enhanced DNA immobilization for the electrochemical detection of sequence-specific DNA, *J. Electroanal. Chem.*, 510, 78 (2001).

Carter S.B., Principles of cell motility, the direction of cell movement and cancer invasion, *Nature*, 208, 1183–1187 (1965).

Chan W.C.W. and S. Nie, Quantum dot bioconjugates for ultrasensitive nonisotopic detection, *Science*, 281, 2016–2018 (1998).

Chen S., J. Zheng, L. Li and S. Jiang, Strong resistance of phosphorylcholine self-assembled monolayers to protein adsorption: Insights into nonfouling properties of zwitterionic materials, *J. Am. Chem. Soc.*, 127, 14473–14478 (2005).

Chiari M., M. Cretich, A. Corti, F. Damin, G. Pirri and R. Longhi, Peptide microarrays for the characterization of antigenic regions of human chromogranin A, *Proteomics*, 5, 3600–3603 (2005).

Choy K., Chemical vapour deposition of coatings, *Prog. Mater. Sci.*, 48, 57–110 (2003).

Cohen S.M.A., W.T.S. Huck, J. Genzer, M. Muller, C. Ober, G.B. Stamm, M. Sukhirukov, I. Szleifer, V.V. Tsukruk, M. Urban, F. Winnik, S. Zauscher, I. Luzinov and S. Minko, Emerging applications of stimuli-responsive polymer materials, *Nat. Mater.*, 9, 101–113 (2010).

Cretich M., F. Damin and M. Chiari, Protein microarray technology: How far off is routine diagnostics?, *Analyst*, 139(3), 528–542 (2014).

Cretich M., G. Pirri, F. Damin, I. Solinas and M. Chiari, A new polymeric coating for protein microarrays, *Anal. Biochem.*, 332, 67–74 (2004).

Cretich M., G. Di Carlo, R. Longhi, C. Gotti, N. Spinella, S. Coffa, C. Galati, L. Renna and M. Chiari, High sensitivity protein assays on microarray silicon *slides*, *Anal. Chem.*, 81, 5197–5203 (2009b).

Cretich M., V. Sedini, F. Damin, G. Di Carlo, C. Oldani and M. Chiari, Protein and peptide arrays: Recent trends and new directions, *Sens. Actuator B*, 132, 258–264 (2008).

Cretich M., V. Sedini, F. Damin, M. Pelliccia, L. Sola and M. Chiari, Coating of nitrocellulose for colorimetric DNA microarrays, *Anal. Biochem.*, 397, 84–88 (2009a).

Crowther J.R., *ELISA: Theory and Practice*, Humana, New Jersey (1995).

Crumbliss A.L., S.C. Perine, J. Stonehuerner, K.R. Tubergen, J. Zhao and R.W. Henkens, Colloidal gold as a biocompatible immobilization matrix suitable for the fabrication of enzyme electrodes by electrodeposition, *Biotechnol. Bioeng.*, 40, 483 (1992).

Dabbousi B.O., J. Rodriguez-Viejo, F.V. Mikulec, J.R. Heine, H. Mattoussi, R. Ober, K.F. Jensen and M.G. Bawendi, (CdSe)ZnS core–shell quantum dots: Synthesis and characterization of a size series of highly luminescent nanocrystallites, *J. Phys. Chem. B*, 101, 9463–9475 (1997).

Daniel M.C. and D. Astruc, Gold nanoparticles: Assembly, supramolecular chemistry, quantum size-related properties, and applications toward biology, catalysis, and nanotechnology, *Chem. Rev.*, 104(1), 293–346 (2004).

Darbandi M., R. Thomann and T. Nann, Single quantum dots in silica spheres by microemulsion synthesis, *Chem. Mater.*, 17, 5720–5725 (2005).

Decher G., *Multilayer Thin Films. Sequential Assembly of Nanocomposite Materials*, Wiley-VCH, Weinheim (2002).

Del Campo A. and I.J. Bruce, Substrate patterning and activation strategies for DNA chip fabrication, *Top. Curr. Chem.*, 260, 77–111 (2005).

Dequaire M., C. Degrand and B. Limoges, An electrochemical metalloimmunoassay based on a colloidal gold label, *Anal. Chem.*, 72, 5521 (2000).

De Saizieu A., U. Certa, J. Warrington, C. Gray, W. Keck and J. Mous, Bacterial transcript imaging by hybridization of total RNA to oligonucleotide arrays, *Nat. Biotechnol.*, 16, 45–48 (1998).

Dilly S.J., M.P. Beecham, S.P. Brown, J.M. Griffin, A.J. Clark, C.D. Griffin, J. Marshall, R.M. Napier, P.C. Taylor and A. Marsh, Novel tertiary amine oxide surfaces that resist nonspecific protein adsorption, *Langmuir*, 22, 8144–8150 (2006).

Dou Y.H., N. Bao and J.J. Xu, Separation of proteins on surface modified poly(dimethylsiloxane) microfluidic devices, *Electrophoresis*, 25, 3024–3031 (2004).

Draper J., I. Luzinov, S. Minko, I. Tokarev and M. Stamm, Mixed polymer brushes by sequential polymer addition: Anchoring layer effect, *Langmuir*, 20, 4064–4075 (2004).

Dubertret B., P. Skourides, D.J. Norris, V. Noireaux, A.H. Brivanlou and A. Libchaber, In vivo imaging of quantum dots encapsulated in phospholipid micelles, *Science*, 298, 1759–1762 (2002).

Efimenko K., W.E. Wallace and J. Genzer, Surface modification of sylgard poly(dimethylsiloxane) network by ultraviolet and ultraviolet/ozone treatment, *J. Colloid Interface Sci.*, 254, 306–315 (2002).

Efros A.L. and M. Rosen, The electronic structure of semiconductor nanocrystals, *Annu. Rev. Mater. Sci.*, 30, 475–521 (2000).

Finetti C., M. Colombo, D. Prosperi, G. Alessio, C. Morasso, L. Sola and M. Chiari, One-pot phase transfer and surface modification of CdSe-ZnS quantum dots using a synthetic functional copolymer, *Chem. Comm.*, 50, 240–242 (2014).

Fink J., C.J. Kielv, D. Bethel and D.J. Schiffrin, Self-organization of nanosized gold particles, *Chem. Mater.*, 10, 922–926 (1998).

Fleer G.J., S.M.A. Cohen, J.M.H.M. Scheutjens, T. Cosgrove and B. Vincent, *Polymers at Interfaces*, Chapman & Hall, London (1993).

Freeman R.G., K.C. Grabar, K.J. Allison, R.M. Bright, J.A. Davis, A.P. Guthrie, M.B. Hommer, M.A. Jackson, P.C. Smith and D.G. Walter, Self-assembled metal colloid monolayers: An approach to SERS substrates, *Science*, 267, 1629–1632 (1995).

Fung E.T., *Protein Arrays: Methods and Protocols, Method. Mol. Cell. Biol.*, Humana Press Totowa, NJ, 264 (2004).

Gagni P., L. Sola, M. Cretich and M. Chiari, Development of a high-sensitivity immunoassay for amyloid-beta 1-42 using a silicon microarray platform, *Biosens. Bioelectron.*, 47, 490–495 (2013).

Gao X. and S. Nie, Doping mesoporous materials with multicolor quantum dots, *J. Phys. Chem. B*, 107, 11575–11578 (2003).

Garcia C.D., B.M. Dressen and A. Henderson, Comparison of surfactants for dynamic surface modification of poly(dimethylsiloxane) microchips, *Electrophoresis*, 26, 703–709 (2005).

Gerion D., F.Q. Chen, B. Kannan, A.H. Fu, W.J. Parak, D.J. Chen, A. Majumdar and A.P. Alivisatos, Room-temperature single-nucleotide polymorphism and multiallele DNA detection using fluorescent nanocrystals and microarrays, *Anal. Chem.*, 75, 4766–4772 (2003).

Gerion D., W.J. Parak, S.C. Williams, D. Zanchet, C.M. Micheel and A.P. Alivisatos, Sorting Fluorescent Nanocrystals with DNA, *J. Am. Chem. Soc.*, 124, 7070–7074 (2002).

Gervais L., N. de Rooij and E. Delamarche, Microfluidics chips for point-of-care immuno-diagnostics, *Adv. Mater.*, 23, 151–176 (2011).

Goldman E.R., A.R. Clapp, G.P. Anderson, H.T. Uyeda, J.M. Mauro, I.L. Medintz and H. Mattoussi, Multiplexed toxin analysis using four colors of quantum dot fluororeagents, *Anal. Chem.*, 76, 684–688 (2004).

Grest G.S., Computer simulations of shear and friction between polymer brushes, *Curr. Opin. Colloid Interface Sci.*, 2, 271–277 (1997).

Groll J., E.V. Amirgoulova, T. Ameringer, C.D. Heyes, C. Röcker, G.U. Nienhaus and M. Möller, Biofunctionalized, ultrathin coatings of cross-linked star-shaped poly(ethylene oxide) allow reversible folding of immobilized proteins, *J. Am. Chem. Soc.*, 126, 4234–4239 (2004).

Guschin D., G. Yershov, A. Zaslavsky, A. Gemmel, V. Shick, D. Proudnikov, P. Arenkov and A.D. Mirzabekov, Manual manufacturing of oligonucleotide, DNA, and protein microchips, *Anal. Biochem.*, 250, 203–211 (1997).

Gygi S.P., Y. Rochon, B.R. Franza and R. Aebersold, Correlation between protein and mRNA abundance in yeast, *Mol. Cell. Biol.*, 19, 1720–1730 (1999).

Halperin A., M. Tirrell and T.P. Lodge, Tethered chains in polymer microstructures, *Adv. Polym. Sci.*, 100, 31 (1992).

Han M., X. Gao, J.Z. Su and S. Nie, Quantum-dot-tagged microbeads for multiplexed optical coding of biomolecules, *Nat. Biotechnol.*, 19, 631–635 (2001).

Hashimoto K., T. Fujisawa, M. Kobayashi and R. Yosomiya, Graft copolymerization of glass fiber and its application, *J. Macromol. Sci. Pure*, A18, 173–190 (1982).

Hayashi G., M. Hagihara, C. Dohno and K. Nakatani, Photoregulation of a peptide–RNA interaction on a gold surface, *J. Am. Chem. Soc.*, 129, 8678 (2007).

He F., Y. Tang, S. Wang, Y. Li and D. Zhu, Fluorescent amplifying recognition for DNA G-quadruplex folding with a cationic conjugated polymer: A platform for homogeneous potassium detection, *J. Am. Chem. Soc.*, 127, 12343–12346 (2005).

Hlady V. and J. Buijs, Protein adsorption on solid surfaces, *Curr. Opin. Biotechnol.*, 7, 72–77 (1996).

Hoffmann J., J. Groll, J. Heuts, H. Rong, D. Klee, G. Ziemer, M. Möller and H.P. Wendel, Blood cell and plasma protein repellent properties of Star-PEG-modified surfaces, *J. Biomater. Sci. Polym. Ed.*, 17, 985–996 (2006).

Holloway A.J., R.K. van Laar, R.W. Tothill and D.D. Bowtell, Options available—From start to finish—For obtaining data from DNA microarrays, *Nat. Genet.*, 32, 481–489 (2002).

Homola J., Surface plasmon resonance sensors for detection of chemical and biological species, *Chem. Rev.*, 108(2), 462–493 (2008).

Hyeon T., S.S. Lee, J. Park, Y. Chung and H.B. Na, Synthesis of highly crystalline and monodisperse maghemite nanocrystallites without a size-selection process, *J. Am. Chem. Soc.*, 123, 12798–12801 (2001).

Jiang W., S. Mardyani, H. Fischer and W.C.W. Chan, Design and characterization of lysine cross-linked mercapto-acid biocompatible quantum dots, *Chem. Mater.*, 18, 872 (2006).

Jones R.A.L. and R.W. Richards, *Polymers at Surfaces and Interfaces*, Cambridge University Press, Cambridge (1999).

Kaiser W. and U. Rant, Conformations of end-tethered DNA molecules on gold surfaces: Influences of applied electric potential, electrolyte screening, and temperature, *J. Am. Chem. Soc.*, 132, 7935–7945 (2010).

Kambhampati D., *Protein Microarray Technology*, Wiley-VCH, Weinheim (2003).

Kambhampati D., P.E. Nielsen and W. Knoll, Investigating the kinetics of DNA–DNA and PNA–DNA interactions using surface plasmon resonance-enhanced fluorescence spectroscopy, *Biosens. Bioelectron.*, 16, 1109–1118 (2001).

Kane R.S., P. Deschatelets and G.M. Whitesides, Kosmotropes form the basis of protein-resistant surfaces, *Langmuir*, 19, 2388–2391 (2003).

Kang Y. and T.A. Taton, Core-shell gold nanoparticles via self-assembly and crosslinking of micellar, block-copolymer shells, *Angew. Chem. Int. Ed.*, 44, 409–412 (2005).

Kaufmann H., J.E. Bailey and M. Fussenegger, Use of antibodies for detection of phosphorylated proteins separated by two-dimensional gel electrophoresis, *Proteomics*, 1, 194–199 (2001).

Kelley S.O., J.K. Barton, N.M. Kackson, L.D. McPherson, A.B. Potter, E.M. Spain, M.J. Allen and M.G. Hill, Orienting DNA helices on gold using applied electric fields, *Langmuir*, 14, 6781–6784 (1998).

Kim S.H., A. Tamrazi, K.E. Carlson and J.A. Katzenellenbogen, A proteomic microarray approach for exploring ligand-initiated nuclear hormone receptor pharmacology, receptor selectivity, and heterodimer functionality, *Mol. Cell. Proteomics*, 4(3), 267–277 (2005).

Kiyonaka S., K. Sada, I. Yoshimura, S. Shinkai, N. Kato and I. Hamachi, Semi-wet peptide/protein array using supramolecular hydrogel, *Nat. Mater.*, 3, 58–64 (2004).

Klein J., Y. Kamiyama, H. Yoshizawa, J.N. Israelachvili, G.H. Fredrickson, P. Pincus and L.J. Fetters, Lubrication forces between surfaces bearing polymer brushes, *Macromolecules*, 26, 5552–5560 (1993).

Klein J., E. Kumacheva, D. Mahalu, D. Perahia and L.J. Fetters, Reduction of frictional forces between solid surfaces bearing polymer brushes, *Nature*, 370, 634–636 (1994).

Kneipp K., Y. Wang, H. Kneipp, L.T. Perelman, I. Itzkan, R. Dasari and M.S. Feld, Single molecule detection using surface enhanced Raman scattering (SERS), *Phys. Rev. Lett.*, 78(9), 1667–1670 (1997).

Knoll W., M. Zizlsperger, T. Liebermann, S. Arnold, A. Badia, M. Liley, D. Piscevic, F.J. Schmitt, J. Spinke and M. Zizlsperger, Streptavidin arrays as supramolecular architectures in surface-plasmon optical sensor formats, *Colloids Surf. A*, 161, 115–137 (2000).

Ko K.S., F.A. Jaipuri and N.L. Pohl, Fluorous-based carbohydrate microarrays, *J. Am. Chem. Soc.*, 127, 13162–13163 (2005).

Kolasinska M., R. Krastev and T. Gutberlet, Layer by layer deposition of polyelectrolytes. Dipping versus spraying, *Langmuir*, 25(2), 1224–1232 (2009).

Kovarik M.L., D.M. Ornoff, A.T. Melvin, N.C. Dobes, Y. Wang, A.J. Dickinson, P.C. Gach, P.K. Shah and N.L. Allbritton, Micro total analysis system: Fundamental advances in applications in the laboratory, clinic, and field, *Anal. Chem.*, 82, 451–472 (2013).

Krug J.T., G.D. Wang, S.R. Emory and S.M. Nie, Efficient Raman enhancement and intermittent light emission observed in single gold nanocrystals, *J. Am. Chem. Soc.*, 121(39), 9208–9214 (1999).

Kushida A., M. Yamato, C. Konno, A. Kikuchi, Y. Sakurai and T. Okano, Decrease in culture temperature releases monolayer endothelial cell sheets together with deposited fibronectin matrix from temperature-responsive culture surfaces, *J. Biomed. Mater. Res.*, 45, 355 (1999).

Lashkari D.A., J.L. DeRisi, J.H. McCusker, A.F. Namath, C. Gentile, S.Y. Hwang, P.O. Brown and R.W. Davis, Yeast microarrays for genome wide parallel genetic and gene expression analysis, *Proc. Natl. Acad. Sci. U.S.A.*, 94, 13057–13062 (1997).

Le Berre V., E. Trevisiol, A. Dagkessamanskaia, A.M. Caminade, J.P. Majoral, B. Meunier and J. François, Dendrimeric coating of glass slides for sensitive DNA microarrays analysis, *Nucleic Acids Res.*, 31, 88 (2003).

Lee H.J., Y. Yan, G. Marriott and R.M. Corn, Quantitative functional analysis of protein complexes on surfaces, *J. Physiol.*, 563, 61–71 (2005).

Lemeer S., R. Ruijtenbeek, M.W.H. Pinkse, C. Jopling, A.J.R. Heck, J. den Hertog and M. Slijper, Endogenous phosphotyrosine signaling in zebrafish embryos, *Mol. Cell. Proteomics*, 6, 2088–2099 (2007).

Li Y., Y. Wang, C. Jia, Y. Ma, Y. Lan and S. Wang, Detection of human papillomavirus genotypes with liquid bead microarray in cervical lesions of northern Chinese patients, *Cancer Genet. Cytogen.*, 182, 12–17 (2008).

Lin C.A.J., R.A. Sperling, J.K. Li, T.Y. Yang, P.Y. Li, M. Zanella, W.H. Chang and W.G.J. Parak, Design of an amphiphilic polymer for nanoparticle coating and functionalization, *Small*, 4, 334–341 (2008).

Lipshutz R.J., S.P. Fodor, T.R. Gingeras and D.J. Lockhart, High density synthetic oligonucleotide arrays, *Nat. Genet.*, 21, 20–24 (1999).

Liu D., A. Bruckbauer, C. Abell, S. Balasubramanian, D.J. Kang, D. Klenerman and D. Zhou, A reversible pH-driven DNA nanoswitch array, *J. Am. Chem. Soc.*, 128, 2067–2071 (2006).

Liu T., J. Zhong, X. Gan, C. Fan, G. Li and N. Matsuda, Wiring electrons of cytochrome c with silver nanoparticles in layered films, *Chemphyschem*, 4, 1364 (2003).

Liu Y., W. Wang, W. Hu, Z. Lu, X. Zhou and C.M. Li, Highly sensitive poly[glycidyl mathacrylate-co-poly(ethylene glycol) methacrylate] brush-based flow-through microarray immunoassay device, *Biomed Microdevices*, 13(4), 769–777 (2011).

Luccardini C., C. Tribet, F. Vial, V. Marchi-Artzner and M. Dahan, Size, Charge, and interactions with giant lipid vesicles of quantum dots coated with an amphiphilic macromolecule, *Langmuir*, 22, 2304–2310 (2006).

Luk Y.Y., M. Kato and M. Mrksich, Self-assembled monolayers of alkanethiolates presenting mannitol groups are inert to protein adsorption and cell attachment, *Langmuir*, 16, 9604–9608 (2000).

MacBeth G., A.N. Koehler and S.L. Schreiber, Printing small-molecules as microarrays and detecting protein-ligand interactions en masse, *J. Am. Chem. Soc.*, 121, 7967–7968 (1999).

Makamba H., J.H. Klm, K. Lim, N. Park and J. Hahn, Surface modification of poly(dimethylsiloxane) microchannels, *Electrophoresis*, 24, 3607–3619 (2003).

Manna L., E.C. Scher and A.P. Alivisatos, Synthesis of soluble and processable rod-, arrow-, teardrop- and tetrapod-shaped CdSe nanocrystals, *J. Am. Chem. Soc.*, 122, 12700–12706 (2000).

Manz A., N. Graber and H.M. Widmer, Miniaturized total chemical analysis systems: A novel concept for chemical sensing, *Sens. Actuators, B-Chem.*, 1, 244–248 (1990).

Mathauer K., F. Embs and G. Wegner, *Comprehensive Polymer Science*, vol. 1, Pergamon Press, Oxford, 449 (1992).

Matsui J., K. Akamatsu, N. Hara, D. Miyoshi, H. Nawafune, K. Tamaki and N. Sugimoto, SPR sensor chip for detection of small molecules using molecularly imprinted polymer with embedded gold nanoparticles, *Anal. Chem.*, 77(13), 4282–4285 (2005).

Mattoussi H., M.J. Mauro, E.R. Goldman, G.P. Anderson, V.C. Sundar, F.V. Mikulec and M.G. Bawendi, Self-assembly of CdSe-ZnS quantum dot bioconjugates using an engineered recombinant protein, *J. Am. Chem. Soc.*, 122, 12142–12150 (2000).

Mendelsohn J.D., S.Y. Yang, J.A. Hiller, A.I. Hochbaum and M.F. Rubner, Rational design of cytophilic and cytophobic polyelectrolyte multilayer thin films, *Biomacromolecules*, 4, 96–106 (2003).

Mendes P.M., Stimuli responsive surfaces for bio-applications, *Chem. Soc. Rev.*, 37, 2512–2529 (2008).

Mendes P.M., K.L. Christman, P. Pathassarathy, E. Schopf, J. Ouyang, Y. Yang, J.A. Preece, H.D. Mayanard, Y. Chen and J.F. Stoddart, Electrochemically controllable conjugation of proteins on surfaces, *Bioconjug. Chem.*, 18, 1919 (2007).

Meng F., Y. Liu, L. Liu and G. Li, Conformational transitions of immobilized DNA chains driven by pH with electrochemical output, *J. Phys. Chem. B*, 113, 894–896 (2009).

Michel R., S. Pasche, M. Textor and D.G. Castner, Influence of PEG architecture on protein adsorption and conformation, *Langmuir*, 21, 12327–12332 (2005).

Molloy M.P., N.D. Phadke, H. Chen, R. Tyldesley, D.E. Garfin, J.R. Maddock and P.C. Andrews, Profiling the alkaline membrane proteome of *Caulobacter crescentus* with two-dimensional electrophoresis and mass spectrometry, *Proteomics*, 2, 899–910 (2002).

Morales-Narvaez E., H. Monton, A. Fomicheva and A. Merkoci, Signal enhancement in antibody microarrays using quantum dots nanocrystals: Application to potential Alzheimer's disease biomarker screening, *Anal. Chem.*, 84, 6821–6827 (2012).

Morasso C., D. Mehn, R. Vanna, M. Bedoni, C.P. García, D. Prosperi, F. Gramatica, A. Campion and P. Kambhampati, Star-like gold nanoparticles as highly active substrate for surface enhanced Raman spectroscopy. Surface-enhanced Raman scattering, *Chem. Soc. Rev.*, 27(4), 241–250 (1998).

Moriarty P., Nanostructured materials, *Rep. Prog. Phys.*, 64, 297–381 (2001).

Mrksich M., G.B. Sigal and G.M. Whitesides, Surface Plasmon Resonance permits in situ measurement of protein adsorption on self-assembled monolayers of alkanethiolates on gold, *Langmuir*, 11, 4383–4385 (1995).

Nann T., Phase-transfer of CdSe@Zns quantum dots using amphiphilic hyperbranched poly-ethylenimine, *Chem. Commun.*, 13, 1735–1736 (2005).

Nath N., J. Hyun, H. Ma and A. Chilkoti, Surface engineering strategies for control of protein and cell interactions, *Surf. Sci.*, 570, 98–110 (2004).

Nichkova M., D. Dosev, A.E. Davies, S.J. Gee, I.M. Kennedy and B.D. Hammock, Quantum dots as reporters in multiplexed immunoassays for biomarkers of exposure to agrochem-icals, *Anal. Lett.*, 40, 1423–1433 (2007).

Nida D.L., N. Nitin, W.W. Yu, V.L. Colvin and R. Richards-Kortum, Photostability of quan-tum dots with amphiphilic polymer-based passivation strategies, *Nanotechnology*, 23, 035701 (2008).

Nie S.M. and S.R. Emery, Probing single molecules and single nanoparticles by surface-enhanced Raman scattering, *Science*, 275(5303), 1102–1106 (1997).

Njoki P.N., I.I.S. Lim, D. Mott, H.Y. Park, B. Khan, S. Mishra, R. Sujakumar, J. Luo and C.J. Zhong, Size correlation of optical and spectroscopic properties for gold nanoparticles, *J. Phys. Chem. C*, 111(40), 14664–14669 (2007).

Ostuni E., R.G. Chapman, R.E. Holmlin, S. Takayama and G.M. Whitesides, A survey of structure—Property relationship of surfaces that resist the adsorption of protein, *Langmuir*, 17, 5605–5620 (2001).

Park J., J. Joo, S.G. Kwon, Y. Jang and T. Hyeon, Synthesis of monodisperse spherical nano-crystals, *Angew. Chem. Int. Ed.*, 46, 4630–4660 (2007).

Pathak S., A.K. Singh, J.R. McElhanon and P.M. Dentinger, Dendrimer-activated surfaces for high density and high activity protein chip applications, *Langmuir*, 20, 6075–6079 (2004).

Patton W.F., Proteome analysis. II. Protein subcellular redistribution: Linking physiology to genomics via the proteome and separation technologies involved, *J. Chromatogr. B*, 722, 203–223 (1999).

Pellegrino T., L. Manna, S. Kudera, T. Liedl, D. Koktysh, A.L. Rogach, S. Keller, J. Radler, G. Natile and W.J. Parak, Hydrophobic nanocrystals coated with an amphiphilic polymer shell: A general route to water soluble nanocrystals, *Nano Lett.*, 4, 703–707 (2004).

Peng Z.A. and X.G. Peng, Mechanisms of the shape evolution of CdSe nanocrystals, *J. Am. Chem. Soc.*, 123, 1389–1395 (2001).

Piehler J., A. Brecht, K.E. Geckeler and G. Gauglitz, Surface modification for direct immuno-probes *Biosens. Bioelectron.*, 11, 579–590 (1996).

Piletsky S., E. Piletska, A. Bossi, N. Turner and A. Turner, Surface functionalization of porous polypropylene membranes with polyaniline for protein immobilization, *Biotechnol. Bioeng.*, 82, 86–92 (2003).

Pirri G., M. Chiari, F. Damin and A. Meo, Microarray glass slides coated with block copolymer brushes obtained by reversible addition chain-transfer polymerization, *Anal. Chem.*, 78, 3118–3124 (2006).

Pirri G., F. Damin, M. Chiari, E. Bontempi and L.E. Depero, Characterization of a polymeric adsorbed coating for DNA microarray glass slides, *Anal. Chem.*, 76, 1352–1358 (2004).

Pirrung M.C., How to make a DNA chip, *Angew. Chem. Int. Ed.*, 41, 1276–1289 (2002).

Platt G.W., F. Damin, M.J. Swann, I. Metton, G. Skorski, M. Cretich and M. Chiari, Allergen immobilization and signal amplification by quantum dots for use in a biosensor assay of IgE in serum, *Biosens. Bioelectron.*, 52, 82–88 (2014).

Ponten J. and L. Stolt, Proliferation control in cloned normal and malignant human cells, *Exp. Cell Res.*, 129, 367–375 (1980).

Potapova I., R. Mruk, S. Prehl, R. Zentel, T. Basché and A. Mews, Semiconductor nanocrystals with multifunctional polymer ligands, *J. Am. Chem. Soc.*, 125, 320–321 (2003).

Prime K.L. and G.M. Whitesides, Adsorption of proteins onto surfaces containing end-attached oligo(ethylene oxide): A model system using self-assembled monolayers, *J. Am. Chem. Soc.*, 115, 10714–10721 (1993).

Prucker O. and J. Rühe, Synthesis of poly(styrene) monolayers attached to high surface area silica gels through self-assembled monolayers of azo initiators, *Macromolecules*, 31, 592–601 (1998a).

Prucker O. and J. Rühe, Mechanism of radical chain polymerizations initiated by azo compounds covalently bound tot he surface of spherical particles, *Macromolecules*, 31, 602–613 (1998b).

Raj C.R., T. Okajima and T. Ohsaka, Gold nanoparticle arrays for the voltammetric sensing of dopamine, *J. Electroanal. Chem.*, 543, 127 (2003).

Rant U., K. Arinaga, S. Fujita, N. Yokoyama, G. Abstreiter and M. Tornow, Dynamic electrical switching of DNA layers on a metal surface, *Nano Lett.*, 4, 2441–2445 (2004).

Rant U., K. Arinaga, S. Scherer, E. Pringsheim, S. Fujita, N. Yokoyama, M. Tornow and G. Abstreiter, Switchable DNA interfaces for highly sensitive detection of label-free DNA targets, *Proc. Natl. Acad. Sci. U.S.A.*, 104, 17364 (2007).

Ratner B.D., A.S. Hoffmann, F.J. Schoen and J.E. Lemons, *Biomaterials Science, An Introduction to Materials in Medicine*, Academic Press, San Diego, CA (1996).

Resch-Genger U., M. Grabolle, S. Cavaliere-Jaricot, R. Nitschke and T. Nann, Quantum dots versus organic dyes as fluorescent labels, *Nat. Methods*, 5, 763–775 (2008).

Rodriguez L.L., P.R.A. Alvarez, F.J.G. de Abajo and M.L.M. Liz, Surface enhanced Raman scattering using star-shaped gold colloidal nanoparticles, *J. Phys. Chem. C*, 114(16), 7336–7340 (2010).

Rogach A.L., D.V. Talapin and H. Weller, Semiconductor nanoparticles. In *Colloids and Colloid Assemblies*, Caruso, F. Ed., Wiley-VCH, Weinheim, 52–95 (2004).

Roy D., J.N. Cambre and B.S. Sumerlin, Future perspectives and recent advances in stimuli-responsive materials, *Prog. Polym. Sci.*, 35, 278–301 (2010).

Rühe J. and W.J. Knoll, Functional polymer brushes, *Macromol. Sci. Rev.*, C42, 91–138 (2002).

Rühe J., V. Novotny, T. Clarke and G.B. Street, Friction and durability characteristics of ultrathin perfluoropolyether lubricant film composed of bonded and mobile molecular layers on diamond-like carbon surfaces, *J. Tribol.-Trans. ASME*, 118, 663 (1996).

Sackmann E.K., A.L. Fulton and D.J. Beebe, The present and future role of microfluidics in biomedical research, *Nature*, 507, 181–189 (2014).

Sagiv J., Organized monolayers by adsorption. I. Formation and structure of oleophobic mixed monolayers on solid surfaces, *J. Am. Chem. Soc.*, 102, 92–98 (1980).

Samuel J.D., T. Brenner, O. Prucker, M. Grumann, J. Ducree, R. Zengerle and J. Ruhe, Tailormade microfluidic devices through photochemical surface modification, *Macromol. Chem. Phys.*, 211, 195–203 (2010).

Santoni V., S. Kieffer, D. Desclaux, F. Masson and T. Rabilloud, Membrane proteomics: Use of additive main effects with multiplicative interaction model to classify plasma membrane proteins according to their solubility and electrophoretic properties, *Electrophoresis*, 21, 3329–3344 (2000).

Sapsford K.E., T. Pons, I.L. Medintz and H. Mattoussi, Biosensing with luminescent semiconductor quantum dots, *Sensors*, 6, 925–953 (2006).

Sapsford K.E., S. Spindel, T. Jennings, G. Tao, R.C. Triulzi, W.R. Algar and I.L. Medintz, Optimizing two-color semiconductor nanocrystal immunoassays in single well microtiter plate formats, *Sensors*, 11, 7879–7891 (2011).

Sarioglu H., F. Lottspeich, T. Walk, G. Jung and C. Eckerskorn, Deamidation as a widespread phenomenon in two-dimensional polyacrylamide gel electrophoresis of human blood plasma proteins, *Electrophoresis*, 21, 2209–2218 (2000).

Schabas G., H. Yusuf, M.G. Moffitt and D. Sinton, Controlled self-assembly of quantum dots and block copolymers in a microfluidic device, *Langmuir*, 24, 637–643 (2008).

Schmid G. and A. Lehnert, The complexation of gold colloids, *Angew. Chem. Int. Ed. Engl.*, 28, 780–781 (1989).

Shevchenko E.V., D.V. Talapin, A.L. Rogach, A. Kornowski, M. Haase and H.J. Weller, Colloidal synthesis and self-assembly of CoPt(3) nanocrystals, *J. Am. Chem. Soc.*, 124, 11480–11485 (2002).

Shu W., D. Liu, M. Watari, C.K. Reiner, T. Strunz, M.E. Welland, S. Balasubramanian and R.A. McKendry, DNA molecular motor driven micromechanical cantilever arrays, *J Am Chem Soc*, 127(48), 17054–17060 (2005).

Silberzan P., L. Léger and D. Ausserré, Silation of silica surfaces. A new method of constructing pure or mixed monolayers, *Langmuir*, 7, 1647–1651 (1991).

Smith A.M., H. Duan, M.N. Rhyner, G. Ruan and S. Nie, A Systematic examination of surface coatings on the optical and chemical properties of semiconductor quantum dots, *Phys. Chem.*, 8, 3895–3903 (2006).

Sola L. and M. Chiari, Modulation of electroosmotic flow in capillary electrophoresis using functional polymer coatings, *J. Chromatogr. A*, 1270, 324–329 (2012).

Sperling A., T. Pellegrino, J.K. Li, W.H. Chang and W.J. Parak, Electrophoretic separation of nanoparticles with a discrete number of functional groups, *Adv. Funct. Mater.*, 16, 943–948 (2006).

Spuhler P.S., J. Knežević, A. Yalçin, Q. Bao, E. Pringsheim, P. Dröge, U. Rant and S.M. Ünlü, Platform for in situ real-time measurement of protein-induced conformational changes of DNA, *Proc. Natl. Acad. Sci. U.S.A.*, 107, 1397–1401 (2010).

Spuhler P.S., L. Sola, X. Zhang, M.R. Monroe, J.T. Greenspun, M. Chiari and S.M. Ünlü, Precisely controlled smart polymer scaffold for nanoscale manipulation of biomolecules, *Anal. Chem.*, 84, 10593–10599 (2012).

Stoughton R.B., Applications of DNA microarrays in biology, *Annu. Rev. Biochem.*, 74, 53–82 (2005).

Sugawara T. and T. Matsuda, Photochemical surface derivatization of a peptide containing Arg-Gly-Asp (RGD), *J. Biomed. Mater. Res.*, 29, 1047–1052 (1995).

Sun S. and H.J. Zeng, Size-controlled synthesis of magnetite nanoparticles, *J. Am. Chem. Soc.*, 124, 8204–8205 (2002).

Taniguchi N., A. Ekuni, J.H. Ko, E. Miyoshi, Y. Ikeda, Y. Ihara, A. Nishikawa, K. Honke and M. Takahashi, A glycomic approach tot he identification and characterization of glycoprotein function in cells transfected with glycosyltransferase genes, *Proteomics*, 1, 239–247 (2001).

Tenne R., Advances in the synthesis of inorganic nanotubes and fullerene-like nanoparticles, *Angew. Chem. Int. Ed.*, 42, 5124–5132 (2003).

Thompson L.F., C.G. Willson and M.J. Bowden, *Introduction to Microlithography*, 2nd Ed., American Chemical Society, Washington, DC (1994).

Thube S.A., B.S. Budhwani and M.P. Atif, DNA microarray technology: The future, *J. Pharm. Res.*, 2, 1823–1833 (2009).

Timofeev E.N., A.D. Kochetkova, A.D. Mirzabekov and V.L. Florentiev, Regioselective immobilization of short oligonucleotides to acrylic copolymer gels, *Nucleic Acids Res.*, 24, 3142–3148 (1996).

Tirrell M., E. Kokkoli and M. Biesalski, The role of surface science in bioengineered materials, *Surf. Sci.*, 500, 61–83 (2002).

Tokareva I., S. Minko, J.H. Fendler and E. Hutter, Nanosensors based on responsive polymer brushes and gold nanoparticles enhanced transmission surface plasmon resonance spectroscopy, *J. Am. Chem. Soc.*, 126, 15950–15951 (2004).

Tsubokawa N., A. Kuroda and Y. Sone, Grafting onto carbon black by the reaction of reactive carbon black having epoxide groups with several polymers, *J. Polym. Sci.*, A27, 1701–1712 (1989a).

Tsubokawa N., K. Maruyama, Y. Sone and M. Shimomura, Graft polymerization of acrylamide from ultrafine silica particles by use of a redox system consisting of ceric ion and reducing groups on the surface, *Polym. J.*, 21, 475–481 (1989b).

Ulman A., *An Introduction to Ultrathin Organic Films*, Academic Press, New York (1991).

Vansant E.F., P. Van Der Voort and K.C. Vranken, *Characterization and Chemical Modification of the Silica Surface, Technology and Engineering*, vol. 1, Elsevier Ed. Oxford, UK (1995).

Vargo T.G., E.J. Bekos, Y.S. Kim, J.P. Ranieri, R. Bellamkonda, P. Aebischer, D.E. Margevich, P.M. Thompson, F.V. Bright and J.A. Gardella Jr., Synthesis and characterization of fluoropolymeric substrata with immobilized minimal peptide sequences for cell adhesion studies. I, *J. Biomed. Mater. Res.*, 29, 767–778 (1995).

Wang A.J., J.J. Xu and H.Y. Chen Proteins modifications of poly(dimethylsiloxane) microfluidic channels for the enhanced microchip electrophoresis, *J. Chrom. A*, 1107, 257–264 (2006).

Wang M., N. Felorzabihi, G. Guerin, J.C. Haley, G.D. Sechloes and M.A. Winnik, Water-soluble CdSe quantum dots passivated by a multidentate diblock copolymer, *Macromolecules*, 40, 6377–6384 (2007).

Wu X., H.J. Liu, J.Q. Liu, K.N. Haley, J.A. Treadway, J.P. Larson, N.F. Ge, F. Peale and M.P. Bruchez, Immunofluorescent labeling of cancer marker Her2 and other cellular targets with semiconductor quantum dots, *Nat. Biotechnol.*, 21, 41–46 (2003).

Xia F., W. Guo, Y. Mao, X. Hou, J. Xue, H. Xia, L. Wang, Y. Song, J. Hang, Q. Ouvang, Y. Wang and L. Jiang, Gating of single synthetic nanopores by proton-driven DNA molecular motors, *J. Am. Chem. Soc.*, 130, 8345–8350 (2008).

Xia Y.N. and G.M. Whitesides, Soft lithography, *Angew. Chem. Int. Ed.*, 37, 551–575 (1998).

Yam C.M., M. Deluge, D. Tang, A. Kumar and C. Cai, Preparation, characterization, resistance to protein adsorption, and specific avidin-biotin binding of poly(amidoamine) dendrimers functionalized with oligo(ethylene glycol) on gold, *J. Colloid Interface Sci.*, 296, 118–130 (2006).

Yang Y., G. Liu, H. Liu, D. Li, C. Fan and D. Liu, An electrochemically actuated reversible DNA switch, *Nano Lett.*, 10, 1393–1397 (2010).

Yoon J.J., Y.S. Nam, J.H. Kim and T.G. Park, Surface immobilization of galactose onto aliphatic biodegradable polymers for hepatocyte culture, *Biotechnol. Bioeng.*, 78, 1–10 (2002).

Yoshikawa C., A. Goto, Y. Tsujii, T. Fukuda, T. Kimura, K. Yamamoto and A. Kishida, Protein repellency of well-defined, concentrated poly(2-hydroxyethyl methacrylate) brushes by the size-exclusion effect, *Macromolecules*, 39, 2284–2290 (2006).

You T., O. Niwa, M. Tomita and S. Hirono, Characterization of platinum nanoparticle-embedded carbon film electrode and its detection of hydrogen peroxide, *Anal. Chem.*, 75, 2080–2085 (2003).

Yu, W.W., E. Chang, J.C. Falkner, J. Zhang, A.M. Al-Somali, C.M. Sayes, J. Johns, R. Drezek and V.L. Colvin, Forming biocompatible and nonaggregated nanocrystals in water using amphiphilic polymers, *J. Am. Chem. Soc.*, 129, 2872–2879 (2007).

Yurke B., A.J. Turberfield, A.P. Mills, F.C. Simmel and J.L. Neumann, A DNA-fuelled molecular machine made of DNA, *Nature*, 406, 605–608 (2000).

Zhou J., A.E. Ellis and N.H. Voelcker, Recent development in PDMS surface modification for microfluidic devices, *Electrophoresis*, 31, 2–16 (2010).

Zhu H. and M. Snyder, Protein chip technology, *Curr. Opinion Chem. Biol.*, 7, 55–63 (2003).

Zhu Q., M. Uttamchandani, D. Li, M.L. Lesaicherre and S.Q. Yao, Enzymatic profiling system in a small-molecule microarray, *Organic Lett.*, 5, 1257–1260 (2003).

Zhuo Y., R. Yuan, Y.Q. Chai, D.P. Tang, Y. Zhang, N. Wang, X.L. Li and Q. Zhu, A reagentless amperometric immunosensor based on gold nanoparticles/thionine/Nafion-membrane-modified gold electrode for determination of a-1-fetoprotein, *Electrochem. Commun.*, 7, 355–360 (2005).

Zilio C., L. Sola, F. Damin, L. Faggioni and M. Chiari, Universal hydrophilic coating of thermoplastic polymers currently used in microfluidics, *Biomed. Microdevices*, 16, 107–114 (2014).

Section IV

Safety of Nanomaterials

15 Nanotoxicity
A Mechanistic Approach

Indarchand Gupta, Swapnil Gaikwad,
Avinash Ingle, Kateryna Kon,
Nelson Duran, and Mahendra Rai

CONTENTS

ABSTRACT

Nanotechnology is developing with fast pace. Many nanotechnology applications are coming forward with several benefits to humans. This is because of the unique characteristics of the nanomaterials. As the number of newer applications increases, the toxicity concerns also increase due to exposure of nanomaterials to human health. As far as exposure to humans are concerned, the nanoparticles enter inside the human body through inhalation, ingestion, and dermal exposure. They tend to get accumulated in the exposed tissue and thereby disturb their homeostasis.

At the cellular level, nanoparticles have been reported to interact with plasma membrane causing disturbance in their normal structure and function. Later on, after getting entry inside the cell, it disrupts the mitochondrial membrane potential, induces reactive oxygen species, and damages the nuclear DNA. Many research groups in the world are trying to explore further these aspects. But the data available till date are insufficient and need more attention. Therefore, toxicity study of nanoparticles is also an important issue to focus on. Taking into consideration the importance of this issue and referring to the available knowledge the present chapter is an effort to discuss mechanism of nanotoxicity in detail.

Keywords: Nanotoxicity, ROS, DNA damage, Mitochondrial damage, Plasma membrane damage

15.1 INTRODUCTION

15.1.1 NANOTECHNOLOGY

Nanoparticles are a type of particles that have characteristically altered properties as compared to their bulk counterpart (Rai et al. 2009). Owing to their electrical, thermal, and mechanical properties, artificially made nanoparticles are highly preferred in order to improve the quality and performance of materials where they are being used (Donaldson et al. 2010; Maynard et al. 2004).

Current trends in nanotechnology have allowed researchers to explore the possible uses of materials at the nanometer level. These materials are increasingly being used for various commercial purposes such as fillers, catalysts, cosmetics, and drug carriers (Nel et al. 2006). Nanobased drug delivery systems can be used to control drug release, reduce drug-related toxicity, and protect drugs from metabolic degradation/ excretion and drug targeting (Das et al. 2010; Mamo et al. 2010; Sharma and Garg 2010; Sutradhar and Amin 2014; Villalonga-Barber et al. 2008; Vyas et al. 2006).

According to the US National Science Foundation, in 2015, the nanotechnology-based product market will be worth more than 1 trillion US dollars. Thus, obviously, the increased use of nanoparticles through a myriad of nanoproducts will sometimes cause unpremeditated exposure to researchers, workers, and consumers (Jiang et al. 2008). In this perspective, many reports that mainly focus on the concerns regarding their potential occupational and public exposure have been published (Gupta et al. 2012; Melo et al. 2014). However, the data presented through all of these studies are unorganized and eventually failed to establish the exact mechanism of all nanoparticles in common. Therefore, through this chapter, we have made an attempt to discuss the recent updates regarding the hazardous effects of various nanoparticles. More importantly, our main focus is to extract and present precise information on the mechanism of toxicity at the cellular level, from various published reports.

15.1.2 NANOTOXICOLOGY

Toxicity is the result of interaction between molecules comprising some form of life and molecules of exogenous chemicals or physical factors (Rozman et al. 2006). It takes account of the effect on whole organisms such as bacteria, animals, or plants, and it includes the study of the effects on organs of an organism or cells as well (Durán et al. 2014). Donaldson et al. (2004) for the first time proposed the term *nanotoxicology* as a branch of nanotechnology dealing with the study of its adverse effects on humans and environment. Despite the recommendations that nanotoxicology will deal with the toxic effects of synthetic nanoparticles, it is also suggested that it should also include the toxic effects of natural nanoparticles present in the atmosphere (Oberdörster 2010; Oberdörster et al. 2005).

As the applications of nanomaterials are increasing in scope and field, reports show an increase in their toxicity, and safety of their use with respect to the human body and the environment remains unclear. Additionally, to date, very little data have been published in this field, and therefore, there is an inadequate understanding of the toxicological properties of various nanomaterials. Nevertheless, most of the published studies have revealed the toxicological aspect of nanomaterials in question, but very few of them discussed the mechanism at the cellular level, underlying the nanomaterial-induced toxicity, that is to say, nanotoxicity (Yan et al. 2013). With the various applications of nanoparticles, nanotoxicity studies are of utmost importance as the scientific community now realizes that measuring their toxicity will help us in the handling of nanoparticles for any of their applications (Sarkar et al. 2014).

15.1.3 Need of Nanotoxicity Study

The continuous growth in the production and application of synthetic nanoparticles in consumer products such as cosmetics (Kessler 2011; Scheringer 2008), agriculture and food (Chen et al. 2014), medicine (Ling and Hyeon 2013), and paints (Al-Kattan et al. 2014) is expected to result in the unintended release of nanoparticles in the environment. This release can then result in various harmful consequences causing threats to humans and the environment. Therefore, as discussed earlier, with the application of nanoparticles, studying the hazards associated with their overuse or release into the surroundings is also important. Although studying such hazards is a great tool to understand the mechanistic aspects of nanotoxicology of new nanomaterials, they are not completely understood (Casals et al. 2012; Fu et al. 2014; Pereira et al. 2013, 2014; Seabra et al. 2014). Henceforth, efforts to know whether nanoparticle properties might explain its toxicity are current areas of research. For that reason, the study of nanotoxicity is of highest importance (Durán et al. 2014; Nel et al. 2006; Rai et al. 2014; Scown et al. 2010), and growing interest to studies in this field is well illustrated by the number of PubMed publications that increased dramatically during the last few years (Figure 15.1).

Nanoparticles are usually categorized on the basis of their sizes, morphology, contents, homogeneity/dispersity, and agglomeration (Tyagi et al. 2011). Although, for each nanoparticle preparation, all of these are important factors, it is also imperative to identify whether all of the nanoparticles are toxic or whether their toxicity depends on any one (or more) of their properties mentioned earlier. Actually, different kinds of nanoparticles such as gold nanoparticles (Connor et al. 2005) and quantum dots (QDs) (Derfus et al. 2004) appear to be nontoxic, while others may have harmful effects especially to humans. These contradicting results are probably a reflection of nanomaterials that are not completely characterized, and now this

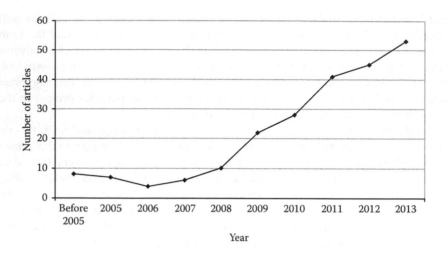

FIGURE 15.1 Dynamics of PubMed publications on nanotoxicology.

important aspect in nanotoxicology is extensively discussed (Coluci et al. 2014; Faria et al. 2012; Martinez et al. 2014; Paula et al. 2014; Stéfani et al. 2011).

Human skin, lungs, and gastrointestinal tract are more prone to the entry of any foreign material and pathogens (Weaver et al. 2013). However, skin is a physical barrier that can efficiently resist the entry of any foreign substance. On the contrary, the lungs and gastrointestinal tracts are not able to match the resistance of skin and, therefore, they are more susceptible. Because of their small sizes, nanoparticles can easily translocate from their entry portal into the circulatory and lymphatic systems, thus reaching the body tissues and organs (Buzea et al. 2007). Some nanoparticles such as multiwalled carbon nanotubes (Glasgow et al. 2014), depending on their composition and size, can cause irreversible damages to cells by oxidative stress and/or organelle injury, thereby affecting the corresponding organ and ultimately the entire body of the exposed organism (Klaper et al. 2014). Despite the fast growth of nanoproducts in the market, latest reports/reviews discuss the hazardous effects of many nanoparticles, most especially silver nanoparticles. Such reviews identified various loopholes concerning toxicokinetics (Christensen et al. 2010; De Lima et al. 2012; Pronk et al. 2009; Sarkar et al. 2014; Stensberg et al. 2011). Similar knowledge gaps were recognized for the probable registration of nanosilver as a material under the EU REACH regulation (Wijnhoven et al. 2009).

The present inadequate knowledge regarding the nanotoxicity to aquatic flora and fauna is attributed to significant gaps in information available for the underlying mechanism. For example, titanium dioxide nanoparticles (TiO_2 NPs) are well known to have photocatalytic properties. Hence, it is suggested that the formation of reactive oxygen species (ROS) (Risom et al. 2005) might involve their toxic action. However, the toxicity studies of TiO_2 NPs on *Daphnia magna* do not correlate their photocatalytic activity with their toxic potential (Hund-Rinke and Simon 2006). This study indicates that a more mechanistic approach is needed to understand the exact mechanism underlying the toxic potential of all types of nanoparticles (Handy et al. 2008a).

15.2 WHAT MAKES NANOPARTICLES TOXIC?

It is well known that nanoparticles have enormous applications in various fields including medicine and pharmacy (Cheraghipour et al. 2013; Knezevic et al. 2013; Xu and Sun 2013). However, there is still little information available about their biocompatibility. It should also be considered that different properties of nanoparticles play an important role in deciding their toxicity. Therefore, when studying any nanoparticle, it is important to assess their activity, size, surface capping, and composition. These are the properties that can contribute a lot to their harmful activity, making them toxic.

15.2.1 Ultrahigh Activity

The ultrahigh reactivity of a nanoparticle depends on its composition and also on its surface coating and charge. According to Meng et al. (2007), the chemical reaction between solid phase and liquid phase always initiates at the surface molecules of the two phases. Therefore, molecules present on the surface of nanoparticles, also called *capping agents*, can directly affect the chemical reactivity of nanoparticles. Furthermore, Meng et al. (2007) also suggested that according to the collision theory, a massive surface area necessarily leads to a higher probability of effective collision, which governs the ultrahigh reactivity during the process of molecular interaction. Therefore, when the particle size decreases to nanolevels, the massive surface area will abruptly increase the rate of chemical reaction. This sudden rise in the speed of the chemical reaction ultimately leads to the higher activity of the material at the nanoscale as compared to the same material at the macroscale. This property will show a similar effect on the toxic action of the nanoparticles.

For example, copper nanoparticles with a diameter 23.5 nm have an average surface area of 2.95×10^5 cm^2/g, whereas copper microparticles with a diameter of 17 μm have a surface area of 3.99×10^2 cm^2/g, which is approximately three orders of magnitudes smaller than the surface area of copper nanoparticles. This ultrahigh activity therefore provokes a hazardous effect, such as metabolic alkalosis and copper ion overload *in vivo* (Meng et al. 2007). However, the mechanism of cellular uptake is imperative in view of various applications of nanoparticles in medicine, cancer diagnosis, and treatment. Still, the precise mechanism of internalization of nanoparticles through endocytosis remains unknown. A study demonstrated the internalization of carboxydextran-coated iron oxide nanoparticles by human mesenchymal stem cells, and the extent of uptake correlated with the amount of carboxyl groups present on the surface of the nanoparticles (Mailander et al. 2008). The cationic D,L-polylactide (PLA)-NPs were reported to enter with larger amounts as compared to anionic PLA-NPs (Dausend et al. 2008; Harush-Frenkel et al. 2007). The uptake of nanoparticles also depends on the thickness of surface coatings (Chang et al. 2006) or the type of cells (Xia et al. 2008).

15.2.2 Size Matters

In any multiphase chemical reaction, the size of reactants plays a key role. As stated in Section 15.2.1, nanoparticle size contributes to their reactivity (Warheit et al. 2007). Many studies have proposed that the smaller the nanoparticles, the higher their reactivity at similar concentrations (Guzman et al. 2012; Raghupathi et al. 2011; Shang et al. 2014; Suttiponparnit et al. 2010). In the same way, it will affect their toxicities at similar concentrations (Oberdörster et al. 2007). Nevertheless, negligible data are available to date depicting the toxic effect of nanoparticle size on biological systems (Handy et al. 2008b).

As for surface coating and charge, the uptake of nanoparticles also depends on their size. This is because the smaller the size, the larger will be the specific surface area that provides them with high chemical reactivity and also intrinsic toxicity (Ada et al. 2010). For example, a study was performed comparing the toxicity of TiO_2 in variable sizes, namely, non-nanosized TiO_2 NP 200 nm in size and nanosized TiO_2 100 nm in size. The study revealed that nanosized TiO_2 had significantly higher acute toxicity approximately twice as that of its bulk counterpart within 96 h exposure (Dabrunz et al. 2011), owing to the fact that 100 nm TiO_2 NP has approximately four times higher surface as compared to 200 nm TiO_2. Likewise, the 25-nm-sized TiO_2 NP has been found to have higher toxicity in terrestrial isopods as compared to 75 nm TiO_2 NP. The similar pattern follows if we go to the smaller TiO_2 nanoparticles (Drobne et al. 2009). Similarly, 1- to 2-nm-sized gold nanoparticles were shown to have elevated toxicity to human and mouse cell line than gold particles 15 nm in diameter (Pan et al. 2007).

A report on size- and coating-dependent toxicity of thoroughly characterized Ag NPs after exposure of human lung cells using coated Ag NPs of different primary particle sizes (10, 40, and 75 nm) as well as 10-nm PVP-coated and 50-nm uncoated Ag NPs was recently published (Gliga et al. 2014). The results showed cytotoxicity only of the 10-nm particles independent of the surface coating. In contrast, all Ag NPs tested caused an increase in overall DNA damage after 24 h (comet assay), indicating an independent mechanism for cytotoxicity and DNA damage. The authors concluded that small Ag NPs (10 nm) are cytotoxic for human lung cells and that the toxicity observed is associated with the rate of intracellular Ag release, a "Trojan horse" effect (Gliga et al. 2014).

Therefore, it is imperative that the smaller particles can attach easily and strongly bind to cell or organism surface, resulting in higher toxicity than particles with bigger size.

15.2.3 Excessive Accumulation

Hitherto, it is a well-established fact that the toxicity of any type of chemical material including pesticides is mainly a function of its exposure dose (Rand and Petrocelli 1985). The same principle also applies to nanomaterials (Ji et al. 2007). For nanomaterials, particle size and particle surface characteristics seem to be less important than that of their concentration in driving the extent of potential toxic effects (Handy et al. 2008b).

Most of the available reports have suggested that the harmful effects of nanoparticles are due to their excessive accumulation (Ji et al. 2007). A main reason for such accumulation includes the excessive usage of nanoparticles and the employment of nanoparticles at concentrations beyond the level they are deemed to be safe. Additionally, the lack of metabolism or degradation of nanoparticles in biological systems also contributes a lot to their accumulation (Braydich-Stolle et al. 2005; Cho et al. 2010; Sanvicens and Marco 2008).

As discussed earlier, nanoparticles have a very high reactivity; therefore, wherever they will be available, they are going to react with the materials or molecules present in their vicinity. Because of the accumulation or aggregation of nanoparticles at certain locations in a biological system, nanoparticles will react with the biomolecules near them. Second, these accumulations will also interfere with the normal metabolism of the cell, tissue, or organ of the concerned plant or animal. This will lead to the complete or partial malfunctioning of the biological system.

15.3 MECHANISM OF NANOTOXICITY

15.3.1 INTERACTION WITH PLASMA MEMBRANE

It is a well-known fact that the plasma membrane encloses the entire cell cytoplasm and thereby keeps the structure intact. It also plays a role in the selective or nonselective transport of different types of molecules. This implies that for any compound to go inside in the cell, it should first interact with its plasma membrane. Therefore, this interaction is of greater importance in keeping the cell under healthy and highly metabolic conditions.

Like any other compounds, nanoparticles also interact with the plasma membrane of a cell to which they are exposed (Leroueil et al. 2007; Verma et al. 2008). They have high reactivity and, therefore, can react with the lipid protein component of the plasma membrane. This interaction can then guide the fate of the concerned cell or the entire tissue or organ where nanoparticles accumulate. These interactions hence alter the cell plasma membrane and will result in the loss of its structure and functions. The loss of its structure will most probably result in its loosening or in the formation of pores at many locations. This will ultimately lead to the leakage of the cell cytoplasm in the surrounding medium (Kim et al. 2009; Napierska et al. 2009), finally resulting in cell death. As assessed by enzyme leakage assay, it was revealed that nanoparticles affect membrane integrity. In one study involving the mechanism of TiO_2 nanoparticles, the ultrathin cross section of the plasma membrane shows the presence of those nanoparticles inside the head and the plasma membrane of buffalo spermatozoa (Pawar and Kaul 2012). Despite direct diffusion though the plasma membrane, nanoparticles can also enter the cell via endocytosis. Endocytosis is the conserved process by which materials, present extracellularly, can be transferred inside the cell with the help of vesicles formed through invagination of the plasma membrane (Conner and Schmid 2003).

The uptake of nanoparticles involves many routes such as phagocytosis, macropinocytosis, clathrin-mediated endocytosis, caveolae-dependent endocytosis, and clathrin/caveolae-independent endocytosis through which nanoparticles can be internalized by cells (Geiser et al. 2005; Paull et al. 2003). Pinocytosis involves macropinocytosis encompassing uptake of particles bigger than 1 μm. Other methods of uptake, as mentioned earlier, are clathrin/caveolae-mediated endocytosis and clathrin/caveolae-independent endocytosis. Caveolae involves 50- to 80-nm-sized invagination of plasma membrane containing cholesterol and sphingolipids, receptors, and caveolins (Lajoie and Nabi 2007; Pelkmans et al. 2002). Endocytosis of various membrane receptors might also involve lipid rafts (Nichols 2003). They provide a platform for the assembly of receptors, adaptors, regulators, and other downstream proteins or signaling complexes and may be joined with caveolae. Clathrin-coated pits (100–200 nm) have been found to be associated with the key protein clathrin and other scaffold proteins such as AP-2 and eps15 (Ehrlich et al. 2004). Macropinocytosis, on the other hand, is a form of endocytosis associated with cell surface ruffling and offers a route for nonselective endocytosis of solute macromolecules. Macropinosomes are between 0.2 and 5 μm in diameter (Swanson and Watts 1995). It is possible that NPs may be taken up by cells via their size selectivity that may match those of endocytic pits.

On a similar pathway, Xu et al. (2009) had made an attempt to find the interaction of TiO_2 nanoparticles and fullerene with the plasma membrane. The study revealed that the lipid raft–disrupting agent Nystatin, which has the property to bind with cholesterol present in cell membranes, disturbs the formation and trafficking of caveolae. Through such observation, this study showed that the endocytosis of the plasma membrane modified the mutagenic response to nanoparticle exposure (Stuart and Brown 2006). Assuming that C60 is lipophilic, it is likely that C60 might interact with lipids present in the plasma membrane and causes toxic effects directly in the absence of cellular uptake (Oberdörster 2004). It is also possible that C60 could interact with cell membrane receptors to trigger or alter intracellular signal transduction pathways. Because of the high energetic adhesive forces close to the surface, nanoparticles are easily agglomerated to form larger particles. Thus, whether single particles or agglomerates are important in the genotoxicity of nanoparticles has not been identified yet.

QDs possess photoemission ability and photostability. Therefore, they have vast applications in the field of biological sciences. Like other nanoparticles, they have also been shown to have toxic properties attributed to their overuse. A study elaborated the mechanism of toxic action of QDs containing cadmium/selenide core with a zinc sulfide shell. The study proposed that lipid rafts of a cell membrane instead of clathrin or caveolae recognize carboxylic coatings of QDs. Later, QDs become internalized into early endosomes and then transferred to late endosomes or lysosomes. The endocytosis of QDs is found to be primarily regulated by a G-protein-coupled receptor–associated pathway and a low-density lipoprotein receptor/scavenger receptor. It is also expected that endocytosis-interfering agents might also play a role but with limited inhibitory effect (Zhang and Monteiro-Riviere 2009).

15.3.2 INTERACTION WITH MITOCHONDRIAL MEMBRANE

Many nanoparticles readily travel throughout the body, are deposited in target organs, enter the cell by penetrating the cell membranes, interact with mitochondria, and thus generate adverse responses.

During normal cell metabolism, especially in the mitochondrion, ROS are generated at a lower level. These ROS are certainly neutralized by antioxidant defenses such as glutathione (GSH) and other antioxidant enzymes (Halliwell and Gutteridge 1999). However, in the state of excessive generation of ROS, the natural antioxidant defenses may be overwhelmed, resulting in the oxidative stress where GSH remains to be depleted and oxidized GSH (GSSG) accumulates. Cells react to this drop in GSH/GSSG ratio by increasing the protective or injurious responses (Bell 2003; Halliwell and Gutteridge 1999; Nel 2005; Xiao et al. 2003).

Piao et al. (2011), while studying the Ag NP–induced harmful effects on human liver cells, found that Ag NPs induced the generation of ROS and suppression of GSH. The ROS generated herein were revealed to impair numerous cell components.

One of these effects included the induction of mitochondria-dependent apoptotic pathway through modulation of Bax and Bcl-2 expressions, causing the disturbance in mitochondrial membrane potential. It followed the release of cytochrome c from mitochondria, ultimately inducing the caspase 9 and caspase 3 pathways. Therefore, any alteration in mitochondrial functioning will definitely affect the normal metabolism of cell and, consequently, affect its viability.

15.3.3 Damaging the Nuclear DNA

In addition to cell and mitochondrial membrane damage, it is also important to consider that some of the nanomaterials interacting with cells might also result in other forms of injury such as DNA damage. As mentioned earlier, nanoparticles have very small sizes, less than 100 nm; they can enter the cell (Park et al. 2007) or cellular organelle and they certainly can penetrate the cell nucleus. Inside the nucleus, they can interact with the DNA and, thereby, they can affect its normal structure and functioning (Chen and von Mikecz 2005). Such studies that define the extent and type of DNA damage including gene mutation (Driscoll et al. 1997; Wang et al. 2007; Warheit et al. 2007), chromosomal damage (Gurr et al. 2005; Kang et al. 2008; Linnainmaa et al. 1997; Rahman et al. 2002; Wang et al. 2007), and DNA strand break (Kang et al. 2008; Wang et al. 2007) are called *genotoxicity studies*. These studies are of great importance in cancer research, especially in the evaluation of the risks associated with potential carcinogens (Trouiller et al. 2009).

Nanoparticle-induced DNA damage was revealed by finding the interaction of TiO_2 nanoparticles with DNA (Gurr et al. 2005). According to this study, TiO_2 NPs might damage the DNA directly. Another way of inducing damage is via an indirect pathway, namely, oxidative stress by the induction of ROS (Federici et al. 2007; Gurr et al. 2005; Kang et al. 2008) and/or inflammatory responses (Chen et al. 2006; de Haar et al. 2006; Grassian et al. 2007; Li et al. 2008; Oberdörster et al. 1994; Zhu et al. 2007), and interaction with DNA phosphate group, but whether TiO_2 NPs are acting as a mutagen has not been proven (Li et al. 2008; Zhu et al. 2007).

As discussed earlier, exposure to nanoparticles induces oxidative stress in the growing cell. During replication, oxidative DNA lesions, namely, 8-OHdG, single-strand breaks, or stalled replication forks, lead to double-strand break repair after replication, resulting in the permanent genome rearrangement by the process of DNA recombination (Reliene and Schiestl 2006). Furthermore, oxidative stress including the role of ROS may also cause DNA deletions (Brennan et al. 1994), whereas a toxicity study of Ag NPs exposed to Jurkat T cells has shown to activate p38 mitogen-activated protein kinase through nuclear factor-2 and nuclear factor-kappaB signaling pathways followed by induction of DNA damage, cell cycle arrest, and apoptosis (Eom and Choi 2010). Similar results were also found while studying the exposure effect of cerium oxide nanoparticles (CeO_2 NPs) on human neuroblastoma cells at doses of 100 and 200 μg/ml. The CeO_2 NPs were also found to follow the same pathway as that of other nanoparticles, that is, causing DNA damage owing to their toxicity and thereby resulting in cell death (Kumari et al. 2014). DNA fragmentation assays have also shown a dose-dependent increase in DNA fragmentation (Pawar and Kaul 2012).

To date, many studies have aimed to present the genotoxic effects of nanoparticles in *in vitro* systems. However, to gather more appropriate data, *in vivo* studies are required. Trouiller et al. (2009) performed the genotoxic study of mice exposed to TiO_2 NPs. Their study revealed that TiO_2 P25 NP induces (i) 8-OHdG, indicating oxidative DNA damage; (ii) formation of γ-H2AX foci, indicating DNA double-strand break; (iii) micronuclei formation, indicating chromosomal damage; (iv) DNA deletions in offspring; and (v) inflammation. All of these results confirm the *in vivo* genotoxicity of TiO_2 NP. Likewise, it is also shown that copper oxide nanoparticles (CuO NPs), zinc oxide nanoparticles (ZnO NPs), $CuZnFe_2O_4$, and carbon nanotube cause DNA damage, which is claimed to be linked to release of Cu ions in the cell medium (Karlsson et al. 2008). As for TiO_2 NPs, nanosized silver also induces micronucleus formation, appearing to cause stronger chromosomal damage (Kawata et al. 2009).

A study of immunocytochemistry of dermal fibroblast exposed to three different nanoparticles such as cerium dioxide, titanium dioxide, and zinc oxide indicated that cell death was most significant with ZnO than with the other nanoparticles. ZnO-treated cells demonstrated double-strand breaks by a significant increase in the

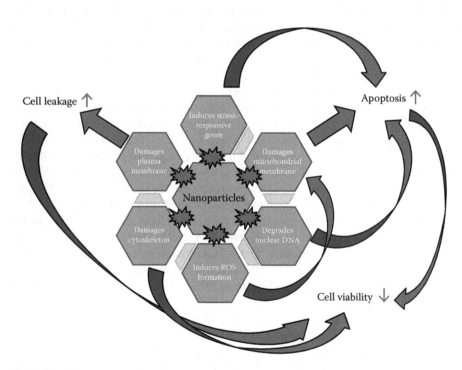

FIGURE 15.2 Schematic to illustrate the interrelations between various cellular responses to various nanoparticle-induced toxicity mechanisms. The NPs, after accumulation at the plasma membrane, disturb its integrity and thus cause the leakage of cellular components. They also damage the cytoskeleton. Furthermore, NPs induce ROS formation, increasing the mitochondrial membrane permeability and damaging the nuclear DNA. Their excessive accumulation also induces the cell to express stress-responsive genes. All of these mechanisms direct the cell for apoptosis, ultimately causing cell death.

presence of γ-H2AX foci, besides Western blot and cell cycle by the phosphorylation of cyclin-dependent kinase 1 (Ramoser et al. 2014).

All of the major pathways causing the toxicity of nanoparticles are summarized in Figure 15.2.

15.4 FUTURE DIRECTIONS

From all of the past studies, it can be said that nanotechnology will play a pivotal role in the present century. The number and type of applications of nanoparticles will rise in the near future. With their applications, issues regarding their handling and release in the environment will also increase, but to date, there is uncertainty regarding the real-life hazards of nanoparticles. Additionally, there is lack of knowledge about the effective protection measures to be taken while handling nanoparticles.

As far as the mechanism of nanotoxicity is concerned, the available data are inadequate. Therefore, there is need for rigorous toxicity evaluation for each nanoparticle using various cell models and biological systems before their extensive use for any type of applications. More studies are required to be performed to gather knowledge about the exact mode of nanoparticle toxicity. Furthermore, the data available are unorganized. Therefore, there is a need to organize and develop a portfolio showing the advantages of certain nanoparticles with their hazardous effect if overused. A detailed investigation of the mechanisms of toxicity will help us design or select the appropriate nanomaterial for application at an appropriate period.

However, further investigations on *in vivo* systems especially in humans are necessary in order to reach a firm conclusion concerning the extent and mechanism of toxicity of nanoparticles and to get a clear picture of their toxicokinetics and tolerance in the system. It can also be expected that a much more detailed knowledge about the chemical basis of nanotoxicity could provide new insights to researchers for the sensible design and production of safer and greener nanomaterials.

15.5 CONCLUSION

As the fabrication and use of nanoparticles are increasing, humans and the environment are more expected to be exposed to nanomaterials via occupational or consumer products. Nevertheless, up to now, toxicity data for most manufactured nanoparticles are limited. Moreover, the toxicity of nanomaterials is greatly correlated to their ultrahigh activity, excessive accumulation, and size/specific surface area. The high reactivity plays a major role in their toxic effect, whereas the size/surface area is also equally important considering their similar activity.

It is now well known that the physicochemical characteristics of nanoparticles might contribute to a greater understanding of nanotoxicology. It is also important to study the potential interactions among nanoparticles' properties while elucidating nanotoxicity. Owing to the significant surface of nanoparticles, they are able to interact with the cell membrane, disturbing its integrity and ultimately causing cell leakage. After entering the cell, nanoparticles can also interact with the mitochondrial membrane, causing the release of cytochrome c. This and other forms of damage to mitochondria are initiated by ROS production, thereby inducing apoptosis in the cell. The nanoparticles can further travel to the cell nucleus where they can damage the genomic DNA, again driving the cell to signal for apoptosis. In combination, or independently, this mechanism results in a reduction in cell viability.

Most of the investigations published to date have mainly focused on *in vitro* studies of the harmful effects of nanoparticles. However, these *in vitro* data can mislead the risk associated with their use. Therefore, for more detailed knowledge, long-term *in vivo* exposures, including humans, are needed in future studies. In conclusion, it can be stated that before the commercialization of nanoparticles, setting up the stringent methods is required for assessing their toxic potential. Identifying the cellular targets of these nanoparticles will definitely help in the design of safer nanoparticles to help protect humans and the environment from the potential hazards they bring.

ACKNOWLEDGMENTS

Mr. I.R. Gupta is thankful to the Council of Scientific and Industrial Research, New Delhi, for providing financial assistance in the form of a Junior Research Fellowship (CSIR-09/996(001)/2009-EMR-I). We also thank University Grants Commission, New Delhi, for providing financial assistance under the UGC-SAP program.

REFERENCES

Ada K., M. Turk, S. Oguztuzun, M. Kilic, M. Demirel, N. Tandogan, E. Ersayar and O. Latif, Cytotoxicity and apoptotic effects of nickel oxide nanoparticles in cultured HeLa cells, *Folia Histochemica et Cytobiologica* 48, 524–529 (2010).

Al-Kattan A., A. Wichser, R. Vonbank, S. Brunner, A. Ulrich, S. Zuin, Y. Arroyo, L. Golanski and B. Nowack, Characterization of materials released into water from paint containing nano-SiO_2, *Chemosphere* S0045-6535(14), 00206–00209 (2014).

Bell A.T., The impact of nanoscience on heterogeneous catalysis, *Science* 299 (5613), 1688–1691 (2003).

Braydich-Stolle L., S. Hussain, J.J. Schlager and M.C. Hofmann, In vitro cytotoxicity of nanoparticles in mammalian germline stem cells, *Toxicological Sciences* 88, 412–419 (2005).

Brennan R.J., B.E. Swoboda and R.H. Schiestl, Oxidative mutagens induce intrachromosomal recombination in yeast, *Mutation Research* 308, 159–167 (1994).

Buzea C., I.I.P. Blandino and K. Robbie, Nanomaterials and nanoparticles: Sources and toxicity, *Biointerphases* 2, MR17–MR172 (2007).

Casals E., E. Gonzalez and V.F. Puntes, Reactivity of inorganic nanoparticles in biological environments: Insights into nanotoxicity mechanisms, *Journal of Physics D: Applied Physics* 45, 443001 (2012).

Chang E., N. Thekkek, W.W. Yu, V.L. Colvin and R. Drezek, Evaluation of quantum dot cytotoxicity based on intracellular uptake, *Small* 12, 1412–1417 (2006).

Chen H., J.N. Seiber and M. Hotze, ACS select on nanotechnology in food and agriculture: A perspective on implications and applications, *Journal Agriculture Food Chemistry* 62, 1209–1212 (2014).

Chen H.W., S.F. Su, C.T. Chien, W.H. Lin, S.L. Yu, C.C. Chou, J.J. Chen and P.C. Yang, Titanium dioxide nanoparticles induce emphysema-like lung injury in mice, *FASEB Journal* 20, 2393–2395 (2006).

Chen M. and A. von Mikecz, Formation of nucleoplasmic protein aggregates impairs nuclear function in response to SiO_2 nanoparticles, *Experimental Cell Research* 305, 51–62 (2005).

Cheraghipour E., A.M. Tamaddon, S. Javadpour and I.J. Bruce, PEG conjugated citrate-capped magnetite nanoparticles for biomedical applications, *Journal of Magnetism and Magnetic Materials* 328, 91–95 (2013).

Cho W.S., M. Cho, J. Jeong, M. Choi, B.S. Han, H.S. Shin, J. Hong, B.H. Chung, J. Jeong and M.H. Cho, Size-dependent tissue kinetics of PEG-coated gold nanoparticles, *Toxicology and Applied Pharmacology* 245(1), 116–123 (2010).

Christensen F.M., H.J. Johnston, V. Stone, R.J. Aitken, S. Hankin, S. Peters and K. Aschberger, Nano-silver—Feasibility and challenges for human health risk assessment based on open literature, *Nanotoxicology* 4(3), 284–295 (2010).

Coluci V.R., D.S.T. Martinez, J.G. Honorio, A.F. de Faria, D.A. Morales, M.S. Skaf, O.L. Alves and G.A. Umbuzeiro, Noncovalent interaction with graphene oxide: The crucial role of oxidative debris, *Journal of Physics and Chemistry C* 118, 2187–2193 (2014).

Conner S.D. and S.L. Schmid, Regulated portals of entry into the cell, *Nature* 422, 37–44 (2003).

Connor E.E., J. Mwamuka, A. Gole, C.J. Murphy and M.D. Wyatt, Gold nanoparticles are taken up by human cells but do not cause acute cytotoxicity, *Small* 1, 325–327 (2005).

Dabrunz A., L. Duester, C. Prasse, F. Seitz, R. Rosenfeldt, C. Schilde, G.E. Schaumann and R. Schulz, Biological surface coating and molting inhibition as mechanisms of TiO_2 nanoparticle toxicity in *Daphnia magna*, *PLoS One* 6, e20112 (2011).

Das N.J., M.M. Amiji, M.F. Bahia and B. Sarmento, Nanotechnology-based systems for the treatment and prevention of HIV/AIDS, *Advances in Drug Delivery Reviews* 62, 458–477 (2010).

Dausend J., A. Musyanovych, M. Dass, P. Walther, H. Schrezenmeier, K. Landfester and V. Mailänder, Uptake mechanism of oppositely charged fluorescent nanoparticles in HeLa cells, *Macromolecular Biosciences* 8, 1135–1143 (2008).

de Haar C., I. Hassing, M. Bol, R. Bleumink and R. Pieters, Ultrafine but not fine particulate matter causes airway inflammation and allergic airway sensitization to co-administered antigen in mice, *Clinical and Experimental Allergy* 36, 1469–1479 (2006).

De Lima R., A.B. Seabra and N. Durán, Silver nanoparticles: A brief review of cytotoxicity and genotoxicity of chemically and biogenically synthesized nanoparticles, *Journal of Applied Toxicology* 32, 867–879 (2012).

Derfus A., W. Chan and S. Bjatia, Proboing the cytotoxicity of semiconductor quantum dots, *Nano Letters*, 4, 11–18 (2004).

Donaldson K., F.A. Murphy, R. Duffin and C.A. Poland, Asbestos, carbon nanotubes and the pleural mesothelium: A review of the hypothesis regarding the role of long fibre retention in the parietal pleura, inflammation and mesothelioma, *Particle and Fibre Toxicology* 7, 5 (2010). Available at http://www.particleandfibretoxicology.com/content/7/1/5.

Donaldson K., V. Stone, C. Tran, W. Kreyling and P.J. Borm, Nanotoxicology, *Occupational and Environmental Medicine* 61, 727–728 (2004).

Driscoll K.E., L.C. Deyo, J.M. Carter, B.W. Howard, D.G. Hassenbein and T.A. Bertram, Effects of particle exposure and particle-elicited inflammatory cells on mutation in rat alveolar epithelial cells, *Carcinogenesis* 18, 423–430 (1997).

Drobne D., A. Jemec and Z.P. Tkalec, In vivo screening to determine hazards of nanoparticles: Nanosized TiO_2, *Environmental Pollution* 157, 1157–1164 (2009).

Durán N., S.S. Guterres and O.L. Alves, *Nanotoxicology: Materials, Methodologies, and Assessments*, 412. Berlin: Springer (2014).

Ehrlich M., W. Boll, A. Van Oijen, R. Hariharan, K. Chandran, M.L. Nibert and T. Kirchhausen, Endocytosis by random initiation and stabilization of clathrin-coated pits, *Cell* 118, 591–605, (2004).

Eom H.J. and J. Choi, p38 MAPK activation, DNA damage, cell cycle arrest and apoptosis as mechanisms of toxicity of silver nanoparticles in Jurkat T cells, *Environmental Science and Technology* 44, 8337–8342 (2010).

Faria A.F., D.S.T. Martinez, A.C.M. Moraes, M.E.H. Maia da Costa, E.B. Barros, A.G.S. Filho, A.J. Paula and O.L. Alves, Unveiling the role of oxidation debris on the surface chemistry of graphene through the anchoring of Ag nanoparticles, *Chemical Material* 24, 4080–4087 (2012).

Federici G., B.J. Shaw and R.D. Handy, Toxicity of titanium dioxide nanoparticles to rainbow trout (*Oncorhynchus mykiss*): Gill injury, oxidative stress, and other physiological effects, *Aquatic Toxicology* 84, 415–430 (2007).

Fu P.P., Q. Xia, H.M. Hwang, P.C. Ray and H. Yu, Mechanisms of nanotoxicity: Generation of reactive oxygen species, *Journal of Food and Drug Analysis* 22, 64–75 (2014).

Geiser M., B. Rothen-Rutishauser, N. Kapp, S. Schürch, W. Kreyling, H. Schulz, M. Semmler, V. Im Hof, J. Heyder and P. Gehr, Ultrafine particles cross cellular membranes by nonphagocytic mechanisms in lungs and in cultured cells, *Environmental Health Perspective* 113, 1555–1560 (2005).

Glasgow G., L. Gardiner, S. Mir, O. Jejelowo and A. Sodipe, The effects of industrial grade, multi walled carbon nanotubes on *Saccharomyces cerevisiae*, *International Journal of Applied Science and Technology* 4(3), 28–33 (2014).

Gliga A.R., S. Skoglund, I.O. Wallinder, B. Fadeel and H.L. Karlsson, Size-dependent cytotoxicity of silver nanoparticles in human lung cells: The role of cellular uptake, agglomeration and Ag release, *Particle and Fibre Toxicology* 11, 11 (2014). Available at http://www.particleandfibretoxicology.com/content/11/1/11.

Grassian V.H., P.T. O'Shaughnessy, A. Adamcakova-Dodd, J.M. Pettibone and P.S. Thorne, Inhalation exposure study of titanium dioxide nanoparticles with a primary particle size of 2 to 5 nm, *Environment Health Perspective* 115, 397–402 (2007).

Gupta I., N. Duran and M. Rai, Nano-silver toxicity: Emerging concerns and consequences in human health, in *Nano-Antimicrobials: Progress and Prospects*, eds. M. Rai and N. Cioffi, 525–548. Berlin: Springer Verlag (2012).

Gurr J.R., A.S. Wang, C.H. Chen and K.Y. Jan, Ultrafine titanium dioxide particles in the absence of photoactivation can induce oxidative damage to human bronchial epithelial cells, *Toxicology* 213, 66–73 (2005).

Guzman M., J. Dille and S. Godet, Synthesis and antibacterial activity of silver nanoparticles against gram-positive and gram-negative bacteria, *Nanomedicine* 8, 37–45 (2012).

Halliwell B. and J.M.C. Gutteridge, *Free Radicals in Biology and Medicine*, Oxford: Clarendon Press (1999).

Handy R., F. von der Kammer, J. Lead, M. Hasellöv, R. Owen and M. Crane, The ecotoxicology and chemistry of manufactured nanoparticles, *Ecotoxicology* 17, 287–314 (2008b).

Handy R.D., R. Owen and E. Valsami-Jones, The ecotoxicology of nanoparticles and nanomaterials: Current status, knowledge gaps, challenges, and future needs, *Ecotoxicology* 17, 315–325 (2008a).

Harush-Frenkel O., N. Debotton, S. Benita and Y. Altschuler, Targeting of NPs to the clathrin-mediated endocytic pathway, *Biochemistry and Biophysics Research Communication* 353, 26–32 (2007).

Hund-Rinke K. and M. Simon, Ecotoxic effect of photocatalytic active nanoparticles (TiO$_2$) on algae and daphnids, *Environmental Science and Pollution Research* 13, 225–232 (2006).

Ji J.H., J.H. Jung, S.S. Kim, J.U. Yoon, J.D. Park, B.S. Choi, Y.H. Chung, I.H. Kwon, J. Jeong, B.S. Han, J.H. Shin, J.H. Sung, K.S. Song and I.J. Yu, Twenty-eight-day inhalation toxicity study of silver nanoparticles in Sprague–Dawley rats, *Inhalation Toxicology* 19, 857–871 (2007).

Jiang J., G. Oberdörster, A. Elder, R. Gelein, P. Mercer and P. Biswas, Does nanoparticle activity depend upon size and crystal phase?, *Nanotoxicology* 2, 33–42 (2008).

Kang S.J., B.M. Kim, Y.J. Lee and H.W. Chung, Titanium dioxide nanoparticles trigger p53-mediated damage response in peripheral blood lymphocytes, *Environmental and Molecular Mutagenesis* 49, 399–405 (2008).

Karlsson H.L., P. Cronholm, J. Gustafsson and L. Möller, Copper oxide nanoparticles are highly toxic: A comparison between metal oxide nanoparticles and carbon nanotubes, *Chemical Research in Toxicology* 21, 1726–1732 (2008).

Kawata K., M. Osawa and S. Okabe, In vitro toxicity of silver nanoparticles at noncytotoxic doses to HepG2 human hepatoma cells, *Environmental Science and Technology* 43, 6046–6051 (2009).

Kessler R., Engineered nanoparticles in consumer products: Understanding a new ingredient, *Environment Health Perspectives* 119, A120–A125 (2011).

Kim S., J.E. Choi, J. Choi, K.H. Chung, K. Park, J. Yi and D.Y. Ryu, Oxidative stress-dependent toxicity of silver nanoparticles in human hepatoma cells, *Toxicology in Vitro* 23, 1076–1084 (2009).

Klaper R., D. Arndt, J. Bozich and G. Dominguez, Molecular interactions of nanomaterials and organisms: Defining biomarkers for toxicity and high-throughput screening using traditional and next-generation sequencing approaches, *Analyst* 139, 882–895 (2014).

Knezevic N.Z., E. Ruiz-Hernández, W.E. Hennink and M. Vallet-Regíde, Magnetic mesoporous silica-based core/shell nanoparticles for biomedical applications, *RSC Advances* 3, 9584–9593 (2013).

Kumari M., S.P. Singh, S. Chinde, M.F. Rahman, M. Mahboob and P. Grover, Toxicity study of cerium oxide nanoparticles in human neuroblastoma cells, *International Journal of Toxicology* 33, 86–97 (2014).

Lajoie P. and I.R. Nabi, Regulation of raft-dependent endocytosis, *Journal of Cellular and Molecular Medicine* 11, 644–653 (2007).

Leroueil P.R., S. Hong, A. Mecke, J.R. Baker Jr., B.G. Orr and M.M.B. Holl, Nanoparticle interaction with biological membranes, *Accounts of Chemical Research* 40, 335–342 (2007).

Li S., H. Zhu, R. Zhu, X. Sun, S. Yao and S. Wang, Impact and mechanism of TiO_2 nanoparticles on DNA synthesis *in vitro*, *Science in China Series B—Chemistry* 51, 367–372 (2008).

Ling D. and T. Hyeon, Chemical design of biocompatible iron oxide nanoparticles for medical applications, *Small* 9, 1450–1466 (2013).

Linnainmaa K., P. Kivipensas and H. Vainio, Toxicity and cytogenetic studies of ultrafine titanium dioxide in cultured rat liver epithelial cells, *Toxicology in Vitro* 11, 329–335 (1997).

Mailander V., M.R. Lorenz, V. Holzapfel, A. Musyanovych, K. Fuchs, M. Wiesneth, P. Walther, K. Landfester and H. Schrezenmeier, Carboxylated superparamagnetic iron oxide particles label cells intracellularly without transfection agents, *Molecular Imaging Biology* 10, 138–146 (2008).

Mamo T., E.A. Moseman, N. Kolishetti, C. Salvador-Morales, J. Shi, D.R. Kuritzkes, R. Langer, U. von Andrian and O.C. Farokhzad, Emerging nanotechnology approaches for HIV/AIDS treatment and prevention, *Nanomedicine (London)* 5, 269–285 (2010).

Martinez D.S.T., A.F. Faria, E. Berni, A.G.S. Filhoa, G. Almeida, A. Caloto-Oliveira, M.J. Grossman, L.R. Durrant, G.A. Umbuzeiro and O.L. Alves, Exploring the use of biosurfactants from *Bacillus subtilis* in bionanotechnology: A potential dispersing agent for carbon nanotube ecotoxicological studies, *Process Biochemistry* 48(7), 1162–1168 (2014).

Maynard A.D., P.A. Baron, M. Foley, A.A. Shvedova, E.R. Kisin and V. Castranova, Exposure to carbon nanotube material: Aerosol release during the handling of unrefined single-walled carbon nanotube material, *Journal of Toxicology and Environmental Health A* 67, 87–107 (2004).

Melo P.S., P.D. Marcato, D.R. de Araújo and N. Durán, In vitro cytotoxicity assays of nanoparticles on different cell lines, in *Nanotoxicology: Nanomedicine and Nanotoxicology*, eds. N. Durán, S.S. Guterres and L. Oswaldo, 111–123. New York: Springer (2014).

Meng H., Z. Chen, G. Xing, H. Yuan, C. Chen, F. Zhao, C. Zhang and Y. Zhao, Ultrahigh reactivity provokes nanotoxicity: Explanation of oral toxicity of nano-copper particles, *Toxicology Letters* 175, 102–110 (2007).

Napierska D., L.C. Thomassen, V. Rabolli, D. Lison, L. Gonzalez, M. Kirsch-Volders, J.A. Martens and P.H. Hoet, Size-dependent cytotoxicity of monodisperse silica nanoparticles in human endothelial cells, *Small* 5, 846–853 (2009).

Nel A., Atmosphere air pollution-related illness: Effects of particles, *Science* 308, 804–806 (2005).

Nel A., T. Xia, L. Madler and N. Li, Toxic potential of materials at the nanolevel, *Science* 311, 622–627 (2006).

Nichols B., Caveosomes and endocytosis of lipid rafts, *Journal of Cellular Science* 116, 4707–4714 (2003).

Oberdörster E., Manufactured nanomaterials (fullerenes, C60) induce oxidative stress in the brain of juvenile largemouth bass, *Environment Health Perspective* 112, 1058–1062 (2004).

Oberdörster G., Concepts of nanotoxicology. *International Conference on Food and Agriculture Applications of Nanotecnologies-NanoAgri* (2010). Available at http://www.fao.org/fileadmin/templates/agns/pdf/NANOAGRI_2010.pdf (accessed on April 13, 2014).

Oberdörster G., E. Oberdörster and J. Oberdörster, Concepts of nanoparticle dose metric and response metric, *Environmental Health Perspective* 115(6), A290 (2007).

Oberdörster G., E. Oberdörster and J. Oberdörster, Nanotoxicology: An emerging discipline evolving from studies of ultrafine particles, *Environmental Health Perspective* 113, 823–839 (2005).

Oberdörster G., J. Ferin and B.E. Lehnert, Correlation between particle size, in vivo particle persistence, and lung injury, *Environmental Health Perspective* 102(Suppl 5), 173–179 (1994).

Pan Y., S. Neuss, A. Leifert, M. Fischler, F. Wen, U. Simon, G. Schmid, W. Brandau and W. Jahnen-Dechent, Size-dependent cytotoxicity of gold nanoparticles, *Small* 3, 1941–1949 (2007).

Park S., Y.K. Lee, M. Jung, K.H. Kim, N. Chung, E.K. Ahn, Y. Lim and K.H. Lee, Cellular toxicity of various inhalable metal nanoparticles on human alveolar epithelial cells, *Inhalation Toxicology* 19, 59–65 (2007).

Paula A.J., C. Silveira, D.S.T. Martinez, A.G. Souza Filho, F.V. Romero, L.C. Fonseca, L. Tasic, O.L. Alves and N. Durán, Topography-driven bionano-interactions on colloidal silica nanoparticles, *ACS Applied Mathematics and Interfaces* 6(5), 3437–3447 (2014).

Paull R., J. Wolfe, P. Hebert and M. Sinkula, Investing in nanotechnology, *Nature Biotechnology* 21, 1144–1147 (2003).

Pawar K. and G. Kaul, Toxicity of titanium oxide nanoparticles causes functionality and DNA damage in buffalo (*Bubalus bubalis*) sperm *in vitro*, *Toxicology and Industrial Health* 30(6), 520–530 (2012).

Pelkmans L., D. Puntener and A. Helenius, Local actin polymerization and dynamin recruitment in SV40-induced internalization of caveolae, *Science* 296, 535–539 (2002).

Pereira M.M., L. Mouton, C. Yéprémian, A. Couté, J. Lo, J.M. Marconcini, L.O. Ladeira, N.R.B. Raposo, H.M. Brandão and R. Brayner, Ecotoxicological effects of carbon nanotubes and cellulose nanofibers in *Chlorella vulgaris*, *Journal of Nanobiotechnology* 12, 15 (2014). doi:10.1186/1477-3155-12-15.

Pereira M.M., N.R. Raposo, R. Brayner, E.M. Teixeira, V. Oliveira, C.C.R. Quintão, L.S. Camargo, L.H. Mattoso and H.M. Brandão, Cytotoxicity and expression of genes involved in the cellular stress response and apoptosis in mammalian fibroblast exposed to cotton cellulose nanofibers, *Nanotechnology* 24(7), 075103 (2013). doi:10.1088/0957-4484/24/7/075103.

Piao M.J., K.A. Kang, I.K. Lee, H.S. Kim, S. Kim, J.Y. Choi, J. Choi and J.W. Hyun, Silver nanoparticles induce oxidative cell damage in human liver cells through inhibition of reduced glutathione and induction of mitochondria-involved apoptosis, *Toxicology Letters* 201, 92–100 (2011).

Pronk M.E.J., S.W.P. Wijnhoven, E.A.J. Bleeker, E.H.W. Heugens, W.J.G.M. Peijnenburg, R. Luttik and B.C. Hakkert, Nanomaterials under REACH. Nanosilver as a case study. Bilthoven, The Netherlands: RIVM. RIVM report601780003 (2009). Available at http://www.rivm.nl/bibliotheek/rapporten/601780003.html.

Raghupathi K.R., R.T. Koodali and A.C. Manna, Size-dependent bacterial growth inhibition and mechanism of antibacterial activity of zinc oxide nanoparticles, *Langmuir* 27(7), 4020–4028 (2011).

Rahman Q., M. Lohani, E. Dopp, H. Pemsel, L. Jonas, D.G. Weiss and D. Schiffmann, Evidence that ultrafine titanium dioxide induces micronuclei and apoptosis in Syrian hamster embryo fibroblasts, *Environment Health Perspective* 110, 797–800 (2002).

Rai M., A. Ingle, I. Gupta, S. Gaikwad, A. Gade, O. Rubilar and N. Durán, Cyto-, Geno-, and ecotoxicity of copper nanoparticles, in *Nanotoxicology*, eds. N. Durán, S. Guterres and O.L. Alves, 325–345. Berlin: Springer (2014).

Rai M., A. Yadav and A. Gade, Silver nanoparticles as a new generation of antimicrobials, *Biotechnology Advances* 27, 76–83 (2009).

Rand G. and S. Petrocelli, *Fundamentals of Aquatic Toxicology: Methods and Applications*, New York: Hemisphere Publishing (1985).

Reliene R. and R.H. Schiestl, Antioxidant N-acetyl cysteine reduces incidence and multiplicity of lymphoma in Atm deficient mice, *DNA Repair* 5, 852–859 (2006).

Risom L., P. Møller and S. Loft, Oxidative stress-induced DNA damage by particulate air pollution, *Mutation Research* 592, 119–137 (2005).

Ramoser A.A., M.F. Criscitiello and C.M. Sayes, Engineered nanoparticles induce DNA damage in primary human skin cells, even at low doses, *Nano Life 04*, 1440001, 13 (2014).

Rozman K.K., W.L. Roth and J. Doull. Influences of dynamics, kinetics, and exposure on toxicity in the lung, in *Toxicology of the Lung*, 4th ed., ed. D.E. Gardner, 195–230. London: Taylor & Francis Group, LLC (2006).

Sanvicens N. and M.P. Marco, Multifunctional nanoparticles—Properties and prospects for their use in human medicine, *Trends in Biotechnology* 26, 425–433 (2008).

Sarkar A., M. Ghosh and P.C. Sil, Nanotoxicity: Oxidative stress mediated toxicity of metal and metal oxide nanoparticles, *Journal of Nanoscience Nanotechnology* 14, 730–743 (2014).

Scheringer M., Environmental risks of nanomaterials, *Nature Nanotechology* 3, 322–323 (2008).

Scown T.M., R. van Aerle and C.R. Tyler, Review: Do engineered nanoparticles pose a significant threat to the aquatic environment?, *Critical Reviews in Toxicology* 40, 653–670 (2010).

Seabra A.B., A.J. Paula, R. de Lima, O.L. Alves and N. Durán, Nanotoxicity of graphene and graphene oxide, *Chemical Research in Toxicology* 27, 159–168 (2014).

Shang L., K. Nienhaus and G.U.H. Nienhaus, Engineered nanoparticles interacting with cells: Size matters, *Journal of Nanobiotechnology* 12, 5 (2014). Available at http://www.jnanobiotechnology.com/content/12/1/5.

Sharma P. and S. Garg, Pure drug and polymer based nanotechnologies for the improved solubility, stability, bioavailability and targeting of anti-HIV drugs, *Advances in Drug Delivery Review* 62, 491–502 (2010).

Stéfani D., A.J. Paula, B.G. Vaz, R.A. Silva, N.F. Andrade, G.Z. Justo, C.V. Ferreira, A.G. Filho, M.N. Eberlin and O.L. Alves, Structural and proactive safety aspects of oxidation debris from multiwalled carbon nanotubes, *Journal of Hazardous Materials* 189, 391–396 (2011).

Stensberg M.C., Q. Wei, E.S. McLamore, D.M. Porterfield, A. Wei and M.S. Sepulveda, Toxicological studies on silver nanoparticles: Challenges and opportunities in assessment, monitoring and imaging, *Nanomedicine* 6, 879–898 (2011).

Stuart A.D. and T.D.K. Brown, Entry of feline calicivirus is dependent on clathrin-mediated endocytosis and acidification in endosomes, *Journal of Virology* 80, 7500–7509 (2006).

Sutradhar K.B. and L. Amin, Nanotechnology in cancer drug delivery and selective targeting. *ISRN Nanotechnology* 2014, 939378 (2014). Available at http://www.hindawi.com/journals/isrn/2014/939378.

Suttiponparnit K., J. Jiang, M. Sahu, S. Suvachittanont, T. Charinpanitkul and P. Biswas, Role of surface area, primary particle size, and crystal phase on titanium dioxide nanoparticle dispersion properties, *Nanoscale Research Letters* 6, 27 (2010). Available at http://www.nanoscalereslett.com/content/6/1/27.

Swanson J.A. and C. Watts, Macropinocytosis, *Trends in Cell Biology* 11, 424–428 (1995).

Trouiller B., R. Reliene, A. Westbrook, P. Solaimani and R.H. Schiest, Titanium dioxide nanoparticles induce DNA damage and genetic instability in vivo in mice, *Cancer Research* 69, 8784–8789 (2009).

Tyagi P.K., Shruti, S. Sarsar and A. Ahuja, Synthesis of metal nanoparticles: A biological prospective for analysis, *International Journal of Pharmacy and Innovation* 2, 48–60 (2011).

Veranth J.M., E.G. Kaser, M.M. Veranth, M. Koch and G.S. Yost, Cytokine responses of human lung cells (BEAS-2B) treated with micron-sized and nanoparticles of metal oxides compared to soil dusts, *Particle Fibre Toxicology* 4, 2 (2007). Available at http://www.ncbi.nlm.nih.gov/pmc/articles/PMC1821039/pdf/1743-8977-4-2.pdf.

Verma A., O. Uzun, Y. Hu, Y. Hu, H.-S. Han, N. Watson, S. Chen, D.J. Irvine and F. Stellacci, Surface structure-regulated cell membrane penetration by monolayer protected nanoparticles, *Nature Material* 7, 588–595 (2008).

Villalonga-Barber C., M. Micha-Screttas, B.R. Steele, A. Georgopoulos and C. Demetzos, Dendrimers as biopharmaceuticals: Synthesis and properties, *Current Topics in Medical Chemistry* 8, 1294–1309 (2008).

Vyas T.K., L. Shah and M.M. Amiji, Nanoparticulate drug carriers for delivery of HIV/AIDS therapy to viral reservoir sites, *Expert Opinion in Drug Delivery* 3, 613–628 (2006).

Wang J.J., B.J. Sanderson and H. Wang, Cyto- and genotoxicity of ultrafine TiO_2 particles in cultured human lymphoblastoid cells, *Mutation Research* 628, 99–106 (2007).

Warheit D.B., R.A. Hoke, C. Finlay, E.M. Donner, K.L. Reed and C.M. Sayes, Development of a base set of toxicity tests using ultrafine TiO_2 particles as a component of nanoparticle risk management, *Toxicology Letters* 171, 99–110 (2007).

Weaver C.T., C.O. Elson, L.A. Fouser and J.K. Kolls, The th17 pathway and inflammatory diseases of the intestines, lungs, and skin, *Annual Review in Pathology* 8, 477–512 (2013).

Wijnhoven S.W.P., W.J.G.M. Peijnenbeurg, C.A. Herberts, W.I. Hagens, A.G. Oomen, E.H.W. Heugens, B. Roszek, J. Bisschops, I. Gosens, D. Van De Meent, S. Dekkers, W.H. De Jong, M. van Zijverden, A.J.A.M. Sips and R.E. Geertsma, Nano-silver—A review of available data and knowledge gaps in human and environmental risk assessment, *Nanotoxicology* 3(2), 109–138 (2009).

Xia T., M. Kovochich, M. Liong, J.I. Zink and A.E. Nel, Cationic polystyrene nanosphere toxicity depends on cell-specific endocytic and mitochondrial injury pathways, *ACS Nano* 2, 85–96 (2008).

Xiao G.G., M. Wang, N. Li, J.A. Loo and A.E. Nel, Use of proteomics to demonstrate a hierarchical oxidative stress response to diesel exhaust particle chemicals in a macrophage cell line, *Journal of Biological Chemistry* 278, 50781–50790 (2003).

Xu A., Y. Chai, T. Nohmi, T.K. Hei, Genotoxic responses to titanium dioxide nanoparticles and fullerene in *gpt* delta transgenic MEF cells, *Particle and Fibre Toxicology*, 6, 3 (2009).

Xu C. and S. Sun, New forms of superparamagnetic nanoparticles for biomedical applications, *Advanced Drug Delivery Reviews* 65, 732–743 (2013).

Yan L., Z. Gu and Y. Zhao, Chemical mechanisms of the toxicological properties of nanomaterials: Generation of intracellular reactive oxygen species, *Chemistry An Asian Journal* 8, 2342–2353 (2013).

Zhang L.W. and N.A. Monteiro-Riviere, Mechanisms of quantum dot nanoparticle cellular uptake, *Toxicological Sciences* 110, 138–155 (2009).

Zhu R.R., S.L. Wang, R. Zhang, X.Y. Sun and S.-D. Yao, A novel toxicological evaluation of TiO_2 nanoparticles on DNA structure, *Chinese Journal of Chemistry* 25, 958–961 (2007).

Index

A

Milton Keynes UK
Ingram Content Group UK Ltd.
UKHW021841071024
449327UK00021B/1530

9 780367 575649